HUMAN OSTEOLOGY
in Archaeology and Forensic Science

To Theya Molleson
and Don Brothwell,
who taught us so much

HUMAN OSTEOLOGY
in Archaeology and Forensic Science

Editors

**Margaret Cox and
Simon Mays**

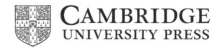

CAMBRIDGE UNIVERSITY PRESS
Cambridge, New York, Melbourne, Madrid, Cape Town, Singapore, São Paulo

Cambridge University Press
The Edinburgh Building, Cambridge CB2 2RU, UK

Published in the United States of America by Cambridge University Press, New York

www.cambridge.org
Information on this title: www.cambridge.org/9780521691468

First published 2000
Reprinted 2002
Digitally reprinted by Cambridge University Press 2006

A catalogue record for this publication is available from the British Library

ISBN-13 978-0-521-69146-8 paperback
ISBN-10 0-521-69146-X paperback

Contents

Acknowledgements x

Author Biographies xi

Preface xxi

CHAPTER 1

Studies on skeletal and dental variation: a view across two centuries 1
Don Brothwell

SECTION I
Juvenile health, growth and development

Introduction 7

CHAPTER 2

Development and ageing of the juvenile skeleton 9
Louise Scheuer and Sue Black

CHAPTER 3

Growth studies of past populations: an overview and an example 23
Louise Humphrey

CHAPTER 4

Non-adult palaeopathology: current status and future potential 39
Mary Lewis

SECTION II
Palaeodemography

Introduction 59

CHAPTER 5

Ageing adults from the skeleton 61
Margaret Cox

CHAPTER 6

Ageing from the dentition 83
David Whittaker

CHAPTER 7

Problems and prospects in palaeodemography 101
Andrew Chamberlain

CHAPTER 8

Sex determination in skeletal remains 117
Simon Mays and Margaret Cox

CHAPTER 9

Assessment of parturition 131
Margaret Cox

SECTION III
Disease in the past

Introduction 143

CHAPTER 10

Infectious disease in biocultural perspective: past, present and future
work in Britain 145
Charlotte Roberts

CHAPTER 11

The palaeopathology of joint disease 163
Juliet Rogers

CHAPTER 12

The diagnosis of metabolic disease in archaeological bone 183
Megan Brickley

CHAPTER 13

Congenital conditions and neoplastic disease in British palaeopathology ... 199

Trevor Anderson

CHAPTER 14

Dental health in British antiquity 227

Chrissie Freeth

CHAPTER 15

Chemical methods in palaeopathology 239

Angela Gernaey and David Minnikin

CHAPTER 16

An introduction to palaeohistopathology 255

Lynne Bell and Kim Piper

SECTION IV
Human variation

Introduction 275

CHAPTER 17

Biodistance studies using craniometric variation in British
archaeological skeletal material 277

Simon Mays

CHAPTER 18

Skeletal non-metric traits and the assessment of inter- and
intra-population diversity: past problems and future potential 289

Andrew Tyrrell

CHAPTER 19

Skeletal indicators of handedness 307

James Steele

CHAPTER 20

Forensic and archaeological reconstruction of the human
face upon the skull 325

Richard Neave

SECTION V
Assaults on the skeleton

Introduction 335

CHAPTER 21

Trauma in biocultural perspective: past, present and future
work in Britain 337
Charlotte Roberts

CHAPTER 22

Evidence for weapon-related trauma in British archaeological samples 357
Anthea Boylston

CHAPTER 23

Bone adaptation and its relationship to physical activity in the past 381
Christopher Knüsel

CHAPTER 24

The analysis of cremated bone 403
Jacqueline McKinley

SECTION VI
Microscopic, biochemical and analytical approaches

Introduction 423

CHAPTER 25

New directions in the analysis of stable isotopes in excavated
bones and teeth 425
Simon Mays

CHAPTER 26

The chemical degradation of bone 439
*Christina Nielsen-Marsh, Angela Gernaey, Gordon Turner-Walker, Robert Hedges,
Alistair Pike and Matthew Collins*

CHAPTER 27

Ancient DNA applications in human osteoarchaeology:
achievements, problems and potential 455
Keri Brown

CHAPTER 28

Analysing human skeletal data 475
John Robb

CHAPTER 29

Forensic osteology in the United Kingdom 491
Sue Black

Index 505

Acknowledgements

The Editors thank the many individuals and organizations who have made this volume possible. Funding was provided by the School of Conservation Sciences, Bournemouth University, and English Heritage, London. Dr Ellen Hambleton acted as subeditor, and we are enormously grateful for her efforts in this regard, and for the patience and perseverance she displayed. The Editors also acknowledge the hard work and expertise of the contributing authors, and are grateful to the referees who reviewed the contributions. Thanks are due to Linda O'Connell for providing the photograph for the front cover.

Author Biographies

Trevor Anderson
Vichy House, 15 St Mary's Street, Canterbury, Kent CT1 2QL, UK

Trevor Anderson received his first degree in Ancient History and Archaeology from the University of Birmingham in 1977. After several years of working with human bones, including Norwegian material, he obtained an MA (with distinction) in Funerary Archaeology and Palaeopathology from the University of Sheffield. For the past 11 years he has been resident osteoarchaeologist with the Canterbury Archaeological Trust, where he has examined thousands of skeletons ranging in date from Neolithic to Victorian. In recent years he has also been employed as a consultant to external UK projects, and has also been involved in the examination of medieval rural populations in Southern Italy. He has published over one-hundred articles and bone reports, which have included the first evidence of cleft lip and palate; endemic syphilis; Freiberg's infarction; Madelung deformity; as well as cranial meningioma and prostatic carcinoma. His main research interests are the history of congenital conditions and neoplastic disease.

Lynne Bell
Department of Palaeontology, The Natural History Museum, Cromwell Road, London SW7 5BD, UK

Dr Lynne Bell is a Wellcome Research Fellow in the Department of Palaeontology at The Natural History Museum, London. Her training is in archaeological science and mineralized tissue biology; she obtained her PhD from the Department of Anatomy, University College London, which detailed microstructural diagenetic change to the mammalian skeleton and its taphonomic significance. Current research projects include DNA preservation within a mineralized cell, and stable light isotopic dietary and spatial tracking. She has published extensively in archaeological, forensic and medical journals.

Sue Black
Department of Forensic Medicine and Science, University of Glasgow, Glasgow G12 8QQ, UK

Dr Sue Black originally studied human anatomy at the University of Aberdeen (1978–87) specializing in the identification of human skeletal remains. She has held positions as a Lecturer in Anatomy, firstly at St Thomas' Hospital, London, and then at UMDS. In 1992 she took up a part-time position as Forensic Osteologist in the Department of Forensic

Medicine and Science, University of Glasgow. Since that date she has worked almost exclusively on forensic casework, which includes work not only in Scotland, but also throughout England and, recently, in Italy, where she worked on a multiple murder case for the Italian Government in Verona. In 1999 she worked with the British Forensic Investigative Team in Kosovo. She has been writing a comprehensive text on the juvenile skeleton entitled *Developmental Juvenile Osteology* with Louise Scheuer (forthcoming, 2000). Under the guidance of the Home Office she is currently compiling a National Register for Forensic Anthropologists to provide a national network of experts.

Anthea Boylston
Calvin Wells Laboratory, Department of Archaeological Sciences, University of Bradford, Bradford BD7 1DP, UK

Anthea Boylston is Contract Organiser for the Calvin Wells Laboratory in the Department of Archaeological Sciences, University of Bradford. She received an MSc in Osteology, Palaeopathology and Funerary Archaeology at the same university in 1991. Since then she has been working on human bone assemblages for a number of archaeological units, including the City of Lincoln Archaeological Unit, the City of Gloucester Archaeology Unit, Humber Archaeology Partnership, Northern Archaeological Associates, Bedfordshire County Council and the British Museum. In 1996 she organized a group of MSc students to assist in the recovery of individuals from a mass grave dating to the Battle of Towton (AD 1461) and is in the process of co-editing a monograph on the results of this excavation.

Megan Brickley
Department of Ancient History and Archaeology, University of Birmingham, Edgbaston, Birmingham B15 2TT, UK

Dr Megan Brickley graduated in Ancient History and Archaeology from the University of Birmingham, and then obtained an MSc in Ancient History and Archaeology of Disease from the Institute of Archaeology, London. Her doctoral research, undertaken jointly between the Institute of Archaeology and the Hard Tissue Research Unit (Department of Anatomy, University College London), was in age-related bone loss and osteoporosis. She is currently Lecturer in Environmental Archaeology at the University of Birmingham. She has a number of publications on techniques for studying bone density and osteoporosis, and is currently running a NERC funded research project to develop a 'standard' to measure bone-loss in archaeological bone.

Don Brothwell
Department of Archaeology, University of York, The King's Manor, York YO1 7EP, UK

Don Brothwell, BSc (Hons), MA, PhD, is Professor of Human Palaeoecology, University of York. Previous posts were at the University of Cambridge, The Natural History Museum, London, and University College London. His research has included studying bog bodies, vitrified forts and ancient foods, but most of his life has been involved with various aspects of skeletal biology. He has over one-hundred publications including numerous research papers and books on the subject of human osteology.

Keri Brown
Department of Biomolecular Sciences, UMIST, Manchester M60 1QD, UK

Keri Brown, BA, MPhil, has been a Research Assistant in the Department of Biomolecular Sciences, UMIST, since 1990 where, in collaboration with Dr Terry Brown, she has carried out research into ancient DNA from animal and human remains. She helped to develop the MSc course in Biomolecular Archaeology, and teaches both archaeology and biomolecular applications. She has a strong background in archaeology, having published research on the Southern Italian Neolithic, and having regularly excavated in Italy and elsewhere. Her grounding in biomolecular archaeological research is equally strong, having published reviews and reports on cremated bone, human and animal bone. In 1996 she was appointed to the Editorial Board of *Ancient Biomolecules*. Her research interests lie in using ancient DNA to uncover aspects of prehistoric social organization previously unobtainable by conventional techniques, such as kinship, sex identification and palaeodisease. She is currently working on ways to improve biomolecular-based methods of sex identification of human remains.

Andrew Chamberlain
Department of Archaeology and Prehistory, University of Sheffield, Northgate House, West St, Sheffield S14 ET, UK

Dr Andrew Chamberlain is a Senior Lecturer in the Department of Archaeology and Prehistory, University of Sheffield. Following undergraduate studies in Geology at the University of Liverpool and graduate training in Archaeological Science at the University of Southampton, he returned to Liverpool to study for a PhD in Human Evolution. Since 1990 he has co-directed the University of Sheffield/Bradford University graduate training programme in Osteology, Palaeopathology and Funerary Archaeology. He is the author of *Human Remains* (British Museum Press, 1994) and many research articles. Research interests include human evolution, palaeodemography and cave archaeology.

Matthew Collins
Department of Fossil Fuels and Environmental Geochemistry, Drummond Building, University of Newcastle, Newcastle upon Tyne NE1 7RU, UK

Dr Matthew Collins co-heads the Ancient Biomolecules Group at the University of Newcastle researching the deterioration of proteins with specific reference to bone. Originally trained as a Zoologist, he conducted PhD research into taphonomy before joining the Geobiochemie Werkgroup of Professor Peter Westbroek in Leiden, The Netherlands, where he was trained in biochemical and immunological methods. He spent time in Glasgow and Bristol (the latter in Professor John Parkes's Geomicrobiology group), before being appointed a lecturer in Biogeochemistry at the NRG (University of Newcastle). His current research interest is in the modelling of protein diagenesis, in particular racemization kinetics.

Margaret Cox
School of Conservation Sciences, Bournemouth University, Talbot Campus, Fern Barrow, Poole BH12 5BB, UK

Dr Margaret Cox obtained a PhD in Archaeology from University College London in 1989. She is Reader in Archaeological Science at Bournemouth University where she has developed an MSc in Forensic Archaeology. She currently works with many police forces in the UK and has worked for the UN in Kosovo. Before joining the School of Conservation Sciences at Bournemouth she was an archaeological consultant with an engineering firm. Before this she was Conservation Archaeologist in the Somerset Levels and Moors. She was Historian and Senior Osteologist for the Christ Church, Spitalfields Project in the 1980s. Previous publications include a co-authored volume on the Christ Church Project (with Theya Molleson) and the editorship of *Grave Concerns: Death and Burial in England 1700–1850* (1998). She is currently writing (with Charlotte Roberts) a book on disease in Britain from prehistory to the present, and another on women's health from the Roman period to the 1930s.

Chrissie Freeth
Calvin Wells Laboratory, Department of Archaeological Sciences, University of Bradford, Bradford BD7 1DP, UK

Chrissie Freeth obtained a BA (Hons) in Archaeology from the University of Bradford, where she is currently writing up her PhD thesis. Her doctoral research focuses on the prevalence of dental diseases in British archaeological populations. Other research interests include the evidence of dental treatment in the past.

Angela Gernaey
Department of Fossil Fuels and Environmental Geochemistry, Drummond Building, University of Newcastle, Newcastle upon Tyne NE1 7RU, UK

Dr Angela Gernaey (formerly Child) co-heads the Ancient Biomolecules Group, University of Newcastle. The main research areas of interest for the group are the preservation of mineralized proteins, and microbial biomarkers for palaeopathological diagnosis. Originally trained as a microbiologist, the subject of her PhD thesis was the microbial degradation of bone protein. The Ancient Biomolecules Group has investigated the chemical degradation of collagen and osteocalcin and is currently looking at the degradation of bone as a composite, with EU funding. Funding has also been obtained to develop microbial lipids as disease biomarkers, in collaboration with Professor David Minnikin. The research concentrates on the diagnosis of ancient tuberculosis and leprosy. She has published articles on the preservation of ancient biomolecules, and the detection of ancient diseases, particularly tuberculosis.

Robert Hedges
Research Laboratory for Archaeology and the History of Art, University of Oxford, 6 Keble Road, Oxford OX1 3QJ, UK

Dr Robert Hedges is Professor in Archaeology at the University of Oxford and Deputy Director of the Research Laboratory for Archaeology and the History of Art in Oxford, where he has been since 1971. Since 1980 he has been Director of the Radiocarbon Accelerator Unit. His main research aims are in the application of physical and chemical techniques to help broaden archaeological knowledge. Previous and current research interests have concentrated on obtaining archaeological information from molecular, and particularly isotopic, evidence. This has emphasized dating (mainly radiocarbon dating by accelerator mass spectrometry, but also uranium series dis-equilibrium dating, especially of bone and teeth), as well as stable isotope signatures of organic material. His research projects have also extended to include attempts to understand the changes in bone during burial, in both organic and inorganic components, and he has tried to develop a physical chemical basis for the interaction between bone and its burial environment. He has published in the areas of preservation and analysis of ancient DNA, ancient proteins, methodologies of dating by radiocarbon and uranium series methods, and the development of stable isotope analysis for the reconstruction of ancient diet.

Louise Humphrey
Human Origins Group, Department of Palaeontology, The Natural History Museum, Cromwell Road, London SW7 5BD, UK

Dr Louise Humphrey is a researcher in the Human Origins Group at The Natural History Museum, London. She is a BSc in Archaeology and a PhD in Biological Anthropology. Research interests include the nature and causes of inter- and intra-specific variation in the relative timing of developmental events in the skeleton and dentition in humans and other primates, and she has publications in this field. This incorporates ongoing research into the relationship between events occurring in early life and subsequent variation in skeletal and dental development, adult morphology and survivorship.

Christopher Knüsel
Calvin Wells Laboratory, Department of Archaeological Sciences, University of Bradford, Bradford BD7 1DP, UK

Dr Christopher Knüsel is lecturer in Biological Anthropology in the Department of Archaeological Sciences, University of Bradford, and is Course Manager for the MSc in Osteology, Palaeopathology, and Funerary Archaeology, run jointly with the University of Sheffield. He came to the University of Bradford as a Leverhulme Research Fellow in 1991. Research interests include skeletal biology, especially with regard to activity-related bone change and orthopaedic disabilities; funerary archaeology, particularly in northern and central Europe in the Iron Age; palaeopathology; and human evolution. He has recently co-authored 'Comparative degenerative joint disease of the vertebral column in the medieval monastic cemetery of the Gilbertine Priory of St. Andrew, Fishergate, York, England', *American Journal of Physical Anthropology*; and 'The man–woman or "Berdache" in Anglo-Saxon England and post-Roman Europe?', in *Social Identity in Early Medieval Britain*.

Mary Lewis
The Calvin Wells Laboratory, Department of Archaeological Sciences, University of Bradford, Bradford BD7 1DP, UK

Mary Lewis is a final year PhD student at the University of Bradford. Her research focuses on the health of non-adults in urban and rural environments from the early medieval to the Industrial period in Britain. In 1993 she received an MSc in Osteology, Palaeopathology and Funerary Archaeology from the Universities of Bradford and Sheffield. Since then she has worked on various projects including the analysis of maxillary sinusitis in urban and rural populations, and in Denmark, examining the health of children from a medieval monastery and leprosy hospital. Research interests cover many aspects of urban–rural health, incorporating research into growth, metabolic and infectious diseases, and non-specific indicators of stress. She has an additional interest in childhood leprosy, its diagnosis and significance in the transmission of the disease in the past. She has co-authored a number of research papers.

Simon Mays
Ancient Monuments Laboratory, English Heritage, Fort Cumberland, Fort Cumberland Road, Eastney, Portsmouth PO4 9LD, UK

Dr Simon Mays obtained a PhD in Archaeology from the University of Southampton in 1987, and he is currently a Human Skeletal Biologist (Senior Scientific Officer) in the Ancient Monuments Laboratory, English Heritage, Portsmouth. His research interests cover all areas of human osteoarchaeology and his book *The Archaeology of Human Bones* (1998) is a key text on the subject. Recent research articles include 'Infanticide in Roman Britain', *Antiquity*; 'Carbon stable isotope ratios in medieval and later human skeletons from Northern England', *Journal of Archaeological Science*; and 'Osteoporosis in earlier human populations', *Journal of Clinical Densitometry*.

Jacqueline McKinley
Wessex Archaeology, Portway House, Old Sarum Park, Salisbury SP4 6EB, UK

Jaqueline McKinley has been a Project Officer (Osteoarchaeologist) at Wessex Archaeology, Salisbury, for the past five years. Her time is divided between running archaeological excavations and the analysis of human remains excavated by Wessex Archaeology and other archaeological organizations. She also regularly lectures on cremation at various university departments. Her archaeological career has included a combination of site and specialist work, working for a variety of different organizations across the UK, and as a freelance archaeologist. Her predominant specialist research interest comprises the study of cremated remains and the mortuary rite of cremation, which has involved observations at modern crematoria and of experimental pyres. Previous publications include *The Anglo-Saxon Cemetery at Spong Hill, North Elmham. Part VIII: The Cremations* (1994), based on the analysis of 2500 cremation burials.

David Minnikin
Department of Chemistry, University of Newcastle, Newcastle upon Tyne NE1 7RU, UK

David Minnikin is Professor of Microbial Chemistry at the University of Newcastle. His current research interests are: structure, role and taxonomic potential of bacterial lipids, particularly those from mycobacteria; the synthesis and evaluation of inhibitors of long-chain fatty acids, such as mycolic acids, to pinpoint new drug targets in *Mycobacterium tuberculosis* and to elucidate the mode of action of existing drugs; and the evaluation of lipids as biomarkers for ancient and modern leprosy and tuberculosis. He has co-authored a number of papers on these subjects, including 'An integrated procedure for the direct detection of characteristic lipids in tuberculosis patients' and 'Identification of the leprosy bacillus and related mycobacteria by analysis of mycocerosate profiles', *Annales de la Societe Belge de Medecine Tropicale*; 'Detecting ancient tuberculosis', *Internet Archaeology*; and 'Demonstration of *Mycobacterium tuberculosis* complex DNA in calcified pleura from remains 1400 years old', *Letters in Applied Microbiology*.

Richard Neave
Unit of Art in Medicine, Stopford Building, University of Manchester, Oxford Road, Manchester M13 9PT, UK

Richard Neave trained as an artist and entered the Middlesex Hospital, London, in 1957 to study medical art. In 1959 he moved to the University of Manchester as the Medical Artist at the Manchester Royal Infirmary. His current appointment is that of Artist in Medicine and Life Sciences in the Faculty of Medicine, Dentistry and Nursing at the University of Manchester. In 1973 he became involved with the reconstruction of human heads and faces on skulls as part of an archaeological study of ancient Egyptian remains. This in turn led to the application of the technique in the forensic area, and such work has continued to expand ever since. His current interest lies particularly in the area of reconstructing heads on skulls mechanically made from digital information acquired from CT scans. Publications include 'Reconstruction of the head of Phillip II of Macedon', *Journal of Hellenic Studies*; 'Reconstruction of the skull and soft tissues of the head and face of Lindow Man', *Canadian Society of Forensic Science Journal*; and (with John Prag) *Making Faces*.

Christina Nielsen-Marsh
Department of Fossil Fuels and Environmental Geochemistry, Drummond Building, University of Newcastle, Newcastle upon Tyne NE1 7RU, UK

Dr Christina Nielsen-Marsh is a Research Associate in Archaeological Science at the University of Newcastle. She currently works as the scientific advisor on archaeological bone analysis for a European-funded project, 'The Degradation of Bone as an Indicator in the Deterioration of the European Archaeological Property'. Alongside this project she has various research interests including the degradation mechanisms of archaeological bone, the development of differential scanning calorimetry and mercury intrusion porosimetry as screening methods for bone survival, and the diagenetic analysis of Central and South American megafauna remains. Before joining the Ancient Biomolecules Group at Newcastle, she worked at the Research Laboratory for Archaeology, University of Oxford, with Robert Hedges where she completed a DPhil in archaeological bone diagenesis.

Alistair Pike
Research Laboratory for Archaeology and the History of Art, University of Oxford, 6 Keble Road, Oxford OX1 3QJ, UK

Alistair Pike is currently a doctoral student at the Research Laboratory for Archaeology, University of Oxford, and the Department of Earth Sciences, Open University. His research interests are directed towards not only uranium uptake in archaeological bone and uranium-series dating, but also span bone diagenesis, burial-environment geochemistry and hydrology, and dating the origins of modern humans. After graduating from the Department of Archaeological Sciences, University of Bradford, he spent two years as a Scientific Officer at English Heritage and a year at the Department of Scientific Research of The British Museum.

Kim Piper
Department of Oral Pathology, St Bartholomew's and the Royal London School of Medicine and Dentistry, Clinical Sciences Research Building, 2 Newark Street, London E1 2AD, UK

Dr Kim Piper is a lecturer in Oral Pathology at St Bartholomew's and the Royal London School of Medicine and Dentistry, Whitechapel, London. Her research interests centre around bone cell biology with work on both osteoclast cell function and regulation of osteoblast cell commitment. Her work as an oral pathologist centres on the diagnosis of pathology in the head and neck, she has long held an interest in palaeohistopathology. She has co-authored research papers on these subjects, including 'Tuberculosis of the mandible in a child', *Journal of Laryngology and Otology*; and 'Volumes of chick and rat osteoclasts cultured on glass', *Calcified Tissue International*.

John Robb
Department of Archaeology, University of Southampton, Southampton SO17 1BF, UK

Dr John Robb was awarded a PhD by the University of Michigan in 1995, and is currently Lecturer in European Prehistory at the University of Southampton. He has worked on human skeletons from Italy, Iran, Palestine, England and the USA. He is particularly interested in using skeletons to investigate social change in later prehistory and in incorporating skeletons into the theoretical interpretation of social relations. Publications include *Material Symbols* (1999), and numerous articles and book chapters. Besides studying human skeletons, he is interested in archaeological theory and is currently excavating prehistoric sites in Calabria, Southern Italy.

Charlotte Roberts
Department of Archaeology, University of Durham, South Road, Durham DH1 3LE, UK

Dr Charlotte Roberts has recently taken up the position of Reader in Archaeology at the University of Durham. Before this she was Senior Lecturer in Biological Anthropology, Department of Archaeological Sciences, University of Bradford. She qualified as a State Registered Nurse in 1978 and obtained a BA in Archaeological Studies from the University of Leicester in 1982, followed by a MA in Environmental Archaeology and Palaeoeconomy from the University of Sheffield in 1983, and in 1988 a PhD in Biological Anthropology (trauma and its treatment in antiquity). Her key research projects include studies of evolution and palaeoepidemiology of infectious disease; sex and gender, environment and climate and their effects on health patterning in the past; recognition and interpretation of disease associated disability and stigma in the archaeological record; biocultural approaches to palaeopathology. She has co-authored a number of key texts, including *The Archaeology of Disease* (2nd edn, 1995) and *Studies in Crime: An Introduction to Forensic Anthropology* (1996).

Juliet Rogers
Rheumatology Unit, Bristol Royal Infirmary, Bristol BS2 8HW, UK

Dr Juliet Rogers is a Senior Research Fellow in Palaeopathology in the Rheumatology Unit, University of Bristol. She is the only palaeopathologist working in a clinical medical department, and as well as being medically qualified, she has a wide experience of working on archaeological material. She has been involved in the recovery and examination of skeletal material from many sites, including Hazelton, Wells and St Oswald's Priory. For the past ten years she has been leading the team undertaking examination of skeletal material and analysis of the data from St Peter's, Barton-on-Humber, one of the largest collections so far recovered in this country. She is currently writing up the results of this work. Research interests include the palaeopathology of joint disease and, in collaboration with Tony Waldron, she has worked on the definition of the palaeopathological diagnostic criteria of these diseases. Together, they have published *Field Guide to Joint Disease in Archaeology* (1994), as well as a series of papers on these diseases. She also runs a series of undergraduate courses at the University of Bristol.

Louise Scheuer
Department of Anatomy and Developmental Biology, Royal Free and University College Medical School, Royal Free Campus, London NW3 2PF, UK

Dr Louise Scheuer is an Honorary Senior Lecturer at the Royal Free and University College Medical School. Her main interests are in the development of the juvenile skeleton, the skeletal biology of past peoples, and forensic osteology. She has taught human anatomy to medical and dental students, run a BSc course in Forensic and Archaeological Osteology and taught osteology to postgraduate groups in London, Bradford, Glasgow and Bournemouth universities, and at the Law Society, London. She also undertakes consultancy work for the Metropolitan and other police forces. Together with Sue Black, she was awarded a Leverhulme Research grant for the conservation and re-evaluation of the St Bride's crypt skeletal collection. Both she and Sue Black have been writing *Developmental Juvenile Osteology* (forthcoming, 2000), a work on the juvenile skeleton.

James Steele
Department of Archaeology, University of Southampton, Highfield, Southampton SO17 1BJ, UK

Dr James Steele is Lecturer in Early Hominid Studies, University of Southampton. He teaches palaeoanthropology and Palaeolithic archaeology at undergraduate level, and convenes the MA in Osteoarchaeology. Research interests include hominid evolution (brain organization, socio-ecology, diet, geographical distribution); initial human dispersals into the Americas; and skeletal markers of handedness. He has published articles on these and related topics in *World Archaeology*, *International Journal of Osteoarchaeology*, etc., and has co-edited (with Stephen Shennan) a book entitled *The Archaeology of Human Ancestry: Power Sex and Tradition* (1996) on reconstructing hominid behaviour.

Gordon Turner-Walker
Institute of Archaeology and Cultural History, Vitenskapsmuseum, Norwegian University of Science and Technology, N–7491 Trondheim, Norway

Dr Gordon Turner-Walker is a researcher in Archaeological Science and Conservation, based at the Vitenskapsmuseum, Norwegian University of Science and Technology (NTNU), Trondheim. He gained a BSc in Astrophysics at Queen Mary College, University of London, before working in field archaeology for several years. In 1989 he completed a Diploma in Archaeological Conservation at the University of Durham, followed by a PhD in the characterization of fossil bone, also at Durham. His primary interests lie in diagenesis studies of ancient bones, and the application of electron microscopy and other imaging techniques to the quantification of post-mortem changes in bone tissue. He is currently a post-doctoral fellow at the University Hospital, undertaking research on the distribution and severity of osteoporosis in the medieval population of Scandinavia.

Andy Tyrrell
Archaeology and Archaeological Science Research School, University of Sheffield, 2 Mappin Street, Sheffield S1 4DT, UK

Dr Andy Tyrrell has recently completed a PhD at the Department of Archaeology and Prehistory, University of Sheffield. He graduated from the University of Bristol in 1992 from the School of Archaeology and Geology and then went on to study for an MSc in Osteology, Palaeopathology and Funerary Archaeology at Sheffield and Bradford universities. He has co-edited (with Bill Frazer) *Social Identity in Early Medieval Britain* (1998). He has also recently been involved in a forensic capacity with the UN ICTY in Bosnia-Herzegovina. Research interests include quantitative anthropological genetics and micro-evolution, early medieval population dynamics, forensic facial reconstruction and other forensic applications of biological anthropology, and ancient and modern attitudes to ethnicity. He has publications in these areas.

David Whittaker
Department of Basic Dental Science, University of Wales College of Medicine, Dental School, Heath Park, Cardiff CF4 4XY, UK

Dr David Whittaker is Reader in Oral Biology and Forensic Dentistry, University of Wales College of Medicine, where he is also Course Director for an MSc in Forensic Dentistry. He has 30 years of experience in this field and appears in Court regularly. He lectures and advises throughout the world, and in his capacity as a Consultant Dental Surgeon examines at under- and postgraduate levels, both in the UK and abroad. He has authored and co-authored more than one-hundred publications in the scientific literature, and is first author of a standard text on Forensic Dentistry. He has also published in the archaeological field, particularly in relation to the Christ Church, Spitalfields, London, project.

Preface

Human remains from archaeological contexts form one of the most important sources of evidence about our past. Human osteoarchaeology, the study of human skeletons from archaeological sites, can provide information on health, demography, diet, activity patterns, physique and genetic aspects of earlier populations. When combined with other archaeological or historical evidence, osteological data can contribute to the study of a broad range of topics including early migrations of peoples, ancient warfare and the study of the effects the rise of social inequality on human health and lifestyles. Osteological analyses also clearly have a wide range of forensic applications, such as aiding the identification of unknown human remains, and resolution of criminal investigations, including war crimes.

In the preparation of this volume, the Editors invited leading specialists to contribute chapters that would review the current status and future potential of a particular field. All contributions were subject to confidential peer-review. The volume begins with an historical overview of osteological research in Britain. The main part of the book is organized into six sections: juvenile health, growth and development; palaeodemography; disease in the past; human variation; assaults on the skeleton; and microscopic, biochemical and analytical approaches.

No textbook can be completely comprehensive, and while we have attempted to cover most of the main areas of research in osteological analysis as practised in north-western Europe, some aspects are not included. Perhaps the most notable omission is the determination of race. We consider that concepts of race are scientifically unsatisfactory, and that they are not useful in archaeological work in a north-west European context. Even in forensic work, race determination is often rendered problematic by the phenomenon of mixed parentage. That aside, we have intended to provide broad coverage of core essentials such as age and sex determination which underpin many other analyses, while at the same time also considering cutting-edge applications such as DNA analyses and chemical methods in palaeopathology, and higher level data analytical techniques used in fields such as palaeodemography.

One of the most significant points to come from many of the chapters is the need to test, refine and develop techniques on collections of skeletons of known ancestry, sex, age and socio-economic background. At present most such collections are from modern contexts, and there is a real need to undertake further methodological research on documented archaeological samples to obtain direct information on the reliability of our methods on earlier human populations.

1

STUDIES ON SKELETAL AND DENTAL VARIATION: A VIEW ACROSS TWO CENTURIES

Don Brothwell

INTRODUCTION

It seems that every few decades there is value in reviewing research and progress in studies on earlier human populations. For the emphasis within a subject may change, with new avenues being explored or new researchers with different interests appearing on the scene. While human bioarchaeological research is broadly based, some of us have been especially involved over the years with human remains from British sites, and it would therefore seem an ideal subject to discuss here.

What follows is a summary overview of the work that has been undertaken on earlier British populations, beginning in the Pleistocene and finishing in the medieval period. This work extends back well over a century and has produced a vast literature. In the space available, an attempt will be made to highlight some of the main themes and results. It will be seen that the investigations have met problems and have raised as many questions as they have answered, but nevertheless they have also contributed to progress concerning the more general biology of past populations.

PLEISTOCENE BRITONS

Perhaps more than in most other parts of the world, claims for British Palaeolithic human fossils have had a controversial history. Investigations of cave sites began early, for instance the sites of Goat's Hole, Paviland and Kent's Cavern, Torquay, which began to be explored between 1823 and 1824.[1] While some finds turned out to be of questionable date, the so-called 'Red Lady' of Paviland is firmly Upper Palaeolithic (about 16 500 BC). By the 1870s, Mousterian artefacts and associated Neanderthal fragments had been found at Pontnewydd cave in Wales and other cave sites were also being explored.

Pleistocene sands and gravels were to contribute significantly, although again not without controversy. Red Crag sands at Foxhall, near Ipswich, produced a modern-looking mandible in 1855, sadly now lost.[2] The 90-foot Thames terrace at Galley Hill, Kent,[3] produced a skeleton in 1888 that interested palaeontologists, but which is now thought likely to be only Neolithic in date. Perhaps the most notable year for problematic finds was in 1912, producing the Halling skeleton from Brick Earth in Kent,[4] and the now infamous Piltdown skull from Sussex.[5] Neither is now seen as Pleistocene, but the Piltdown bones have at least provided a fine example of the scientific detection of a palaeontological fraud.[6]

Fortunately, the discovery of part of a 250 000-year-old human skull in a 100-foot Thames terrace at Swanscombe in 1935,[7] and recently teeth and part of a 500 000-year-old tibia at Boxgrove in Sussex[8] provides tantalizing but incomplete evidence of late *Homo erectus*, and a more advanced pre-Neanderthal form of hominid. While it is to the credit of English Heritage that considerable funds were made available to excavate areas of the Boxgrove quarry site, it raises two important issues for us all. First, United Nations-supported international law to stop quarrying at such world important hominid sites is long overdue. There is no doubt that many stone tools, much faunal material and perhaps more hominid remains have been lost at the Boxgrove site before the eventual termination of quarrying. The second issue is that, because of the removal of deep gravel deposits from critical parts of the site, the environment of some preserved potential hominid-yielding deposits has been transformed, and there is thus now great danger of accelerated weathering and decay.

It should be said that the biological significance of the Boxgrove hominid tibia is that its cortical robustness supports other evidence of a strongly built European *H. erectus* physique. On the other hand, the Swanscombe skull helps to establish significant cranial remodelling within the next 200 000 years, with increasing vault height and upper parietal bossing (a significant advance on the erectine level). The most controversial feature is perhaps the skull thickness, still viewed by some as a primitive trait, but which can surely only be used as an indicator of environmental stress.

HOLOCENE POPULATIONS

Let me now move on to studies on more recent British populations. Under the stimulus of antiquarianism, many excavations took place in the 19th century, although some were little more than plundering and treasure hunting. Fortunately, as a result of the influence of anatomists and other medical specialists, human remains were often saved for study, especially the skull. Thomas Bateman, for example, digging between 1848 and 1858, initiated a skeletal collection that remains today in Sheffield. Others followed, and some reported on and illustrated the cranial material, and even T. H. Huxley became involved.[9] Indeed, in 1865 Drs Barnard Davis and John Thurnam produced a large volume, *Crania Britannica*, considering 260 skulls of Neolithic to medieval date, pointing out that there were osteometric changes through time.[10]

Methodology was already being considered, and new techniques of recording explored. John Grattan, for instance, developed a contouring method as an alternative or extension of conventional measurement. More rigorous mathematical treatment of osteometric data was also needed, and Karl Pearson at University College London took up this challenge. For the next 40 years, his journal *Biometrika* was to provide detailed osteometric analysis, both of specific cemeteries and reviewing geographic areas.[11,12] To embrace multiple measurements in considering biological affinities of different populations, he devised the *coefficient of racial likeness* (CRL) – useful in its time, but now replaced by D^2, canonical analysis and principal component analysis. For all its faults, the CRL confirmed and extended on the conclusions of 19th-century biologists that there were micro-evolutionary differences between earlier British populations.

Surprisingly, following the Second World War, there were very few similar studies of British material and this work was largely kept alive by Dr Jack Trevor at the University of Cambridge. There is still a neglect of osteometric studies, but a real need to determine further the degree of regional variation and the finer details of changes through time. Contrary to the views of some prehistorians, the differences in physique tentatively established between the early Neolithic and Bronze Age peoples of Britain demonstrates that there was a considerable influx of distinctive Beaker/Food Vessel people into the country (see Mays, chapter 17, in this volume). What is more puzzling and demands far more investigation is that there are also noticeable changes from Anglo-Saxon to Norman times.[13]

There is still the possibility that osteometric measurements may at times assist in dating problematic skeletal samples. Such a series was excavated from one of the Five Knolls barrows in Bedfordshire[14] and was thought to be early Saxon, but the skeletal analysis eventually showed their affinities were with medieval groups; they are probably medieval gallows victims.

Regarding non-metric traits, the potential for using them is similarly far from realised (see Tyrell, chapter 18, in this volume). They were neglected until the late 1950s, and while some fluctuate in frequency through time, and can be used multifactorially to evaluate population distances between groups, there is an urgent need to consider their aetiology in more detail. While some traits may be under simple genetic control, oral tori in particular seem to be especially enigmatic and could be environmentally determined. As so often happens, these traits have been drawn into the basic methodology of investigating skeletons, and are even used to suggest family clustering in cemeteries,[15] which makes their further study even more urgent. It is correct to call these traits 'epigenetic' as none show simple Mendelian inheritance. Rather, they are the expression of genes affecting development, but are also influenced by environmental factors.

STUDIES ON DISEASE

Although early in the 20th century British anatomists and anthropologists were contributing significantly to the study of the health status of the ancient Egyptians, there was a puzzling absence of the same kind of detailed studies on early British populations. Pathology had, of course, been noted (reviewed by Brothwell[16]), but not in a systematic and comparative way. Again, it was not until the second half of this century that a range of studies on the evidence for disease appeared and, much to my concern, have somewhat overwhelmed other skeletal and dental research. So the literature on the palaeopathology of early British populations is now vast and growing, but in fact specific lines of research are still poorly funded. For instance, investigations on the survival of microbial DNA in different burial environments demand further research.

But for all the problems, a history of some diseases in early British groups is beginning to take shape. We now have quite a wide range of evidence, from clubfoot and Down's syndrome representing congenital abnormality, to increasing evidence of malignant tumours and even surgery. There is still much to debate. The impact and, indeed, the correct identification of environmental stressors on the skeleton are an area of current British research interest. For instance, was the Bronze Age child from Wiltshire,[17] with thickened skull and areas of surface remodelling, a victim of anaemia or rickets? How complex is the aetiology of orbital cribra? How can we distinguish the major factors causing Harris lines or zones of enamel hypoplasia? Perhaps osteoporosis, cortical bone loss, can be more simply investigated, and it has recently been searched for in early Londoners and a medieval village population (both with success[18]). But frequencies are low, compared with those which can occur for orbital cribra or Harris Lines.

The most neglected of the environmentally determined conditions is surely hypothyroidism. Regions of Britain are known to have been iodine-deficient in the past. We also know that iodine deficiency may cause not only cretinism in a population, but also less severe growth disturbance, so why have we not taken account of this in skeletal samples from goitrogenic areas?

Since the early days of skeletal biology, the classification and understanding of joint diseases has greatly improved, and most of the forms of arthropathy have been identified in human remains. Perhaps of special note is the fact that archaeological material has contributed significantly to establishing rheumatoid arthritis[19] as rare before post-medieval times, in the UK at least. Only in recent centuries has it reached epidemic proportions.

There are still interesting research problems concerned with joint diseases. We still neglect brucellosis arthritis, although it could display distinctive joint changes and may well have been common. And what of Schmorl's nodes? This anomaly was seen in the CT scans of the Lindow II bog body, and while the vertebral herniations are not usually clinically important, they *are* common in past populations, and can occur by later adolescence, and are surely indicators of biomechanical stress. At least, they deserve more detailed investigation.

Discriminating between different patterns of bone change caused by a number of major infectious diseases has gained the attention of researchers over the years.[20] Mycobacterial diseases, and especially leprosy,[21] had a significant impact on British medieval populations, and in fact extended well beyond the areas where leper hospitals were established. Its appearance in the south of England as far west as the Scilly Isles by later Roman-Dark Age times as well as in the far north, in the Norse community of the Orkney Islands (9th–12th century AD), suggests to me that there was not a single region of entry, but at least a kind of pincer movement, from both south and north.

The pathogens that have especially interested me are those causing treponemal diseases, including venereal syphilis. Three of the four clinical conditions produce bone changes and offer a special challenge in piecing together their micro-evolutionary history and relationships. In 1926, a site at Spitalfields Market in London produced a skull with advanced tertiary syphilis.[22] Unfortunately, it turned out to have a post-medieval date, but further discoveries have now been made, the first with a firm pre-Columbian date in York.[23] There is not space here to elaborate on the discoveries of probable treponemal disease in the UK or elsewhere, except to say that archaeology is beginning to contribute to an understanding of treponemal evolution. My own current view is that venereal syphilis is a late medieval, *newly evolved* form, probably derived from endemic syphilis in Southwest Asia. Its late appearance into Britain fits the hypothesis that the pathogen was late in adapting to populations living in colder northern European climates and societies, and had to become more aggressive and venereal in transmission.[24]

In some respects, prospects continue to improve for the study of ancient populations, whether in the UK or elsewhere, with CT scans, DNA analysis, and improved computer technology (see Brown, chapter 27, in this volume). In other respects, however, there may be growing problems. Funding is getting more difficult to find. Restrictions on X-raying living individuals, or in other respects being less able to study certain diseases in living peoples because they have become uncommon or extinct, limits studies on skeletal and dental changes. Growing restrictions on animal experimentation also make aspects of comparative pathology perhaps less promising for the future.

The cloud on the horizon, which will probably not go away, is the reburial issue. At a personal level the present author has had two British cemetery samples removed for reburial before full study, and the situation could get worse. There is therefore good cause to review where our studies have got to and which aspects deserve our special research efforts before it is too late!

REFERENCES

1   Oakley KP. The problem of man's antiquity. An historical survey. *Bulletin of The British Museum (Natural History): Geology Series* 1964; **2**: 85–155.

2   Collyer RH. The fossil human jaw from Suffolk. *Anthropology Review* 1867; **5**: 221.

3   Newton ET. On a human skull and limb bones found in the Palaeolithic terrace gravel at Galley Hill, Kent. *Quarterly Journal of the Geological Society of London* 1895; **15**: 246–263.

4   Keith A. *The Antiquity of Man*. London: Williams & Norgate, 1915.

5   Dawson C, Woodward AS. On the discovery of a Palaeolithic human skull and mandible in a flint-bearing gravel overlying the Wealdon (Hastings beds) at Piltdown, Fletching (Sussex). *Quarterly Journal of the Geological Society of London* 1913; **69**: 117–144.

6   Weiner JS, Oakley KP, Le Gros Clark WE. The solution of the Piltdown problem. *Bulletin of The British Museum (Natural History): Geology Series* 1953; **2**: 141–146.

7   Ovey CD (ed.). *The Swanscombe Skull: A Survey of Research on a Pleistocene Site*. London, Royal Anthropological Institute, 1964.

8   Roberts MB. Excavation of the lower Palaeolithic site at Amey's Earthen Pit, Boxgrove, West Sussex: a preliminary report. *Proceedings of the Prehistoric Society* 1986; **52**: 215–245.

9   Huxley TH. Notes upon the human remains from Keiss. In: S Laing, *Pre-historic Remains of Caithness*. London: Williams & Norgate, 1866: pp. 83–148.

10   Davis BJ, Thurnam J. *Crania Britannica*. London: Taylor & Francis, 1865.

11   Macdonell WR. A study of the variation and correlation of the human skull, with special reference to English crania. *Biometrika* 1904; **3**: 191–244.

12   Morant GMA. First study of the craniology of England and Scotland from Neolithic to early historic times, with special reference to the Anglo-Saxon skulls in London Museums. *Biometrika* 1926; **18**: 56–98.

13   Brothwell D, Krzanowski W. Evidence of biological differences between early British populations from Neolithic to medieval times, as revealed by eleven commonly available cranial vault measurements. *Journal of Archaeological Science* 1974; **1**: 249–260.

14   Dingwall D, Young M. The skulls from excavations at Dunstable, Bedfordshire. *Biometrika* 1933; **25**: 147–157.

15   Stead S. The human bones. In: IM Stead (ed.), *Iron Age Cemeteries in East Yorkshire*. London: English Heritage, 1991: pp. 126–139.

16   Brothwell D. The palaeopathology of early British man: an essay on the problems of diagnosis and analysis. *Journal of the Royal Anthropological Institute of Great Britain and Ireland* 1961; **91**: 318–344.

17   Brothwell D. The human remains from Avebery barrow G55, with special reference to the further evidence of a childhood deficiency disease in the Bronze Age. *Wiltshire Archaeology and Natural History Magazine* 1992; **85**: 141–144.

18   Mays SA. Age-dependent cortical bone loss in a medieval population. *International Journal of Osteoarchaeology* 1996; **6**: 144–154.

19   Rogers J, Waldron T, Dieppe P, Watt I. Anthropathies in palaeopathology: the basis of classification according to most probable cause. *Journal of Archaeological Science* 1987; **14**: 179–193.

20   Roberts C, Manchester K. *The Archaeology of Disease* (2nd edn). Stroud: Sutton, 1995.

21   Manchester K, Roberts C. The palaeopathology of leprosy in Britain: a review. *World Archaeology* 1989; **21**: 265–272.

22   Morant GM, Hoadley MF. A study of the recently excavated Spitalfields crania. *Biometrika* 1931; **23**: 191–248.

23   Dawes JD, Magilton JR. *The Cemetery of St. Helen-on-the-Walls, Aldwark*. The Archaeology of York, 12/1. York: Council for British Archaeology, 1980.

24   Brothwell DR. Microevolutionary change in the human pathogenic treponemes: an alternative hypothesis. *International Journal of Systematic Bacteriology* 1981; **31**: 82–87.

Section I

Juvenile health, growth and development

The study of immature human skeletal remains has arguably been a rather neglected area of osteoarchaeology. In part this reflects the often incomplete and fragmentary nature of such material, but it is also a manifestation of what has until recently been a broader neglect of the study of childhood in the past. However, as the chapters in this section illustrate, osteological studies of juvenile remains have the potential to make important contributions to the study of the archaeology of childhood, particularly in terms of growth, health and mortality. They also provide sensitive indicators of the general health of the population from which they came.

Determination of age at death is, of course, the foundation of most osteological analyses of immature remains, and Louise Scheuer and Sue Black begin this section with a discussion of methods for age determination in immature remains, and the processes of skeletal development and maturation upon which they are based. Louise Humphrey discusses the value of growth studies of archaeological material. Although growth rates are important indicators of the well-being of a population, results need to be interpreted with caution. Using a case study approach, she demonstrates the value of using a combination of different methodologies when comparing growth rates between populations. The health of juveniles is discussed by Mary Lewis, who considers the role of pathologies indicative of dental disease, specific and non-specific infections and metabolic disease in understanding children's lives in the past. The importance of assessing trauma is discussed, particularly in relation to such practices as child abuse or child labour. Such issues extend in importance beyond their obvious palaeopathological significance to indicate cultural values and practices. All authors in this section discuss the importance of recognizing the limitations of immature skeletal samples for making inferences about the past populations.

2

DEVELOPMENT AND AGEING OF THE JUVENILE SKELETON

Louise Scheuer and Sue Black

INTRODUCTION

Death rates and life expectancies as revealed by a demographic profile are often used as a reflection of the health and well-being of a population. When attempting to reconstruct the lifestyle of past peoples, who are represented only by their skeletal remains, there are particular problems which are absent from the study of living populations.

It is rare for the sex and ages at death of the individuals that comprise a skeletal assemblage to be known and normally one of the principal tasks in the analysis of skeletal remains is to establish these two basic biological parameters. Another unknown factor is how far the remains constitute a representative sample of the population of which they formed a part. This has the potential to bias the age at death profile of the original population. The determination of sex, age at death and representativeness of the immature component of a skeletal assemblage requires a somewhat different approach from that in the adult and this chapter aims to examine some of the factors that affect their analysis in juveniles.

TERMINOLOGY

The terminology applied to different periods of an individual lifespan varies both in different countries, and as used by clinicians, evolutionary biologists and skeletal biologists and this can lead to confusion. Accepted definitions of the periods from the beginning of life at fertilization through the childhood years are shown in Table 1.

After this time usage begins to vary. *Puberty* is generally taken to be a physiological term describing the beginning of secondary sexual change, usually ranging from 10 to 14 years in girls and 12–16 years in boys. *Adolescence* is used by some authors interchangeably with puberty but by others to describe the behavioural and psychological changes that accompany it. Some paediatricians describe adolescence as the period from 13 to 19 years of age.[1]

Table 1 – Periods from fertilization through childhood.

Embryo	First 2 months of intra-uterine life
Foetus	Third month to birth
Perinate	Around the time of birth
Neonate	Birth to the end of the first month
Infant	Birth to the end of the first year
Early childhood	To the end of the fifth year
Late childhood	About 6 years to puberty

Two schemes commonly used by skeletal biologists vary in the terminology applied to the period between the end of childhood (14–15 years) and adult life which they defined as the time of closure of the spheno-occipital synchondrosis. Acsádi and Nemeskéri[2] call the period *juvenile* and Ferembach *et al.*,[3] for the Workshop of European Anthropologists, call the same period *adolescence*. However, the age ranges of between 17 and 25 years for the closure of the spheno-occipital synchondrosis that are quoted in most standard anatomical texts are almost certainly too late.[4–6] Recourse to the original literature describing the results of inspection of dry skulls, cadavers, histological and radiological investigations report this as occurring much earlier, on average between 11 and 15 years.[7–13] On this definition the whole of the juvenile or adolescent age range as defined by the two schemes would be eliminated.

In the UK and North America the terms *immature* and *sub-* or *non-adult* are sometimes used to describe any age that is not truly adult. Also in more recent publications the term *juvenile* is increasingly used in their place.[14–21] Here *juvenile* describes the whole age range from early embryonic to adult life. The terms in Table 1 are used for the earlier part of the range and *puberty* and *adolescence* are used interchangeably to describe the time of secondary sexual change. *Young adult* is applied to the period between the cessation of growth in height, signalled by fusion of the long bone epiphyses, to the final fusion of the late-fusing epiphyses such as those of the vertebral column, clavicle, iliac crest and jugular growth plate.

SAMPLING

It is unlikely that the number of skeletons in an assemblage will approximate to the total number of the population who lived and died in the vicinity of the burial place. Burial in a particular place is affected by a variety of factors including social and economic conditions and religious beliefs. After burial, subsequent skeletonization and preservation of bones are in turn affected by physical conditions and these may include temperature, type of soil, coffin design and disturbance by humans and predators. Even when an excavation is carefully planned, it is not always possible to recover all of the material in a good enough condition to contribute useful information towards sexing and ageing of individual skeletons. As a result, the age profile of the initial population will always remain uncertain. Some of the factors affecting sampling and their effects on recovery and reconstruction are discussed in more detail elsewhere.[22–24]

REPRESENTATIVENESS

It is a common observation that the number of juveniles is often lower than might be expected for a particular time and place and this can seriously bias the age profile drawn from any analysis of the assemblage.[25–28] Occasionally this supposition can be corroborated by documentary evidence. For example, it is clear from examination of the burial registers that the proportions of adults to children interred in the crypt of St Bride's Church, Fleet Street, London and the St Bride's cemetery are quite different. Therefore, any conclusions concerning the numbers of child deaths in the parish drawn from the age at death profile of the crypt collection alone would be invalid.[28] One known reason for the low number of juveniles is the custom of selectively excluding infants and young children from the main adult burial site for cultural, religious or economic reasons.[14,16,25,28] It has also been argued that the reason for low numbers of juveniles, especially infants, is due to the special physicochemical properties of their relatively fragile bones leading to poor preservation.[29–32] However, Sundick[33] believed that the principal reasons for low retrieval rate were deficiencies of skill on the part of the excavators and failure to recognize small, unfused parts of the immature skeleton rather than the nature of the material. Certainly detailed knowledge of the anatomy of the developing skeleton will lead to better awareness of the expected number of different elements and so improve recovery of juveniles.

Several methods have recently been tested in attempts to make use of juvenile material, which was previously thought to be too damaged to include in an analysis and so compensate in some way for small numbers of immature remains. Measurements of fragments of long bones, rather than total length, from Anglo-Saxon remains have been used successfully in a growth study[15], and a similar method increased sample size in an analysis of prehistoric Ontario skeletons by > 100%. Experience with two very different samples led to the recommendation of a population-specific model.[34] Another standardized method for analysing growth used any long bone that represented a single individual. This was included on a single plot to maximize information from all material vailable.[31]

GROWTH, SEXING AND AGEING

Growth consists of two factors: an increase in size and the attainment of consecutive levels of maturity but these two aspects do not necessarily advance in synchrony. For example, a boy of 6 years may be several centimetres taller than his friend of the same age. Similarly, two girls, both aged 14 years, can be at different stages of skeletal and sexual maturity.

Many factors affect the growth of the skeleton, and there is a great range of variability between different populations, between the sexes and between individuals of the same population. Part of this variation is genetically based but in many populations children subjected to adverse environmental pressures, chiefly those of undernutrition and exposure to disease, exhibit a slower rate of growth than their optimum potential.[35,36] Rates of increase in size and increase in maturity differ between the sexes and this is evident even before birth.[37,38] There are also differences in the timing of ossification of bones,[39] of bone mineral density,[40] peak bone mass[41] and mineralization and emergence of teeth.[42–46] As puberty approaches, differential hormone secretion increases sexual dimorphism. The timing of the adolescent growth spurt varies between individuals of the same sex (early and late maturers) but in general, girls are about 2 years in advance of boys in maturity at the same chronological age.[47]

The actual sex and age at death of the members of an archaeological collection are rarely known, the only sizeable collections in the UK where this is so being the documented remains from St Bride's Church, Fleet Street and from Christ Church, Spitalfields, both in London. Even here, caution must be exercized as various factors can combine to alter what appears to be, at first sight, a well-documented fact. Bones from different skeletons can become commingled after excavation and it has been found that so-called documented facts are sometimes concealed for personal reasons.[28,48]

In the majority of skeletal collections it is not possible to establish actual chronological age and the concept of biological age has to be used as an indicator of how far along the developmental continuum an individual has progressed. However, because a large component of growth variation is sex dependent, and it is not possible to sex juveniles with any degree of reliability, any estimated age category is necessarily wider than it would have been had the sex been known.

SEXING

The difficulty of determining sex is arguably the biggest problem in the analysis of the juvenile portion of the age range and needs to be considered briefly. A sizeable literature on sexual dimorphism in juveniles has accumulated, centred on those regions of the skeleton such as the pelvis, cranium, mandible and teeth that show most sexual dimorphism in the adult.[49–55] Although there are undoubtedly skeletal morphological differences between the sexes from an early age, they do not reach a high enough level for reliable determination of sex until after the pubertal modifications have taken place (see Mays and Cox, chapter 8, in this volume).

AGEING

Biological age may be expressed as either dental or skeletal age. Dental age is expressed either from the time of emergence of the teeth into the mouth or from the stages of mineralization of the teeth. In juveniles, the estimation of skeletal age uses both the times of appearance and fusion of ossification centres and the size and morphology of the bones of the skeleton.

Dental ageing

Ageing from the teeth has several advantages over skeletal ageing. First, teeth survive inhumation better than bones, which makes dental ageing especially relevant to palaeontologists and skeletal biologists. Teeth are often the only structures representing some fossil species and in more recent skeletal assemblages they may be the least damaged. Second, the growth and development of the teeth takes place over almost the whole of the juvenile age range starting in the embryonic period and nearing completion during the late adolescent and early adult period. Skeletal development tends to occur in punctuated fits and starts and as a consequence there are certain barren periods where skeletal ageing is difficult. Finally, it is well recognized that in living populations, for a given chronological age, dental age exhibits less variation than does skeletal age.[56-58] In a small archaeological sample of known chronological age where age estimation has been tested, the estimated dental age diverged less from actual age than estimated skeletal age.[59] Ageing from the teeth is considered further elsewhere (see Whittaker, chapter 6, in this volume).

Skeletal ageing

In general, size appears to be more affected by adverse circumstances than is maturity, and the majority of studies have therefore recorded diaphyseal measurements of the major long bones. Sources with which these data may be compared are derived from two completely different data sets. First, longitudinal radiological growth studies of healthy living children that were originally compiled as standards for normal growth data for screening and other clinical studies. For example, those from the Brush Foundation, the Fels Institute, the University of Colorado, USA, and the Harpenden and Oxford Growth Studies in the UK. Those recorded by Maresh[60] have become the most commonly used for comparison with archaeological samples. The other sort of data is from dry bone measurements from archaeological samples where age has been estimated, usually from dental development. This material is likely to be composed of the remains of individuals who suffered under a variety of adverse circumstances.[15,21,25,33,61-79]

Skeletal assemblages are necessarily cross-sectional in nature and it is obvious that these data originate from different temporal periods, geographical locations and gene pools. Ideally, an appropriate sample for comparison should be drawn from a similar background to the material studied but this is rarely possible. An age at death estimated from a single bone compared with a number of different standards can vary widely.[80] There are many practical and theoretical problems associated with this sort of comparison which can make inferences drawn from differences in bone size between populations erroneous. One rather extreme view is that any demographic profile of unknown remains is bound to reflect the range of the sample with which it is compared.[81,82] Some of the problems involved in size comparisons and attempts to solve them are discussed elsewhere (see Humphrey, chapter 3, in this volume).

The most comprehensive study of foetal osteology is that by Fazekas and Kósa.[49] It contains much valuable information including measurements of most bones of the skeleton from 3 lunar months to birth. However, the age/bone size correlations involve a circular argument as their material was, for the most part, of undocumented age. Foetuses were grouped according to crown–heel length and each group was assigned an age in half lunar month intervals. Their 'regression diagrams' (graphs) are of body length as the independent variable against bone length as the dependent variable. While there is undoubtedly a close correlation between foetal age and size, all the bones, especially those of the limbs, and particularly those of the lower limb that actually contribute to body length, inevitably show a high correlation and lie very close to a straight line. Modified regression diagrams show age in lunar months superimposed onto these graphs.

Most of the other available data from the prenatal period relate to diaphyseal lengths. There is a relatively large database for comparison with gestational age drawn from measurements on alizarin-stained foetuses, dry bone, standard radiological and ultrasound views.[83–98] It should be remembered, however, that age *per se* in the prenatal period is always an estimate and does not exist with the same certainty as postnatally.

Maturity, as opposed to size, may be assessed from the morphology of the individual bones, or bone elements. However, the efficient use of this method requires an appreciation of the way in which bones grow and in addition, a detailed knowledge of the development of all parts of the skeleton.[99]

Mammalian bone arises from the differentiation of primitive mesenchymal tissue in a variety of different ways. At some sites bone develops directly in mesenchyme via a process known as intramembranous formation. In others, a cartilaginous template of the future bone element is formed as an intermediary element and this is then destroyed and replaced by bone in a process called endochondral formation. A third type is displayed by a few bones that start intramembranously and then acquire secondary cartilaginous sites.

In general, the bones of the calvarium and face are formed intramembranously while most of the skull base, the vertebral column and the bones of the limbs and their girdles are formed endochondrally. It has been suggested that intramembranous formation results in a faster production of bone in order to cover the rapidly expanding brain.[100,101] The clavicle, mandible and some sutural areas of the skull are formed by a mixture of the two types of bone formation.

Osteogenesis normally starts in the mesenchymal connective tissue precursor at a constant locus, which is known as the primary centre, and this expands until the precursor is totally replaced by bone. Most long bones and many other irregular bones also develop secondary centres known as epiphyses. They are situated at the ends of long bones, or at traction sites associated with irregular bones. The primary centres of the majority of bones form in prenatal life and most secondary centres appear in postnatal life, although a few develop before birth. Secondary centres are separated from the primary centre by an area of cartilage, the growth plate (epiphyseal plate or physis) which is an organized area of cartilage proliferation that provides growth of the bone.

Not all bones have secondary centres, the notable exceptions being the skull and small bones of the wrist and ankle. In the majority of skull bones the primary centre forms the entire bone, but in some of the complex bones (such as the occipital, temporal and sphenoid) several primary centres form, which are separated by cartilaginous growth plates. The carpal and tarsal bones have primary centres that expand until they fill out the original cartilage template.

There is a wide time span stretching from the perinatal period to early adult life during which secondary centres develop, but the order and chronological appearance is well documented for the majority. Once a bone has reached its final size, the growth plate narrows and is totally replaced by bone as epiphyseal fusion occurs. In the major long bones, those epiphyses that commence ossification in early childhood fuse after those that start ossification later. These are situated at the growing end of the bone, that is, the shoulder and the wrist in the upper limb and around the knee in the lower limb.

In theory, it is possible to age a juvenile skeleton by observation of the primary or secondary centre at one of its three phases of development. First, the time at which the centre appears; second, by the morphology and size of the centre; and finally, the time at which primary and secondary centres fuse with each other. However, only the morphology and size of centres and their time of fusion with each other are of much practical use in most archaeological contexts.

Appearance of ossification centres

Most centres for the skull, vertebral column and the primary centres of major long bones and their girdles commence ossification during the embryonic or foetal periods of life. Information on their appearance is based on studies using histological sections, alizarin-stained whole foetuses and radiological examination. They are identified by their anatomical position, rather than their distinctive morphology, and so require soft tissue to hold them in place. Secondary centres develop within cartilaginous templates during postnatal life and, with a few exceptions, commences ossification as rather nondescript spherical or ovoid nodules. Even in the unlikely event of recovery, newly formed centres of ossification are not identifiable in isolation. Therefore, this phase of bone formation is of little use in ageing from skeletal remains, the only exception being the investigation of mummified remains where radiography may identify bony tissue *in situ*.

Morphology and size of ossification centres

The second phase of bone development occurs when an ossification centre has increased in size, or altered in shape sufficiently, so that it may be recognized in isolation and distinguished from other bones. It is at this stage that the bone, or bone element, may be used to advantage in ageing. The critical period for each centre varies greatly depending on the part of the skeleton under consideration. Most of the bones of the skull, the vertebral centra and arches, ribs, and major long bones of the limbs are recognizable from mid-fetal life onwards. Some of the tarsal bones and the early forming long bone epiphyses may be identified in the first few years of life but those of the carpus and later developing epiphyses do not reach a recognizable stage until well into the childhood years. Many of these centres, including long bone shafts develop their own particular changes that may be useful for ageing. There is also a distinctive group of secondary centres of the scapula, clavicle and pelvis that do not develop until late adolescence and the early adult period (see Cox, chapter 5, in this volume). Age estimation will be determined with greater accuracy using those bone elements that undergo distinct changes within a relatively short time.

Apart from atlases of the major joints which are standard two-dimensional views of diaphyses and epiphyses,[39,102–104] there is very little information concerning the morphological changes that occur during development in either primary or secondary ossification centres. Fazekas and Kósa[49] comment briefly on the appearance of bones in the perinatal period, and the size and morphology of the component parts of the occipital bone have been related to age.[105,106] Otherwise there is at present no significant body of information except for isolated accounts scattered in the clinical, mainly radiological, literature and this has remained until now a neglected area of osteology.[99]

One of the major reasons for the lack of information is undoubtedly the difficulty of obtaining juvenile material. Post-mortem specimens are fortunately rare, and rightly diffi-cult to obtain, because of the sensitivity and obvious emotional consequences of a child's death. In archaeological skeletal collections, the later developing epiphyses are particularly rare which is partly due to the age profile of most of the samples. Children succumb to disease and malnutrition in the early years of life but usually, if they survive for about the first 5 years, few die in later childhood years between the ages of 6 and 12 years. This in part explains why, for example, it is fairly common to find epiphyses of the proximal humerus, distal radius, proximal femur and tibia but hardly ever elbow or trochanteric epiphyses. Even with adult material, retrieval of certain parts is lower than expected and it was suggested that one of the factors was lack of awareness of the anatomy[107] on the part of the excavators. For example, retrieval of hyoid bones and ossified laryngeal elements is greatly improved if the cervical and upper thoracic regions are carefully scrutinized before any disturbance or lifting of larger bones.

Fusion of ossification centres

The third phase of bone development is when fusion occurs between one or more primary centres, or between a primary centre and its epiphyses. The time at which this takes place varies greatly, partly in response to the function of the soft tissues with which the bones are associated. For example, the primary centres of the temporal and sphenoid bones fuse around the time of birth and those of the vertebral column and the occipital bone are complete by about the age of 6 years as these skeletal elements reflect the precocious devel-opment of the human central nervous system. By contrast, bones of the locomotor system, especially those of the male, do not complete fusion until the late adolescent or early adult period which coincides with the delayed spurt in muscle growth.

Data on this phase of development has been obtained from observations on dry bone[108–111] and from radiographic studies[39,102–104] and accounts of timing between the two methods often differ. In dry bone studies, fusion is observed by noting bridges of bone on the periphery of the epiphyseal/metaphyseal junction, whereas radiographs often describe fusion beginning in the centre of the epiphyseal plate. Reported times of fusion are variable, especially those of later fusing bones, as variability always increases with age. This is partly due to increasing effects of environmental as opposed to genetic effects, and also by variation in the onset of the adolescent growth spurt. Again, the difficulties in sexing juvenile remains until sexual dimor-phism is well advanced, necessarily complicates the use of fusion times during this period of life. As with any other phase of bone development, changes occurring within a relatively short time span are of most use for accuracy of ageing.

CONCLUSIONS

The major problem associated with ageing the skeletal remains of juveniles is the ineffec-tiveness of most methods of sexing in this age range. New methods will undoubtedly be devised, but the material on which they are tested must be a documented sample. Most studies do detail their sexing methods but there is sometimes a tendency to refer to confirmation of sex where both the original and the derived data were observed from anatomical parameters thus slipping into a circular argument. These studies have a certain value in themselves but should more properly be described as concordances between different skeletal methods. The other main difficulty lies in the choice of an appropriate sample with which to compare any markers that reflect defects of growth and development. Unless carefully chosen, there is a risk of squeezing the newly observed sample into a reflection of the comparison. In addition to these problems, there are many living populations on which there is no metric or morphological data, thus reducing the database for comparisons.

Truly documented samples are one of the most valuable resources to which a skeletal biologist has access. Such collections are very limited and must be treasured and maintained in good order. Improved methods of establishing biological parameters will undoubtedly be developed and may be tested upon them. Even then, caution must be used when applying standards derived from relatively recent material to ancient human remains, because the archaeological sample may not show the same relationship between chronological and skeletal age as that displayed by the reference sample. Only then can relevant and meaningful conclusions be drawn from the skeletal remains of past peoples.

REFERENCES

1   Forfar JO. Demography, vital statistics and the pattern of disease in childhood. In: Campbell AGM, McIntosh N (eds), *Forfar and Arneil's Textbook of Pediatrics* (5th edn). Edinburgh: Churchill Livingstone, 1998.

2   Acsádi G, Nemeskéri J. *History of Human Lifespan and Mortality*. Budapest: Akadémiai Kiado, 1970.

3   Ferembach D, Schwidetsky I, Stloukal M. Recommendations of age and sex diagnoses of skeletons. *Journal of Human Evolution* 1980; **9**: 517–549.

4   Frazer JE. *The Anatomy of the Human Skeleton* (5th edn). London: Churchill, 1948.

5   Grant JCB. *A Method of Anatomy* (4th edn). London: Baillière, Tindall & Cox, 1948.

6   Williams PL, Bannister LH, Berry MM, Collins P, Dyson M, Dussek JE, Ferguson MWJ. *Gray's Anatomy* (38th edn). Edinburgh: Churchill Livingstone, 1995.

7   Irwin GL. Roentgen determination of the time of closure of the spheno-occipital synchondrosis. *Radiology* 1960; **75**: 450–453.

8   Powell TV, Brodie AG. Closure of the spheno-occipital synchondrosis. *Anatomical Record* 1964; **147**: 15–23.

9   Konie JC. Comparative value of X-rays of the spheno-occipital synchondrosis and of the wrist for skeletal age assessment. *Angle Orthodondist* 1964; **34**: 303–313.

10 Melsen B. Time of closure of the spheno-occipital synchondrosis determined on dry skulls – a radiographic craniometric study. *Acta Odontologica Scandinavica* 1968; **27**: 73–90.

11 Melsen B. Time and mode of closure of the spheno-occipital synchondrosis determined on human autopsy material. *Acta Anatomica* 1972; **83**: 112–118.

12 Ingervall B, Thilander B. The human spheno-occipital synchondrosis. I – The time of closure appraised macroscopically. *Acta Odontologica Scandinavica* 1972; **30**: 349–356.

13 Sahni D, Jit I, Neelam, Suri S. Time of fusion of the basisphenoid with the basilar part of the occipital bone in northwest Indian subjects. *Forensic Science International* 1998; **98**: 41–45.

14 Saunders SR. Subadult skeletons and growth related studies. In: Saunders SR, Katzenberg MA (eds), *Skeletal Biology of Past Peoples: Research Methods*. New York: Wiley-Liss, 1992: pp. 1–20.

15 Hoppa RD. Evaluating human skeletal growth: an Anglo-Saxon example. *International Journal of Osteoarchaeology* 1992; **2**: 275–288.

16 Molleson T, Cox M. *The Spitalfields Project*, vol. 2: *The Anthropology – The Middling Sort*. Research Report 86. York: Council for British Archaeology, 1993.

17 Saunders SR, Hoppa RD. Growth deficit in survivors and non-survivors: biological mortality bias in subadult skeletal samples. *Yearbook of Physical Anthropology* 1993; **36**: 127–151.

18 Saunders SR, Hoppa RD, Southern R. Diaphyseal growth in a nineteenth century skeletal sample of subadults from St. Thomas' Church, Belleville, Ontario. *International Journal of Osteoarchaeology* 1993; **3**: 265–281.

19 Huda TFJ, Bowman JE. Age determination from dental microstructure in juveniles. *American Journal of Physical Anthropology* 1995; **97**: 135–150.

20 Lampl M, Johnston FE. Problems in the aging of skeletal juveniles: perspectives from maturation assessments of living children. *American Journal of Physical Anthropology* 1996; **101**: 345–355.

21 Steyn M, Henneberg M. Skeletal growth of children from the Iron Age site at K2 (South Africa). *American Journal of Physical Anthropology* 1996; **100**: 389–396.

22 Boddington A. Chaos, disturbance and decay in an Anglo-Saxon cemetery. In: Boddington A, Garland AN, Janaway RC (eds), *Death, Decay and Reconstruction: Approaches to Archaeology and Forensic Science*. Manchester: Manchester University Press, 1987: pp. 27–42.

23 Henderson J. Factors determining the state of preservation of human remains. In: Boddington A, Garland AN, Janaway RC (eds), *Death, Decay and Reconstruction: Approaches to Archaeology and Forensic Science*. Manchester: Manchester University Press, 1987: pp. 43–54.

24 Waldron T. *Counting the Dead – The Epidemiology of Past Populations*. Chichester: Wiley, 1994: pp. 10–27

25 Saunders SR, Melbye FJ. Subadult mortality and skeletal indicators of health in late Woodland Ontario Iroquois. *Canadian Journal of Archaeology* 1990; **14**: 61–74.

26 Cox M. *Life and Death in Spitalfields 1700–1850*. York: Council for British Archaeology, 1996: p. 20

27 Scheuer JL, Bowman JE. Correlation of documentary and skeletal evidence in the St. Bride's Crypt population. In: Saunders SR, Herring A (eds), *Grave Reflections: Portraying the Past through Cemetery Studies*. Toronto: Canadian Scholars' Press, 1995: pp. 49–70.

28 Scheuer L. Age at death and cause of death of the people buried in St. Bride's Church, Fleet Street, London. In: Cox M (ed.), *Grave Concerns: Death and Burial in England 1700–1850*. Research Report 113. York: Council for British Archaeology, 1998: pp. 100–111.

29 Kerley ER. Forensic anthropology and crimes involving children. *Journal of Forensic Science* 1976; **21**: 333–339.

30 Johnston FE, Zimmer LO. Assessment of growth and age in the immature skeleton. In: Isçan MY, Kennedy KAR (eds), *Reconstruction of Life from the Skeleton*. New York: Liss, 1989: pp. 11–21.

31 Goode H, Waldron T, Rogers J. Bone growth in juveniles: a methodological note. *International Journal of Osteoarchaeology* 1993; **3**: 321–323.

32 Guy H, Masset C, Baud C-A. Infant taphonomy. *International Journal of Osteoarchaeology* 1997; **7**: 221–229.

33 Sundick RI. Human skeletal growth and age determination. *Homo* 1978; **29**: 228–249.

34 Hoppa RD, Gruspier KL. Estimating epiphyseal length from fragmentary subadult skeletal remains: implications for paleodemographic reconstructions of a southern Ontario ossuary. *American Journal of Physical Anthropology* 1996; **100**: 341–354.

35 Bogin, B. Rural-to-urban migration. In: Mascie-Taylor, CGN, Lasker GW (eds), *Biological Aspects of Human Migration*. Cambridge: Cambridge University Press, 1988: pp. 90–129.

36 Eveleth PB, Tanner JM. *Worldwide Variation in Human Growth* (2nd edn). Cambridge: Cambridge University Press, 1990.

37 Choi SC, Trotter M. A statistical study of the multivariate structure and race–sex differences of American White and Negro fetal skeletons. *American Journal of Physical Anthropology* 1970; **33**: 307–312.

38 Pedersen JF. Fetal crown–rump length measurement by ultrasound in normal pregnancy. *British Journal of Obstetrics and Gynaecology* 1982; **89**: 926–930.

39   Pyle SI, Hoerr NL. *Radiographic Atlas of Skeletal Development of the Knee*. Springfield: Charles C Thomas, 1955.

40   Miller JZ, Slemenda CW, Meany FJ, Reister TK, Hui S, Johnston CC. The relationship of bone mineral density and anthropomorphic variables in healthy male and female children. *Bone and Mineral* 1991; **14**: 137–152.

41   Specker BL, Brazero LW, Tsang RC, Levin R, Searcy J, Steichen J. Bone mineral content in children 1–6 years of age. *American Journal of Diseases of Children* 1987; **141**: 343–344.

42   Garn SM, Burdi AR. Prenatal ordering and postnatal sequence in dental development. *Journal of Dental Research* 1971; **50**: 1407–1414.

43   Robinow M, Richards TW, Anderson M. The eruption of deciduous teeth. *Growth* 1942; **6**: 127–133.

44   Fanning EA. A longitudinal study of tooth formation and root resorption. *New Zealand Dental Journal* 1961; **57**: 202–217.

45   Haavikko K. The physiological resorption of the roots of deciduous teeth in Helsinki children. *Proceedings of the Finnish Dental Society* 1973; **69**: 93–98.

46   Nyström M, Haataja J, Kataja M, Evälahti M, Peck L, Kleemola-Kujala E. Dental maturity in Finnish children, estimated from the development of seven permanent mandibular teeth. *Acta Odontologica Scandinavica* 1986; **44**: 193–198.

47   Tanner JM. *Growth at Adolescence* (2nd edn). Oxford: Blackwell, 1962.

48   Cox M, Molleson T, Waldron T. Preconception and conception: the lessons of a 19th century suicide. *Journal of Archaeological Science* 1990; **17**: 573–581.

49   Fazekas I Gy, Kósa F. *Forensic Fetal Osteology*. Budapest: Akadémiai Kiadó, 1978.

50   Schutkowski H. Sex determination of fetal and neonate skeletons by means of discriminant analysis. *International Journal of Anthropology* 1987; **2**: 347–352.

51   Schutkowski H. Sex determination of infant and juvenile skeletons: 1. Morphognostic features. *American Journal of Physical Anthropology* 1993; **90**: 199–205.

52   Weaver DS. Sex differences in the ilia of a known sex and age sample of fetal and infant skeletons. *American Journal of Physical Anthropology* 1980; **52**: 191–195.

53   Hunt DR. Sex determination in the subadult ilia: an indirect test of Weaver's non-metric sexing method. *Journal of Forensic Sciences* 1990; **35**: 881–885.

54   Mittler DM, Sheridan SG. Sex determination in subadults using auricular surface morphology: a forensic science perspective. *Journal of Forensic Sciences* 1992; **37**: 1068–1075.

55   Molleson T, Cruse K, Mays S. Some sexually dimorphic features of the human juvenile skull and their value in sex determination in immature juvenile remains. *Journal of Archaeological Science* 1998; **25**: 719–728.

56   Lewis AB, Garn SM. The relationship between tooth formation and other maturational factors. *Angle Orthodondist* 1960; **30**: 70–77.

57   Demirjian A. Dentition. In: Falkner F, Tanner JM (eds), *Human Growth*, vol. 2: *Postnatal Growth* (2nd edn). London: Baillière Tindall, 1986: pp. 413–444.

58   Smith BH. Standards of human tooth formation and dental age assessment. In: Kelley MA, Larsen CS (eds), *Advances in Dental Anthropology*. New York: Wiley-Liss, 1991: pp. 143–168.

59   Bowman JE, MacLaughlin SM, Scheuer JL. The relationship between biological and chronological age in the juveniles from St. Bride's Church, Fleet Street. *Annals of Human Biology* 1992; **19**: 216.

60   Maresh MM. Measurements from roentgenograms. In: McCammon RW (ed.), *Human Growth and Development*. Springfield: Charles C Thomas, 1970: pp. 157–200.

61   Johnston FE. Growth of long bones of infants and young children at Indian Knoll. *American Journal of Physical Anthropology* 1962; **20**: 249–254.

62   Walker PL. The linear growth of long bones in Late Woodland Indian children. *Proceedings of the Indiana Academy of Science* 1969; **78**: 83–87.

63   Armelagos GJ, Mielke JH, Owen KH, Van Gerven DP, Dewey JR, Mahler PA. Bone growth and development in prehistoric populations from Sudanese Nubia. *Journal of Human Evolution* 1972; **1**: 89–119.

64   Y'Edynak G. Long bone growth in western Eskimo and Aleut skeletons. *American Journal of Physical Anthropology* 1976; **45**: 569–574.

65   Merchant VL, Ubelaker DH. Skeletal growth of the protohistoric Arikara. *American Journal of Physical Anthropology* 1977; **46**: 61–72.

66   Stloukal M, Hanáková H. Die Länge der Längsknochen altslawischer bevölkerungen – Unter besonderer Berücksichtigung von Wachstumsfragen. *Homo* 1978; **29**: 53–69.

67   Hummert JR, van Gerven DP. Skeletal growth in a medieval population from Sudanese Nubia. *American Journal of Physical Anthropology* 1983; **60**: 471–478.

68   Owsley DW, Bradtmiller B. Mortality of pregnant females in Arikara villages: osteological evidence. *American Journal of Physical Anthropology* 1983; **61**: 331–336.

69   Jantz RL, Owsley DW. Long bone growth variation among Arikara skeletal populations. *American Journal of Physical Anthropology* 1984; **63**: 13–20.

70   Mays SA. The relationship between Harris line formation and bone growth and development. *Journal of Archaeological Science* 1985; **12**: 207–220.

71   Mensforth RP. Relative tibia long bone growth in the Libben and Bt–5 prehistoric skeletal populations. *American Journal of Physical Anthropology* 1985; **68**: 247–262.

72   Owsley DW, Jantz RL. Long bone lengths and gestational age distributions of post-contact period Arikara Indian perinatal infant skeletons. *American Journal of Physical Anthropology* 1985; **68**: 321–328.

73   Storey R. Perinatal mortality at pre-Columbian Teotihuacan. *American Journal of Physical Anthropology* 1986; **69**: 541–548.

74   Molleson TI. Social implications of mortality patterns of juveniles from Poundbury Camp, Romano-British cemetery. *Anthropologischer Anzeiger* 1989; **47**: 27–38.

75   Lovejoy CO, Russell KF, Harrison ML. Long bone growth velocity in the Libben population. *American Journal of Human Biology* 1990; **2**: 533–541.

76   Wall CE. Evidence of weaning stress and catch-up growth in the long bones of a central California Amerindian sample. *Annals of Human Biology* 1991; **18**: 9–22.

77   Miles AEW, Bulman JS. Growth curves of immature bones from a Scottish Island population of sixteenth to mid-nineteenth century: limb bone diaphyses and some bones of the hand and foot. *International Journal of Osteoarchaeology* 1994; **4**: 121–136.

78   Mays S. The relationship between Harris lines and other aspects of skeletal development in adults and juveniles. *Journal of Archaeological Science* 1995; **22**: 511–520.

79   Ribot I, Roberts C. A study of non-specific stress indicators and skeletal growth in two medieval subadult populations. *Journal of Archaeological Science* 1996; **23**: 67–79.

80   Ubelaker DH. The estimation of age at death from immature human bone. In: Isçan MY (ed.), *Age Markers in the Human Skeleton*. Springfield: Charles C Thomas, 1989: pp. 55–70.

81   Bocquet-Appel J-P, Massett C. Farewell to palaeodemography. *Journal of Human Evolution* 1982; **11**: 321–333.

82   Bocquet-Appel J-P, Massett C. Matters of moment. *Journal of Human Evolution* 1985; **14**: 107–111.

83   Balthazard V, Dervieux F. Études anthropologiques sur le foetus humain. *Annales de Médicine Légales* 1921; **1**: 37–42.

84   Hesdorffer MB, Scammon RE. Growth of long-bones of human fetus as illustrated by the tibia. *Proceedings of the Society for Experimental Biology and Medicine* 1928; **25**: 638–641.

85   Moss ML, Noback CR, Robertson GG. Growth of certain human fetal cranial bones. *American Journal of Anatomy* 1956; **98**: 191–204.

86   Olivier G, Pineau H. Nouvelle détermination de la taille foetalle d'après les longeurs diaphysaires des os longs. *Annales de Médicine Légales* 1960; **40**: 141–144.

87   Olivier G. Précision sur la détermination de l'âge d'un foetus d'après sa taille ou la longuer de ses diaphyses. *Médicine Légale et Dommage Corporel* 1974; **7**: 297–299.

88   Keleman E, Jánossa M, Calvo W, Fliedner TM. Developmental age estimated by bone-length measurement in human fetuses. *Anatomical Record* 1984; **209**: 547–552.

89   Bareggi R, Grill V, Zweyer M, Sandrucci MA, Narducci P, Forabosco A. The growth of long bones in human embryological and fetal upper limbs and its relationship to other developmental patterns. *Anatomy and Embryology* 1994; **189**: 19–24.

90   Bareggi R, Grill V, Zweyer M, Sandrucci MA, Martelli AM, Narducci P, Forabosco A. On the assessment of the growth patterns in human fetal limbs: longitudinal measurements and allometric analysis. *Early Human Development* 1996; **45**: 11–25.

91   Scheuer JL, Musgrave JH, Evans SP. The estimation of late fetal and perinatal age from limb bone length by linear and logarithmic regression. *Annals of Human Biology* 1980; **7**: 257–265.

92   Bagnall KM, Harris PF, Jones PRM. Radiographic study of the longitudinal growth of primary ossification centers in limb long bones of the human fetus. *Anatomical Record* 1982; **203**: 293–299.

93   Jeanty P, Kirkpatrick C, Dramaix-Wilmet M, Struyven J. Ultrasonic evaluation of fetal limb growth. *Radiology* 1981; **140**: 165–168.

94   O'Brien GD, Queenan JT, Campbell S. Assessment of gestational age in the second trimester by real-time ultrasound measurement of the femur length. *American Journal of Obstetrics and Gynecology* 1981; **139**: 540–545.

95   Filly RA, Golbus MS. Ultrasonography of the normal and pathologic fetal skeleton. *Radiologic Clinics of North America* 1982; **20**: 311–323.

96   Seeds JW, Cefalo RC. Relationship of fetal limb lengths to both biparietal diameter and gestational age. *Obstetrics and Gynecology* 1982; **60**: 680–685.

97   Jeanty P, Romero R. *Obstetrical Ultrasound*. New York: McGraw Hill, 1983.

98   Bertino E, Di Battista E, Bossi A, Pagliano M, Fabris C, Aicardi G, Milani S. Fetal growth velocity: kinetic, clinical, and biological aspects. *Archives of Disease in Childhood* 1996; **74**: F10–15.

99   Scheuer L, Black S. *Developmental Juvenile Osteology*. London: Academic Press, 2000.

100 Holden L. *Human Osteology* (6th edn). London: Churchill, 1882.

101 Last RJ. *Anatomy, Regional and Applied* (5th edn). Edinburgh: Churchill Livingstone, 1973.

102 Greulich WW, Pyle SI. *Radiographic Atlas of Skeletal Development of the Hand and Wrist*. Stanford: Stanford University Press, 1959.

103 Brodeur AE, Silberstein MJ, Graviss ER. *Radiology of the Pediatric Elbow*. Boston: Hall Medical, 1981.

104 Hoerr NL, Pyle SI, Francis CC. *Radiographic Atlas of Skeletal Development of the Foot and Ankle: A Standard of Reference*. Springfield: Charles C Thomas, 1962.

105 Redfield A. A new aid to aging immature skeletons: development of the occipital bone. *American Journal of Physical Anthropology* 1970; **33**: 207–220.

106 Scheuer JL, MacLaughlin-Black SM. Age estimation from the pars basilaris of the fetal and juvenile occipital bone. *International Journal of Osteoarchaeology* 1994; **4**: 377–380.

107 Waldron T. The relative survival of the human skeleton: implications for palaeopathology. In: : Boddington A, Garland AN, Janaway RC (eds), *Death, Decay and Reconstruction: Approaches to Archaeology and Forensic Science*. Manchester: Manchester University Press, 1987: pp. 55–64.

108 Stevenson PH. Age order of epiphyseal union in man. *American Journal of Physical Anthropology* 1924; **7**: 53–93.

109 Todd TW. The roentgenographic record of differentiation in the pubic bone. *American Journal of Physical Anthropology* 1930; **14**: 255–271.

110 Stewart TD. Sequence of epiphyseal union, third molar eruption and suture closure in Eskimos and American Indians. *American Journal of Physical Anthropology* 1934; **19**: 433–452.

111 McKern TW, Stewart TD. Skeletal age changes in young American males, analysed from the standpoint of age identification. *HQ Quartermaster Research Development Command*; Technical Report EP–45. Natick, Massachusetts, 1957

3

GROWTH STUDIES OF PAST POPULATIONS: AN OVERVIEW AND AN EXAMPLE

Louise Humphrey

INTRODUCTION

In 1962, Johnston[1] presented the first study of skeletal growth in a past population, using measurements of long bones of children from Indian Knoll. Since then, an impressive array of studies of long bone growth in archaeological populations has been published. This chapter examines why analysis of the growth of past populations is useful as an indicator of the well-being of a population and how the methods and objectives of growth studies from skeletal samples have changed and evolved over the past four decades.

Studies of the growth of children from different socio-economic backgrounds, secular trends in body weight and stature, and studies showing the effects of unemployment, famine and warfare on child growth underscore the importance of growth rates as indicator of the health and well-being of a population.[2-4] The most common causes of developmental retardation and poor growth are inadequate nutrition and exposure to infectious disease, or the synergistic interaction of poor nutrition and infection.[2,3] Parameters which could have a significant impact on types of environmental stress factors to which a population is exposed, and the short- and long-term ability of the population to buffer itself against such stress factors, include a change in subsistence patterns, technological innovation (affecting, for example, food production, storage and preparation or sanitation), changing social structures, political unrest, environmental degradation and climatic disasters or fluctuation.[5-11] The analysis of skeletal growth in a past population will not in itself allow us to infer the cause of developmental stress suffered by individuals within that population. Interpretation of growth data within a wider context, including additional skeletal and dental investigations and independent archaeological evidence, can in some cases allow hypotheses to be generated concerning the nature of the environmental stress that caused disruption of the normal course of development.

Individuals subjected to elevated levels of environmental stress may exhibit a slower rate of bone growth, diminished adult size, delayed skeletal and dental maturation, and a prolonged growth period.[11] Within a population it may be difficult to identify stressed individuals using developmental data, since they will not always stand out against a background of normal developmental variation. At the population level, variation in each of these parameters is commonly used to infer variation in the magnitude of environmental stress experienced by different groups. However, such interpretations must also be made against a background of normal variation in the developmental schedules and adult body size of different human populations. Within a population it is reasonable to infer that changes in mean adult stature, or in mean long bone length for a particular age category, reflect an improvement or deterioration of environmental circumstances. This inference is less secure for comparisons between samples from different archaeological sites or between an archaeological sample and a non-archaeological comparative sample. Comparison of samples from different temporal horizons within an archaeological site should also be undertaken cautiously, particularly if there is a possibility of population discontinuity.

There are several additional practical and theoretical difficulties associated with the study of growth in past populations, and many of these issues have been extensively reviewed elsewhere.[12-16] Practical difficulties include poor or biased preservation and recovery, small sample size and variable temporal resolution (the sample may span several generations or even centuries). Numerous factors can introduce error into the estimation of chronological age, particularly in older children and young adults. Among these factors is the lack of appropriate ageing standards for many populations, and variation in the timing of dental and skeletal development between individuals within a population, including sexual differences. Data on the growth of past populations are by necessity cross-sectional (i.e. each data point reflects the growth attainment of a different individual measured at a single moment in time) and the resulting growth profile differs in several crucial respects from the growth curve of any individual within the population represented. In particular, it is not possible accurately to model the age, rate and duration of events, such as the adolescent growth, which vary in their timing between individuals using cross-sectional data. Analytical procedures must also make allowance for the transition from measurements of diaphyseal length to measurements of total long bone length resulting from fusion of the epiphyses of the long bones during the later period of growth. The extent to which mortality bias may influence the outcome of growth studies using past populations continues to be debated.[17,18]

A summary of published reports of the skeletal growth of past populations is presented in Table 1, which briefly describes the stated or inferred aims of each of these contributions. The earliest studies were concerned mainly with the provision of data on the relationship between long bone length and dental development that could be used for ageing subadult skeletal remains from similar archaeological samples if the dentition were insufficiently preserved for this purpose.[1,19] These and subsequent studies have analysed the skeletal growth of groups which are temporally, geographically and ecologically varied (Table 1). Comparisons between the growth patterns of such diverse populations are difficult to interpret, since multiple environmental and genetic factors may be contributing to the observed differences. In studies of living populations it is possible partially to unravel the separate effects of environmental and hereditary factors on adult stature by, for example, studying related populations growing up in different countries.[20] However, it remains to be seen whether this type of controlled study will ever be possible for a past population.

Table 1 – Published studies of human skeletal growth in earlier populations.

Author	Year	Ref	Sample	Period	Purpose
Johnston	1962	1	Indian Knoll, Kentucky, USA	Archaic	Evaluation of the long bone growth of a prehistoric population, compared with a modern population. Production of standards for age estimation of Native American infants using long bone lengths
Walker	1969	19	Yokem Mound, Illinois, USA	Late Woodland circa AD1200	Construction of growth charts for estimating the age of children from closely related groups
Armelagos *et al.*	1972	21	Wadi Halfa, Lower Nubia	350 BC–AD 1400	Comparison of growth velocity at different stages of development with a modern sample
Y'Ednak	1976	34	Western Eskimo and Aleut, Alaska, USA	Pre–19th- century AD	Evaluation of the development of typical adult body proportions and of sex differences in skeletal growth
Merchant and Ubelaker	1977	30	Arikara, South Dakota, USA	First half of eighteenth century AD	Investigation of the variation in results generated using different dental ageing techniques. Comparison of Arikara growth data with data from other Native American skeletal samples
Stloukal and Hanáková	1978	22	Ancient Slavic	9th century AD	Provision of data for age estimation and comparison of stature estimates with modern children
Sundick	1978	13	Indian Knoll, Kentucky, USA	Archaic	Comparison of the growth of two skeletal samples and provision of data for age estimation for two different populations
Sundick	1978	13	Altenerding, Germany	6th–7th centuries AD	Comparison of the growth of two skeletal samples and provision of data for age estimation for two different populations
Hummert and van Gerven	1983	6	Kulubnarti, Upper Nubia	Medieval AD550–1450	Comparison growth of children from early and late Christian cemeteries
Cook	1984	8	Illinois Valley Series, USA	Woodland and Mississippian	Evaluation of the effects of intensification of food production. Comparison of the growth of children of differential social status
Jantz and Owsley	1984	9	Arikara, South Dakota, USA	AD 1600–1832	Evaluation of change through time, covering three distinct cultural variants
Mensforth	1985	10	Libben, Ohio, USA	Late Woodland AD 800–1100	Evaluation of the extent to which growth differences between these two sites reflect demographic and epidemiological differences
Mensforth	1985	10	Carston Annis Bt–5, Kentucky, USA	Late Archaic 3992–2655 BC	Evaluation of the extent to which growth differences between these two sites reflect demographic and epidemiological differences
Mays	1985	36	Poundbury, Dorset, UK	Romano British	Evaluation of the relationship between the occurrence of Harris lines and skeletal growth
Lovejoy *et al.*	1990	23	Libben, Ohio USA	Late Woodland AD 800–1100	Comparison with modern sample

Table 1 – continued

Author	Year	Ref	Sample	Period	Purpose
Wall	1991	31	Central Californian series, USA	Early, middle & late Periods 4250–300 BP	Comparison with skeletal samples and evaluation of the effects of weaning
Hoppa	1992	32	Raunds, Northants. UK	Anglo-Saxon 10th century AD	Comparison with other skeletal samples, age estimation
Saunders *et al.*	1993	18	St Thomas's Church, Ontario, Canada	19th century AD	Comparison with modern and skeletal samples
Molleson and Cox	1993	25	Christ Church, Spitalfields, London, UK	18th–19th centuries AD	Comparison with modern sample
Farwell and Molleson	1993	26	Poundbury, Dorset, UK	Romano British	Comparison with modern sample and discussion of social implications
Miles and Bulman	1994 1995	27, 33	Ensay, Scotland, UK	16th–mid 19th centuries AD	Comparison with modern and skeletal samples
Mays	1995	37	Wharram Percy, North Yorkshire, UK	11th–16th centuries AD	Evaluation of the relationship between the occurrence of Harris lines and other developmental stress indicators
Steyn and Henneberg	1996	28	K2, Northern Transvaal, South Africa	Iron Age AD1000–1200	Comparison with modern and skeletal samples
Ribot and Roberts	1996	38	Raunds, Northants. UK	Anglo-Saxon 8th–10th centuries AD	Comparison of growth status of individuals with and without non-specific stress indicators
Ribot and Roberts	1996	38	Chichester, Sussex, UK	16th and 17th centuries AD	Comparison of growth status of individuals with and without non-specific stress indicators
Mays	1998	29	Wharram Percy, North Yorkshire, UK	11th–16th centuries AD	Calculation of stature and comparison with modern and historical data
Humphrey	1998	35	London crypt sample, UK	18th–19th centuries AD	Comparison of growth of different skeletal dimensions and analysis of male and female differences in the growth in the post-cranial skeleton,

Many authors have documented differences in long bone growth between one or more past populations and a modern comparative sample, and have offered an interpretation of these differences in terms of the underlying environmental or genetic causes.[1,21–29] More recently, as published data on the growth of past populations have accumulated, authors have compared their growth data to that from other past populations, using data from published studies on populations from similar geographical areas or origins,[10,24,30,31] or distantly related groups.[27,28,33] Part of the variation seen in the growth profiles of past populations is likely to be the result of methodological factors, including sample composition and variation in the techniques used for acquiring and evaluating growth data. Even the application of different dental ageing techniques to the same sample can generate markedly different growth profiles.[30] Analytical methods and dental ageing techniques could in theory be standardized for all studies, but there is a general tendency for researchers to aim to improve upon methods used in previous studies. A further problem relates to the use of dental development to infer age at death. Tooth formation and emergence schedules differ between populations and a set of developmental standards derived from one population may result in biased age estimates if used with a different population. Some authors have adjusted dental ageing techniques in an attempt to correct for these biases,[9,23] but it is possible that this has merely added to the confusion.

Opportunities to carry out carefully controlled comparative growth studies in past populations, for which methods are standardized and a single environmental factor is variable, are limited for practical reasons. Nevertheless, this type of study represents a theoretical ideal, and if the majority of parameters are known to be constant, and appropriate samples are available within a clearly stratified framework from a single population, this type of study is possible. Several studies have compared the growth of samples of individuals from different chronological horizons of the same site or a closely affiliated set of sites in order to test carefully framed hypotheses concerning the nature or causes of variation in growth patterns.[6,8,9] Other studies have examined variation in skeletal growth between subgroups within a contemporaneous sample from a single population such as differences between males and females,[34,35] or variation in relation to inferred social status.[8] Another example of this type of carefully controlled study is the comparison of growth in subgroups exhibiting different levels of skeletal and dental stress indicators.[36–38]

Skeletal growth studies do not indicate whether differences in the magnitude of environmental stress between populations are the result of variation in the severity of environmental stress or differences in the frequency or duration of exposure. Additional study of other indicators of dental and skeletal stress may help to distinguish between different types of developmental disruption. Mays[36,37] demonstrated that it is possible to distinguish between chronic and acute environmental stress, by examining lines of arrested growth in the long bones (Harris lines) in relation to skeletal growth attainment, so as to determine whether catch up growth occurred. Unlike bone, tooth enamel preserves a permanent record of developmental disturbances, which result in defective enamel structure, and can be used more reliably for retrospective analysis of developmental stress. Hillson and Bond[39] have demonstrated that the chronology, duration and frequency of stress events that cause enamel defects can be evaluated by reference to incremental structures within the tooth enamel. The application of this technique to skeletal samples from past populations will allow detailed analyses of the relationship between developmental stress and skeletal growth to be undertaken, and may provide a means of understanding the basis of skeletal growth disruption in earlier populations. As an example, Skinner *et al.*[40] proposed that recurrent enamel defects with regular periodicity could be an indicator of seasonal stress.

DEVELOPMENTAL STRESS INDICATORS

The skeleton and dentition can provide direct and indirect evidence of developmental stress.[7,11] Direct evidence of childhood deprivation is provided by non-specific stress indicators such as developmental defects in tooth enamel, orbital and vault lesions and subperiosteal new bone formation and lines of arrested growth.[36,41] Stress indicators such as these can be reliably documented for a single skeleton. Other, indirect evidence of developmental stress can only be observed in a comparative context. These include reduced adult stature, small skeletal size, small tooth size, fluctuating asymmetry, poor growth, prolonged growth, and delayed maturation. The following section examines three different ways in which developmental stress can be inferred from the growth and maturation of the skeleton.

Small size for age

Studies of living children have convincingly demonstrated that small size for age is an indicator of impoverished environmental circumstances,[2,3] and variation in skeletal size relative to dental age is commonly used as a method of inferring differential levels of environmental stress by researchers of past populations.[6,8–10,24,31,32] Typically skeletal growth comparisons are based on the size attained at specific developmental ages or age groups, and data are normally presented as a graph of skeletal size plotted against dental age. This type of study will indicate whether children were smaller or larger than children of the same age from a comparative sample at a particular stage of dental development, and whether there is a trend for size differences to increase or decrease across the period of study.

Prolonged skeletal growth

Studies of well-nourished and undernourished children in developing countries demonstrate that skeletal maturation is delayed in undernourished children and that the duration of growth is prolonged.[2] Historical evidence for the age of growth cessation in military recruits confirms that the duration of growth is affected by economic, climatic and social variables and that prolonged growth is an indicator of impoverished environmental circumstances.[42] In such cases, the size difference between two samples may be lower in adults than would be predicted on the basis of subadult size.

The cessation of the growth in length of a long bone normally coincides with the fusion of the epiphyses, and if epiphyseal fusion is delayed growth can continue until fusion occurs.[2,43] The age of cessation of long bone growth in a past population cannot normally be inferred directly from skeletal evidence owing to small sample size, intra-population variation (including sex differences), and the difficulty of obtaining accurate independent age estimates for individuals in the appropriate age range. Variation in the duration of skeletal growth can be inferred indirectly by comparison of the percentage of adult size achieved at different ages. A consistent pattern of variation in the percentage of adult size attained at successive ages between two groups is indicative of a difference in the duration of growth.

Comparison of the percentage of adult size attained standardizes the endpoint of growth of each of the groups being compared.[35,44] This standardization has the effect of correcting for differences in the adult size of the samples being compared (e.g. differences between males and females, populations or species) as well as for any size variation caused by slight differences in measurement techniques. For population comparisons, it is suggested that variation in the percentage of adult size attained at a given age is a more appropriate indicator of health than variation in actual skeletal size, which may simply reflect a difference in growth potential between two groups. It is possible though, that there is a genetic component to variation in the average duration of skeletal growth between populations. The timing and intensity of the adolescent growth spurt may also vary between populations and this could affect the interpretation of growth data, particularly during the adolescent period. The standardization corrects for the environmentally caused component of adult size differences in the groups being compared in addition to differences that are genetically based. Comparisons based on the percentage of adult size may therefore be less sensitive as indicators of the health of a population than comparisons based on actual size.

To calculate the percentage of adult size attained, the average size of the adult population has to be used as an estimate of adult size for each individual in the sample, since the actual size that each individual would have achieved is obviously not known. Many published growth studies do not present data on adult size, and as a result data cannot be re-evaluated using this method. Adult long bone lengths include the distal and proximal ends of the bone whereas juvenile measurements usually exclude the unfused epiphyses. If comparisons are restricted to younger age groups and none of the individuals have fused epiphyses, it does not matter whether the percentage of adult size is calculated using total long bone length or diaphysis length, provided the same technique is applied to each population being compared. If the comparisons are extended into an age range in which some of the individuals have fused epiphyses, the measurements should be adjusted to allow for the size of the proximal and/or distal epiphyses.[35]

Delayed skeletal maturation relative to dental development

A second method that uses delayed development to infer developmental stress in a past population is the occurrence of a disparity between age estimates derived from skeletal maturation and those based on dental development.[45] This technique is based on the well-documented observation that skeletal development is more responsive to environmental stress than dental development.[46] The presence of a large proportion of individuals exhibiting delayed skeletal development relative to dental development is interpreted as an indicator of environmental stress. This is an interesting approach but in practice it may have a fairly limited application.

To be useful for estimating age at death from the skeleton, particular stages of dental and skeletal development need to be unambiguously defined and their age of occurrence needs to be well documented in modern populations. In practice, skeletal maturation is most useful as an indicator of age at death in older juveniles and young adults, during the period of fusion of the epiphyses of the long bones, clavicle, scapula and pelvis. Other events are too poorly documented in known populations, too widely spaced in time to be useful for age estimation, or not applicable to skeletal samples. The age range for which it is possible to estimate age from skeletal maturation therefore coincides with the period in which dental age estimates become less accurate. The reliability of this technique is affected by the amount of variation in dental and skeletal developmental schedules within and between populations, and could be influenced by sample composition. It is possible, for example, that the presence of a high proportion of individuals exhibiting delayed skeletal maturation relative to dental development could be the result of a biased sex ratio, since sex differences in the timing of skeletal maturation are greater than sex differences in the timing of dental development.[47]

COMPARATIVE METHODS

The majority of growth studies of past populations incorporate measurements of the diaphyseal length of one or more of the long bones. Long bone growth can be evaluated by reference to the long bone growth of recent children or the growth of other samples from past populations. Comparative data on the growth of other past populations are widely available in the literature but these studies have employed a variety of different methods for estimating age at death and have used a range of statistical techniques. To minimize the error introduced by methodological variation, it is advisable to replicate the methods used for age estimation and the statistical treatment of the data used to generate the published results as closely as possible.

Comparative data on the growth of the long bones in recent populations are derived from measurements from radiographs of living children of known chronological age. Mixed longitudinal data for the lengths of the long bones, using measurements from repeated radiographs of the arm and leg, were collected during several comprehensive growth studies carried out earlier this century before the dangers of repeated exposure to radiation were realised. The data presented by Maresh[48] in 1955 are most commonly used as a modern comparative sample[1,21,23-27,34]. These data are based on a radiographic study of Denver children aged between 2 months and 18 years. Measurements for the six long bones are presented without epiphyses from 2 months to 12 years, and with epiphyses from 10 to 16 years, as the 50th percentile (midpoint) of successive age classes together with the 10th and 90th percentiles. Separate data are presented for males and females. Maresh[49] published an updated version of the growth statistics generated from the Denver growth study in 1970, and extended the data to 18 years in males and 17 years in females. These data are presented as means and standard deviations for successive age categories as well as percentiles. In archaeological samples, the sample size in each age range is often small, and in this situation the midpoint of the sample is unlikely to be an accurate measure of the population average. The data for means are more suitable than growth percentiles for comparison with data collected from archaeological samples, for which data are normally presented as means for successive age classes.

In a research context, there is no need to convert long bone lengths into stature. Conversion merely introduces another layer of possible inaccuracy since stature estimates are based on population averages for the relationship between long bone length and stature. The relationship between stature and long bone length is likely to vary between populations, and further error will be introduced if the conversion is derived from data from an inappropriate population. In the context of understanding the daily lives of past peoples and transmitting that information to a wider audience, information about the growth of children in the past needs to be presented in a readily accessible way. Long bone measurements can be used to estimate stature, using mathematical relationships derived from a series of radiographs of long bones belonging to of children of known stature.[50] A simple way in which to express the extent of growth deficiencies of children in the past is to illustrate that, for example, a child of 11 years old was only as tall as an average modern child of 8 years old. Another context in which it is useful to convert long bone measurements into stature estimates is for comparison with historical data on the stature of children in previous centuries.[29]

GROWTH IN THE LONDON CRYPT SAMPLE

Below, two different techniques are used to compare the growth of subadults from a recent population of living children and an earlier population represented by a skeletal sample. The comparisons are based on measurements of femur diaphyseal length for children aged between birth and 12 years. Data for the recent sample are summary statistics derived from measurements of radiographs of femur length from a mixed longitudinal sample of children from the Denver Growth Study.[49] Data for the past population are measurements of femur diaphyseal length of 55 individuals, buried in the crypts of Christ Church, Spitalfields, and the churches of St Brides and St Barnabas in the 18th and 19th centuries (the London crypt sample). The age at death of these individuals was derived from information on associated coffin plates and further documentary evidence. Although the sex of each individual in the London crypt sample is known, males and females were not analysed separately in this study since the sex of juveniles is not typically known for archaeological assemblages.

The first technique examines variation in femur diaphyseal length at different ages in the two samples. This is carried out using both raw data and residuals calculated from the mean femur length attained by children of the same chronological age in the Denver sample. Mean femur length of the Denver children was calculated as half of the sum of the male and female means for each age category. A curve was fitted to these values to describe the data mathematically. The mean femur length of the Denver sample can be determined at each age required using the equation for the fitted line, and the residual can be calculated from that value. The residuals calculated using this method are more accurate than would be the case if the comparative data had to be put into one of the half-yearly age categories for which data are available.

The purpose of fitting a curve to the data was to provide an accurate mathematical description of the distribution of data points rather than to describe the underlying pattern of growth with a realistic biological model. The fit of the equation was evaluated in terms of the distribution of residual values of known data points (corresponding to the actual means for the Denver sample in children aged 2, 4 and 6 months, and at 6 monthly intervals thereafter) about the fitted line. An equation provides an accurate description of the data points if the residual values (i.e. the differences between the observed values of a series and those predicted by the model) are low and randomly distributed with respect to age. Standard logistic and polynomial equations were tested in addition to models that were specifically developed to describe growth.[35,51] A five phased polynomial equation of the form $a + bx + cx^2 + dx^3 + ex^4 + fx^5$, where x = age and $a = y$ intercept, gave the most accurate description of the data. Previous experience indicates that the polynomial equation can yield erratic results for human growth data including a tendency for size to decline with age, particularly if sample sizes are small. The polynomial equation lacks an asymptote (i.e. it does not approach a fixed value defined by parameters in the equation) and therefore continues to fluctuate in the age range at which growth is complete. Despite these deficiencies, the polynomial works well in this case since the data are based on a comprehensive sample, and cover a period of continuous growth. Lines illustrating ± 1 and 2 SD from the mean were generated using the mean of the male and female SD of the Denver sample.[49]

In Figure 1a, femur diaphysis length is plotted against chronological age for each individual in the London crypt sample. Lines illustrating the mean size of the Denver sample at successive chronological ages and the range of sizes encompassed by 1 and 2 SD from the mean are shown for comparative purposes. The difference between the London crypt sample and the Denver samples can be seen more clearly in Figure 1b, in which the same data are displayed as residuals from a line describing the mean size of children in the Denver sample at successive chronological ages. With the exception of four children aged < 8 months old, the entire London crypt sample has femur lengths that are > 1 SD below the mean size of children of the same age derived from the Denver growth study. By the age of 15 months, the majority of London children have femur lengths that are > 2 SD below the mean size of the Denver sample. The trend, indicated by the distribution of data points, is a crude indication of the growth pattern of individuals within the population represented by the London crypt sample. Compared with the Denver sample, the London children exhibit a marked deficit in growth in the first 15 months of life. After this age, the difference between the mean femur lengths of the Denver and London samples increases more gradually and the general trend indicated by the data points is only slightly steeper than the line illustrating –2 SD from the mean. There is no evidence for catch up growth, indicating that the children from the London crypt sample do not recover from an initial disruption to growth in femoral length during the later stages of growth.

The second method applied to the same growth data examines variation in the percentage of adult femur length attained at different ages in the two samples. For this analysis, the percentage of adult size attained was calculated using mean adult femur length including the epiphyses as an estimate of adult size in each population. No attempt was made to calculate final diaphyseal length by subtracting the size of the epiphyses from total femur length since comparable data on epiphyseal size are not available for the two populations. For the London crypt sample, adult femur length was estimated as the mean of adult male and female femur length, measured on a sample of adults from Christ Church, Spitalfields and St Brides Church. For the Denver sample, adult size was estimated as the mean of male

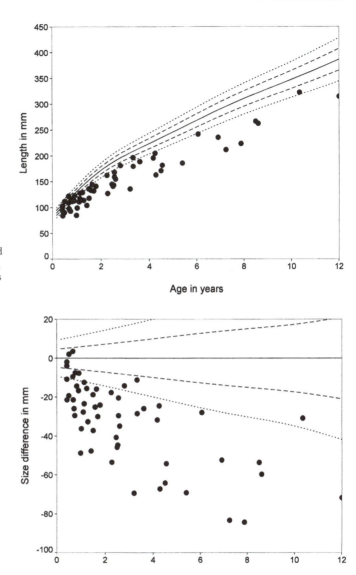

Figure 1a – Femur diaphysis length plotted against chronological age in the London crypt sample (black circles) and the Denver sample (solid line = sample mean, dashed lines = plus and minus one standard deviation, dotted lines = plus and minus two standard deviations).

Figure 1b – Differences in femur diaphysis length from the mean value in the Denver sample against chronological age. The differences for are calculated as residuals from the curve fitted to the mean values for femur diaphysis length in the Denver sample at successive chronological ages. Symbols are the same as figure 1a.

femur length at age 18 years and female femur length at age 16 years. Growth in the female sample appears to be complete at this age since mean femur length at 16 years is slightly lower than at 15.5 years and slightly higher than at 17 years (these are based on smaller samples). Male femur length increases by < 3 mm between 17 and 18 years so male femur length at 18 years may be a slight underestimate of adult male femur length.

The percentage of adult size attained by each individual from the London crypt sample is plotted against chronological age in Figure 2a, together with lines illustrating the percentage of adult size attained at successive chronological ages for the mean and ± 1 and 2 SD from the mean of the Denver sample. In Figure 2b, the same data are displayed as residuals from

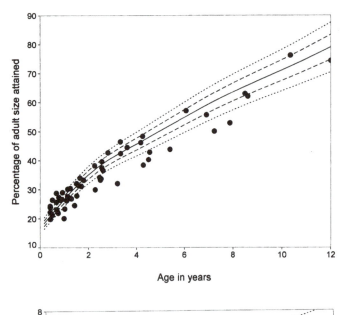

Figure 2a – Percentage of adult femur length attained plotted against chronological age in the London crypt sample and the Denver sample. Symbols are the same as figure 1a.

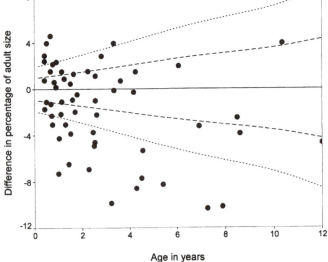

Figure 2b – Differences in the percentage of adult femur length attained from the mean value in the Denver sample against chronological age. The differences are calculataed as residuals from the curve fitted to the mean values for the percentage of adult femur length attained in the Denver sample at successive chronological ages. Symbols are the same as figure 1a.

a line describing the mean percentage of adult size attained at successive chronological ages by children in the Denver sample. The data points for individuals from the London crypt sample are distributed both above and below the lines representing ± 2 SD from the mean for the percentage of adult size attained at successive ages in the Denver sample, and about 60% of data points lie within the range defined by these lines. The distribution of data points suggests an overall tendency towards more prolonged growth in femoral length in the London crypt population than in the population sampled for the Denver growth study. Out of a total of 55 individuals, 22 lie above the mean and 33 fall below it, but this difference is not statistically significant (chi-square = 2.291, d.f. = 1).

The tendency for children from the London crypt sample to have attained a lower percentage of adult size than those in the Denver sample appears to increase with age. During the first 2 years there are about equal numbers of children from the London crypt sample lying above and below the mean of the Denver sample, but in subsequent groups there is a marked imbalance with more of the London children lying below the mean of the Denver sample. Despite this pattern, which could be interpreted as a weak evidence of growth prolongation, the result of this analysis is ambiguous. An alternative explanation for the distribution of data points shown in Figure 2a and b is that the children exhibiting severe growth retardation represented a distinct group who had been exposed to chronic environmental stress before death and whose growth was not typical of the sample as a whole. Nine children represented by the data points lying furthest below the line representing –2 SD from the mean, and aged between 12 months and 8 years of age, can be singled out as displaying particularly severe growth retardation. Additional analysis of skeletal and dental stress indicators would be necessary to determine whether these individuals had been exposed to a different pattern of stress from that experienced by the other individuals used for this growth analysis.

Summary

Small adult size, skeletal growth deficits and prolonged skeletal growth can each be used as indicators of environmental stress in a past population. Adults from the London crypt sample have shorter femora than the oldest age groups represented by the Denver sample, but the extent to which this difference reflects impoverished environmental circumstances rather than a genetic difference in growth potential is not immediately clear. In terms of actual femur length, the children from the London crypt sample are typically smaller than the mean size of children from the Denver sample by the age of 8 months, and show a marked deficit in growth by the age of 15 months. The difference in adult size between the two populations can be largely attributed to events occurring in the first 15 months of life, rather than a gradual divergence of growth patterns occurring throughout the growth period. It therefore seems likely that a significant part of the difference in adult size between the two populations is the result of impoverished living conditions experienced by the London children during infancy.

It is tempting to relate the development of a growth deficit during infancy to inadequate nutritional intake and increased exposure to pathogens during the weaning period.[25,52] The difference in the distribution of femoral lengths in the Denver sample and the London crypt sample is less marked when the data are evaluated in terms of the percentage of adult size attained. There is a weak tendency for children from the London crypt sample to have achieved less than the mean percentage of adult size attained by children from the Denver sample at the same chronological age. However, there is insufficient evidence to argue convincingly that growth was prolonged in the population represented by the London crypt sample. The combination of methods used in this study allows the growth difference between the London crypt sample and the Denver sample to be more thoroughly investigated than would be possible with any single comparative technique. A clearer picture would emerge if sample size was increased (by including unidentified individuals), and a complementary study of direct dental and skeletal stress indicators was undertaken.

ACKNOWLEDGEMENTS

I thank Margaret Cox and Simon Mays for inviting me to contribute to this volume. Thanks to Theya Molleson, Louise Scheuer and Jacqui Bowman for permission to study skeletal material used in this study and for their insights into the biology of Londoners in the past, and to two anonymous referees for helpful comments on this paper.

REFERENCES

1   Johnston FE. Growth of the long bones of infants and young children at Indian Knoll. *American Journal of Physical Anthropology* 1962; **20**; 249–254.

2   Bogin B. *Patterns of Human Growth.* Cambridge: Cambridge University Press, 1988.

3   Eveleth PB, Tanner JM. *Worldwide Variation in Human Growth* (2nd edn), Cambridge: Cambridge University Press, 1990.

4   Floud R, Wachter K, Gregory A. *Height, Health and History: Nutritional Status in the United Kingdom, 1750–1980.* Cambridge: Cambridge University Press, 1990.

5   Rudney JD. Skeletal indicators of growth disturbance in a series of ancient Lower Nubian populations: changes over time. *American Journal of Physical Anthropology* 1983; **60**; 463–470.

6   Hummert JR, Van Gerven DP. Skeletal growth in a medieval population from Sudanese Nubia. *American Journal of Physical Anthropology* 1983; **60**; 471–478.

7   Goodman AH, Martin DL, Armelagos GJ, Clarke G. Indications of stress from bone and teeth. In: Cohen MN, Armelagos GJ (eds), *Palaeopathology at the Origins of Agriculture.* Orlando: Academic Press, 1984: pp. 13–49.

8   Cook DC. Subsistence and health in the Lower Illinois Valley: Osteological evidence. In: Cohen MN, Armelagos GJ (eds), *Palaeopathology at the Origins of Agriculture.* Orlando: Academic Press, 1984: pp. 235–269.

9   Jantz RL, Owsley DW. Long bone growth variation among Arikara skeletal populations. *American Journal of Physical Anthropology* 1984; **63**; 13–20.

10 Mensforth RP. Relative tibia long bone growth in the Libben and Bt–5 prehistoric skeletal populations. *American Journal of Physical Anthropology* 1985; **68**; 247–262.

11 Larsen CS. *Bioarchaeology: Interpreting Behaviour from the Human Skeleton.* Cambridge: Cambridge University Press, 1997.

12 Johnston FE. The growth of the skeleton in earlier peoples. In: Brothwell DR (ed.), *The Skeletal Biology of Earlier Human Populations.* Oxford: Pergamon, 1968: pp. 57–66.

13 Sundick RI. Human skeletal growth and age determination. *Homo* 1978; **29**; 228–248.

14 Walker PL Johnson JR, Lambert PM. Age and sex biases in the preservation of human skeletal remains. *American Journal of Physical Anthropology* 1988; **76**; 183–188.

15 Saunders SR. Subadult skeletons and growth related studies. In: Saunders SR, Katzenberg MA (eds), *Skeletal Biology of Past Peoples: Research Methods.* New York: Wiley-Liss, 1992: pp. 1–19.

16 Humphrey LT. Interpretation of the growth of past populations. In: Sofaer-Derevenski, JR (ed.), *Children and Material Culture.* London: Routledge (in press).

17 Wood JW, Milner GR, Harpending HC, Weiss KM. The osteological paradox: problems of inferring prehistoric health from skeletal samples. *Current Anthropology* 1992; **33**; 343–370.

18 Saunders SR, Hoppa RD. Growth deficit in survivors and non-survivors: biological mortality bias in subadult skeletal samples. *Yearbook of Physical Anthropology* 1993; **36**; 127–151.

19 Walker PL. The linear growth of long bones in Late Woodland Indian children. *Proceedings of the Indiana Academy of Sciences* 1969; **78**; 83–87.

20 Frisancho RA, Guire K, Babler, W, Borkan G, Way, A. Nutritional influence of childhood development and genetic control of adolescent growth of Quechuas and Mestizos from the Peruvian Lowlands. *American Journal of Physical Anthropology* 1980; **52**; 367–375.

21   Armelagos GJ, Mielke JH, Owen KH, Van Gerven DP, Dewey JR, Mahler PE. Bone growth and development in prehistoric populations from Sudanese Nubia. *Journal of Human Evolution* 1972; **1**; 89–119.

22   Stloukal M, Hanáková H. Die Länge der Längsknochen altslawischer Bevölkerungen – unter besonderer Berücksichtigung von wachstumsfragen. *Homo* 1978; **29**; 53–69.

23   Lovejoy CO, Russell KF, Harrison ML. Long bone growth velocity in the Libben population. *American Journal of Human Biology* 1990; **2**; 533–542.

24   Saunders S, Hoppa R, Southern R. Diaphyseal growth in a nineteenth century skeletal sample of subadults from St Thomas' Church, Belleville, Ontario. *International Journal of Osteoarchaeology* 1993; **3**; 265–281.

25   Molleson T, Cox M. *The Spitalfields project*, vol. 2: *The Middling Sort*. Council for British Archaeology Research Report 86, 1993.

26   Farwell DE, Molleson TI. *Poundbury*, vol. 2: *The Cemeteries*. Monograph Series No. 11. Dorchester: Dorset Natural History and Archaeological Society, 1993.

27   Miles AEW, Bulman JS. Growth curves of immature bones from a Scottish island population of sixteenth to mid-nineteenth century: limb-bone diaphyses and some bones of the hand and foot. *International Journal of Osteoarchaeology* 1994; **4**; 121–136.

28   Steyn M, Henneberg M. Skeletal growth of children from the Iron Age site at K2 (South Africa). *American Journal of Physical Anthropology* 1996; **100**; 389–396.

29   Mays SA. *The Archaeology of Human Bones.* London: Routledge, 1998.

30   Merchant VL, Ubelaker DH. Skeletal growth of the protohistoric Arikara. *American Journal of Physical Anthropology* 1977; **46**; 61–72.

31   Wall CE. Evidence of weaning stress and catch-up growth in the long bones of a central Californian Amerindian sample. *Annals of Human Biology* 1991; **18**; 9–22.

32   Hoppa RD. Evaluating human skeletal growth: an Anglo-Saxon example. *International Journal of Osteoarchaeology* 1992; **2**; 275–288.

33   Miles AEW, Bulman JS. Growth curves of immature bones from a Scottish island population of sixteenth to mid-nineteenth century: shoulder girdle, ilium, pubis and ischium. *International Journal of Osteoarchaeology* 1995; **5**; 15–27.

34   Y'Edynak G. Long bone growth in Western Eskimo and Aleut skeletons. *American Journal of Physical Anthropology* 1976; **45**; 569–574.

35   Humphrey LT. Patterns of growth in the modern human skeleton. *American Journal of Physical Anthropology* 1998; **105**; 57–72.

36   Mays SA. The relationship between Harris line formation and bone growth and development. *Journal of Archaeological Science* 1985; **12**; 207–220.

37   Mays SA. The relationship between Harris lines and other aspects of skeletal development in adults and juveniles. *Journal of Archaeological Science* 1995; **22**; 511–520.

38   Ribot I, Roberts C. A study of non-specific stress indicators and skeletal growth in two mediaeval subadult populations. *Journal of Archaeological Science* 1996; **23**; 67–79.

39   Hillson S, Bond S. Relationship of enamel hypoplasia to the pattern of tooth crown growth: a discussion. *American Journal of Physical Anthropology* 1997; **104**; 89–103.

40   Skinner MF, Dupras TL, Moyà-Solà S. Periodicity of linear hypoplasia among Miocene *Dryopithecus* from Spain. *Journal of Palaeopathology* 1995; **7**; 195–222.

41   Lewis M, Roberts, C. Growing pains: the interpretation of stress indicators. *International Journal of Osteoarchaeology* 1997; **7**; 581–586.

42   Steegmann AT. 18th Century British military stature: growth cessation, selective recruiting, selective trends, nutrition at birth, cold and occupation. *Human Biology* 1985; **57**; 77–95.

43   Roche AF. Bone Growth and Maturation. In: Falkner F, Tanner JM (eds), *Human Growth*, vol. 2: *Postnatal Growth and Neurobiology* (2nd edn), New York: Plenum, 1986: pp. 25–60.

44   Humphrey LT. Relative mandibular growth in humans, gorillas and chimpanzees. In: Hoppa R, FitzGerald C (eds), *Human Growth in the Past: Studies from Bones and Teeth.* Cambridge: Cambridge University Press 1999: 56–87

45   Prendergast Moore K, Thorp S, Van Gerven DP. Pattern of dental eruption, skeletal maturation and stress in a Medieval Population from Sudanese Nubia. *Human Evolution* 1986; **1**; 325–330.

46   Demirjian A, Dentition. In: Falkner F, Tanner JM (eds), *Human Growth*, vol. 2: *Postnatal Growth and Neurobiology* (2nd edn), New York: Plenum, 1986: pp. 269–298.

47   Roche AF. *Growth, Maturation and Body Composition: The Fels Longitudinal Study 1929–1991*. Cambridge: Cambridge University Press, 1992.

48   Maresh MM. Linear growth of long bones of extremities from infancy through adolescence. *American Journal of Diseases in Childhood* 1955; **89**; 725–742.

49   Maresh MM. Measurements from roentgenograms. In: McCammon RW (ed.), *Human Growth and Development*. Springfield: Charles C Thomas, 1970: pp. 157–200.

50   Feldesman MR. Femur/stature ratio and estimates of stature in children. *American Journal of Physical Anthropology* 1992; **87**; 447–459.

51   Jolicouer P, Pontier J, Pernin O, Sempé M. A lifetime asymptotic growth curve for human height. *Biometrics* 1988; **44**; 995–1003.

52   Fildes VA. The culture and biology of breastfeeding: an historical review of Western Europe. In: Stuart-Macadam P, Dettwyler KA (eds), *Breastfeeding: Biocultural Perspectives*. New York: Aldine de Gruyter, 1995: pp. 101–126.

4

NON-ADULT PALAEOPATHOLOGY: CURRENT STATUS AND FUTURE POTENTIAL

Mary Lewis

INTRODUCTION

Data from non-adult skeletal material are widely believed to represent the most demographically variable and sensitive barometer of biocultural change.[1,2] Patterns of infant and child mortality have been shown to have a profound effect on the crude death rates of a population and, when coupled with evidence of childhood morbidity, have become accepted as a measure of population fitness.[3] In other words, the health and survival of the offspring indicate the level to which a population has adapted to the environment in which it lives. However, despite this recognition, the study of non-adult remains in biological anthropology has been limited. Small sample sizes and poor preservation has led researchers to concentrate on adult skeletal material for insights into population health and adaptation. This paper will examine some of the advantages and limitations in analysing non-adult material, and discuss the current nature of research into past child health in British populations.

There are many advantages to the study of health based on non-adult material. Age estimates of non-adults are derived using age specific markers (see Scheuer and Black, chapter 2, in this volume), mainly of the dentition (see Whittaker, chapter 6, in this volume). The timing and outcome of these events is thought to be linked to a genetic blueprint, unlike the more variable degenerative age indicators of adulthood.[4] For this reason, non-adult skeletons allow for a more precise skeletal age estimation than is possible for adults. The study of 'growth' rather than a static adult stature means that the age at which children fall behind or recover their growth trajectory can be examined. Many indicators of stress on the skeleton and dentition develop during childhood and bone lesions may remodel and disappear as the individual gets older. Therefore, the true prevalence of lesions such as cribra orbitalia or Harris lines can be more accurately assessed in younger individuals. Interpretation of these lesions is problematic and some authors have argued that they only occur in individuals who were strong enough to survive a stress episode.[5] The precise age at which these lesions develop can also help us answer questions about the nature of stress and survival.[6] Nevertheless, it should be remembered that children in an archaeological sample represent the 'non-survivors' from any given population, and their pattern of growth or frequency of lesions might not reflect that of the children who went on to survive into adulthood.[5,7]

The early death of these individuals provides other challenges in the study of non-adult palaeopathology. Chronic diseases need time to develop, but the children that enter the archaeological record have usually died in the acute stages of disease, before the skeleton has had time to respond. At the present time, studies that concentrate on non-adult material are hindered by the inability to make reliable sex estimations, due to absence of the secondary sexual characteristics evident on the adult skull and pelvis. Although sexual dimorphism has been identified *in utero*, there is still disagreement about the validity of quantifying morphological traits in the non-adult skeleton.[8,9] However, the application of DNA analysis in determining the sex of non-adult skeletal material has begun to be used[10] and hopefully, future work in non-adult palaeopathology will begin to focus on sex, and perhaps gender differences in health and survival.

PROBLEMS OF PRESERVATION AND RECOVERY

Preservation is perhaps one of the most frustrating limitations in non-adult palaeopathology, as a complete, well-preserved skeleton is a pre-requisite for the diagnosis of pathological conditions. Furthermore, without the recovery of the epiphyses, that will later fuse to become adult joint surfaces, the cause of a problem, such as paralysis, cannot be fully ascertained. Without the joint it is often impossible to determine if the condition was the result of trauma, infection, a circulatory problem or whether it was congenital.

Differential preservation during burial, archaeological methods of excavation, and cultural factors that dictate how and where children are buried, are often cited as reasons for the small numbers of non-adults retrieved from excavations.[11] It has been suggested that growing bones, with a high organic and low mineral content, are particularly susceptible to taphonomic processes, and that non-adult remains simply do not survive in the ground.[12] However, during an analysis of a group of skeletons from Belleville, Ontario, Saunders[13] found that non-adult skeletal remains were preserved as well as, if not better than the adult skeletons. Molleson[14], reporting on the non-adult material from Poundbury, Dorset, supported this view. It is possible that infant burials were placed in shallower graves, which are more susceptible to disturbances by subsequent burials, ploughing or cemetery clearances. In addition, factors such as the age of the non-adult and soil pH have been proved to have an effect on preservation.[15,16] However, the skill of the excavator is vital in the retrieval of the remains. Immature skeletons may be more susceptible to colour change in the ground (Figure 1) and the epiphyses can mimic small stones and this can easily be missed by the untrained eye. Foetal bones may lie within the abdominal cavity of an adult female and these tiny bones may be overlooked in a hurried excavation when sieving is not possible. Ageing of these younger individuals can also be hindered by the loss of the fragile developing dental crowns during cleaning and storage.

When using data derived from cemetery samples it is important to remember that we are actually measuring *burial rates* and not *mortality rates*. Cultural practices may dictate if, and

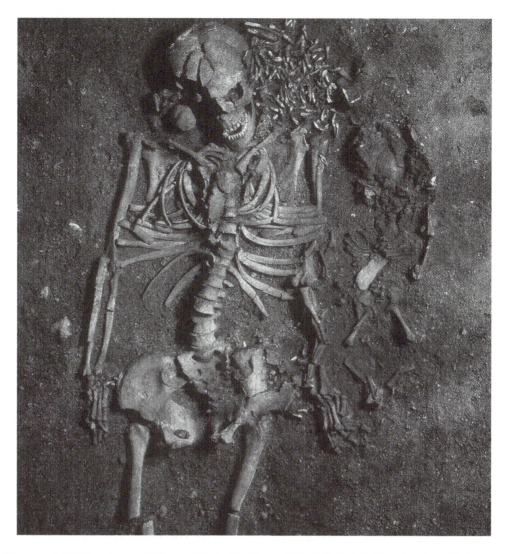

Figure 1 – Woman and child from the mesolithic site of Vedbaek in Denmark (Ertebølle Period). Reproduced with kind permission from the Nationalmuseet, Copenhagen.

where, certain individuals were placed within a cemetery; non-adults are often clustered, and if the whole area of the cemetery is not excavated this could lead to an under-representation of the youngest members of the society. For example, at St Helen-on-the-Walls, York, only two-thirds of the cemetery was uncovered, leaving the north west corner unexcavated.[17] The striking under-enumeration of infants ($n = 12$) suggests that they could have been buried at this corner of the site. In some cases, the lack of non-adults in many Anglo-Saxon cemeteries has led some researchers to suggest that infants were buried elsewhere in the settlement.[18,19] Evidence of separate burial sites for infants in the UK is lacking, but special cemeteries for infants have been discovered in early medieval Italy.[20] During the medieval period in England, unbaptized and illegitimate babies could have been omitted from cemeteries.[11] Later, in the 18th and early 19th centuries, the practice of using wet-nurses meant that children from towns and cities, who died while being nursed, were often buried in the countryside rather than being returned home.[21] This type of infant migration should be taken into account when attempting to interpret mortality levels.

Problems with the recovery of non-adult skeletons mean that the samples are often too small to allow a significant examination of the morbidity and mortality of the group to be carried out. When attempts are made, comparisons between groups are hindered by the lack of consistency in age categories. In Europe, individuals classed as non-adults range from 1 to 20 years of age depending on the osteologist's preference and 'infants' may include any individual aged up to 4 years. The correct clinical use of the term infant only includes individuals up to 1 year of age.

PRINCIPLES OF NON-ADULT PALAEOPATHOLOGY

There are many conditions commonly recorded on the adult skeleton that can be identified on non-adult remains, with the exception of neonatal material. Dental disease, specific and non-specific infections, indicators of stress, trauma and metabolic diseases have all been recorded.

The nature of the fragile periosteum in non-adults can result in more severe pathological lesions than seen in adults. The periosteum is the fibrous sheath that covers all the bones of the skeleton, with the exception of the endocranial surface of the skull and the joints. The sheath has two layers; the outer layer consists of a white fibrous tissue with a few fat cells and the inner layer is made up of a dense network of fine elastic fibres.[22] This layer retains its osteoblastic capacity throughout life and is vulnerable to traumatic separation and haemorrhage. The periosteum is bound to the cortex by Sharpey's fibres, which are less numerous and shorter in children, due to the need for the bone underneath to change its morphology during the growth process. This leaves the sheath particularly susceptible to rupture.[23] In adults, the invasion of a foreign organism causes inflammation and may result in involvement of the periosteum, which stimulates the osteoblasts to deposit osteoid on the extracortical surface of the adjacent bone. The firm attachment of the periosteum to the cortex in adults limits the spread of infection and new bone formation (Figure 2a). However, in non-adults, the periosteum may be stripped from the entire length of the shaft resulting in hypertrophy of the affected bone (Figure 2b). Children are more susceptible to bone infection, due to the abundant blood supply in the red bone marrow at the ends of the long bones. A good blood supply is essential to maintain rapid growth in these areas but also transports foreign organisms to these sites, many of which rely on an abundance of iron to achieve their full growth and replication potential.[24]

Although the recognition of severe infections, such as osteomyelitis or sclerosing osteomyelitis is relatively straightforward,[25-27] the diagnosis of periostitis in non-adult skeletal remains is more problematic. In the long bones, appositional growth involves the deposition of immature disorganized bone on the periosteal surface. This new bone is macroscopically identical to the 'woven' bone deposited during an infection or after trauma.

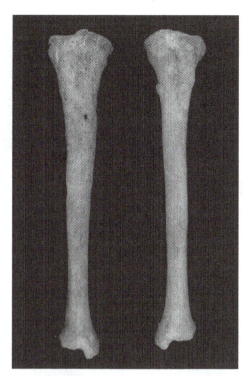

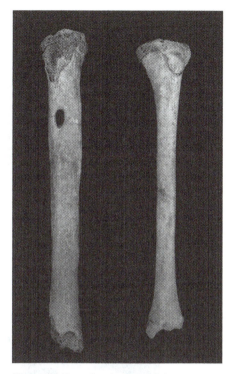

Figure 2a – Osteomyelitis in an adult individual. The periosteum is more firmly attached and has limited the spread of the infection.

Figure 2b – Extensive osteomyelitis in a non-adult.

Therefore, in the youngest individuals, it is almost impossible to distinguish between normal and abnormal bone, and in some cases a diagnosis of this lesion in non-adults under the age of two years is not attempted.[28] In the few studies that mention non-adult periostitis, it is recognized as a unilateral, isolated patch of bone raised above the cortex.[3,29,30] However, if the inflammation is the result of a more widespread infection, the diffuse deposits of periostitis will be indistinguishable from normal rapid appositional growth. New bone formation in the form of grey woven bone, has also been identified on the endocranial surfaces of the skull (Figure 3) and in some instances may represent a normal appearance in the infant.[22] However, intra-cranial haemorrhage can occur in pre-term infants and may also be responsible for some of these lesions.[31] Studies of non-adults dying from chronic tuberculous meningitis in Lithuania have revealed 'corn-sized' depressions on the endocranial surface, thought to be the result of calcified tubercles.[32–35] Birth trauma, child abuse, syphilis, rickets, scurvy, hypervitaminosis A and infantile cortical hyperostosis (Caffey's disease) can all occur in the new-born and infant but are rarely recognized in archaeological material.[36–43] Without further investigation into the nature of these deposits, and a precise guide of where and at what age growth occurs in the skull and long bones, we may never identify the true extent of inflammatory episodes in a child's life.

During childhood, active growth produces a rapid turnover of bone, which can both aid and hinder the diagnosis of certain conditions. Rickets (vitamin D deficiency) becomes

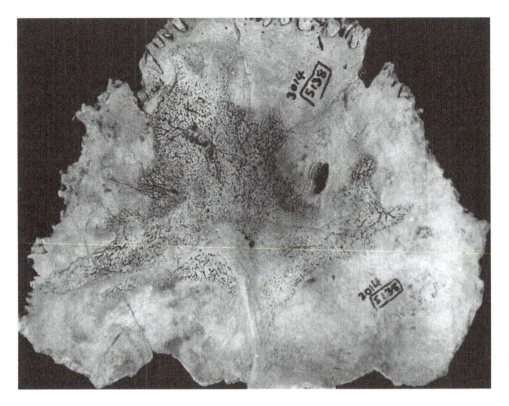

Figure 3 – Endocranial new bone formation on the occipital of a non-adult from Raunds Furnells, Northamptonshire.

apparent as large quantities of inferior new bone rapidly replace the previously ossified cortex. The adult form of the disease, osteomalacia, is less evident as bone turnover occurs at a much slower rate. Once rickets has been resolved, accelerated ('catch-up') growth allows the inferior bone to be quickly replaced by normal tissue causing both the macroscopic and radiographic signs of the disease to disappear within 3–4 months.[44] In addition, the identification of fractures in non-adult skeletons is rare compared with the rates seen in adult samples. It seems unlikely that children did not suffer trauma in the past and the real explanation may be that they developed greenstick fractures (a partial break of the bone shaft). The highly plastic nature of non-adult bones commonly produces fractures of this type that do not result in deformation and heal quickly.[45]

TYPES OF PALAEOPATHOLOGICAL INFORMATION

The types of palaeopathological data that can be retrieved from non-adult material are both direct and indirect. The presence of foetuses within, or expelled from, the abdominal cavity of an adult female can provide indirect evidence of obstetric health hazards, such as obstructed labour, infection or haemorrhage. The child may have been inappropriately positioned in the womb or there may be pelvic obstruction, e.g. the mother may have had deformities associated with vitamin D deficiency. Congenital syphilis and tuberculosis, as well as more acute conditions, can induce spontaneous abortion and may account for some of the foetal remains in a sample. Wells[46,47] carried out a survey of obstetric casualties in Europe and presented cases from Kingsworthy in Hampshire and St Nicholas Shambles, London. More recently, Farwell and Molleson[48] reported on a Romano-British case from Poundbury, and Boylston *et al.*[49] highlighted an example of an obstetric hazard from Barton-upon-Humber.

Mays[50,51] examined the age at death of perinatal infants in Romano-British samples and suggested that the unusually large number of neonates, dying around the time of birth, was indicative of infanticide. This practice may be another possible reason why so few children are recovered from cemeteries during this period. Special burial areas or exposure may account for the loss of their remains. For example Smith and Kahila[52] reported on nearly 100 infants deposited in a sewer in Late Roman Israel. Child homicide was not confined to the Roman period, and documentary evidence for the burning, drowning, suffocation and poisoning of children is also available from the medieval period,[53] and the 18th and 19th centuries.[54,55]

The prevalence of indicators of stress, and adults harbouring deformities from childhood infections can also provide indirect information on childhood disease. A shortened limb in an adult individual suggests that trauma or infection resulted in damage to the growth plate during childhood that prevented the limb reaching full adult size. In addition, there is the added advantage that we can sex adults and thus produce projected information on the preferential treatment of boys and girls within that society.

The most commonly used direct methods for assessing morbidity in non-adults are growth curves and age at death profiles. Less commonly, stress indicators and metabolic diseases are incorporated. Growth curves are constructed to assess the level of growth or identify stunting, in relation to a modern standard (see Humphrey, chapter 3, in this volume). Age at death profiles generally show an increase in mortality between two and four years of age, and this finding is generally associated with the weaning period. The presence of active cribra orbitalia, dental enamel defects and Harris lines in children from this age group, have been used to support this hypothesis (see Katzenberg *et al.*[56] for a fuller discussion). However, the aetiology of these conditions is not fully understood and some of the problems associated with them need to be highlighted.

Cribra orbitalia and porotic hyperostosis

Cribra orbitalia and porotic hyperostosis are commonly associated with iron deficiency anaemia and are the result of a thinning of the outer table of the skull and expansion of the inner diploic space.[57] This is thought to occur during childhood when the diploic space is filled with enlarging red bone marrow, producing bone changes which, once the condition is resolved, will remodel.[58] Malnutrition, chronic blood loss, dietary deficiency, and an increased pathogen load have all been cited as causes of anaemia.[3,59,60]

The relationship between orbital and vault lesions is rarely disputed in North American studies, as the lesions are often found to occur together and 'porotic hyperostosis' is a term used to describe them both. In Europe however, cribra orbitalia is much more frequent than porotic hyperostosis, which is rarely recorded despite the occurrence of severe orbital lesions. This has lead to speculation in the UK that the lesions are not necessarily linked and may have different aetiologies.[61] When recording cribra orbitalia, care should be taken to distinguish healed (filled holes with rounded edges) from active lesions (sharp edged, or 'hair-on-end') but in many cases there may be a mix of both lesions, indicating that the problem has re-occurred.

Porotic hyperostosis, involving both the vault and orbits, is seen in thalassaemia and sickle cell anaemia but can be distinguished from acquired iron deficiency anaemia by additional post-cranial lesions.[62] Vault and orbital lesions are also common in rickets and scurvy but are slightly different in expression, these lesions are the result of new bone deposition on the outer table, rather than an expansion of the diploic space.[63] Nevertheless, both rickets and scurvy are associated with anaemia and both types of lesions may be present.

Dental enamel hypoplasias

Dental enamel hypoplasias, seen as pits or furrows on the enamel surface, are a popular stress indicator as they do not remodel and provide a chronological record of childhood stress from birth to about 12 years of age (Figure 4). Numerous conditions have been shown to cause these defects including fever, starvation, congenital infections and low birth weight.[31,65–67] Enamel hypoplasias are the most widely used stress indicators for assessing the age of weaning in different populations. The age at which a defect is formed is usually calculated by taking a measurement of the defect from the cemento-enamel junction and estimating the number of years the crown takes to develop.[68] Numerous studies of North American and European populations from many periods, have shown a peak in the age of defect formation between two and four years, and this has been interpreted as representing

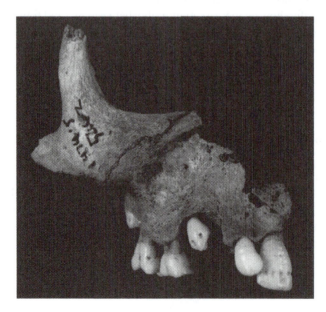

Figure 4 – Dental enamel hypoplasias on the developing dentition of a non-adult from St Helen-on-the-Walls, York.

stress at the time of weaning.[69–73] However, this idea has been disputed, and in 1994 Blakey *et al.*[74] showed that the highest frequency of defects in their African-American slave population was up to 3 years after they were documented to have weaned their children. More recently, Hillson and Bond[75] suggested that the position of the defect on the crown is more an expression of the pattern of enamel layers than the timing of a stress episode.

Harris lines

Harris lines, or transverse lines of increased radio-opacity, occurring in the growing bones of non-adults are a popular, but problematic, indicator of non-specific stress. An episode of acute or chronic stress will result in a slowing of the cartilage growth plate and the deposition of a thin layer of bone, visible on X-ray.[76,77]

The use of Harris lines to estimate the frequency of stress episodes is fraught with problems. Marshall[78] argued that the number of lines in a child's radius did not relate to the number of insults they had suffered in the past. Gindhart[79] showed that diseases were only followed by a line in 25% of cases and 10% of the lines occurred when no stressful episode was documented. Males and females have different rates of remodelling, and mild stresses, such as a child's first day at school, or a stress as severe as malnutrition, may cause a cessation of growth and the development of a line.[80] It has yet to be decided whether the thickness of a line is a measure of the severity or longevity of the stress episode,[81] or whether it relates to individual variability in the thickness of the cartilage plate and the speed of chondroblast recovery. In addition, to develop a line the individual would need to recover from the stress, and hence Harris lines might not be visible in the weaker members of society.[82] The recording of these lesions also provides problems. Hughes *et al.*[83] have argued that the type and side of the bone examined could affect the prevalence of the lines recorded in a skeletal sample. They concluded that while the distal tibia showed lines more frequently than any other bone, the lesions were not bilateral and those from the left side had greater numbers. Other authors have pointed out problems in counting the frequencies of the lines by the same and different researchers.[84,85]

STATUS OF NON-ADULT PALAEOPATHOLOGY IN THE UK

Studies of purely non-adult samples are limited in both Europe and the USA. In Britain, the examination of large groups of non-adults to answer particular archaeological questions is rare and research usually concentrates on a specific sample rather than a comparison of children from different populations and periods. In addition, many cases of specific and non-specific infection are recorded as case studies. Molleson and co-workers [14,86,87] have reported extensively on the 400 non-adults recovered from Poundbury Camp, and have discussed preservation problems, ages at death and reported on a number of pathologies. These include a congenitally deaf child, an infant with cut marks thought to indicate an embryotomy, and up to 24 cases of infantile cortical hyperostosis. Mays[88] also studied the non-adults from Poundbury Camp and tested the association of growth, cortical thickness and Harris lines. Studies examining the impact of childhood stress on growth have been carried out by Wiggins[89] on non-adults from Barton-on-Humber, and by Ribot and Roberts[28] who compared the prevalence of stress indicators with growth curves from a later medieval and an Anglo-Saxon population. Interestingly, none of these studies have shown that stress indicators significantly affect the growth of the non-adult. Work on growth and age at death of non-adults from particular populations in Britain have been carried out by Molleson and Cox,[90] Miles and Bulman[91] and Humphrey[92] but so far little work has been done to compare these children with other British groups.

Studies of dental disease as a measure of nutritional stress have also been carried out on non-adult remains. O'Sullivan et al.[93] surveyed 221 non-adults from 12 different sites in England and found an association between caries and cribra orbitalia. However, although the prevalence of enamel hypoplasias on deciduous teeth in North American archaeological populations has been discussed in the light of prenatal stress[94,95] no such data have been compiled for British populations.

FUTURE POTENTIAL OF NON-ADULT PALAEOPATHOLOGY

Comparisons of non-adults from different periods and geographical areas are essential if we are to start addressing archaeological and historical questions about changes in society's attitudes towards children, their adaptation to contrasting environments and general child health and care.

Recently, Crawford has attempted to address the question of 'child worth'.[96] She took examples of chronic diseases in Anglo-Saxon non-adults, and adults who survived childhood illnesses, as evidence that people invested time to care for sick children. In this Crawford was challenging the now discredited notion, introduced by Aries in 1960,[97] that parents did not invest emotionally in their children because child mortality was so high. Additional evidence for the special care of infants (by one person at least) comes from Barton-upon-Humber and Buckland[49] where crude feeding vessels have been found in children's graves. Evidence for the treatment and care of sick children is otherwise limited.

Knight[98] reviewed documentary evidence for Caffey's disease, and argued that many cases were actually examples of child abuse. This type of treatment has an unspoken history but lesions indicative of "battered baby syndrome" should be identifiable on skeletal material. Multiple fractures at different stages of healing are identified clinically in the vertebrae, ribs, skull and long bones. Periostitis may be evident on the arms and legs, as the result of stretching and shearing of the periosteum during violent shaking.[23] Attempts to identify this behaviour have been carried out in the USA,[30,99] but the non-specific nature of the lesions makes diagnosis difficult and more research is needed.

Reactive new bone, usually located around the meningeal vessels on the endocranial surface of the skull in non-adults, is a relatively new area of investigation into childhood disease. These features either appear as layers of new bone on the original cortical surface, expanding around meningeal vessels, as 'hair-on-end' extensions of the inner diploe around the vessels, or as 'capillary-like' impressions extending into the inner table of the cranium. These lesions are commonly found on the occipital bone, outlining the cruciate eminence, but have also been recorded on the parietal and frontal bones and appear to follow the areas of venous drainage. The various appearances of endocranial lesions may indicate different aetiologies such as meningitis, epidural haematomas, birth trauma, neoplasms, scurvy or tuberculosis but, as yet, the precise aetiology of these lesions is unknown.[32,100-102] As meningitis is often a childhood disease, the distribution of these lesions in the different age categories would be of interest, but more work on the nature of these lesions is needed.

The change from agricultural to industrial environments is documented to have had a major impact on child health. Tuberculosis was spread by the import of infected cow's milk and meat, and by overcrowded conditions, and rickets and scurvy became endemic (Figure 5). However, osteological evidence of these diseases in the past is surprisingly rare, and it is important to understand more about the nature of the conditions and how they manifest on the skeleton, especially in children. Tuberculosis is a childhood disease. The initial infection may lie dormant in a healthy individual after a brief inflammatory response, and become pathological later in life when the immune status becomes compromised, following re-infection or as a result of trauma to the affected bone or joint. However, in a more vulnerable individual it can lead to acute or miliary tuberculosis, where infection spreads throughout the body via the bloodstream, and is usually fatal.[23,62]

Although skeletal tuberculosis only occurs in about 3–5% of people with the disease, it is more common in non-adults due to the abundant blood supply of the growing bones that

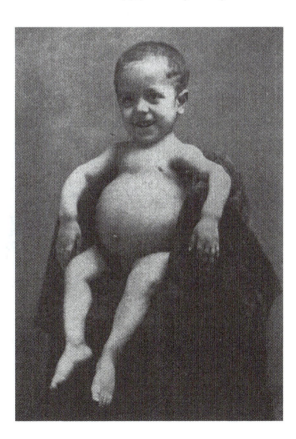

Figure 5 – Two-and-a-half-year-old child with rickets from 19th-century England. The distended abdomen, constricted chest and swelling of the wrists and ankles are characteristic of the disease. Reproduced from Holt.[64]

attracts the bacilli. Tuberculosis most commonly affects the spine, hip, and knee, and in infants also affects the tubular bones of the hands and feet (*'spina ventosa'*) due to their highly vascular nature. These lesions are not frequently seen and may heal with little or no sign of deformity.[62,103] Nevertheless, non-adults with evidence of pulmonary tuberculosis have been identified at Christ Church, Spitalfields (Figure 6)[90] and Abingdon.[104] In the future, rates of pulmonary and/or gastrointestinal tuberculosis may help to answer questions about the transmission of the disease and whether children were more susceptible to the gastrointestinal form as a result of infected milk, or equally susceptible to the pulmonary disease in the industrial environment.

Despite the endemic nature of rickets and scurvy in the Industrial period, the diagnosis of these conditions has, until recently, been neglected with older studies recording the prevalence of enamel hypoplasias as evidence for the disease.[105] Nevertheless, diagnostic techniques are becoming more sophisticated; Ortner and Mays[106] describe eight cases of rickets in rural Wharram Percy, one case was discovered at Jewbury in York[107] and about 20 cases were reported at Spitalfields.[90] The early changes of rickets are subtle and usually begin with an expansion and fraying of the rib ends and distal radius. The extreme bowing deformities are later manifestations and occur when the child applies weight to the affected limbs. However, the disease can render children immobile and, as they are susceptible to fatal respiratory and gastrointestinal infections as a result of the disease,[108] they may not live long enough to develop the most obvious signs.

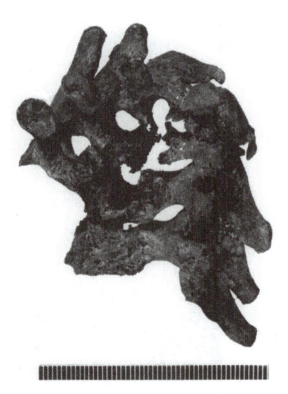

Figure 6 – Pott's disease (*tuberculous kyphosis*) in a non-adult from Christ Church Spitalfields, London. Reproduced with kind permission from the Natural History Museum, London.

Scurvy is not reported as frequently as rickets and this may be due to the fact that rickets and scurvy can occur together both today and in the past, a condition commonly known as 'Barlow's disease'.[109] The skeletal changes of rickets may mask the periosteal reactions resulting from haemorrhage characteristic of scurvy. However, changes to the sphenoid, maxilla and orbits are specific to vitamin C deficiency.[110] Improved diagnostic techniques will aid in distinguishing rickets from scurvy and other conditions such as Caffey's disease (Figure 7).

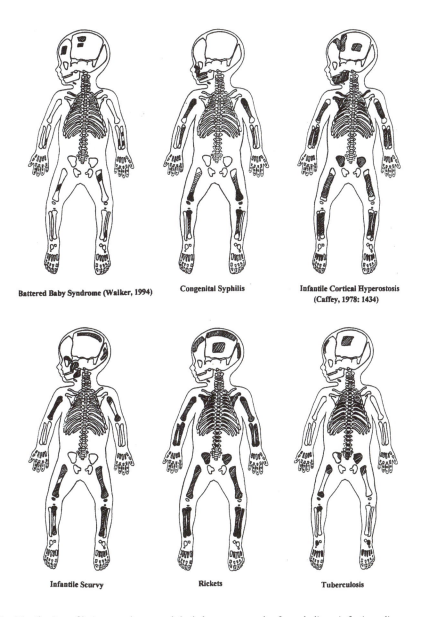

Figure 7 – Distribution of lesions on the non-adult skeleton as a result of metabolic or infectious disease.

The recognition of congenital syphilis, from dental and skeletal stigmata, may help to resolve the arguments of whether the endemic form of the disease was present in the Old World before 1493. In Europe, new evidence for the presence of congenital syphilis, and hence venereal syphilis, is now being put forward. Cases of congenital syphilis have been reported in a 9–10-year-old child from 17th-century Hungary[111] and a possible case of late congenital syphilis was reported in 14th–17th-century Poland.[112] Two pre-Columbian cases from Europe have also been described and directly question the Columbian theory.[113,114]

CONCLUSIONS

Although previously neglected, the potential for future research into non-adult palaeopathology is very exciting. As more archaeologists are trained to recognize and recover these small remains there are many areas still to be investigated. Improved DNA techniques may help us assign a sex to non-adults and allow us to address sex and gender issues and develop the questions of male:female preferential treatment, infanticide and natural susceptibility to disease. Stable isotope analysis, and examination of strontium/calcium ratios to pinpoint weaning ages has been carried out on many samples[115–120] but, as yet, has not been investigated in British populations. We need to analyse the timing and pattern of growth in children to help distinguish periostitis from normal new bone and finally identify neonatal and infant diseases using both long bone and skull lesions. Improved methods for the identification of rickets and scurvy are needed to develop a fuller picture of the conditions in both pre- and post-industrial societies. Fracture patterns, although limited by remodelling, may help identify child abuse or accidents, and may perhaps suggest the type of labour they were engaged in, for instance, at what time were children put to work and does this pattern change in different periods?

Once the problems of preservation and diagnosis have been resolved, broader questions about the treatment and health of children from different times and societies can begin to be answered, and further insights into the adaptation of a population to environmental change will be possible.

ACKNOWLEDGEMENTS

The contents of this paper are the result of PhD research funded by the University of Bradford. I thank Charlotte Roberts (University of Bradford) and two anonymous reviewers for their advice on the text, and Theya Molleson (Natural History Museum, London) for Figure 6. I am grateful to Jean Brown (University of Bradford) for producing the photographs.

REFERENCES

1   Van Gerven DP, Armelagos GJ. 'Farewell to paleodemography?' Rumors of its death have been greatly exaggerated. *Journal of Human Evolution* 1983; **12**: 353–360.

2   Roth EA. Applications of demography models to paleodemography. In: Saunders SR, Katzenberg MA (eds), *Skeletal Biology of Past Peoples: Research Methods*. New York: Wiley-Liss, 1992: pp. 175–188.

3   Mensforth RP, Lovejoy OC, Lallo JW, Armelagos GJ. The role of constitutional factors, diet and infectious disease in the etiology of porotic hyperostosis and periosteal reactions in prehistoric infants and children. *Medical Anthropology* 1978; **2(1)**: 1–59.

4   Rallison ML. *Growth Disorders in Infants, Children and Adolescents.* New York: Wiley, 1986.

5   Wood JW, Milner GR, Harpending HC, Weiss KM. The osteological paradox. problems of inferring prehistoric health from skeletal samples. *Current Anthropology* 1992; **33(4)**: 343–370.

6   Goodman AH. On the interpretation of health from skeletal remains. *Current Anthropology* 1993; **34(3)**: 281–288.

7   Saunders SR, Hoppa RD. Growth deficit in survivors and non-survivors: biological mortality bias in subadult skeletal samples. *Yearbook of Physical Anthropology* 1993; **36**: 127–151.

8   Schutkowski H. Sex determination of infant and juvenile skeletons: 1. Morphognostic features. *American Journal of Physical Anthropology* 1993; **90**: 199–205.

9   Holcomb SMC, Konigsberg LM. Statistical study of sexual dimorphism in the human fetal sciatic notch. *American Journal of Physical Anthropology.* 1995; **97(2)**: 113–126.

10   Colson IB, Richards MB, Bailey JF, Sykes BC, Hedges REM. DNA analysis of seven human skeletons excavated from the Terp of Wijnaldum. *Journal of Archaeological Sciences* 1997; **24**: 911–917.

11   Daniell C. *Death and Burial in Medieval England 1066–1550.* London: Routledge, 1997.

12   Johnston FE, Zimmer LO. Assessment of growth and age in the immature skeleton. In: Isçan MY, Kennedy KAR (eds), *Reconstruction of Life from the Skeleton.* New York: Alan R Liss, 1989: pp. 11–21.

13   Saunders SR. Subadult skeletons and growth related studies. In: Saunders SR, Katzenberg MA (eds), *Skeletal Biology of Past Populations: Advances in Research Methods.* New York: Wiley-Liss, 1992: pp. 1–20.

14   Molleson TI. Social implications of mortality patterns of juveniles from Poundbury Camp, Romano-British cemetery. *Anthropologischer Anzeiger* 1989; **47(1)**: 27–38.

15   Gordon CG, Buikstra JE. Soil pH, Bone preservation, and sampling bias at mortuary sites. *American Antiquity* 1981; **48**: 566–571.

16   Guy H, Masset C, Baud C-A. Infant taphonomy. *International Journal of Osteoarchaeology* 1997; **7**: 221–229.

17   Dawes JD, Magilton JR. *The Cemetery of St. Helen-on-the-Walls, Aldwark.* London: Council for British Archaeology, 1980.

18   Harman M, Molleson TI, Price JL. Burials, bodies and beheadings in Romano-British and Anglo-Saxon cemeteries. *Bulletin of the British Museum of Natural History (Geol.)* 1981; **35(3)**: 145–188.

19   Sherlock SJ, Welch MG. *An Anglo-Saxon Cemetery at Norton, Cleveland.* Research Report Number 82. London: Council for British Archaeology, 1992.

20   Becker MJ. Children's cemeteries: Early Christianity, not disease. *Paleopathology Newsletter* 1995; **80**: 10–11.

21   Fildes V. The English wet-nurse and her role in infant care 1538–1800. *Medical History* 1988; **32**: 142–173.

22   Williams PL, Warwick R. *Gray's Anatomy* (36th edn). Edinburgh: Churchill Livingston, 1980.

23   Caffey J (ed.), *Pediatric X-ray Diagnosis* (7th edn). Chicago: Year Book Medical, 1978.

24   Ulijaszek SJ. Nutritional status and susceptibility to infectious disease. In: Harrison GA, Waterlow JC (eds), *Diet and Disease in Traditional and Developing Societies.* Society for the Study of Human Biology. Symposium 30. Cambridge: Cambridge University Press, 1990: pp. 137–154.

25   Canci A, Tarli SMB, Repetto E. Osteomyelitis of probable haematogenous origin in a Bronze Age child from Toppo Daguzzo (Basilicata, Southern Italy). *International Journal of Osteoarchaeology* 1991; **1**: 135–139.

26   Anderson T, Carter AR. An unusual osteitic reaction in a young medieval child. *International Journal of Osteoarchaeology* 1995; **5**: 192–195.

27   Malgosa A, Aluja M, Isidro A. Pathological evidence in newborn children from the sixteenth century in Huelva (Spain). *International Journal of Osteoarchaeology* 1996; **6**: 388–396.

28   Ribot I, Roberts C. A study of non-specific stress indicators and skeletal growth in two mediaeval subadult populations. *Journal of Archaeological Science* 1996; **23**: 67–79.

29   Anderson T, Carter AR. Periosteal reaction in a new born child from Sheppey, Kent. *International Journal of Osteoarchaeology* 1994; **4**: 47–48.

30   Walker PL. Skeletal evidence for child abuse in earlier populations. *Proceedings of the Tenth European Meeting of the Paleopathology Association, Göttingen, Germany. Homo Supplement* 1994; p. 139.

31   Seow KW. Dental enamel defects in low birthweight children. *Journal of Paleopathology Monographic Publication* 1992; **2**: 321–330.

32   Jankauskas R, Schultz M. Meningeal reactions in a late medieval–early modern child population from Alytus, Lithuania. *Journal of Paleopathology* 1995; **7(2)**: 106.

33   Jankauskas R. Tuberculosis in Lithuania: palaeopathological and historical correlations. In: Pálfi G, Dutour O, Deák J (eds), *ICEPT Proceedings of the Evolution and Palaeoepidemiology of Tuberculosis*. Szeged: Tuberculosis Foundation, 1997.

34   Teschler-Nicola M. Epidemiology of tuberculosis in an early mediaeval population from Gars/Thunau Lower Austria. In: Pálfi G, Dutour O, Deák J (eds), *ICEPT Proceedings of the Evolution and Palaeoepidemiology of Tuberculosis*. Szeged: Tuberculosis Foundation, 1997.

35   Teschler-Nicola M. Differential diagnosis of tuberculosis: the diagnostic value of endocranial features. In: Pálfi G, Dutour O, Deák J (eds), *ICEPT Proceedings of the Evolution and Palaeoepidemiology of Tuberculosis*. Szeged: Tuberculosis Foundation, 1997.

36   Snedecor S, Knapp. R, Wilson H. Traumatic ossifying periostitis of the newborn. *Surgical Gynecological Obstetrics* 1935; **61**: 385–387.

37   Barba WP, Freriks DJ. The familial occurrence of infantile cortical hyperostosis in *utero. Journal of Pediatrics* 1953; **42(2)**: 141–150.

38   Caffey J, Silverman WA. Infantile cortical hyperostoses. Preliminary report on a new syndrome. *American Journal of Roentgenology and Radium Therapy* 1945; **54(1)**: 1–16.

39   Malmberg N. Occurrence and significance of early periosteal proliferation in the diaphyses of premature infants. *Acta Paediatrica* 1944–5; **32**: 626–633.

40   Swerdloff BA, Ozonoff MB, Gyepes MT. Late recurrence of infantile cortical hyperostosis (Caffey's Disease). *American Journal of Roentgenology* 1970; **108**: 461–467.

41   Blank E. Recurrent Caffey's cortical hyperostosis and persistent deformity. *Pediatrics* 1975; **55(6)**: 856–860.

42   Tufts E, Blank E, Dickerson D. Periosteal thickening as a manifestation of trauma in infancy. *Child Abuse and Neglect.* 1982; **6**: 359–364.

43   Walker PL, Cook DC, Lambert PM. Skeletal evidence of child abuse. Unpublished MS, 1997.

44   Harris HA. *Bone Growth in Health and Disease*. London: Oxford University Press, 1933.

45   Roberts C, Manchester K. *The Archaeology of Disease* (2nd edn). Stroud: Sutton, 1995.

46   Wells C. Ancient obstetric hazards and female mortality. *Bulletin for the New York Academy of Medicine* 1975; **51(11)**: 1235–1249.

47   Wells C. A medieval burial of a pregnant woman. *The Practitioner* 1978; **221**: 442–444.

48   Farwell DE, Molleson TI. *Excavations at Poundbury 1966–80*, vol. 2: *The Cemeteries*. Monograph Series No. 11. Dorset: Dorset Natural History and Archaeological Society, 1993.

49   Boylston A, Wiggins R, Foreman M, Roberts C. Difficult births and brief lives at Castledyke, Barton-upon-Humber, England. In: Cockburn E (ed.), *Proceedings of the Twenty-third Annual Meeting of the Paleopathology Association*. Durham, North Carolina, 1996: p. 16.

50   Mays S. Infanticide in Roman Britain. *Antiquity* 1993; **67**: 883–888.

51   Mays S. Killing the unwanted child. *British Archaeology* 1995; **2**: 8–9.

52   Smith P, Kahila G. Identification of infanticide in archaeological sites: a case study from the Late Roman–Early Byzantine Periods at Ashkelon, Israel. *Journal of Archaeological Sciences* 1992; **19**: 667–675.

53   Damme C. Infanticide: the worth of an infant under law. *Medical History* 1978; **22**: 1–24.

54   Sauer R. Infanticide and abortion in nineteenth-century Britain. *Population Studies* 1978; **32(1)**: 81–93.

55   Forbes TR. Deadly parents: child homicide in eighteenth and nineteenth century England. *Journal of History of Medicine and Allied Sciences* 1986; **41**: 175–199.

56   Katzenberg AM, Herring AD, Saunders SR. Weaning and infant mortality: evaluating the skeletal evidence. *Yearbook of Physical Anthropology* 1996; **39(23)**: 177–199.

57 Ponec DJ, Resnick D. On the etiology and pathogenesis of porotic hyperostosis of the skull. *Investigative Radiology* 1984; **19(4)**: 313–317.

58 Stuart-Macadam P. Iron deficiency anaemia: exploring the difference. In: Grauer AL, Stuart-Macadam P (eds), *Sex and Gender in Paleopathological Perspective*. Cambridge: Cambridge University Press, 1998: pp. 45–63.

59 Stuart-Macadam P, Kent S. *Diet, Demography and Disease: Changing Perspectives on Anemia*. New York: Aldine de Gruyter, 1992.

60 Weinberg ED. Iron withholding in prevention of disease. In: Stuart-Macadam P, Kent S (eds), *Diet, Demography and Disease: Changing Perspectives on Anemia*. New York: Aldine de Gruyer, 1992: pp. 105–150.

61 Wiggins R. Porotic hyperostosis, cribra orbitalia, enamel hypoplasia, periosteal reaction and metopism: a correlation of their prevalence and an assessment of the nature of porotic hyperostosis in three British archaeological populations. MSc dissertation, University of Bradford, 1991.

62 Ortner DJ, Putschar WGJ. *Identification of Pathological Conditions in Human Skeletal Remains* (2nd edn). Smithsonian Contributions to Anthropology 28, Washington, DC: Smithsonian Institution Press, 1985.

63 Lanzkowsky P. Radiological features of iron-deficiency anemia. *American Journal of Diseases in Children* 1968; **116**: 16–29.

64 Holt LM. *The Diseases of Infancy and Childhood* (3rd edn). London: Sidney Appleton, 1906; p. 259 (plate V).

65 Sarnat BG, Schour I. Enamel hypoplasia (chronological enamel aplasia) in relation to systemic disease: a chronologic, morphologic and etiologic classification. *Journal of the American Dental Association* 1941; **28**: 1989–2000.

66 Kreshover SJ. Metabolic disturbances in tooth formation. *Annual of the New York Academy of Sciences*. 1960; **85**: 161–167.

67 Goodman AH, Rose JC. Assessment of systemic physiological perturbations from dental enamel hypoplasias and associated histological structures. *Yearbook of Physical Anthropology* 1990; **33**: 59–110.

68 Goodman AH, Rose JC. Dental enamel hypoplasias as indicators of nutritional status. In: Kelley MA, Larsen C (eds), *Advances in Dental Anthropology*. New York: Wiley-Liss, 1991: pp. 279–293.

69 Swardstedt T. *Odontological Aspects of a Medieval Population from the Province of Jamtland/Mid-Sweden*. Stockholm: Tiden Barnangen, AB, 1966.

70 Goodman AH, Armelagos GJ, Rose JC. The chronological distribution of enamel hypoplasias from prehistoric Dickson Mounds populations. *American Journal of Physical Anthropology* 1984; **65**: 259–266.

71 Corruccini RS, Handler JS, Jacobi KP. Chronological distribution of enamel hypoplasia and weaning in a Caribbean slave population. *Human Biology* 1985; **57**: 699–711.

72 Lanphear K, M. Frequency and distribution of enamel hypoplasias in a historic skeletal sample. *American Journal of Physical Anthropology* 1990; **81**: 35–43.

73 Moggi-Cecchi J, Pacciani E, Pinto-Cisternas J. Enamel hypoplasia and age at weaning in 19th century Florence, Italy. *American Journal of Physical Anthropology* 1994; **93**: 299–306.

74 Blakey ML, Leslie TE, Reidy JP. Frequency and chronological distribution of dental enamel hypoplasia in enslaved African Americans: a test of the weaning hypothesis. *American Journal of Physical Anthropology* 1994; **95**: 371–383.

75 Hillson S, Bond S. Relationship of enamel hypoplasia to the pattern of tooth crown growth: a discussion. *American Journal of Physical Anthropology* 1997; **104**(1): 89–103.

76 Park EA, Richter CP. Transverse lines in bone: the mechanism of their development. *Bulletin of the Johns Hopkins Hospital* 1953; **93**: 234–248.

77 Acheson RM. Effects of starvation, septicaemia and chronic illness on the growth cartilage plate and metaphysis of the immature rat. *Journal of Anatomy* 1959; **93(1)**: 123–134.

78 Marshall WA. Problems in relating the presence of transverse lines in the radius to the occurrence of disease. In: Brothwell DR (ed.), *The Skeletal Biology of Past Human Populations*. London: Pergamon, 1968: pp. 245–261.

79 Gindhart SP. The frequency of appearance of transverse lines in the tibia in relation to childhood illnesses. *American Journal of Physical Anthropology* 1969; **31**: 17–22.

80 Dreizen S, Spirakis CN, Stone RE. The influence of age and nutritional status on 'bone scar' formation in the distal end of the growing radius. *American Journal of Physical Anthropology* 1964; **22**: 295–306.

81 Huss-Ashmore R, Goodman AH, Armelagos GJ. Nutritional inference from paleopathology. In: Schiffer B (ed.), *Advances in Archaeological Method and Theory*. New York: Academic Press, 1982: pp. 395–474.

82 Park EA. The imprinting of nutritional disturbances on the growing bone. *Pediatrics* 1964; **33(6)**: 815–862.

83 Hughes C, Heylings DJA, Power C. Transverse (Harris) lines in Irish archaeological remains. *American Journal of Physical Anthropology* 1996; 101(1): 115–131.

84 Macchiarelli R, Bondioli L, Censi L, Kristoff Hernaez M, Salvadei L, Sperduti A. Intra- and interobserver concordance in scoring Harris lines: a test on bone sections and radiographs. *American Journal of Physical Anthropology* 1994; **95**: 77–83.

85 Grolleau-Raoux J-L, Crubezy E, Rouge D, Brugne J-F, Saunders S. Harris lines: A study of age-associated bias in counting and interpretation. *American Journal of Physical Anthropology* 1997; 103(2): 209–217.

86 Molleson T, Cox M. A neonate with cut bones from Poundbury Camp, 4th century AD, England. *Bulletin de la Société Royal Belge d'Anthropologie et de Préhistoire* 1988; **99**: 53–59.

87 Molleson TI. Mortality patterns in the Romano-British cemetery at Poundbury Camp near Dorchester. In: Bassett S (ed.), *Death in Towns: Urban Responses to the Dying and the Dead, 100–1600*. Leicester: Leicester University Press, 1992: pp. 43–55.

88 Mays S. The Relationship between Harris line formation and bone growth and development. *Journal of Archaeological Sciences* 1985; **12**: 207–220.

89 Wiggins R. Skeletal stress indicators and long bone length for age in the subadult population from St. Peter's Church, Barton on Humber: an ongoing study. In: Cockburn E (ed.), *Proceedings of the Eleventh European Meeting of the Paleopathology Association*. Maastricht 1996: p. 22.

90 Molleson T, Cox M. *The Spitalfields Project*, vol. 2: *The Middling Sort*. Research Report. 86. York: Council for British Archaeology, 1993.

91 Miles AEW, Bulman JS. Growth curves of immature bones from a Scottish island population of sixteenth to mid-nineteenth century: limb-bone diaphysis and some bones of the hand and foot. *International Journal of Osteoarchaeology* 1994; **4**: 121–136.

92 Humphrey LT. Growth patterns in the modern human skeleton. *American Journal of Physical Anthropology* 1998; **105**(1): 57–72.

93 O'Sullivan EA, Williams SA, Curzon MEJ. Dental caries in relation to nutritional stress in early English child populations. *Pediatric Dentistry* 1992; **14(1)**: 26–29.

94 Cook DC, Buikstra JE. Health and differential survival in prehistoric populations: prenatal dental defects. *American Journal of Physical Anthropology* 1979; **51**: 649–664.

95 Blakey ML, Armelagos GJ. Deciduous enamel defects in prehistoric Americans from Dickson Mounds: prenatal and postnatal stress. *American Journal of Physical Anthropology* 1985; **66**: 371–380.

96 Crawford S. Illness and cure in Anglo-Saxon England. Paper presented at the University of Birmingham, September 1998.

97 Aries P. *Centuries of Childhood*. London: Cape, 1960.

98 Knight B. The history of child abuse. In: Cule J, Turner T (eds), *Child Care Through the Ages*. Cardiff: British Society for the History of Medicine, 1986: pp. 109–119.

99 Walker PL. Is the Battered-Child Syndrome a modern phenomenon? Unpublished MS 1997.

100 Griffith JPC. *The Diseases of Infants and Children*. London: WB Saunders 1919.

101 Schultz M. *Vestiges of Non-specific Inflammation in Prehistoric and Historic Skulls: A Contribution to Palaeopathology*. Aesch: Anthropolgische Beiträge, 1993; Band 4B (Abbildungen).

102 Kreutz K, Teichmann G, Schultz M. Palaeoepidemiology of inflammatory processes of the skull: a comparative study of two early medieval infant populations. *Journal of Paleopathology* 1995; **7(2)**: 108.

103 Lincoln EM, Sewell EM. *Tuberculosis in Children*. New York: McGraw-Hill, 1963.

104 Ortner D, Bush H. Destructive lesions of the spine in a 17th century child's skeleton from Abingdon, Oxfordshire. *Journal of Paleopathology* 1993; **5(3)**: 143–152.

105 Wells C. Prehistoric and historical changes in nutritional diseases and associated conditions. *Progress in Food and Nutritional Science* 1975; **1**(11): 729–779.

106 Ortner D, Mays S. Dry-bone manifestations of rickets in infancy and early childhood. *International Journal of Osteoarchaeology* 1998; **8**: 45–55.

107 Lilley SM, Stroud G, Brothwell DR, Williamson MH (eds), *The Jewish Burial Ground at Jewbury*. York: Council for British Archaeology, 1994.

108 Sheldon. *Diseases of Infancy and Childhood* (4th edn). London: Churchill, 1943.

109 Barlow T. On cases described as 'acute rickets' which are probably a combination of scurvy and rickets. *Archives of Diseases in Childhood* 1935; **10**: 223–252.

110 Ortner D, Ericksen MF. Bone changes in the human skull probably resulting from scurvy in infancy and childhood. *International Journal of Osteoarchaeology* 1997; **7**: 212–220.

111 Ferencz M, Jozsa L. Congenital syphilis on a medieval skeleton. *Anthropologie* 1992; **30(1)**: 95–98.

112 Gladykowska-Rzeczycka JJ, Krenz M. Extensive change within a subadult skeleton from a medieval cemetery of Slaboszewo, Mogilno District, Poland. *Journal of Paleopathology* 1995; **7(3)**: 177–184.

113 Palfi G, Dutour O, Borreani M, Brun J-P, Berato J. Pre-Columbian congenital syphilis from the late antiquity in France. *International Journal of Osteoarchaeology* 1992; **2**: 245–261.

114 Henneberg M, Henneberg RJ. Treponematosis in an ancient Greek colony of Metaponto, Southern Italy, 580–250 BCE. In: Dutour O, Pálfi G, Berato J, Brun J-P (eds), *L'origine de la syphilis en Europe avant ou après 1493?* Paris: Centre Archéologique du Var, editions Errance, 1994: pp. 92–98.

115 Sillen A, Smith P. Weaning patterns are reflected in strontium–calcium ratios of juvenile skeletons. *Journal of Archaeological Sciences* 1984; **11**: 237–245.

116 Hühne-Osterloh G, Grupe G. Causes of infant mortality in the middle ages revealed by chemical and palaeopathological analyses of skeletal remains. *Zeitschrift für Morphologie und Anthropologie* 1989; **77(3)**: 247–258.

117 Herring DA, Saunders SR, Katzenberg MA. Investigating the weaning process in past populations. *American Journal of Physical Anthropology* 1998; **105**(4): 425–439.

118 Wright LE. Stable carbon and oxygen isotopes in human tooth enamel: identifying breastfeeding and weaning in prehistory. *American Journal of Physical Anthropology* 1998; **106**(1): 1–18.

119 Katzenberg MA, Saunders S, R, Fitzgerald WR. Age differences in stable carbon and nitrogen isotope ratios in a population of prehistoric maize horticulturists. *American Journal of Physical Anthropology* 1993; **90**: 267–281.

120 Katzenberg MA, Pfeiffer S. Nitrogen isotope evidence for weaning age in a nineteenth century Canadian skeletal sample. In: Grauer AL (ed.), *Bodies of Evidence: Reconstructing History Through Skeletal Analysis*. New York: Wiley-Liss, 1995: pp. 221–235.

Section II

Palaeodemography

Determination of sex and age at death are fundamental, both for personal identification in forensic cases and for palaeodemographic and other analyses based on archaeological cemetery data. In the opening chapter in this section, Margaret Cox discusses issues concerned with age determination in ancient skeletons within a more general archaeological framework. She goes on to give a critical appraisal of some of the osteological methods currently available for determining age at death in the adult skeleton. David Whittaker then discusses age determination from the dentition. He considers a variety of techniques, paying particular attention to those based on microscopic and chemical analyses of dental remains. He draws attention to some important methodological issues in these areas which need to be tackled. These include post-depositional changes in dental hard tissues and the problem of the extent to which methods derived from modern populations can be applied to determining age in archaeological groups where diet and general way of life were very different. Andrew Chamberlain explores the rationale behind the use of some statistical methods and life-tables in palaeodemography. He draws attention to the way in which the age structure of a reference sample can influence the adult age at death profile generated from an archaeological assemblage, and he advocates Bayesian statistical methods as a means of circumventing this bias. Margaret Cox, however, emphasizes a more fundamental problem with age determination in adult remains when she reminds us that currently used ageing techniques are in general rather poor indicators of age in the adult, and that many aspects of the biology of skeletal ageing are poorly understood; consequently, so are the extrinsic factors that may affect the relationship between currently used skeletal age indicators and chronological age.

Simon Mays and Margaret Cox consider sex determination in adults and juveniles. The reliability of the various techniques is discussed, with particular emphasis given to the problematic area of sexing immature remains.

In the final chapter in this section, Margaret Cox discusses the determination of parity from female skeletal material. Despite the cultural and demographic importance of a consideration of fertility, parity assessment is an area often given rather short shrift in textbooks of biological anthropology. She examines various aspects of skeletal morphology that have been suggested as indicators of parity status and concludes that the morphology of the pubic tubercle may be the most promising indicator.

5

AGEING ADULTS FROM THE SKELETON

Margaret Cox

INTRODUCTION AND CULTURAL FRAMEWORK

The determination of age at death of adults in archaeological assemblages is unquestionably an important component of scientific archaeology, biological anthropology and palaeodemography. It is crucially important in understanding the biocultural and epidemiological significance of trauma and disease. However, this need is arguably influenced and heightened by the fact that archaeologists and anthropologists encumber their analysis and understanding of the past and past lives with their own cultural values. Western Europe, as we enter the new millennium, is a conglomeration of cultures, all of which demonstrate an obsession with chronological age.

Age determines many aspects of our lives from beginning to end. If an infant is not born at about the 40th week of gestation, parturition will usually be induced; children attend school at four, are examined for academic progress at a variety of specific but ever-changing ages, can leave school, smoke, and have lawful heterosexual sex at 16, drive a car at 17, can marry without parental consent at 18 years (in England and Wales). State pensions are payable from 65, etc. Combined with that, Western culture values youth and beauty far more than the attributes of experience and old age despite the fact that as the century has progressed the life expectancy of all socio-economic classes has increased.

In light of this complex scenario, it is worth considering how 'ageing' fits into archaeological theory. Tilley[1] has raised the spectre that archaeology, of which biological anthropology can be considered a part, presently sustains contemporary social order rather than realising its emancipatory potential. He suggests that archaeology has become a science involved in the technical control of the past, a commodification, one which affirms present values. This implies that by accepting, or even creating, an anthropology which confirms that life in the past[2] was mean and lean, biological anthropologists might be affirming the value of the capitalist policies and values of the West in the later 20th century.

As representatives of our culture and time, our obsession with age fuels a drive to determine accurate age at death for past populations. As Hershkovitz *et al.* note, 'it has been one of anthropology's more ambitious interests'.[3] However, for much of our ancestry, the majority have been illiterate and innumerate and consequently age was probably neither known, with any exactitude, nor relevant. What mattered to individuals and communities was biological status and physical condition. That a child was weaned, could sit or walk rendered him or her (and their mother) available to undertake certain physical tasks, such as scaring crows in rural England over much of the last three millennia and beyond, or spinning silk in 18th-century Spitalfields.[4] Puberty would have meant a crucial change in a juvenile's status, just as it still does in much of the Third World. Once fecund, a female's fertility was likely to have been a precious commodity and her treatment within society would have been different. Similarly, the significance of the menopause would have been considerable.

Physical maturation would have been linked to physical output or conversely input to the needs of the community. It would have been closely linked to health in terms of status and functionality; the absence of either being a considerable loss to both self and community. It is interesting to note that, with few exceptions,[5,6] little has been published examining the assessment of skeletal indicators of puberty or menopause, and that when examining archaeological samples few osteologists report on the level of physical contribution to society that individuals might have made. Despite this they continue to replicate age at death statistics which, while reading between the lines, many clearly believe to be rather meaningless.

As a product of the later 20th century, this paper will consciously demonstrate that what it strives to achieve reflects current rather than past preoccupations. It represents an attempt to understand the past on our terms. This chapter will examine methods developed to assess the age of adults using only their osteological remains. Age determination using dental parameters will be considered by Whittaker (chapter 6, in this volume). Scheuer and Black (chapter 2, in this volume) examine juvenile ageing and Chamberlain (chapter 7, in this volume) discusses palaeodemographic reconstruction using statistical modelling and such tools as life-tables. Specific methods that have been the subject of thorough and critical analysis elsewhere will be treated in less depth than those which have not.

Recent research trends

'The days of our age are threescore years and ten; though men be so strong that they may come to fourscore years.'[7] Before the 1980s palaeodemographic analysis consistently and unquestioningly reported high levels of young adult mortality with few individuals apparently living beyond their fifth decade: 'for many sites, everyone is reported to have died before 45 or 50 years of age'.[8] This has been despite one of the oldest comments upon human longevity known to us (above), a statement supported by numerous Roman tombstones celebrating long-lived dedicatees, and reference to many centenarians in the London Bills of Mortality during the 17th, 18th and 19th centuries. This trend in ageing largely reflected the low upper age limits of contemporary skeletal ageing methods.[9-11] By their application, they predetermined the age range and mean of any sample to which they were applied. The designation and acceptance by practitioners of such low upper age limits, however, reflected contemporary misconceptions about longevity in past populations. Perspectives began to change in the 1980s with thought provoking papers such as those by Bocquet-Appel and Masset.[12-14] Such work exacerbated the doubt that existed in the minds of experienced practitioners who, time and time again, saw evidence of pathological conditions known to affect only the elderly, in skeletons aged using traditional macroscopic techniques, at about 35 years of age.

A response to this affirmation of doubt was evident in the abundance of papers examining the use of multifactorial determination of age at death.[5,15–17] Basically, what such authors sought to demonstrate was, that by using all available methods, the result would be more meaningful than when only one method of ageing was applied, even though most of the methods involved were known to be inaccurate. At the same time great pains were taken to try and refine and improve upon some of the early schema.[18]

Methodological considerations

A major consideration when applying methods aimed at deducing age at death from skeletal material is that all such methods were developed from analysis of either archaeological material[19] or that from modern willed body or dissection room samples, or a combination of the two. Yet with very few exceptions[20–22] archaeological samples are of unknown sex and age. Consequently, their use served to replicate fundamental conceptual errors underlying the authors' preconceptions about life spans in the past. Furthermore, many modern samples exhibit socio-economic and genetic bias, which may affect biological trends. Many samples were small, some had a skewed age distribution, disproportionate representation of the sexes and ancestry, and some were subject to the specific removal of biological outliers (these issues are discussed further below).

Some contemporary skeletal assemblages are partly derived from material lacking documentary proof of age, sex etc. The Hamann–Todd collection for example contains individual skeletons for which sex and age were derived from soft tissue attributes. While the former can be ascertained relatively straightforwardly, the latter cannot. It should also be considered that many methods are tested against the ages derived from the application of other (potentially flawed) ageing methods, rather than *known* age. This results in the propagation of systematic errors rather than establishing methods based on reliable and independent criteria – if indeed such is realistically achievable given the differences in rates of senescence observable between and within living families and communities.

An ill-understood bias in ageing was brought to the attention of anthropologists in 1982 and 1985 by Bocquet-Appel and Masset.[12,13] Their concerns were reiterated in 1996.[14] They argue that developing an ageing method on a sample will result in the replication of the original sample's mortality profile in samples to which the method is applied. These ideas provoked considerable response in the USA.[23–25] Nevertheless, several researchers argue that whatever the precise mechanisms involved, methodological bias is serious, leading particularly to an under-representation of the over 40s in our interpretation of the archaeological record.[26–28] Such researchers are currently applying such statistical models as 'maximum likelihood estimation techniques' in an attempt to remove this bias.

This chapter will review methods currently employed for the estimation of age at death in skeletal material, where possible examining the biological basis of each and considering the significance of the suitability of samples upon which methods were initially developed and subsequently tested. This is of particular significance in forensic cases, as the wide variety of ageing methods discussed below were primarily developed for use on samples not individuals. Systematic errors within each method are less significant among the 'sample' than when dealing with 'individuals' and this is clearly of considerable importance in the forensic context.

Fundamental to all osteological ageing characteristics is the fact that bone in the living is a dynamic tissue subject to renewal, repair and remodelling in response to a host of stressors and stimuli. Bone can adapt its form to a limited extent to cope with physical demands made upon it, and it can repair itself in response to trauma and disease. Bone health and status in adults is maintained by a balanced relationship between osteoblasts and osteoclasts, a relationship that changes with such factors as levels of exercise as well as increasing age. Physical ageing processes centre on progressive denaturation of protein in collagen fibrils[29] and the death of non-replaceable neurons and other cells. Ageing changes include hypertrophy and can involve atrophy.

When anthropologists estimate the age at death of an individual or sample of skeletons, they are attempting to determine chronological age from physiological changes reflective of either developmental or degenerative processes. Clearly, the former is a relatively constant, linear and predictable progression but, importantly, the latter is not. Variables that increase the complexity of this difficult area of research and application include random individual variation in maturation and degeneration, and the systematic effects of environmental, nutritional and genetic factors on growth and senescence. It was certainly no understatement when Maples[30] commented that 'age determination is ultimately an art, not a precise science'.

During the early years of an individual's life, estimating age is relatively straightforward. The development of dentition and the appearance and the fusion of growth centres of bone offer relatively dependable indicators of age and occur within a comparatively short age range. Fortunately, some of these continue into our legal definition of adulthood (over 18 years), and these are included in this discussion. Once skeletal maturation is complete, it is far more difficult to assess age because few growth processes continue during this phase of life. This leaves age estimation dependent, almost entirely, on processes of degeneration and remodelling which occur at differing rates between and within different populations and samples. Variation in the level of age-related change in different parts of the same skeleton can be exacerbated by a number of factors[31] and is not an uncommon occurrence. These include genetic influences, growth, health status, occupation, life-style, nutrition and endocrine function.

AGEING METHODS

Currently employed methods of ageing adults using skeletal material are based on four principal criteria. First, for young adults, the final stages of skeletal maturation which take place into the late 20s. Second, morphological changes to joints where movement is either limited or non-existent. These comprise cranial suture closure and rib-end, auricular surface and pubic symphysis morphology. With this category of age-related change, the biological relationship with chronological age is generally ill understood.[32] Third is examination of continued ossification of hyaline cartilage, e.g. laryngeal and plastron. Finally, there are changes to bone structure including involutional bone loss and osteon frequency. A further category of methodology is that of multifactorial application of several of the methods falling within the above categories. These are discussed below.

Final stages of skeletal maturation

Several areas of the skeleton complete maturation during the late second and third decades of life and consequently have value in identifying those dying in early adulthood. These include the iliac crest, ventral rings of the vertebrae, fusion of the medial clavicle and petroexoccipital articulation. The spheno-occipital synchondrosis is also discussed.

Iliac crest

The first of these to achieve maturation is the iliac crest. This is discussed in numerous general studies on skeletal maturation (on samples of known age) and was considered to be complete by the age of 15 years by such as Francis.[33] However, the value of such studies was limited by being based on samples with a maximum age of 15. Employing the clinical data and roentgenograms compiled during the Cleveland Longitudinal Study of Growth and Development (1927–42), Scoles et al.'s study,[6] based on a healthy and normal sample of 474 females and 322 males aged from 10 to 19 is more useful. This demonstrated that complete fusion of the iliac crest apophysis occurred at a mean age of 18 years and 1 month for females (SD 12 months) and 18 years and 6 months for males (SD 7 months). It also pointed out that generally, the onset of menses preceded the appearance of iliac crest apophysis by a few months. This study also confirmed the value of assessment of maturation of this element using Risser's five-stage system of recording sequential appearance and subsequent fusion of the apophysis.[6]

Ventral rings of the vertebrae

The superior and inferior ventral rings of the vertebrae are among the last bony elements to fuse and consequently have some utility in ascribing age in young adults. Among others, this was examined in 1957 by McKern and Stewart,[9] who found a progressive union of the thoracic vertebral rings up to the age of 25 in a young male sample ($n = 259$). Albert and Maples[34] examined this progression in a sample of 55, which included males and females (Negroid and Caucasian) from autopsies. This small sample shows fusion within ± 2.55 years, a range that would almost certainly increase with a larger sample. These results support those of McKern and Stewart in suggesting that complete fusion occurs about 24–25 years and that, as would be expected, fusion seems to occur earlier in females than in males.

Petroexoccipital articulation

Fusion of the jugular growth plate (petroexoccipital articulation) is an area that has received recent attention.[35–37] Examining 98 crania from the Utrecht collection,[36] Maat and Mastwijk found no fusion in individuals under 22 years ($n = 4$) with unilateral fusion occurring between 22 and 34 years ($n = 7$). Bilateral fusion had occurred in females by 34 and males by 36. However, evaluation of a larger sample ($n = 1869$ Hamann–Todd collection) by Hershkovitz et al.[37] demonstrated that closure can occur up to the age of 50, and that in up to 9% of cases it did not occur at all. The latter study clearly demonstrated the inherent problems that arise when devising methods on small sample sizes (i.e. ranges of human variation are reduced). However, it should be remembered that the 'known' ages of some of this collection might have been deduced from biological criteria.

Medial clavicle

Age changes in the clavicle are extremely useful as it is the first bone to commence ossification and the last to complete epiphyseal fusion.[38] In individuals who are post-pubertal, changes in the morphology of the medial epiphyseal complex are useful ageing indicators generally occurring between 16 and 30 years of age. Black and Scheuer's evaluation of a five-phase system of medial epiphyseal fusion on archaeological material of known age from London and modern material from Lisbon ($n = 43$)[38] demonstrated that as the last stage of epiphyseal fusion in the human, the method is particularly useful for ageing young adults ($n = 16$ for 21–25 years; $n = 24$ for 26–30 years), indicating that in this sample fusion was always complete by 29 years with the archaeological material completing fusion before the modern material. Similar results were obtained on the Libben material.[5] However, Webb and Suchey,[39] examining 859 individuals (of all ages) from a medical examiner's collection note that the Caucasoid sample had 100% fusion by 28 years and the Negroid sample by 34 years.

Spheno-occipital synchondrosis

The main anatomical texts report fusion of the spheno-occipital synchondrosis at between 18 and 25 years.[40] However, reference to individual studies suggests that this is not the case and that closure usually occurs during late adolescence rather than early adulthood.[41–46] Powell and Brodie's[43] work was based upon the largest sample ($n = 205$).

Clavicular and vertebral ring maturation, iliac crest apophysis and closure of the petroexoccipital articulation all represent different biological processes. In light of the results discussed above, should a large documented sample of young to middle-aged adults become available then further evaluation of these methods would be prudent.

Morphological change at joints with limited or no movement

The search for methods determining the age of death of adults, using changes to joint surfaces, began with assessment of cranial suture closure, moving to morphological change of the pubic symphysis, sternal rib ends and the auricular surface of the innominate.

Cranial suture closure

Historically, the skull was the first part of the skeleton to be systematically investigated for the estimation of age at death,[32] reflecting the pre-eminence this skeletal element had in the minds of early anthropologists. Studies of cranial suture closure conducted in the latter half of the 19th century and early this century found a positive correlation with age.[47] However, Dwight[48] noted the extreme variability in the order and timing of closure, and von

Lenhössek[49] found sex differences characterized by later closure in females. Researchers considered that the capricious nature of this site precluded any precise estimation of age from being undertaken.

In the 1920s, Todd and Lyon[50-53] conducted a series of studies in Negroid and Caucasian American males from the Hamann–Todd collection. Their approach resulted in a closure formula for cranial sutures. Endocranial sutures were more dependable than ectocranial, but the authors expressed misgivings about the accuracy of these. When Caucasoid and Negroid were compared, interracial differences were observed.[51-53] Surprisingly, despite their reservations, the authors concluded that there was one modal type of human suture closure and that separate standards were not necessary!

In 1937, Cattaneo [cited in 47] studied 100 Argentine skulls and noted that cranial suture closure was only a suggestive indicator of age. Hrdlicka[54] concluded that ectocranial suture closure was unreliable, as did Singer.[55] McKern and Stewart[9] found the onset and progress of suture closure to be erratic and unreliable.

Despite such results, research continued. In 1960, Nemeskéri et al.[56] developed a five-phase assessment of obliteration to evaluate the progress of closure in 16 sections of vault sutures. They considered that endocranial suture closure (the recording of which is not always practically possible) could be useful, but only as part of the Complex Method. Perizonius[57] used 79 Dutch crania to test this method and concluded that further investigation of this process was required if such a method was to be useful. Meindl and Lovejoy[58] re-evaluated endocranial suture closure in a slightly different way in an attempt to establish more precise criteria, which they maintained was useful particularly for older age ranges. In a sample of Negroid and Caucasoid North Americans ($n = 256$) from the Hamann–Todd collection, they considered the latero-anterior region of the cranium to be the most consistent in the pattern of suture fusion but that any relationship with age was only general. They also concluded that suture closure could be of value if used in conjunction with other skeletal age markers. Using more of the same sample with material from the Terry collection, Hershkovitz et al.[3] concluded that in their sample of 3638 crania, sagittal suture closure is independent of age, sexually biased and has minimal stress association.

Masset's[59] approach focused on examining systematic statistical errors reflecting sex differences, the age structure of the reference population in relation to the unknown group, and the attraction to the middle age range when combining individual estimates into an age structure. He concluded that while cranial sutures could not be used for precise individual age estimation, they were of benefit in revealing major demographic shifts over time in a particular cemetery. But, that while many systematic errors could be resolved, the resultant age distribution could not essentially deviate from that of the reference population.

Little attention has been paid to the closure of the maxillary sutures. Mann et al.[60] found that a trend was apparent in a very small sample of 36 maxillae including males and females. However, ranges appear very large and overlap is considerable in this small sample.

Examination of suture closure on two archaeological samples of known race, sex and age (documented) produced further discouraging results. Molleson and Cox[20] found the method to overage young adults (under about 40 years) and underage older adults (over about 40 years) when it was applied to the Christ Church, Spitalfields sample. Analysis of this material focused upon the reliability of the Complex Method[61] and cranial suture closure proved to be the least effective of the four methods when examined in isolation. In a more detailed analysis of this material, Key et al.[32] found that the Ascadi and Nemskéri method could distinguish young from middle aged from older crania but that it could not assign specific ages in years to individuals. They found Meindl and Lovejoy's[58] method to show strong sexual dimorphism, in that it was more useful for females than males, but overall that there was a very low correlation in the entire sample. Examining Perizonius'[57] method they found a good correspondence in the under 50s between endocranial closure and age but none in the over 50s.

Saunders et al.[22] examining documented archaeological material from St Thomas', Belleville, Ontario, used Meindl and Lovejoy's[58] method as described above and reported that predicted ages matched actual ages very poorly. No age under 30 or, more importantly, over 50 was predicted with accuracy, yet the biggest proportion of this sample was in fact aged over 60.[22]

As Key et al.[32] concluded, methods derived from one sample cannot necessarily be applied to another; and there can be considerable sexual dimorphism in rates of closure.[55,62,63] Key et al.[32] devised a new and simplified method using the Spitalfields sample, one which assesses under/over 50 year age groups, and tested it on a known age modern sample. On those to which they applied their method they achieved 70% accuracy for males and 65% accuracy for females. However, their test involved removing from that sample cases where patterns of closure were different from those observed at Spitalfields. Todd[64] selected material for use in determining age-related trends and he devalued his results by artificially reducing the age range of specific trends. Quite rightly, this practice has been condemned,[65] as it reduces sample variability and the practical application of a method to other material. What Key et al. have done must be subject to similar comment and, issues of inter-/intra-observer error in selection aside, such practice limits the extent of applicability and, consequently, usefulness of a method. Nevertheless, a method that can identify the over 50s would be extremely useful in light of their general invisibility in the archaeological record.

It is worth ending this subsection with a comment that applies to each of those methods discussed in this chapter. While it is known that cranial sutures can (but do not always) progressively close (though not necessarily at a reliable rate) and become obliterated, the underlying biological processes determining if and when closure occurs are not under-stood. Consequently, we have no understanding of if, or which, extrinsic factors can affect closure rates and cannot meaningfully or safely apply this method to archaeological mate-rial. In summary, despite attempts to 'find the secret ageing formula …',[3] the research described above unequivocally suggests that cranial suture closure is not a reliable method of ageing adults. This is particularly unfortunate as the cranial bones generally survive better[66] than many other skeletal elements to which ageing significance has been ascribed.

Pubic symphysis morphology

Todd[64] was the first to examine changes to the symphyseal face of the pubis. The reliability of the ages of some of Todd's sample is uncertain and a further problem with this method lies in the fact that he removed individuals falling outside recognized criteria for their ages from his sample. This reduced the variability of the sample and the age span for each category of change he described. McKern and Stewart[9] reappraised this method in the 1950s based on US servicemen killed in the Korean War. The restricted and young age span of this sample was a problem as was the lack of female standards. Gilbert and McKern produced a schema for females in 1973[10] based on a small sample of reliably documented individuals but which was found to be wanting by Suchey.[67] Work has continued on Todd's method[68,69] on a large autopsy sample. Nemeskéri et al.[56] independently produced a scheme of changes which when tested against the US methods produced different results[18] but generally aged large numbers of individuals within the 45–60 age group.

On a practical level, pubic symphyses rarely survive in large numbers in archaeological samples,[66,70] its anterior position and anatomical make-up rendering it prone to weathering and mechanical damage. This can be a serious drawback mitigating against its use. Of greater importance is the fact that most up to date schema have incredibly large age ranges for the different stages. Brooks and Suchey's[69] work produced age ranges (at 95% confidence) which, with the exception of stage I, fall within very large ranges (e.g. stage IV = 26–70 years for males; 23–57 years for females), and which have enormous overlap (e.g. stage V = 25–83 years for males; 27–66 years for females).

When tested on documented archaeological material this method produced variable but generally unimpressive results. Assessment of pubic symphysis morphology with chronological age on the Spitalfields sample[20,71] produced disappointing results. The methods of Todd,[63] McKern and Stewart, and Gilbert and McKern[9,10] were shown to underage some 80% of those aged over 45 years by at least 10 years. Ascadi and Nemeskéri's[15] method produced different results which were only accurate for the 40–60 age group to within ± 10 years, and which over-aged the under 40s and under-aged the over 70s. This may well reflect the fact that the Spitalfields sample more closely reflects the mortality profile of the sample upon which Ascadi and Nemeskéri developed their method. Saunders et al.[22] were disturbed by their results using the Brooks and Suchey's method[69] on the Belleville, Ontario sample. It performed very poorly in terms of intra- and inter-observer error and the authors were also unimpressed by its inherent levels of inaccuracy. As noted above, the ranges are so broad with such enormous areas of overlap as to be almost meaningless.

Rib end morphology

Ribs articulate with the sternum by lengths of cartilage which are considered by Işcan et al.[31,72,73] to become increasingly irregular in morphology as age increases. They have classified these changes using the right fourth rib into eight distinct phases for both sexes, related to age ranges. Their sample was of modern autopsy material (n = 277) and the authors found a rate of low inter-observer error in their studies, regardless of experience.

Examination of this method on archaeological material is seriously hampered by the need to identify the fourth rib. Ribs are often incomplete and fragmentary in archaeological material. In the 1980s, experienced anthropologists found it very difficult and time consuming to identify this element in the Spitalfields sample. Interestingly, Loth[74] found this less of a problem, perhaps indicating that efficient use of this method requires a greater than usual familiarity with rib morphology.

Loth tested this method on 36 males and 38 females from Christ Church, 44 of which were aged over 60 years. This paper is marred by several historical inaccuracies and relevant omissions, such as a failure to consider historical indicators of the age of menarche in the sample. The latter weakens her suggestion that a late menarche contributed to the under-ageing of some age groups. This is unlikely when some females are known to have under-gone parturition in their very early teens, for example 12 and 14 years.[20] Overall, results were within the same decade for the under 18-year-olds ($n = 13$) and 40–49-year-olds ($n = 6$). The 18–29 ($n = 8$), 30–39 ($n = 6$) and 50–59 ($n = 10$) -year-olds were all over-aged and the over 60s were all under-aged. Analysis of inaccuracy showed the males were aged more accurately than the females, with the greatest levels of inaccuracy for males in their 50s and for females in their 40s. Usefully, this study suggests that in 97% of individuals with a surviving rib 3, 4 and 5, the bony changes were falling within the same phase.

Reflecting problems with bone condition and identification, Saunders et al. found this method could only be examined on 27 of the Ontario sample. It was most accurate in those below 30 and between 40 and 59, thereafter under-ageing individuals with amounts increasing with real age. This method also showed the greatest degree of inter-observer disparity of all methods applied to this sample.[22]

As an archaeological ageing method, sternal rib-end morphology is seriously impaired by its reliance upon one of the least well preserved skeletal elements in archaeological material.[66] Its credibility will be enhanced when it is demonstrated to be both useful and accurate by researchers other than those responsible for the development of the methodology.

Auricular surface of the ilium

Although age-related changes to the auricular surface were first noted by Sashin[75] and later by Kobayashi,[76] they were first schematically associated with eight age ranges by Lovejoy et al.[16] A single scheme was recommended for all racial groups and both sexes but evaluation of this method is hampered by the fact that 75–82% of their test sample were of unknown age, sex, race and parity status.[18] As discussed by Jackes,[18] these changes are highly correlated with changes to the pubic symphysis. The method was in part developed on the Todd collection, despite awareness of the fact that the sample was biased by systematic rejection of those extending sample variability.[65]

Bedford et al.[77] considered this method to be superior to the pubic symphysis.[78,79] Murray and Murray's assessment of the method[80] found it wanting in terms of its use as a single indicator of age with age ranges too large for forensic applications. Their results ($n = 200$) suggested that changes to the auricular surface appeared independent of sex and race. The former reflecting that because the sacroiliac joints are not load-bearing, there is limited sexual dimorphism expressed in the auricular surface.

If this method has been tested on the Spitalfields sample, the results are unpublished. Evaluation on the Ontario sample ($n = 49$), indicated that its reliability decreased with age (by under-ageing), particularly from the mid–30s, becoming progressively less accurate thereafter.[22] Rogers is reported to have obtained similar results.[22]

The biological process of change to this diathrodial joint is little understood. It is considered that surface changes are primarily a consequence of an increase in the proportion of fibro-cartilage as a consequence of ageing[75] There is little doubt that this joint surface survives better than the pubic symphysis in archaeological material. However, its usefulness as a method can be limited by the tendency for males aged over 50 to exhibit ankylosis of this joint, and some aspects are impaired when a deep pre-auricular sulcus is present. Further, it can be prone to inter-observer error.[22] Clearly, this method needs further evaluation on large documented samples.

Ossification of hyaline cartilage

Plastron

Roentgenograms of the plastron (chest plate – comprising the 1st to 7th costal cartilages, terminal ends of the sternal ribs, sternum and sternal clavicles) have been examined for assessment of age-related change.[81–83] Vastine et al.[82] established a strong genetic link, and Stewart[83] established broad phases of ossification up to the age of 35 years. This is clearly a type of analysis that is easier to undertake in forensic cases where the body or skeleton is still articulated. Nevertheless, the underlying biology provides useful data with potential value for use with disarticulated archaeological material. The plastron comprises both synchon-droses and diathroses.

A more recent study by McCormick and Stewart[84] examined X-rays of 1965 modern cadavers of known race, sex and age. The sample was multiracial though mostly Caucasoid, and comprised 671 females and 1318 males. Age ranged from 15 to 99 years and from 20 to 74 each 5-year group was represented by at least 100 individuals. It demonstrated that age could be determined within 5 years of real age in 55% of the sample and within 25% of real age in 95%. It was least precise in the over 60s but usefully allowed a 99% accuracy in sex prediction. Negroids could be selected on the basis of the lack of osteoporotic changes to the sternum. The authors have produced a range of phases of change for both sexes for each decade from under 20 to over 70. This method holds promise for archaeological application but requires assessment of how best to adapt it for use on disarticulated material.

Laryngeal cartilages

Ossification of the laryngeal cartilages (i.e. thyroid, cricoid and arytenoid) and age is a subject which has a considerable antiquity.[85] Keen and Wainright[86] and Harrison and Denny[87] considered such change to be endochondral ossification. Approaches include macroscopic, histological and radiographic analyses[86,88] of samples of different racial groups and both sexes.[89] Most studies are based upon small dissecting room or autopsy samples and generally produce results which, while suggesting broad trends, are not particularly helpful in determining age with any degree of accuracy.[90]

Subject to considerable further work, examination of ossified hyaline cartilage, particularly from the plastron, has the potential to be useful in determining age in archaeological assemblages. However, both archaeologists and osteologists will have to improve their ability to recognize such material in a disturbed and fragmented state.

Bone microstructure and involution

Several authors have reviewed the literature concerned with examining age at death from bone histomorphometry[91–93] and the reader is referred to those works. Results from various assessments of methods vary enormously in part reflecting the size and site of the sample and the relationship of the assessment sample with that upon which the method was devised.[12,13] There appears to be a strong relationship between bone remodelling rates and a range of genetic and environmental factors.[91] Further, the application of the method to archaeological material is subject to the degree of diagenetic change the bone has undergone.[94,95]

Recent work has concentrated on the clavicle in association with either the femur or ribs.[96–98] Walker and Lovejoy[96] first noted the advantages of the clavicle over other elements using radiographic assessment of 130 individuals from the Hamann–Todd collection. Stout and Paine[97] found the rib and clavicle in combination to be effective in ageing a sample of 40 autopsy specimens aged between 13 and 62 years most of which were males (32) and 32 of which were Caucasoid. Obviously a sample of this type is going to only exhibit a very limited range of variability for assessment. However, when tested on a sample of 83 individuals of known age from a 19th-century Swiss cemetery (age profile not stated), the method is reported to be accurate to 5.5 years.

A method for estimating age using cortical histomorphometry of the sternal end of the fourth rib is reported[99] as a solution to dealing with fragmented archaeological material. What the authors ignore is both the poor survival of ribs in archaeological samples and that their often fragmentary nature renders their individual identification extremely difficult.

Semiautomatic image analysis of cross-sections of 101 femoral diaphyseal bone sections (from forensic material aged between 18 and 87) by Wallin et al.. reported a SD of 12.58 years.[100] The authors reported that such analysis is less precise than suggested by the literature. Macchiarelli and Bondioli drew a similar conclusion.[101] They undertook linear densitometry and digital image processing of proximal femur radiographs on a sample of 66 individuals aged between 19 and 71 years from the Terry collection. Following earlier work[102] Feik et al. looked at cortical porosity of the entire mid-shaft femur[103] in a sample of 180 modern Australians of known age, sex and weight. Each chronological year was represented by at least one individual of each sex, showing age-related sex differences in the pattern of bone loss. They concluded that the largest contribution to bone loss was through an increase in medullary area from endosteal resorption and that variability in the development of total subperiosteal porosity was apparent in elderly individuals of similar chronological age. Their data suggested that regression analysis showed a significant relationship between both medullary area and intracortical void as a fraction of total subperiosteal area with age. However, variation was such that the method was considered to have little value as a predictor of age in forensic cases.

Cool et al.[104] assessed the value of histological examination of the occipital bone for estimation of age at death in a sample of 18 male autopsy subjects aged between 21 and 70. They concluded by acknowledging that observable changes do occur with increasing age, but that the amount of random variation in the parameters examined precluded their use for accurate prediction of age.

The relationship between involutional bone loss and age is one that has received attention in both modern and archaeological material. Such studies date from the late 19th century[105] and clearly demonstrate that a large number of variables can potentially contribute to the rate and extent of this process. Sex is probably one of the most important[106] but this is complicated by race[102] and a wide range of extrinsic factors including genetics, nutrition and life style. Mays[107] examined this using radiogrammetry in an undocumented medieval sample ($n = 137$) aged into three broad age ranges using conventional methods. He found that older females were suffering from a significant loss of cortical bone. However, when so many of the variables that factor into osteoporotic change can be unknown for an archaeological sample, care has to be taken when interpreting such data.

Multifactorial methods

The perceived advantages of using multifactorial approaches in assigning age at death to archaeological material rest upon the minimization of errors of individual indicators. Jackes[18] considers the multifactorial approach to ageing in considerable critical detail and the reader is referred to that paper. Such methods have existed since 1960.[56] Ascadi and Nemeskéri[15] advocated the use of four sites; Lovejoy et al.[16] suggested five and also advocated the use of seriation instead of grouping individuals into age brackets.

This author finds it very difficult to be convinced by the arguments put forward for the use of multifactorial approaches when there are so many inherent problems within the samples used to develop the individual methods involved. In addition to this is the fact that most methods have been developed on a small number of samples, particularly the Hamann–Todd collection and many of those methods have been assessed for reliability on the same sample.[16] Lovejoy et al.[16] discussed the problems inherent with the Todd sample in depth but failed to appreciate the significance of the fact that many original ages for individuals were rejected because they were out of line with anatomical parameters considered to reflect senescence. This is tantamount to determining the accuracy of the ages of material to be used to devise *biological* age at death by *biological* criteria – which surely defeats the object of the assessment in the first place.

Evaluation of the reliability of such methods on archaeological material is confined to examining the Complex Method[61] on the Spitalfields material and the Lovejoy et al.[16] method on the Ontario sample. The Complex Method claimed an accuracy rate of estimated age falling within 5 years of real age in 80–85% of cases. However, at Spitalfields (387 individuals of known age) it was found wanting, with < 30% of adults aged to within 5 years and a systematic error whereby most older adults were under-aged and younger ones over-aged.[20]

Saunders *et al.* [22] found Lovejoy *et al.*'s[16] method performed badly on the smaller Canadian sample (*n* = 80). Interestingly, contrary to these results, Bedford *et al.*[77] found the Lovejoy *et al.* method worked well on the Grant collection (modern, low socio-economic status material with death certificates (*n* = 55), only one of which was female) producing a smaller error than with individual methods. An important feature of this study was that, unusually, the sample played no part in the development of any of the individual methods being tested.

Bedford *et al.* found the pubic symphysis performed best in ageing younger adults and the auricular surface in older adults. They also found that their method, which involved seriation and principal component analysis, performed better than the individual methods involved. Clearly the results of this analysis can only be considered in relation to males. However, the margin of error evident in this sample demonstrated that Lovejoy *et al.*'s method is not accurate enough to be meaningfully applied to forensic material and with respect to archaeological material the margin of error is not insignificant. The implications for palaeodemography are not inconsequential even though such data can be manipulated and modelled statistically.

Other methods

Arachnoid granulation

A recently explored method of age estimation that does not fall within the above criteria, is based upon arachnoid granulation. The radiographic literature noted that these endocranial indentations increase with age, and Barber *et al.*[108] investigated whether this had a predictive capacity when observed macroscopically. The number of indentations was counted on both the left and right parietal bones in 14 post-mortem calvaria from individuals (of known age) and in an undocumented archaeological sample (*n* = 100) from Barton-upon-Humber (where age was procured by conventional anthropological methods). Correlation of the number of indentations counted with the age assigned gave highly significant ($p < 0.001$) results and from this an equation was calculated to determine the age of an individual to within ± 10 years. This method was then tested on a non-European sample (*n* = 105) of African-Americans of known age at death from the Terry collection. Once again, results showed a high correlation with age ($p < 0.001$), although there was a notable difference in the regression equation constructed for both males and females in comparison with the European sample on which the original model was produced. This led to the recommendation that in order to achieve the most accurate method for age prediction utilizing this technique, different models should be produced for each spatially or racially different population.

This method merits further research on large documented samples. Its reliability and application remains to be demonstrated and should be tempered by the fact that the original scheme was developed on a European sample of which the ages of 88% were biologically determined (therefore estimates). If systemic, genetic and environmental processes influence biological ageing changes in individuals and samples, then it follows that to base a method on such a small sample will simply propagate the same systemic errors.

Extraneous variables

All of the methods discussed above are further complicated by recent results obtained by Belkin *et al.*[109] They assessed the magnitude of environmental effects, particularly temperature and humidity on thermoregulation and consequently basal metabolism rate and circulatory and endocrine functions. This study was based upon a modern sample of known age (18–99 years) from 31 samples from Eurasia (*n* = about 7500). Examination of hand radiographs for osteophytes, involution, osteosclerosis and non-traumatic articular deformities indicated significant correlations with increasing age. However, this was significantly affected by both temperature and relative humidity, which affected rates of bone destruction and loss. The implications of such work for assessment of age in archaeological samples are very important considering the extent of both temporal and spatial climate changes since the end of the last glaciation.

CONCLUSION

It is a fact of modern scholarship that aspects of our preoccupation with determining age at death with accuracy are a reflection of the preoccupation with age which dominates our culture. Nevertheless, it is entirely legitimate to pursue the quest to ascribe age at death with confidence and accuracy in order to address a range of archaeological and anthropological areas of inquiry. If we are to understand such issues as palaeodemography, population dynamics, mortality rates, and the aetiology of disease and trauma we need to determine age at death. Clearly, the need to assess accurate age at death with confidence for forensic reasons is even more urgent as such analysis seeks to serve fundamental issues such as justice rather than those more esoteric.

Subject to the important predeterminants of condition and completeness, what can be reliably undertaken within the framework of research described above? In light of current research it does seem reasonable to conclude that we can identify young adults (under about 30 years) within archaeological and forensic assemblages. For older adults, it seems that ascribed ages can fall within unacceptably large age brackets with a considerable and unacceptable degree of overlap. This problem might be resolvable using statistical modelling in larger samples, but becomes more acute with smaller samples and is unacceptable in individuals. Assessment of methods on the small number of documented archaeological samples available to us suggests that current methods tend to overage the 30–40-year age group and underage the older groups by unacceptably large margins.

The reasons for our difficulties lie in two main areas. One is the fact that we are attempting to predictively correlate non-linear biological changes – largely processes we do not fully understand, which are influenced by genetics, life-style and environment, with a linear and constant phenomenon – passing time. Given the vast range of variation within and between families, samples and populations, this may not be possible within meaningful confidence limits that provide useful data capable of addressing our research agendas. Second, by necessity, there has been an over-reliance upon a small number of samples of material, some of which are not entirely or even largely comprised of reliably documented ages, to both develop and test methodologies. In the last decade or so, more reliable material has become available largely from autopsy rooms. However, generally such sample sizes are small, particularly when broken down into subsets of ancestry, sex and parity status. Further, the arguments for sample bias influencing application outcomes cannot be ignored and need to be constructively addressed.

What of the future? To resolve the issue of the reliability of current skeletal methods for ageing adults, it is imperative that large samples of reliably documented skeletal material become available. Such a scenario is unlikely which makes a case for the reassessment of the reliability of existing samples by independent researchers and, if necessary, the creation of large samples by the amalgamation of a number of small ones. Ideally, for the UK such a sample must include equal numbers of all ages, all ancestral groups, both sexes and all socio-economic groups. In the UK most of our skeletal material is from the historic period and much of that comprises non-homogenous material. Consider for example Romano-British cemeteries which have the potential to include people from or descended from, most of Europe, North Africa and the Near East, people undertaking a wide range of occupations and falling within a wide socio-economic spectrum. Concurrent to that, further research needs to be undertaken to examine the biological processes underlying 'age-related' change[110] and the influence thereon of genetic and environmental variables. Without this, the issue of applying methods developed upon modern material to archaeological (and forensic) material, which can be of unknown or at best uncertain genetic and environmental context, is questionable. This is a challenging area of osteological research which demands to be addressed and must be so if we are to do justice to the wealth of archaeological material that is available for analysis.

ACKNOWLEDGEMENTS

The cranial suture component of this paper is derived but extended from an unpublished paper, 'Ageing and sexing the skull: the anthropologists' contribution', presented at the Cranio-Facial Reconstruction Conference, held at Windsor in July 1997. Linda O'Connell is thanked for input to that paper. References on iliac crest fusion, spheno-occipital synchondrosis and the ossification of hyaline cartilage have been made available from the forthcoming textbook *Developmental Juvenile Osteology* by Louise Scheuer and Sue Black (Academic Press), to whom I am immensely grateful. Thanks are also due to referees for useful and constructive comments, and to Denise McGinley for proving an able research assistant.

REFERENCES

1 Tilley C. Archaeology as socio-economic action in the present. In: Whitley DS (ed.), *Reader in Archaeological Theory: Post-Processual and Cognitive Approaches.* London: Routledge, 1998: pp. 315–330.

2 Lowenthal D. *The Past is a Foreign Country.* Cambridge: Cambridge University Press, 1985.

3 Hershkovitz I, Latimer B, Dutour O, Jellema LM, Wish-Baratz S, Rothschild C, Rothschild BM. Why do we fail in ageing the skull from the sagittal suture? *American Journal of Physical Anthropology* 1997; **103**: 393–399.

4 Cox M. *Life and Death in Spitalfields: 1700–1859.* York: Council for British Archaeology, 1996.

5 Mensforth RP, Lovejoy CO. Anatomical, physiological and epidemiological correlates of the ageing process: a confirmation of multifactorial age determination in the Libben skeletal population. *American Journal of Physical Anthropology* 1985; **68**: 87–106.

6   Scoles PV, Salverno R, Villalba K, Riew D. Relationship of the iliac crest to skeletal and chronological age. *Journal of Pediatric Orthopaedics* 1988; **8**: 639–644.

7   Psalm **90**:10.

8   Weiss KM. Demographic models for anthropology. *Memoirs of the Society for American Archaeology* 1973; 27.

9   McKern TW, Stewart TW. *Skeletal Age Changes in Young American Males. Analysed from the Standpoint of Age Identification*. Environmental Protection Research Division Technical Report No. EP–45 (Quartermaster Research and Development Centre, US Army, Natick, MA, 1957.

10 Gilbert BM, McKern TW. A method for ageing the female os pubis. *American Journal of Physical Anthropology* 1973; **38**: 31–38.

11 Brothwell DR. *Digging up Bones* (3rd edn). London: British Museum (Natural History), 1981.

12 Bocquet-Appel JP, Masset C. Farewell to palaeodemography. *Journal of Human Evolution* 1982; **11**: 321–333.

13 Bocquet-Appel JP, Masset C. Palaeodemography: Resurrection or ghost? *Journal of Human Evolution* 1985; **14**: 107–111.

14 Bocquet-Appel JP, Masset C. Palaeodemography: expectancy and false hope. *American Journal of Physical Anthropology* 1996; **99**: 571–583.

15 Ascadi G, Nemeskéri J. *History of Human Life Span and Mortality*. Budapest: Akademiai Kiado, 1970.

16 Lovejoy CO, Meindl RS, Mensforth RP, Barton TJ. Multifactorial determination of skeletal age at death: a method and blind tests of its accuracy. *American Journal of Physical Anthropology* 1985; **68**: 1–14.

17 Isçan MY. Research strategies in age estimation: the multiregional approach. In: Isçan MY (ed.), *Age Markers in the Human Skeleton*. Springfield: Charles C Thomas, 1989: pp. 325–339.

18 Jackes M. Palaeodemography: problems and techniques. In: Saunders SR, Katzenberg MA (eds), *Skeletal Biology of Past Peoples*. New York: Wiley, 1992: pp. 189–224.

19 Miles AEW. The dentition in the assessment of individual age in skeletal material. In: Brothwell DR (ed.), *Dental Anthropology*. Oxford: Pergamon, 1962.

20 Molleson T, Cox M. *The Spitalfields Project*, vol. 2: *The Anthropology. The Middling Sort*. Research Report 86. York: Council for British Archaeology, 1993.

21 Scheuer L. Age at death and cause of death of the people buried in St. Bride's Church, Fleet Street, London. In: Cox M (ed.), *Grave Concerns: Death and Burial on Post-Medieval England 1700–1850*. Research Report 113. York: Council for British Archaeology, 1998: pp. 100–111.

22 Saunders SR, Fitzgerald C, Rogers T, Dudar C, McKillop H. A test of several methods of skeletal age estimation using a documented archaeological sample. *Canadian Society of Forensic Science Journal* 1992; **25**: 97–117.

23 Van Gerven DP, Armelagos GJ. 'Farewell to Palaeodemography?' Rumours of its death have been greatly exaggerated. *Journal of Human Evolution* 1983; **12**: 353–360.

24 Buikstra JE, Konigsberg LW. Palaeodemography: critiques and controversies. *American Anthropologist* 1985; **87**: 316–333.

25 Green DL, Van Gerven DP, Armelagos GJ. Life and death in ancient populations: bones of contention in palaeodemography. *Human Evolution* 1986; **1**: 193–207.

26 Konigsberg LW, Frankenberg SR. Estimation of age structure in anthropological demography. *American Journal of Physical Anthropology* 1992; **89**: 235–256.

27 Skythe A, Boldsen JL. A method for construction of standards for determination of skeletal age at death. *American Journal of Physical Anthropology* 1993; 16 (suppl.): 182.

28 Paine RR, Harpending HC. Effect of sample bias on palaeodemographic fertility estimates. *American Journal of Physical Anthropology* 1998; **105**: 231–240.

29 Angel JL, Suchey JM, Isçan MY, Zimmerman MR. Age at death estimated from the skeleton and viscera. In: Zimmerman MR, Angel JL (eds), *Dating and Age Determination of Biological Materials*. London: Croom Helm, 1986.

30 Maples WR. The practical application of age estimation techniques. In: Isçan MY (ed.), *Age Markers in the Human Skeleton*. Springfield: Charles C Thomas, 1989: pp. 319–324.

31   Işcan MY. Assessment of age at death in the human skeleton. In: Işcan, MY (ed.), *Age Markers in the Human Skeleton*. Springfield: Charles C Thomas, 1989: pp. 5–18.

32   Key CA, Aiello LC, Molleson TI. Cranial suture closure and its implications for age estimation. *International Journal of Osteoarchaeology* 1994; **4**: 193–207.

33   Francis CC. The appearance of centres of ossification from 6 to 15 years. *American Journal of Physical Anthropology* 1940; **27**: 127–138.

34   Albert AM, Maples WR. Stages of epiphyseal union for thoracic and lumbar vertebral centra as a method of age determination for teenage and young adult skeletons. *Journal of Forensic Sciences* 1995; **40**: 623–633.

35   Maat GJR, Mastwijk RW. Ossification status of the jugular growth plate as an aid for age at death determination of skeletons. *International Journal of Anthropology* 1994; **9**: 219.

36   Maat GJR, Mastwijk RW. Fusion status of the jugular growth plate: an aid for age at death determination. *International Journal of Osteoarchaeology* 1995; **5**: 163–167.

37   Hershkovitz I, Latimer B, Dutour O, Jellema LM, Wish-Baratz S, Rothschild C, Rothschild BM. The elusive petroexoccipital articulation. *American Journal of Physical Anthropology* 1997; **103**: 365–373.

38   Black S, Scheuer L. Age changes in the clavicle: from the early neonatal period to skeletal maturity. *International Journal of Osteoarchaeology* 1996; **6**: 425–434.

39   Webb PAO, Suchey JM. Epiphyseal union of the anterior iliac crest and medial clavicle in a modern multi-racial sample of American males and females. *American Journal of Physical Anthropology* 1985; **68**: 457–466.

40   Williams PL, Warwick R, Dyson M, Bannister LH. *Gray's Anatomy*. Edinburgh: Churchill Livingtone, 1989.

41   Latham RA. Observations on the growth of the cranial base in the human skull. *Journal of Anatomy* 1966; **100**: 435.

42   Latham RA. The sella point and postnatal growth of the human cranium base. *American Journal of Orthodontics* 1972; **61**: 156–162.

43   Powell TV, Brodie AG. Closure of the spheno-occipital synchondrosis. *Anatomical Record* 1963; **147**: 15–23.

44   Melsen B. Time of closure of the spheno-occipital synchondrosis determined on dried skulls. *Acta Odontologica Scandinavica* 1969; **27**: 73–90.

45   Irwin GL. Roentgen determination of the time of closure of the spheno-occipital synchondrosis. *Radiology* 1960; **75**: 450–453.

46   Ingervall B, Thilander B. The human spheno-occipital synchondrosis I. The time of closure observed macroscopically. *Acta Odontologica Scandinavica* 1972; **30**: 349–356.

47   Işcan MY, Loth SR. Osteological manifestations of age in the adult. In: Işcan MY, Kennedy KAR (eds), *Reconstruction of Life from the Skeleton*. Springfield: Charles C Thomas, 1989.

48   Dwight T. The closure of the sutures as a sign of age. *Boston Medical and Surgical Journal* 1890; **122**: 389–535.

49   Lenhössek M von. Über Nahtverknocherung im Kindesalter. *Archiv für Anthropologie : Organ der Deutschen Gesellschaft für Anthropologie, Ethnologie und Urgeschichte, Neue Folge* 1917; **15**: 164–180.

50   Todd TW, Lyon DW. Jr. Endocranial suture closure, its progress and age relationship. Part I. Adult males of white stock. *American Journal of Physical Anthropology* 1924; **7**: 325–384.

51   Todd TW, Lyon DW. Jr. Cranial suture closure, its progress and age relationship. Part II. Ectocranial closure in adult males of white stock. *American Journal of Physical Anthropology* 1925; **8**: 23–45.

52   Todd TW, Lyon DW. Jr. Cranial suture closure, its progress and age relationship. Part III. Endocranial closure in adult males of Negro stock. *American Journal of Physical Anthropology* 1925b; **8**: 47–71.

53   Todd TW, Lyon DW. Jr. Cranial suture closure, its progress and age relationship. Part IV. Ectocranial suture closure in adult males of Negro stock. *American Journal of Physical Anthropology* 1925c; **8**: 149–168.

54   Hrdlicka A. *Practical Anthropometry*. Philadelphia: Wistar Institute, 1939.

55   Singer R. Estimation of age from cranial suture closure: a report on its unreliability. *Journal of Forensic Medicine* 1953; **1**: 52–59.

56   Nemeskéri J, Harsányi L, Acsádi G. Methoden zur diagnose des lebensalters von skelettfunden. *Anthropologischer Anzeiger* 1960; **24**: 70–95.

57 Perizonius WRK. Closing and non-closing sutures in 256 crania of known age and sex from Amsterdam (AD 1883–1909). *Journal of Human Evolution* 1984; **13**: 201–216.

58 Meindl RS, Lovejoy, CO. Ectocranial suture closure: a revised method for the determination of skeletal age at death based on the lateral-anterior sutures. *American Journal of Physical Anthropology* 1985; **68**: 57–66.

59 Masset C. Age estimation on the basis of cranial sutures. In: Işcan MY (ed.), *Age Markers in the Human Skeleton*. Springfield: Charles C Thomas, 1989: pp. 71–103.

60 Mann RW, Symes SA, Bass WM. Maxillary suture obliteration: Ageing the human skeleton based on intact fragmentary maxilla. *Journal of Forensic Sciences* 1987; **32**: 48–157.

61 Workshop of European Anthropologists. Recommendations for age and sex diagnoses of skeletons. *Journal of Human Evolution* 1980; **9**: 517–549.

62 Senyurel MSA. Note on the duration of life of the ancient inhabitants of Anatolia. *American Journal of Physical Anthropology* 1947; **5**: 55–66.

63 Brooks ST. Skeletal age at death: the reliability of cranial and pubic indicators. *American Journal of Physical Anthropology* 1955; **13**: 567–595.

64 Todd TW. Age changes in the pubic bone I. The male white pubis. *American Journal of Physical Anthropology* 1920; **3**: 285–339.

65 Mays SA. *The Archaeology of Human Bones*. London: Routledge, 1998.

66 Waldron T. The relative survival of the human skeleton: implications for palaeodemography. In: Boddington A, Garland AN, Janaway RC (eds), *Death, Decay and Reconstruction*. Manchester: Manchester University Press, 1987: pp. 55–64.

67 Suchey JM. Problems in the ageing of females using the os pubis. *American Journal of Physical Anthropology* 1979; **51**: 467–471.

68 Katz D, Suchey JM. Age determination of the male os pubis. *American Journal of Physical Anthropology* 1986; **69**: 427–436.

69 Brooks ST, Suchey JM Skeletal age determination based on the os pubis: a comparison of the Acsadi–Nemeskéri and Suchey–Brooks methods. *Human Evolution* 1990; **5**: 227–238.

70 Pfeiffer S. Morbidity and mortality in the Uxbridge ossuary. *Canadian Journal of Anthropology* 1986; **5**: 23–31.

71 Aiello LC, Molleson T. Are microscopic ageing techniques more accurate than macroscopic ageing techniques? *Journal of Archaeological Science* 1993; **20**: 689–704.

72 Işcan MY, Loth SR. Determination of age from sternal rib in white males. A test of the phase method. *Journal of Forensic Sciences* 1984; **31**: 122–132.

73 Işcan MY, Loth SR, Scheuerman EH. Determination of age from the sternal rib in white females. A test of the phase method. *Journal of Forensic Sciences* 1985; **31**: 990–999.

74 Loth SR. Age assessment of the Spitalfields cemetery population by rib phase analysis. *American Journal of Human Biology* 1995; **7**: 465–471.

75 Sashin D. A critical analysis of the anatomy and the pathological changes of the sacro-iliac joints. *Journal of Bone and Joint Surgery* 1930; **12**: 891–910.

76 Kobayashi K. Trends in human life based upon human skeletons from prehistoric to modern times in Japan. *Journal of Faculty of Science University of Tokyo* 1967; Sect 3: 107–162.

77 Bedford ME, Russell KF, Lovejoy CO, Meindl RS, Simpson SW, Stuart-Macadam PL. Test of the multifactorial ageing method using skeletons with known ages-at-death from the Grant collection. *American Journal of Physical Anthropology* 1993; **91**: 287–297.

78 Meindl RS, Lovejoy CO. Age changes in the pelvis: implications for palaeodemography. In: Işcan MY (ed.), *Age Markers in the Human Skeleton*. Springfield: Charles C Thomas, 1989: pp. 137–168.

79 Meindl RS, Lovejoy CO, Mensforth RP, Walker RA. A revised method of age determination using the os pubis, with a review and tests of accuracy of other current methods of pubic symphyseal ageing. *American Journal of Physical Anthropology* 1985; **68**: 29–45.

80 Murray KA, Murray T. A test of the auricular surface ageing techniques. *Journal of Forensic Sciences* 1991; **36**: 1162–1169.

81 King JB. Calcification of the costal cartilages. *British Journal of Radiology* 1939; **12**: 2–12.

82 Vastine JH, Vastine MF, Arango O. Genetic influence on osseous development with particular reference to the deposition of calcium in the costal cartilages. *American Journal of Roentgenology and Radium Therapy* 1946; **59**: 213–221.

83 Stewart TD. Metamorphosis of the joints of the sternum in relation to age changes in other bones. *American Journal of Physical Anthropology* 1954; **12**: 519–529.

84 McCormick WF, Stewart JH. Age related changes in the human plastron: a roentgenographic and morphological study. *Journal of Forensic Sciences* 1988; **33**: 100–120.

85 Roncallo P. Research about ossification and conformation of the thyroid cartilage in men. *Acta Otolaryngologica* 1948; **36**: 111–134.

86 Keen JA, Wainwright J. Ossification of the thyroid, cricoid and arytenoid cartilages. *South African Journal of Laboratory and Clinical Medicine* 1958; **4**: 83–108.

87 Harrison DFN, Denny S. Ossification within the primate larynx. *Acta Otolaryngologica* 1983; **95**: 440–446.

88 Curtis DJ, Allman RM, Brion J, Holborow MS, Brahman SL. Calcification and ossification in the artenoid cartilage: incidence and patterns. *Journal of Forensic Sciences* 1985; **30**: 1113–1118 .

89 Hately W, Evison G, Samuel E. The pattern of ossification of the laryngeal cartilages: a radiological study. *British Journal of Radiology* 1965; **38**: 585–591.

90 Turk LM, Hogg DA. Age changes in the human laryngeal cartilages. *Clinical Anatomy* 1993; **6**: 154–162.

91 Stout SD. Methods of determining age at death using bone microstructure. In: Saunders SR, Katzenberg MA (eds), *Skeletal Biology of Past Peoples*. New York: Wiley, 1992: pp. 21–35.

92 Stout SD. The use of cortical bone histology to estimate age at death. In: Işcan MY (ed.), *Age Markers in the Human Skeleton*. Springfield: Charles C Thomas, 1989: pp. 195–207.

93 Ubelaker D. Estimation of age at death from histology of human bone. In: Zimmerman MR, Angel JL (eds), *Dating and Age Determination of Biological Materials*. London: Croom Helm, 1986: pp. 240–247.

94 Garland AN. A histological study of archaeological bone decomposition. In: Boddington A, Garland AN, Janaway RC (eds), *Death, Decay and Reconstruction*. Manchester: Manchester University Press, 1987: pp. 109–126.

95 Boddington A. From bones to population: the problem of numbers. In: Boddington A, Garland AN, Janaway RC (eds), *Death, Decay and Reconstruction*. Manchester: Manchester University Press, 1987: pp. 180–197.

96 Walker RA, Lovejoy CO. Radiographic changes in the clavicle and proximal femur and their use in the determination of skeletal age at death. *American Journal of Physical Anthropology* 1985; **68**: 67–78.

97 Stout SD, Paine RR. Histological age estimation using rib and clavicle. *American Journal of Physical Anthropology* 1992; **87**: 111–115.

98 Stout SD, Parro MA, Perotti B. Brief communication: A test and correction of the clavicle method of Stout and Paine for histological age estimation of skeletal remains. *American Journal of Physical Anthropology* 1996; **100**: 139–142.

99 Stout SD, Dietze WH, Işcan MY, Loth SR. Estimation of age at death using cortical histomorphometry of the sternal end of the fourth rib. *Journal of Forensic Sciences* 1994; **39**: 778–784.

100 Wallin JA, Tkocz I, Kristensen G. Microscopic age determination of human skeletons including an unknown but calculable variable. *International Journal of Osteoarchaeology* 1994; **4**: 353–362.

101 Macchiarelli R, Bondoli L. Linear densitometry and digital image processing of the proximal femur radiographs: implications for archaeological and forensic anthropology. *American Journal of Physical Anthropology* 1994; **93**: 109–122.

102 Eriksen MF. Ageing changes in the medullary cavity of the proximal femur in American blacks and whites. *American Journal of Physical Anthropology* 1979; **51**: 563–569.

103 Feik SA, Thomas CDL, Clement JG. Age-related changes in cortical porosity of the mid-shaft of the human femur. *Journal of Anatomy* 1997; **191**: 407–416.

104 Cool SM, Hendrikz JK, Wood WB. Microscopic age changes in the human occipital bone. *Journal of Forensic Sciences* 1995; **40**: 789–796.

105 Schranz D. Age determination from the internal structure of the humerus. *American Journal of Physical Anthropology* 1959; **17**: 273–277.

106 Bartley MH, Arnold JS. Sex differences in human skeletal involution. *Nature* 1967; **214**: 908–909.

107 Mays SA. Age-dependent cortical bone loss in a medieval population. *International Journal of Osteoarchaeology* 1996; **6**: 144–154.

108 Barber G, Shepstone L, Rogers J. A methodology for estimating age at death using arachnoid granulation counts. *American Journal of Physical Anthropology* 1995; 20 (suppl.): 61.

109 Belkin V, Livshits G, Otremski I, Kobyliansky E. Ageing bone score and climatic factors. *American Journal of Physical Anthropology* 1998; **106**: 349–359.

110 Lovejoy CO, Meindl RS, Tague RG, Latimer B. The comparative senescent biology of the homioid pelvis and its implications for the use of age at death indicators in the human skeleton. In: Paine RP. *Integrating Demography: Multidisciplinary Approaches to Prehistoric Population.* Occasional Paper No. 24. Centre for Archaeological Investigations, 1997: pp. 43–63.

6

AGEING FROM THE DENTITION

David Whittaker

INTRODUCTION

Determining the age at death of human remains has long been a challenge for the forensic pathologist and forensic dentist. It is a central issue in correct identification of an unknown body and the more accurately it can be determined the more likely is a positive identification. Most of the techniques available have been developed in relation to contemporary material of a forensic nature, but there has also been an increasing interest in determining age at death in archaeological remains of a single individual, or in population studies where demographic considerations are paramount. It is one of the more difficult problems in forensic or archaeological endeavours and is still an imprecise and developing subject area.

Quantitative studies on disease processes have been difficult to interpret in archaeological samples because of the problems of accurate age at death determination. Many of the methods that have been applied to post-cranial and cranial skeletal remains are limited because of individual variation and because pathological conditions during the life of an individual may extensively modify the information which may be derived from osteological examination. Bones and soft tissues are subject to the influence of disease processes and also have a natural turnover, which is not necessarily related to the chronological age of the individual (see Cox, chapter 5, in this volume).

In a biological sense the teeth are unique structures in mammalian and primate development. They not only follow a well-understood sequential developmental pattern from the foetal stage until the end of the second decade in humans, but also once the tissues are mineralized they have a minimal biological turnover so that information built into them during their growth stages remains unchanged throughout the life of the individual and indeed beyond death.

The application of any forensic techniques to archaeological material requires some assumptions to be made. These centre on the difficulty of determining whether growth rates, dietary influences, disease processes and general environmental conditions in ancient populations would have resulted in a comparable sequence of events to that seen in modern day civilizations. For these reasons age determination in archaeological remains must be approached with great caution and should be used in conjunction with all other methods available and measured against historical records whenever these are available. There is evidence that age determination from the dentition provides the most accurate method yet available but is more likely to result in a ranking order of age in a given population rather than in accurate age determination of any one individual. As in all other methods of age estimation, there is a tendency for incorrect ageing in the older individuals, particularly resulting in an under estimate of age after about 50 years.

AGEING THE HUMAN FOETUS

During the 9 months from conception to birth the deciduous dentition undergoes a sequential development which is well documented and may be reliably used for age determination. The tooth germs for the anterior deciduous teeth commence soft tissue development from the dental lamina at about 6 weeks after conception, but it is not until mineralization of the tooth germs has commenced that this sequence becomes useful in archaeological material reduced to skeletal remains. The mandible or maxilla of a human foetus found associated with adult female skeletal remains may be examined initially by radiographic techniques. Such methods may not be applicable to all the adult members of a population for reasons of cost. However, they are extremely useful in a small number of foetal remnants and are capable of imaging not only the bony crypts for the developing permanent teeth, but also give an indication of the extent of mineralization of each of the 20 deciduous teeth developing within the jaws.

Mineralization of these teeth commences in the anterior region at about 4 months after conception and continues throughout foetal life and into young childhood (Figure 1). Not only do the teeth develop sequentially from the midline to the posterior region of the jaws, but also each tooth develops in a sequential manner. Mineralization begins at the cusp tips which initially remain separated, but as time progresses they fuse together to produce the overall shape of the deciduous crown. It is therefore possible from a radiograph to determine to within a matter of weeks the age of a foetal jaw by mapping the presence of the tooth crypts and the extent of mineralization of individual incisal edges and cusps within these crypts. This pattern of mineralization has been documented[1] and each deciduous tooth has been represented in a diagrammatic form indicating the extent of cuspal mineralization. Although these data were developed from excision and microscopic examination of developing tooth germs, they are useful in comparing the extent of development on radiographs from archaeological remains, and will give a reasonably accurate estimate of gestation time in a given foetus. A useful landmark is a study of the crypt containing the developing first permanent molar, since this begins to mineralize in the mesio-buccal cusp area at or just before birth. In well-preserved material it is therefore possible to produce an independent estimate of gestation age from each of 20 developing and mineralizing deciduous teeth and from the four permanent molars.

The event of birth itself results in physiological changes in the cells which are laying down the hard tissues of the teeth, and recovery of cellular activity takes some days or weeks after birth. The rods or prisms of the enamel are being sequentially laid down during this period

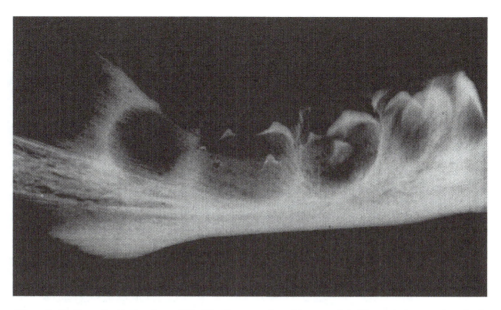

Figure 1 – Radiograph of a foetal mandible. The four cusp tips of the second deciduous molar are mineralized but not fused.

and their structure is changed by the event of birth in such a way that a permanent, accentuated incremental growth line is laid down within the enamel and dentine of the tooth.[2] This is known as the neonatal line and, if it can be demonstrated in the young infant's teeth, will indicate that birth had occurred and that the child died post-natally. In archaeological material individual teeth may be removed from the developing mandible or maxilla and sections prepared to demonstrate the presence or absence of this so-called neonatal line. If the child dies within a short period of birth it may be necessary to use higher resolution techniques such as scanning electron microscopy[3] to demonstrate that this phenomenon had occurred (Figure 2)

INFANT REMAINS

From birth until about 2.5 years of age the mineralization pattern of the deciduous teeth continues and the eruption sequence of the deciduous teeth is well documented.[4] Beyond eruption the roots continue to develop for about a further 2 years. The age at death of an infant may therefore be estimated with reasonable accuracy by studying the deciduous teeth which have erupted, and if necessary, by X-ray or by carefully removing them from the jaw, studying the extent of root development. During this period following birth the permanent dentition will also have commenced mineralization, so a large number of individual items may be used to produce separate estimates of age and a mean produced (Figure 3). There are some tables of this sequence of development available in the literature[5,6] but it has to be admitted that many have been produced on small samples of material and their applicability to archaeological material must be viewed with caution. A useful review of available data has recently been published.[7]

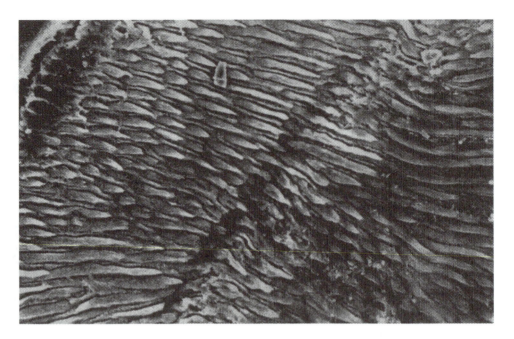

Figure 2 – Scanning electron micrograph of a neonatal line. Disturbance of mineralization is evident in the enamel rods.

The clinical eruption of all the deciduous teeth is complete by about 2.5 years after birth and then, apart from growth of the jaws and development of the permanent dentition within them, the clinical appearance remains constant until the age of about 6 years. At this stage the first permanent molars erupt behind the deciduous dentition and the roots of these teeth are complete some 3 years later at about the age of 9 years. Between the age of 6 and 9 the anterior deciduous teeth are resorbing and being exfoliated and replaced by the anterior permanent teeth. The sequence of eruption of these teeth is somewhat irregular and tables are available from contemporary material which, again, can be applied to archaeological remains but with caution. By the age of 12 years all of the deciduous teeth will have resorbed and exfoliated and will have been replaced by the permanent dentition as far back as the second permanent molars. At about the age of 8 years the third permanent molars are beginning to mineralize but they will not erupt until about the age of 18, resulting in root completion by about the age of 21 years. The inaccuracies in using third molars for age estimation have been reviewed.[8] Direct observation of juvenile archaeological material will therefore enable a reasonably approximate age at death determination to be made up to the end of the second decade, and if radiographs can be used an even more accurate determination may be made.[9] This relatively reliable sequence of events highlights the importance of recovery of juvenile material from any large archaeological population, since age determination is well established and reasonably accurate and provides a baseline against which older material may be measured.

During these first two decades many skeletal age changes are occurring and these have been considered elsewhere (see Scheuer and Black, chapter 2, in this volume). They should be used in conjunction with the sequential development and mineralization of both the deciduous and permanent dentitions when age estimates are made.

AGEING THE ADULT FROM THE TEETH

At the end of the second decade the crowns and roots of all of the permanent teeth have completed their development and therefore only subtle changes will occur over the next 50 or more years. Most of these changes are related to function of the dentition, and only a few are directly attributable to true age changes.

Attrition of the teeth

Many of the techniques used in archaeological ageing are based upon continuing attrition of the dentition commencing with the enamel and progressing to the dentine and eventually to the pulp. If the attrition is at a slow rate then secondary dentine may be laid down at a rate sufficient to keep ahead of the attrition and so prevent the pulp chamber from being exposed. However, if attrition occurs rapidly then secondary dentine formation may be unable to cope with the situation and this will result in exposure of the pulp chamber, infection of the pulp and loss of vitality of the tooth. The infection will usually progress to the apex of the tooth, spread into the peri-apical tissues and result in a peri-apical abscess and eventual discharge through the alveolar bone and through the gingival tissues into the mouth. Other scenarios involve the tracking of infection beyond muscle attachments and into the deeper tissues of the oral cavity, the worst scenarios being infection tracking into the retro-molar areas and eventually into the laryngeal tissues of the neck or via veins into the cranial cavity. This potentially fatal situation is rarely seen in modern humans but may well have been a cause of death in less technologically advanced societies.

The attrition of the occlusal surfaces of the teeth is accompanied by wear of the approximal surfaces. However, the phenomenon of mesial drift ensures that even though the teeth are being shortened in antero-posterior length, the teeth behind drift forwards to maintain the contact areas between adjacent teeth (Figure 3). This means that with increasing age the posterior molars will move forwards and the arch will become shorter. Attrition in the teeth of earlier civilizations has been variously attributed to coarse or fibrous food, sand or grit particles in the diet, or more recently to phytoliths or silica particles contained within the vegetable matter being eaten. Gustafson[10] pointed out that attrition *per se* was a rather inaccurate method of age estimation because too many unknown factors influence it, and the quality of the diet and its contents are unknown in most circumstances. A scholarly contribution in this area was provided by Brothwell[11] who developed a simplified method for age grouping based on patterns of dentine islands on the occlusal surfaces of molar teeth. The method is based on that of Miles[12] in which he recognized that by studying juvenile dentitions from a given population it was possible to make an estimate of the rate of attrition in that population. This is because the first permanent molar erupts at the age of 6 years, the second permanent molar at 12 years and the third permanent molar at 18 years. The juveniles from a population can therefore be aged with reasonable accuracy. The extent of wear over a 6- or 12-year period in the first molar and over a 6-year period in the second molar,

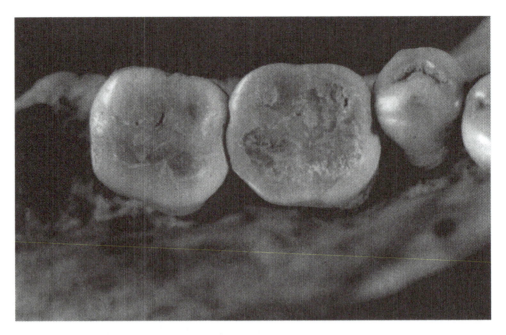

Figure 3 – Approximal attrition resulting in mesial drift of molar teeth and shortening of arch length.

will give an indication of the rate of dental attrition. The assumption then has to be made that the attrition and therefore presumably the diet will remain constant throughout life and from this continuing wear a reasonably accurate age at death may be made in older members of the same population. Combinations of the method of Miles and Brothwell have been used in ageing archaeological material for the past 30 or more years. Kieser *et al.*[13] tested the accuracy of the method on a living population with a culture similar to those encountered in archaeological studies. There was a high correlation between age estimates made from maxillae and mandibles, and also with the true age of the individuals (i.e. between 0.58 and 0.95). Data are available from 235 Danish medieval skulls,[14] 52 of which were in various states of mixed dentition and could therefore be used to establish the criteria of wear in the early years of the population. It was shown that assessments of age at death could be made fairly accurately for the age range 5–30 years but with decreasing accuracy until about 40 years of age.

More recently the technique has been applied to 880 people living in rural and urban areas of the People's Republic of China. Song and Jia[15] added multiple stepwise regression analysis to their study of the statistical examination of data derived from attrition of the occlusal surfaces of the teeth. They argued that if such methods are used, a reasonably accurate estimate of age could be made. There is still some doubt about this however, and the Brothwell chart method (which is based on the Miles method of ageing) was applied to a group of Chinese skulls in which the age at death was known. The specimens covered an age range from 16 to 60 years and the data were analysed by regression methods.[16] Results showed that molar teeth do indeed continue to wear throughout the life of the individual and the first molar teeth wear significantly more quickly than the second molars. It was concluded that this simple ordinal score method for recording dental wear gave an inaccurate estimate of the individual skull's age at death and there was a very wide deviation at the 5% confidence level. Solheim and Sundnes[17] found that age estimation based on the Miles method was slightly less reliable than when apical translucency was used.

In spite of all of these limitations there is, at the present time, no alternative way of estimating the age at death of adult skulls without destroying some of the material.

Age determination from individual teeth

While there is an understandable reluctance for archaeologists to allow destruction of such important items in the skeletal material as teeth, there are techniques available for copying these teeth and replacing them in the mandible or maxilla and thus retaining the normal appearance and structure of the jaws.

Apical translucency

Where destruction of tooth material is allowable the technique of Gustafson,[5] which was originally developed for ageing forensic specimens, may also be applied to archaeological material. When first described the technique involved bucco-lingual longitudinal sections through undemineralized teeth. From these sections, points were awarded for the extent of occlusal or incisal attrition, the extent of secondary dentine formation in the pulp chamber, the apical migration of the attachment of the gingival tissues, the amount of secondary cementum formed, the extent of resorption of the apices and finally, the extent of sclerotic dentine or translucent apical dentine extending from the apex up towards the crown of the tooth. Gustafson produced regression lines from teeth of known age and the total number of points awarded to a particular tooth were checked against these regression lines. It quickly became apparent that the use of all of these changes was unnecessary since most of them were related more to pathological change than to true age, and it is now accepted that the extent of root translucency near to the apex of a tooth is the single most important factor in estimating the age of an individual.[18] It is apparent that there were significant statistical errors in the original articles concerning this method and that more accurate estimates of age can be achieved using other statistical techniques.

The recession of the periodontal ligament has been studied[19] and it was shown that periodontal recession tended to be more rapid in males than in females and that as a sole indicator of age it was not sufficiently accurate to be used in forensic investigations. Only a weak correlation was found between age and the extent of periodontal recession. In any case in skeletal archaeological material it may be difficult to estimate where the soft tissues would have been attached. However, used in conjunction with other methods and using multiple regression statistical analysis it may be a useful technique for age estimation.

The value of secondary dentine deposition has been investigated as one of the several parameters in methods for age estimation. Teeth were prepared by splitting them longitudinally into halves and the area of the coronal pulp and the width of the root and pulp chambers were measured in a stereo-microscope.[20] Pearson correlation coefficients between age and the extent of secondary dentine were derived for various methods of measuring this particular phenomenon. Multiple regression analysis showed that by combining several types of measurements, such as length of secondary dentine, area of secondary dentine and the change in size of the pulp chamber, the correlation with age could be increased. While accepting that multiple regression analysis with as many factors as possible may produce better ageing, there are practical limitations on the amount of time and expense that can be applied to teeth from individuals from large populations.

At the present time the single most acceptable method of ageing in archaeological material using destruction of teeth is a modification of the Gustafson method which uses, as the sole criterion, the amount of root dentine translucency (RDT). Many modifications have been applied to the method in attempts to increase the accuracy.[21] A method using half sectioning of teeth rather than thin sectioning was studied by Solheim[20] and he, in a sample of ten pairs of contralateral teeth, compared age estimates with those obtained by conventional thin sectioning methods. Age calculations were performed according to the methods of Bang and Ramm[21] and Dalitz,[22] and these showed that the half tooth technique was easy to perform and the cut surface produced was suitable for measurements of the factors used in age calculations. There was a tendency for higher measurements to be found using the half tooth technique but the differences were not significant. It was concluded that the methods used for calculating age based on thin sections can be applied successfully to the half tooth technique or to the use of thicker sections.[23] It may well be that such a method is far more applicable to archaeological investigation than the more sophisticated, expensive and diffi-cult thin sectioning technique described previously.

There has been much controversy as to whether length measurements of RDT or area measurements of RDT form the most suitable method of age estimation. Comparison of area measurements[22] with the findings obtained by the use of the methods of Bang and Ramm[21] and of Johanson[24] yielded useful data. Five hundred teeth were used, 50 of each tooth type, but excluding the molars. In step-wise multiple regression analyses the area of translucent dentine was preferred to other types of measurement of the translucency.[25] However, in another study[26] on 1000 teeth excluding molars, the length of the translucent zone measured on unsectioned teeth produced the closest relation to age. Slightly larger translucent areas were found in teeth from males, in darker teeth and in teeth with increased thickness of cementum. The increase in the translucent zone with advancing age was almost linear and not affected by periodontal destruction. The range of accuracy of these age estimations has varied considerably in most of the published studies. RDT was studied in 70 histological sections from teeth from 46 individuals of known sex and age.[27] The ratio of length of root translucency to the total root length in millimetres was calculated and it was reported that the error of the age estimates obtained were at least 5 years either way. It has been claimed that image analysis techniques[28] provide much more precise measurements of the parameters involved in age determination.

A recent study of RDT in 306 single rooted teeth, which were unsectioned and simply tran-silluminated, has been carried out.[29] Information from the transparency of the root and the level of attachment of the periodontal tissues was combined and it was claimed that the mean error between the actual and estimated age was ± 10 years on the working sample and ± 8 years on a controlled sample of forensic cases. Upper incisors showed a better precision than other single rooted teeth and the accuracy was not sex-related. In a comparison of the original sectioning technique of Gustafson and this non-invasive method the data suggested that the whole tooth method might be more accurate. It is certainly fast, easy to use and reasonably accurate, except for cases of individuals under the age of 40 where other methods might be preferred.

Controversy still exists as to the best selection of tooth for modified Gustafson age estimations. Most of the studies support the view that single rooted teeth should be used, although one or two prefer using molars. The problem with the latter is that there is still no clear information as to differences that may occur between the two roots of bi-rooted teeth and the three roots of multi-rooted teeth. There is also some controversy around the issue of whether vital or non-vital teeth produce more or less RDT (vitality, in this context, refers to whether the pulp is living or necrotic). It was observed[25] that the percentage of translucent dentine in non-vital teeth was less than that seen in vital teeth in corresponding ages. However, some workers[30,31] concluded that obliteration of the dentinal tubules is not dependent on the vital odontoblast. Recent work has supported this latter view.[32] When variables of length as a percentage of root length and area as a percentage of root area were plotted against age following digitalization of data, it was shown that there was more apical translucency present in all types of non-vital teeth when compared with vital teeth at any given age.

There is very little information available concerning any variations that may occur between racial types. In a study of 198 single rooted teeth from Caucasian-Malay, Chinese-Malay and Indian-Malay races[33] it was shown that racial differences other than age may be important in the formation of sclerotic apical dentine. The effect of racial origin should therefore be considered when using sclerosis as a means of age determination either in forensic or archaeological cases.

In techniques developed from the Gustafson method almost all available data have been derived from contemporary material. It is still not clear how accurately the method may be applied to archaeological material. There are undoubtedly problems of a taphonomic nature and it is not clear how accurately changes within the dentine due to burial conditions and those due to true ageing may be distinguished. Experienced operators may distinguish microscopically between RDT and taphonomic changes but there is evidence that when image analytical techniques are used[34] the correlation between measurements and age are extremely low. Anecdotally the method appears to produce reasonably accurate ageing when used in conjunction with other information such as post-cranial osteological changes and attrition of the teeth. However, there is no doubt that extensive investigations of populations which are ancient but of known age at death need to be carried out.

Dentinal tubules

Attempts have been made to examine other parameters related to age changes in the teeth that are susceptible to relatively easy measurement. One of these is based upon the biological observations that dentinal tubules become narrower as age progresses because of the deposition of highly mineralized intra-tubular dentine. The exact relationship of this material to the sclerotic dentine obliterating the tubules in the apical region and utilized in the

Gustafson technique is not entirely clear. The number of tubules per mm² in human teeth has been estimated.[35] No attempt was made to relate these counts to proximity to the tooth apex but it was noted that numbers seemed to be lower in this region. A relationship was suggested between the number of tubules seen at the dentine pre-dentine junction and the age of the tooth[36] but the correlation does not appear to be precise. In 173 central incisors from 18- to 83-year-old individuals the dentinal tubule diameters, along with root transparency, were the most reliable parameters on the basis of image analysis for determining the age of the individual.[37] However, there was limited effectiveness of these parameters in age estimation because of individual variations caused by genetic factors. The extent of peritubular or intra-tubular dentine has been studied in central and lateral human incisors from 50 individuals.[38] The results did not demonstrate a significant relationship between age and reduction in the number of tubules. It appears therefore that this method is as yet unacceptable for use in age determination studies.

Pulp chamber

Another, non-invasive approach to age determination is to measure the height and width of the pulp chamber of teeth on radiographs.[39] In 100 individuals there appeared to be a definite relationship between the age of an individual and the size of the dental pulp chamber. It was concluded that these measurements could not be used as a reliable method of age determination. This study was carried out on contemporary individuals and it seems likely that quantitative radiographic techniques of this nature would be even less applicable to the archaeological situation. A similar study carried out on 500 subjects using the mandibular anterior teeth[40] showed a significant change in size of the pulp chambers with advancing age. The most useful measurements were the total length of the pulp chamber and it's width at the cervical margin of the tooth. There were statistical differences in these measurements between most of the age groups studied, and the authors concluded that the method was incapable of determining accurate age of an individual but might well be useful to place individuals in age groupings. Further work in this area is clearly indicated. A recent clinical investigation looked at 100 dental patients attending clinics in the Dental Faculty in Oslo.[41] Radiographs of six different types of teeth from both mandible and maxilla were analysed and the following ratios of dental pulp size were calculated; pulp/root length, pulp/tooth length, tooth/root length and pulp/root width at three different levels within the tooth. The technique showed considerable promise and it was concluded that measurements on dental radiographs are a non-invasive technique for estimating the age of adults both living and dead in both forensic work and archaeological studies, but cautioned that the method should be tested on independent samples.

Ageing from cemental annulations

It has been known for some time that age at death may be determined by studying cemental annulations in carnivores, in ungulates and in rodents and lagomorphs.[42] Both ground and demineralized sections of monkey material have been studied,[43] and it was concluded that the age of primates could be determined accurately using growth layers in cementum (Figure 4). Similar results were obtained on *Macaca mulatta*[44] and some regard the technique as being the most accurate method for ageing adult primates that has yet been tested. It is

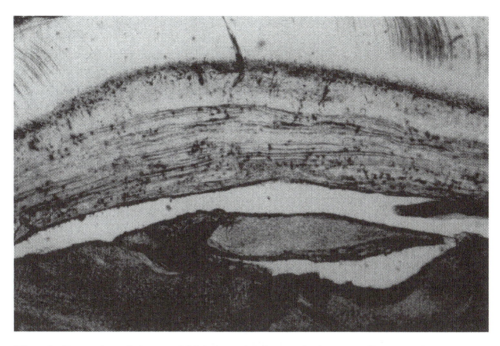

Figure 4 – Cemental annulations are visible in ground or demineralized sections of human teeth.

perhaps not remarkable that in animals that hibernate or exist in an environment and dietary situation, which changes in relation to the seasons, annulations in cementum may be related to the passage of the years. It is difficult however to postulate that a similar situation might occur in humans. Using teeth from only three cadavers it has been claimed that the annulation count of cementum was a means of determining the age of the body.[45] Using a sample of 42 human mandibular canines and first premolar pairs of teeth and using both demineralized and stained mineralized sections[46] it was claimed that, providing several sections are examined per tooth, the cementum ring counts are measurable to a highly repeatable extent. The method provided a level of age estimation which was repeatably more accurate than that reported for the pubic symphysis or auricular surface ageing techniques. The method was evaluated in 80 clinically extracted premolars using demineralized haematoxylin stained sections.[47] The claimed correlation with age was $r = 0.78$ for the entire sample and $r = 0.86$ for a subsample where periodontal disease was excluded. It was concluded that the hypothesis of annual deposition of cemental rings may be useful in determining age of human material. Support for this view came from a study using 31 teeth of known age and using demineralized sections.[48] A correlation was claimed between the number of cemental lines and age and it was suggested that given a large enough specimen size a computer generated formula for age prediction might be possible.

Other investigators have taken contrary views. Using 100 extracted human teeth and ground undemineralized sections, simple regression analysis of the data indicated that determining chronological age in man from cemental annulations is not possible.[49] However, a recent paper by Stein and Corcoran using non-demineralized sections from teeth extracted from 42 patients[50] showed high correlation coefficients between the patients' predicted age using cementum annulations and their actual age. However, this became less accurate in persons older than 55 years. A recent report[51] using demineralized sections, indicated that the correlation coefficient between counted lines and age was as high as 0.84. It was suggested that the method be used only in individuals of more than 50 years of age.

Biochemical methods of age determination

In both forensic and archaeological situations, methods of age estimation using attrition, or changes in dentine, pulp chamber or cementum can only be approximate. Attempts have been made to define changes in tissues that are true indicators of increasing age. One of the early attempts measured calcium and phosphorus weight concentrations as well as their ratio. They were determined by electron probe microanalysis both in intra- and inter-tubular dentine from 25 adults of varying age.[52] A close correlation was shown with both calcium and phosphate weight ratios of the teeth and age, and it was claimed that this would allow individual age determination to be performed in both forensic and palaeoanthropological studies. It is important that further studies of this nature are carried out to confirm this hypothesis.

A more useful approach, which has been developed since 1970, is based on amino acid racemization. It is dependent upon the fact that protein bound amino acids have a three-dimensional configuration which is called by convention the left-handed enantiomer. These L-amino acids are exclusively used by animals and plants during biosynthesis of proteins and once they are bonded into structures such as teeth or the cornea, which have very little biological turnover, the amino acids begin to rotate by a process known as racemization. Eventually the tissues would be composed of 50% L-enantiomers and 50% D-enantiomers. The rate of this racemization is accurately known and is highly temperature-dependent.

The first studies on human teeth appear to have been those carried out by Bada and Brown[53] who pointed out that calculations result in the determination of the age of the tooth as distinct from the age of the individual. The developmental age of the teeth therefore need to be added to the racemization date to age the individual. The method has been applied to teeth from various animals but has also been studied in man[54] where it was demonstrated that amino acids removed from primary dentine gave a more accurate representation of age than did those from secondary dentine which behaved in an irregular manner.

Errors resulting from various experimental conditions have been assessed.[55] These included the sample weight, time and temperature of hydrolysis, concentration of hydrochloric acid to remove the amino acids and other chemical parameters. It was found that the temperature of hydrolysis was the most influential and that alteration of values of other factors did not largely affect the estimation of age. This study was carried out on teeth from recently deceased individuals. The same investigators considered aspartic acid extracted from enamel and dentine in the same tooth and reconfirmed that dentine is superior to enamel in making accurate age estimations from the teeth.[56] Not only total amino acids but their fractionated substances such as insoluble collagen and soluble peptide have been tested. It was concluded that the use of total amino acids can lead to a higher reliability in age estimation.[57] Workers in this field have compared the utilization of aspartic acid, glutamic acid and alanine in similar studies and have concluded that glutamic acid and alanine gave considerably slower racemization velocities when compared with aspartic acid.[58] Most of the measurements of L- and D-aspartic acid ratios have been carried out using gas chromatography or amino acid analysers, but more recently high-performance liquid chromatography has been employed with satisfactory results.[59,60] The same technique has been applied to human cementum, which appears to remain stable throughout the life of the individual,[61] and has also been demonstrated in a case of pink teeth, which is a phenomenon caused by breakdown products of the pulp in certain forensic cases.[62]

It was pointed out in the early days[63] that post-mortem conditions can be crucial to the accuracy of racemization age at death measurements. One specimen studied had been subjected to 51 days of open-air exposure and exhibited a vastly inflated racemization age. Another study on post-mortem change, even in the absence of adipocere formation, gave an estimate of age within 2 years of the age of the individual.[64] In spite of this the only study carried out on a true archaeological population concluded that on fresh material age determinations at death could reliably be made to within ± 4 years in modern forensic teeth, but those obtained from archaeological material gave much less reliable results.[59] Further investigations have attempted to study some of the post-mortem changes affecting accuracy of racemization studies but these are still in progress.[65]

While racemization studies, particularly using amino acids are capable of highly accurate determinations of age at death in contemporary recently dead material, there are further studies required before this technique may be reliably employed in archaeological investigations. Even then, the method may be useful only when burial conditions are of a particular type and where calculations can be made to determine the rate of racemization likely to have occurred since death.

THE PRESENT POSITION

Human teeth are the least destructible part of the body. They develop sequentially from the midline posteriorly but also within the structure of a single tooth and they have a minimal biological turnover, ensuring that information contained within them remains to be accessed. It is no small wonder that teeth have been studied in relation to ageing phenomena for most of this century. In the first two decades of life it has proved possible to relate the sequence of development of the dentition with reasonable accuracy to the biological age of the individual. However, it is becoming apparent that there are considerable variations of a racial nature and also in relation to earlier maturity as general health improves. Extrapolation from contemporary data to archaeological material must therefore be exercized with caution even in the first two decades of life.

From the early 20s until death the problem of ageing of skeletal material even in forensic situations becomes much more difficult. Attempts have been made in recent years to apply modern forensic techniques to the archaeological situation but great caution still needs to be exercized in interpreting such data. In adult forensic material the age at death cannot reliably be estimated to closer than the nearest 15 years using attrition rates, and even then only when juveniles can be used as a rate of wear standard. Measurements of apical translucency (RDT) can be expected in experienced hands to produce estimates within ± 7 years and racemization studies may, in ideal circumstances, be within ± 3 years. Unfortunately data for archaeological material are not well tested against known age. Where quasi-historical material of known age has been studied,[13] attrition rates on molar teeth should be capable of yielding estimates within ± 3 years, but it is generally agreed that in actual archaeological material attrition studies are less reliable than methods using RDT.

Using RDT and image analysis Sengupta *et al.*[34] found that if taphonomically changed teeth were excluded, estimates of age were only accurate in 27% of cases. However, there is evidence that assessment of RDT using microscopic examination by an experienced operator can yield accuracies of ± 8 years in those individual archaeological cases where age at death is known from other sources, although this opinion is based on a very small sample. Racemization techniques in ancient teeth yielded disappointing results[59] of ± 24 years at the 95% confidence level. It appears, therefore, that RDT measurements analysed by an experienced observer are the most accurate method of determining age at death from archaeologically derived material.

It is important that known individuals with an historical background, which can be verified in other ways from the historical record, be examined using such methodologies as are available. Only in this way will further information gradually accrue which will enable us to solve the problems of age determination in ancient populations and to be comfortable that taphonomic and diagenetic effects have been given due allowance.

REFERENCES

1   Kraus BS, Jordan RE. *The Human Dentition Before Birth*. Philadelphia: Lea & Febiger, 1965.

2   Webber DF, Eisenmann DR. Microscopy of the neonatal line in developing human enamel. *American Journal of Anatomy* 1971; **132**: 375–391.

3   Whittaker DK, Richards D. Scanning electron microscopy of the neonatal line in human enamel. *Archives of Oral Biology* 1978; **23**: 45–50.

4   Schour I, Massler M. The development of the human dentition. *Journal of the American Dental Association* 1941; **20**: 379–427.

5   Gustafson G. *Forensic Odontology*. London: Staples, 1966.

6   Moorees CFA, Fanning EA, Hunt EE. Age variation of formation stages for ten permanent teeth. *Journal of Dental Research* 1963; **42**: 264–273.

7   Ciaparelli L. In: Clark DH (ed.), *Practical Forensic Odontology*. Oxford: Wright, 1992; pp. 22–42.

8   Kullman L, Johanson G, Akesson L. Root development of the lower third molar and its relation to chronological age. *Swedish Dental Journal* 1992; **16**: 161–167.

9   Dermirjian A, Goldstein H, Tanner JM. A new system of dental age assessment. *Human Biology* 1978; **45**: 211–217.

10 Gustafson G. Age determination on teeth. *Journal of the American Dental Association* 1950; **41**: 45–54.

11 Brothwell DR. *Digging Up Bones* (2nd edn). London: British Museum, 1972; pp. 67–70.

12 Miles AEW. The dentition in the assessment of individual age in skeletal material. In: DR Brothwell (ed.), *Dental Anthropology*. Oxford: Pergamon, 1963; pp. 191–209.

13 Kieser JA, Preston CB, Evans WG. Skeletal age at death: an evaluation of the Miles method of ageing. *Journal of Archaeological Science* 1983; **10**: 9–12.

14 Helm S, Prydso U. Assessment of age at death from mandibular molar attrition in medieval Danes. *Scandinavian Journal of Dental Research* 1979; **87**: 79–90.

15 Song HW, Jia JT. The estimation of tooth age from attrition of the occlusal surface. *Medicine, Science and the Law* 1989; **29**: 69–73.

16 Santini A, Land M, Raab GM. The accuracy of simple ordinal scoring of tooth attrition in age assessment. *Forensic Science International* 1990; **48**: 175–184.

17 Solheim T, Sundnes PK. Dental age estimation of Norwegian adults – a comparison of different methods. *Forensic Science International* 1980; **16**: 7–17.

18 Maples WR, Rice PM. Some difficulties in the Gustafson dental age estimations. *Journal of Forensic Science* 1979; **24**: 168–172.

19 Solheim T. Recession of periodontal ligament as an indicator of age. *Journal of Forensic Odonto-Stomatology* 1992; **10**: 32–42.

20 Solheim T. Dental age estimation. An alternative technique for tooth sectioning. *American Journal of Forensic Medicine and Pathology* 1984; **5**: 181–184.

21 Bang G, Ramm E. Determination of age in humans from root dentine transparency. *Acta Odontologica Scandinavica* 1970; **28**: 3–35.

22 Dalitz GD. Age determination of adult human remains by teeth examination. *Journal of Forensic Science Society* 1963; **3**: 11–21.

23 Metzger Z, Buchner A, Gorsky M. Gustafson's method for age determination from teeth – a modification for the use of dentists in identification teams. *Journal of Forensic Science* 1980; **25**: 742–749.

24 Johnson CC. Transparent dentine in age estimation. *Oral Surgery, Oral Medicine and Oral Pathology* 1968; **25**: 834–838.

25 Lorentsen M, Solheim T. Age assessment based on translucent dentine. *Journal of Forensic Odonto-Stomatology* 1989; **7**: 3–9.

26 Solheim T. Dental root translucency as an indicator of age. *Scandinavian Journal of Dental Research* 1989; **97**: 189–197.

27 Drusini A, Volpe A, Dovigo S. Age determination in human adults by dental histology. *Zeitschrift für Morphologie und Anthropologie* 1990; **78**: 169–174.

28 Lopez-Nicolas M, Canteras M, Luna A. Age estimation by IBAS image analysis of teeth. *Forensic Science International* 1990; **45**: 143–150.

29 Lamendin H, Baccino E, Humbert JF, Tavernier JC, Zerilli A. A simple technique for age estimation in adult corpses: the two criteria dental method. *Journal of Forensic Science* 1992; **37**:1373–1379.

30 Furseth R. The structure of peripheral root dentine in young human premolars. *Scandinavian Journal of Dental Research* 1974; **82**: 557–561.

31 Holland GR. An ultrastructural survey of cat dentinal tubules. *Journal of Anatomy* 1976; **122**: 1–13.

32 Thomas GJ, Whittaker DK, Embery G. A comparative study of translucent apical dentine in vital and non-vital human teeth. *Archives of Oral Biology* 1994; **39**: 29–34.

33 Whittaker DK, Bakri MM. Racial variations in the extent of tooth root translucency in ageing individuals. *Archives of Oral Biology* 1996; **41**: 15–19.

34 Sengupta A, Whittaker DK, Shellis P. Differences in estimating age using root dentine translucency in human teeth of varying antiquities. *Archives of Oral Biology* (in press).

35 Garberoglio R, Brannstrom M. Scanning electron microscopic investigation of human dentinal tubules. *Archives of Oral Biology* 1976; **21**: 355–356.

36 Whittaker DK, Kneale MJ. The dentine–predentine interface in human teeth. A scanning electron microscope study. *British Dental Journal* 1979; **146**: 43–46.

37 Lopez-Nicolas M, Morales A, Luna A. Morphometric study of teeth in age calculation. *Journal of Forensic Odonto-Stomatology* 1993; **11**: 1–8.

38 Lampe H, Roetzscher K. Forensic odontology: age determination from adult human teeth. *Medicine and Law* 1994; **13**: 623–628.

39 Solheim T. Amount of secondary dentin as an indicator of age. *Scandinavian Journal of Dental Research* 1992; **100**: 193–199.

40 Morse DR, Esposito JV, Schoor RS. A radiographic study of ageing changes of the dental pulp and dentine in normal teeth. *Quintessence International* 1993; **24**: 329–333.

41 Kvaal SI, Kolltveit KM, Thomsen IO, Solheim T. Age estimation of adults from dental radiographs. *Forensic Science International* 1995; **74**: 175–185.

42 Sergeant DE, Pimlott DH. Age determination in moose from sectioned incisor teeth. *Journal of Wildlife Management* 1959; **23**: 315–321.

43 Wada K, Ohtani N, Hachiya N. Determination of age in the Japanese monkey from growth layers in the dental cementum. *Primates* 1978; **19**: 775–784.

44 Kay RF, Rasmussen DT, Beard KC. Cementum annulus counts provide a means for age determination in *Macaca mulatta* (primates anthropoidea). *Folia Primatologica* 1984; **42**: 85–95.

45 Stott GG, Sis RF, Levy BM. Cemental annulation as an age criterion in forensic dentistry. *Journal of Dental Research* 1982; **61**: 814–817.

46 Charles DK, Condon K, Cheverud JM, Buikstra JE. Cementum annulation and age determination in *Homo sapiens*. I. Tooth variability and observer error. *American Journal of Physical Anthropology* 1986; **71**: 311–320.

47 Condon K, Charles DK, Cheverud JM, Buikstra JE. Cementum annulation and age determination in *Homo sapiens*. II. Estimates and accuracy. *American Journal of Physical Anthropology* 1986; **71**: 321–330.

48 Lipsinic FE, Paunovich E, Houston GD, Robison SF. Correlation of age and incremental lines in the cementum of human teeth. *Journal of Forensic Science* 1986; **31**: 982–989.

49 Miller CS, Dove SB, Cottone JA. Failure of use of cemental annulations in teeth to determine the age of humans. *Journal of Forensic Science* 1988; **33**: 137–143.

50 Stein TJ, Corcoran JF. Pararadicular cementum deposition as a criterion for age estimation in human beings. *Oral Surgery, Oral Medicine and Oral Pathology* 1994; **77**: 266–270.

51 Kvaal SI, Solheim T. Incremental lines in human dental cementum in relation to age. *European Journal of Oral Sciences* 1995; **103**: 225–230.

52 Kosa F, Antal A, Farkas I. Electron probe microanalysis of human teeth for the determination of individual age. *Medicine, Science and the Law* 1990; **30**: 109–114.

53 Bada JL, Brown SE. Amino acid racemisation in living animals: biochronological applications. *Trends in Biochemical Sciences* 1980; **5**: 1–3.

54 Saleh N, Deutsch D, Gil-Au E. Racemisation of aspartic acid in the extracellular matrix proteins of primary and secondary dentine. *Calcified Tissue International* 1993; **53**: 103–110.

55 Ohtani S, Yamamoto K. Estimation of ages from racemisation of an amino acid in teeth – assessment of errors under various experimental conditions. *Japanese Journal of Legal Medicine* 1991; **45**: 124–127.

56 Ohtani S, Yamamoto K. Estimation of age from a tooth by means of racemisation of an amino acid, especially aspartic acid – comparison of enamel and dentin. *Journal of Forensic Science* 1992; **37**: 1061–1067.

57 Marumo T. Age estimation by amino acid racemisation in dentine – application of fractionation and extraction. *Kanagawa Shigaku* 1989; **24**: 290–300.

58 Ohtani S, Yamamoto K. Age estimation by amino acid racemisation in teeth – a comparison of aspartic acid with glutamic acid and alanine as indicators. *Japanese Journal of Legal Medicine* 1991; **45**: 119–123.

59 Gillard RD, Hardman SM, Pollard AM, Sutton PA, Whittaker DK. Determinations of age at death in archaeological populations using the D/L ratio of aspartic acid in dental collagen. *Archaeometry* 1990; **90**: 637–644.

60 Mornstad H, Pfeiffer H, Teivens A. Estimation of dental age using HPLC-technique to determine the degree of aspartic acid racemisation. *Journal of Forensic Science* 1994; **39**: 1425–1431.

61 Ohtani S. Studies on age estimation using racemisation of aspartic acid in cementum. *Journal of Forensic Science* 1995; **40**: 805–807.

62   Ohtani S, Yamada Y, Yamamoto I. Improvement of age estimation using amino acid racemisation in a case of pink teeth. *American Journal of Forensic Medicine and Pathology* 1998; **19**: 77–79.

63   Masters PM. Age at death determinations for autopsied remains based on aspartic acid racemisation in tooth dentine: importance of postmortem conditions. *Forensic Science International* 1986; **32**: 179–184.

64   Ohtani S, Utsunomiya J, Minoshima T, Yamamoto K. Tooth based age estimation of an adipocerated cadaver using the amino acid racemisation method. *Japanese Journal of Legal Medicine* 1994; **48**: 279–281.

65   Child AM, Gillard RD, Hardman SM, Pollard AM, Sutton PA, Whittaker DK. Preliminary microbiological investigations of some problems relating to age at death determinations in archaeological teeth. *Proceedings of the Australian Archaeometry Conference* 1991; **1**: 312 abstracts.

7

PROBLEMS AND PROSPECTS IN PALAEODEMOGRAPHY

Andrew Chamberlain

INTRODUCTION

Demography is the study of the structure and dynamics of populations, and *palaeodemography* is distinguished from 'regular' demography only in that the populations under study are those of the past rather than the present day. Demography considers the population as a singular object for quantitative analysis, and seeks to explain variations in population size, population density, age and sex structure, mortality, fertility and migration. Dynamic changes in populations (temporal changes in population size and/or structure) can be complex because they depend on the separate but interacting factors of fertility, mortality and migration. In all populations these factors vary substantially across age and sex categories, and they also themselves change over time.

There are theoretical and methodological reasons why archaeologists and anthropologists have taken a close interest in palaeodemography. Qualitative demographic models have frequently played an important role in theoretical archaeology, and demographic processes such as population growth and migration have been invoked as causative agents of cultural change, especially by advocates of the 'New Archaeology' in the 1960s and 1970s.[1-3] Among many other examples, population growth has been implicated as a primary factor in the replacement of Neanderthals (*Homo neanderthalensis*) by anatomically modern *H. sapiens*,[4] in the peopling of the Americas in the late Pleistocene[5] and in the wave of advance model for the spread of agriculture in the European Neolithic.[6] Migration, encompassing both the deliberate and wholesale translocation of communities as well as the gradual colonization of marginal territory as a passive consequence of population growth, is in itself a perennial and often controversial issue for debate in archaeology.[7-9] On the methodological front, it has been emphasized that it is samples and populations, not individuals, that are the proper subject for biological anthropologists to study.[10] This leads the investigator inevitably to a consideration of the determinants of population structure and population history.

Despite the recognized importance of the topic, there is no quick and easy route by which population size and structure can be inferred from archaeological data. A multitude of confounding factors, including the differential deposition, preservation and recovery of skeletal remains, conspire to render osteological samples incomplete and unrepresentative, while indirect evidence for population numbers such as settlement size and measures of resource availability are open to a variety of conflicting interpretations. In addition to these problems of data quality (which are encountered in many other archaeological datasets) palaeodemography has had to grapple with its own special methodological problems. In particular, problems include the imprecision and inaccuracy of age estimation methods (see Cox, chapter 5, in this volume) and the sometimes questionable practice of applying stable and stationary demographic models to past populations.

The purpose here is to outline some quantitative methods and developing new approaches that are particularly appropriate to the study of archaeological samples of human skeletal remains. It is sometimes claimed that palaeodemographic analysis of skeletal samples is 'futile',[11] or that it can only be undertaken on large and unbiased samples,[12] or that palaeodemography makes unrealistic assumptions about population stability.[13] None of these caveats is necessarily true, and it is important that archaeologists and skeletal biologists are not discouraged from attempting to draw careful demographic inferences from such evidence as is available for study.

MODEL LIFE TABLES AND REAL POPULATIONS

At its simplest, a closed population (closed, that is, to immigration and emigration of living individuals) is augmented by new births and depleted by new deaths. The actual numbers of births and deaths occurring in a given interval of time depend on four parameters: the age-specific fertility and age-specific mortality schedules for the population, the age structure of the population, and the overall size of the population. Although fertility, and to a lesser extent mortality, are partly determined by individual behaviour, in practice individual reproductive decisions and exposure to risk of mortality are distributed around stable central tendencies and each population tends to exhibit constant or slowly changing fertility and mortality. If age-specific fertility and mortality remain constant, the population will converge within a few generations (typically 50–100 years, for human populations) on a stable age structure.[14] Thus, any given closed population will show in its age structure the cumulative effects of up to a century of intrinsic demographic events. Stable populations are idealized constructs because no real population maintains unchanging fertility and mortality schedules for long periods (and few real-life populations are truly closed to migration). However, pre-industrial human populations may approximate stable populations, as the rapid and permanent changes in fertility and mortality rates associated with demographic transitions appear to be a recent historical phenomenon.[15]

As the assumption of stable age structure has been highlighted as a major weakness of palaeodemographic analysis,[11,13] it is useful to examine demographic data from accurately censused hunter-gatherer and farming populations to see whether they diverge from the model life table schedules that summarize the mortality experience of typical or ideal populations. The most widely used model life tables are those compiled by the Office of Population Research at Princeton University.[16] These regional tables are based on over 300 censused populations, mainly from developed countries and with an emphasis on European populations. The tables are grouped into four series, designated 'North', 'South', 'East' and 'West', to indicate the areas within Europe where the different mortality patterns are typically found. The average mortality pattern, and the one which is most widely and frequently used in human palaeodemography, is given by the 'West' series of model life tables. These are thought to give the most reliable results at the high levels of mortality that characterize present day populations in some developing countries.[16] The Princeton model life tables are organized according to differing levels of female life expectancy at birth, with the lowest life expectancy set at 20 years (Level 1) and the highest at 80 years (Level 25). Each increment in level corresponds to an increase in female life expectancy at birth of 2.5 years. Most of the differences between the mortality levels are accounted for by variation in infant and childhood mortality.

Figure 1 illustrates survivorship curves calculated from demographic data for four hunter-gatherer populations, compared with Princeton model life table populations with low and moderate life expectancies at birth (respectively these are 'West' Level 3, e_0 = 25 years, and 'West' Level 15, e_0 = 55 years).

Figure 2 provides similar comparisons for four modern pre-industrial and predominantly rural populations. Although the mortality is on average higher (and hence survivorship is lower) in the modern pre-industrial populations, all of the curves lie within the upper and lower bounds provided by the model life table survivorship curves. These kinds of comparisons between 'real' and model life table demographic data indicate that the regular patterns

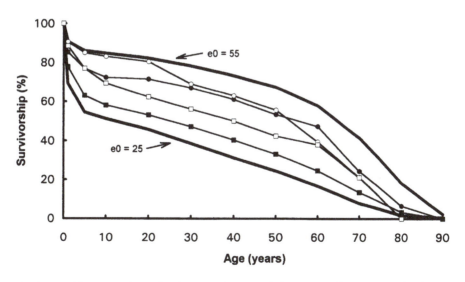

Figure 1 – Age-specific survivorship in four hunter-gatherer populations (narrow lines) compared with survivorship in two of the Princeton 'West' model stable populations (broad lines). The model populations have low life expectancy at birth, e_0 = 25 years, and moderate life expectancy at birth, e_0 = 55 years. From top downwards the hunter gatherer populations are the Yanomamo (open circles), !Kung (filled circles), Ache (open squares) and Hadza (filled squares).

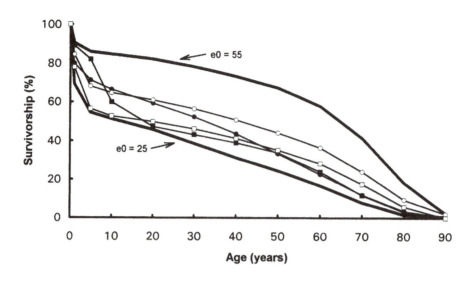

Figure 2 – Age-specific survivorship in four modern pre-industrial populations compared with survivorship in model life table populations. From top downwards the pre-industrial populations are 18th-century Carlisle, England (open circles), early 20th-century Ceylon (filled circles), 18th-century Japan (open squares) and 16th-century Devon, England (filled squares). The model populations (broad lines) are the same as in Figure 1.

of age-specific mortality that have been incorporated in the Princeton model life tables are representative of the mortality experience of a broad range of populations in different continents and practising very different subsistence strategies.

BIAS IN SAMPLES AND METHODS

Biases in demographic data from archaeological samples can be detected by the method of 'pattern matching', an approach analogous to that outlined above in which the distributions of demographic data in different populations or population samples are compared. Thus, archaeological data can be compared with model life table mortality schedules to reveal discrepancies between the demographic structures of the archaeological samples and the reference populations.[17,18] This technique requires a uniformitarian assumption that the age structure of the archaeological population must have originally resembled that of one of the model stable populations. As seen above, there are strong grounds for reasoning that human populations in the past had similar age structures to those documented in the present day.

A major potential source of bias in palaeodemographic data is the under-representation of the youngest age classes, which is a feature of some assemblages of human skeletal remains from archaeological contexts. The shortfall in numbers of children, particularly infants and young children, can occur even when large samples of skeletons are recovered from the cemeteries of communities in which deceased individuals of all ages are expected to have received normative funerary rites.[19,20] Depending on the precise circumstances of burial at particular sites, the skeletal remains of infants and children may have a lower preservation potential (children's skeletons are smaller, their bones are less resistant to physical damage and bioturbation, and their graves are more easily disturbed or truncated) and a lower likelihood of recovery (children's remains are less easily recognized, they may have less elaborate graves, and they may be overlooked when commingled with the remains of adults).[21] The pattern of under-representation of infants in archaeological assemblages is not confined to human examples; archaeozoological samples of the skeletal remains of wild and domestic mammals may also show lower than expected numbers in the youngest age classes.[22]

Another very common but subtle bias has emerged from comparing adult mortality in archaeological samples with the mortality observed in historically documented populations and with the patterns of mortality in model stable populations. Archaeological samples that have been aged using skeletal morphological indicators often show a peak of mortality in the young and middle adult years, usually in the interval between 30 and 45 years (Figure 3b). This pattern, which is often accompanied by an absence of, or at least very few, individuals aged > 60 years, is seen in analyses of skeletal samples from all regions of the world, from prehistoric through to modern times, but is not found in model life tables or in historical demographic data (Figure 3a). The source of this 'middle-aged spread' appears to lie in the systematic bias towards under-ageing adults that is a feature of some anthropological methods for estimating adult age at death from skeletal indicators (see below).

PROBLEMS IN AGE ESTIMATION

Accurate and unbiased estimation of sex and age at death are, of course, a prerequisite for successful palaeodemographic reconstruction.[11] Age at death can be estimated with varying degrees of reliability by observing the state of one or more morphological indicators that tend to fall within a chronological age range. From this an estimate of age with its associated range of error can be derived from the state of the morphological indicator. Age estimation methods that are applicable to juvenile and adult skeletons are discussed elsewhere (see Scheuer and Black, chapter 2; Cox, chapter 5; and Whittaker, chapter 6, in this volume). The quantitative relationship between age and morphological indicator is usually determined using a reference series consisting of identified individuals each of whose age at death and indicator state is either known or assessed from a range of other biological criteria. By means of a uniformitarian assumption (that the underlying biological basis of the age/indicator relationship is constant across samples and populations) the age of any unknown or target individual can then be estimated from observations of its morphological indicator. Where the age/indicator relationship varies among samples, for example between male and female skeletons, or between samples from different geographical regions, then ideally, sample-specific ageing methods should be developed.

Much of the incentive to develop methods of determining age at death from the skeleton has come from the requirements of forensic anthropology,[23,24] and workers have tended to apply these methods to archaeological material without adapting them to the special circumstances of palaeodemography. First, in reconstructing the age distribution of an archaeological sample the palaeodemographer is not primarily interested in accurate age

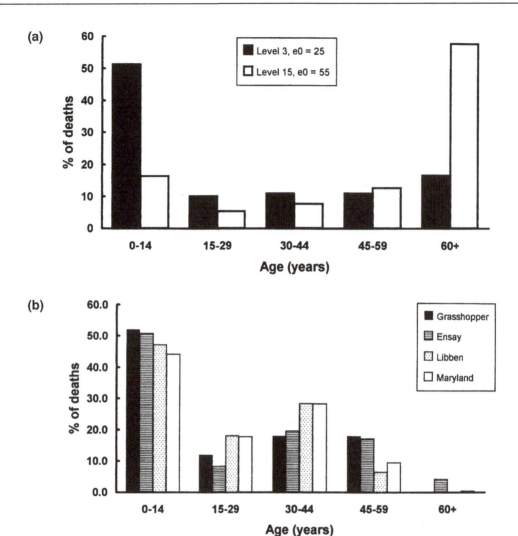

Figure 3 – (a) Age-specific mortality aggregated in 15-year age categories for model stable populations with low life expectancy at birth, $e_0 = 25$ years, and moderate life expectancy at birth, $e_0 = 55$ years. (b) Age-specific mortality in archaeological samples calculated from skeletal indicators of age at death. The skeletal samples are from Grasshopper Pueblo, a prehistoric cemetery in the American Southwest; Libben, a prehistoric cemetery in the Great Lakes region of America; Late Woodland period ossuaries in Maryland; and Ensay, a post-medieval rural cemetery in Scotland. All archaeological samples differ from the model life table populations (a) in showing an apparent peak of mortality in the early and middle adult years, rather than in the oldest age category (especially noticeable in the Libben and Maryland samples). This pattern of mortality has not been found in any historically documented population, and is attributable instead to systematic bias in skeletal estimation of adult age at death.

estimates for target individuals, but intends instead to recover the *distribution* of ages that is responsible for the spread of indicator data observed in the study sample.[25–27] This differs from the objective of a forensic investigation, in which regression or calibration techniques are used to obtain the best point estimate of the age of a single target individual. A second problem with traditional methods of age estimation in palaeodemography is that the resultant age estimates are frequently affected by the age structure of the reference sample.[11,28–30] Known-age skeletal reference series have been assembled using different protocols, including the aggregation of data from medical examiners' autopsies (e.g. the Suchey–Brooks pubic symphysis ageing system[31] and the Iscan/Loth sternal rib-end system[32]), bodies available for anatomical dissection (e.g. the Todd and the Terry skeletal collections[33]) and cemetery samples with historical records of age at death (e.g. Christ Church, Spitalfields, London[34] and St Thomas' Church, Belleville, Ontario[35]). The ages at death among medical examiners' autopsy cases can be dominated by large numbers of young adults, whereas the dissecting room samples have adult deaths that are concentrated in the older age categories.[31]

The following section outlines a Bayesian approach[36] to palaeodemographic age estimation that is simple yet effective in removing the influence of the age structure of the skeletal reference population.

BAYESIAN ESTIMATION METHODS IN PALAEODEMOGRAPHY

The influence of the age structure of the reference series on the estimation of age from skeletal samples can be eliminated by using Bayesian statistical methods.[28–30] A strict implementation of Bayesian methods for *continuous* data would require the use of advanced techniques of numerical analysis,[36] but for ordinal-scale age categories and skeletal age indicators divided into discrete states (which are the norm in biological anthropology) the Bayesian approach becomes simple and straightforward.

Applying Bayes' theorem, the posterior probability of the individual belonging to a specific age category 'A', given the state of the individual's skeletal indicator 'I', is equal to the prior probability of age multiplied by the standardized likelihood of the skeletal indicator:

$$p(A|I) = \frac{p(I|A)}{p(I)} \times p_{prior}(A)$$

where $p(I|A)$ is the conditional probability of I, given A. $p(I)$ = sum of $[p(I|A) \times p_{prior}(A)]$ across all categories of A, and $p_{prior}(A)$ is the prior probability of age category A.

In other words, the probability of being in a particular age category A, given a particular state of the indicator I, is equal to the conditional probability of possessing that indicator state, given the age category, divided by the overall probability of possessing the indicator state, multiplied by the prior probability of being in the age category. Crucial to this approach is the selection of appropriate prior probabilities ('priors') for each age category $[p_{prior}(A)]$, and here there are several options. The use of the reference series as a source of priors can usually be ruled out for the reasons given above (reference series rarely exhibit unbiased age distributions because they are usually constructed by 'availability' sampling). Similarly, the approach advocated by Konigsberg and Frankenberg,[27] in which the priors are obtained iteratively from the distribution of indicator states in the archaeological sample (the 'target' series) by an expectation-maximization algorithm, cannot be recommended. While Konigsberg and Frankenberg's method is an effective way of removing the biasing effects of reference series age structure, it is computationally difficult, and it relies on the target series being an unbiased sample of its parent population. Age estimates obtained by their method cannot, therefore, be used in a pattern-matching exercise to detect and quantify sampling bias in the target series.

The remaining options are to assume a uniform prior probability of age (sometimes called an 'uninformative prior'[27]) or to select fixed model priors based on age-at-death distributions taken from a family of stable populations (such as the Princeton model life tables) or from ethnographic or historical demographic sources. Uninformative priors are appropriate in sex estimation, where the default presumption is that deaths are derived from approximately balanced sex populations, but are often inappropriate in age estimation. Most populations exhibit a large variance in age-specific probability of death, with the result that certain age categories, for example the youngest and the oldest, are more frequently represented in natural mortuary assemblages.

The implementation of Bayesian age estimation for adult skeletal remains is illustrated below using data originally collected by Suchey and Brooks on the age-related morphological changes at the pubic symphysis. Table 1 gives the age-specific distribution of six morphological stages of the pubic symphysis in a reference series of 273 females whose age was documented from birth and death certificates.[31,37] This data set, together with a corresponding data set from 739 male pubic symphyses forms the reference series on which the widely used Suchey–Brooks system of age determination is based. The reference series was obtained from routine autopsies conducted during the late 1970s in Los Angeles. It comprises a diverse sample of individuals from a range of ethnic and socio-economic backgrounds, but the age distribution of the sample is biased towards young adults. This age bias is present because the individuals in the reference series died from homicide, suicide, accident and unexpected natural death, which are the only circumstances under which the

Table 1 – Numbers of individuals according to age (10-year categories) and pubic symphyseal stage in a reference series of 273 adult females. Data are from Brooks and Suchey.[37]

Age (years)	Stage I	Stage II	Stage III	Stage IV	Stage V	Stage VI	Row totals
15–24	47	26	10	0	0	0	83
25–34	1	18	26	17	7	0	69
35–44	0	3	5	14	13	4	39
45–54	0	0	2	4	11	13	30
55–64	0	0	1	2	8	19	30
65–74	0	0	0	2	1	10	13
75–84	0	0	0	0	3	2	5
85–94	0	0	0	0	1	3	4
Column totals	48	47	44	39	44	51	273

performance of a medical examiner's autopsy was mandated. The proportion of adolescents/young adults in the female reference series (those aged 15–34 years, encompassing the first two age categories) is 56%. This figure is considerably higher than the expected proportions of 33% aged 15–34 years if the sample had the age structure of a high-mortality model life table ('West' model, Level 1: $e_0 = 20$), or 25% under the assumption of uniform prior probability of age at death, or 12% for a medium mortality model life table ('West' model, Level 13: $e_0 = 50$).

The contingency table of age versus indicator state was converted into tables of posterior probabilities for the assignment of ages to target individuals using four separate sets of prior probabilities of age (Table 2). The priors chosen were: (1) 'Reference priors', taken from the age distribution of the Suchey–Brooks reference series; (2) 'Uniform priors', in which each of the eight age categories was assigned an equal prior probability of 0.125; and (3) and (4) 'Model priors', taken respectively from the age structures of the Level 1 ($e_0 = 20$) and Level 13 ($e_0 = 50$) 'West' model life tables for females.[16] The methods of calculating the posterior probabilities of age directly from the contingency table (Table 1) are as follows: (*cell* = contents of cell in contingency table; *column* = column total; *row* = row total; Σ = sum down column; $p_{prior}(A_{20})$ = fixed age-specific prior probability from model life table with e_0 = 20; $p_{prior}(A_{50})$ = fixed age-specific prior probability from model life table with e_0 = 50).

	Method	Calculation
1	Reference Prior	$p(A|I)$ = cell/column
2	Uniform Prior	$p(A|I)$ = (cell/row)/Σ(cell/row)
3	Model Prior ($e_0 = 20$)	$p(A|I) = p_{prior}(A_{20}) \times$ (cell/row)/$\Sigma(p_{prior}(A_{20}) \times$ cell/row)
4	Model Prior ($e_0 = 50$)	$p(A|I) = p_{prior}(A_{50}) \times$ (cell/row)/$\Sigma(p_{prior}(A_{50}) \times$ cell/row)

Table 3 lists the posterior probabilities of age, given pubic symphysis stage, for each of the four sets of priors (reference priors, uniform priors, and model priors with $e_0 = 20$ and 50). Each posterior probability table provides, for the six separate skeletal indicator states, probability density functions that can be used to assign ages to unknown or target individuals.

Table 2 – Prior probabilities of age corresponding to different population mortality structures. Reference priors are from the age structure of the Suchey–Brooks pubic symphysis reference series; uniform priors assign equal prior probabilities to each age category; model priors assign prior probabilities of age according to the mortality distributions documented in model life tables for adult females.[16]

Age (years)	Reference Priors	Uniform Priors	Model priors, $e_0 = 20$	Model priors, $e_0 = 50$
15–24	0.304	0.125	0.159	0.051
25–34	0.253	0.125	0.174	0.065
35–44	0.143	0.125	0.162	0.076
45–54	0.110	0.125	0.149	0.099
55–64	0.110	0.125	0.166	0.158
65–74	0.048	0.125	0.136	0.239
75–84	0.018	0.125	0.050	0.235
85–94	0.014	0.125	0.004	0.077

Table 3 – Posterior probabilities of age, given pubic symphysis stage, incorporating estimates of the prior probability of age derived from (a) the age distribution of the Suchey–Brooks reference series, (b) a uniform age distribution, (c) the mortality structures of the Level 1 ($e_0 = 20$) and (d) the Level 13 ($e_0 = 50$) 'West' model life tables for females.

(a) p(Age) given stage, reference priors.

Stage age (years)	I	II	III	IV	V	VI
15–24	0.98	0.55	0.23	0	0	0
25–34	0.02	0.38	0.59	0.44	0.16	0
35–44	0	0.06	0.11	0.36	0.30	0.08
45–54	0	0	0.05	0.10	0.25	0.25
55–64	0	0	0.02	0.05	0.18	0.37
65–74	0	0	0	0.05	0.02	0.20
75–84	0	0	0	0	0.07	0.04
85–94	0	0	0	0	0.02	0.06

(b) p(Age) given stage, uniform priors.

Stage age (years)	I	II	III	IV	V	VI
15–24	0.98	0.48	0.17	0	0	0
25–34	0.02	0.40	0.52	0.26	0.05	0
35–44	0	0.12	0.18	0.37	0.17	0.03
45–54	0	0	0.09	0.13	0.18	0.14
55–64	0	0	0.05	0.07	0.13	0.20
65–74	0	0	0	0.16	0.04	0.25
75–84	0	0	0	0	0.30	0.13
85–94	0	0	0	0	0.12	0.24

(c) p(Age) given stage, model priors ($e_0 = 20$)

Stage age (years)	I	II	III	IV	V	VI
15–24	0.98	0.46	0.16	0	0	0
25–34	0.02	0.42	0.54	0.28	0.08	0
35–44	0	0.12	0.17	0.38	0.25	0.05
45–54	0	0	0.08	0.13	0.26	0.21
55–64	0	0	0.05	0.07	0.21	0.33
65–74	0	0	0	0.14	0.05	0.33
75–84	0	0	0	0	0.14	0.06
85–94	0	0	0	0	0.01	0.01

(d) p(Age) given stage, model priors ($e_0 = 50$)

Stage age (years)	I	II	III	IV	V	VI
15–24	0.97	0.41	0.11	0	0	0
25–34	0.03	0.44	0.47	0.15	0.02	0
35–44	0	0.15	0.19	0.26	0.09	0.02
45–54	0	0	0.13	0.13	0.13	0.09
55–64	0	0	0.10	0.10	0.15	0.21
65–74	0	0	0	0.35	0.06	0.38
75–84	0	0	0	0	0.49	0.19
85–94	0	0	0	0	0.07	0.12

For example, using Table 3b in which the priors are uniform, an individual with a pubic symphysis scored as Stage II would have a probability of 0.48 of being aged 15–24 years, a probability of 0.40 of being aged 25–34 years, and a probability of 0.12 of being aged 35–44 years (note that the sum of the probabilities for each symphysis stage equals unity). In practice, in a specific palaeodemographic analysis there might be ten individuals exhibiting Stage II, in which case five individuals would be assigned to the first age category, four to the second category and one to the third category.

The different sets of prior probabilities of age have a marked influence on the posterior probabilities, particularly for the more advanced pubic symphysis stages IV–VI. Using priors from the reference series (Table 3a) there is a low probability of the individual being aged > 64 years *regardless of the pubic symphysis indicator state*, whereas the posterior probabilities that incorporate uniform and model life table priors (Tables 3b and d) assign greater probabilities to the higher age categories. The priors from the high mortality ($e_0 = 20$) model life table generate posterior probabilities of age that are close to those obtained using reference priors, reflecting the fact that the prior probabilities of age in the reference series and in the high mortality life table are weighted towards the younger age categories (Table 2).

For the first two pubic symphysis stages (Stages I and II) the choice of different priors has little effect on the posterior probabilities of age. This is because there is a narrow dispersion of ages for each of these indicator stages in the original data set (Table 1), whereas in the more advanced pubic symphysis stages the spread of ages is wider, and the effect of the choice of prior is correspondingly greater.

An example of how the posterior probabilities of age are influenced by alternative age estimation methods is shown in Figure 4.

The pubic symphyses of a sample of skeletons from the 18th/19th-century AD burial ground at the former Infirmary site in Newcastle, UK, were assessed using the standard Suchey–Brooks age estimation method, in which the mean age for the relevant pubic symphysis stage is assigned to each skeleton. This generated a peaked distribution of estimated ages at death, centred on the age category 35–44, and no individuals were aged > 64 years. By using a Bayesian method, with prior probabilities of age taken from a high mortality model life table, a broader distribution of estimated ages was obtained for the skeletal sample. For all but one of the age categories the Bayesian age estimation method provided a closer match with the known distribution of ages recorded in the burial register for this cemetery.

It is recommended that existing reference data sets for skeletal age estimation are modified for palaeodemographic purposes so as to incorporate prior probabilities of age that correspond more closely to the real (and, by inference, archaeological) world. Most archaeological populations probably had either moderate or high crude rates of mortality, and the prior probabilities of age can be based on appropriate families of model life tables. In some circumstances, however, it cannot be assumed that the skeletal assemblage derives from the effects of normal attritional mortality. For example, in cases of catastrophic mortality, which may occur in natural disasters, in genocidal mass mortality and in highly virulent epidemics (such as deaths from bubonic plague), the age structure of the skeletal assemblage will

Figure 4 – Distribution of estimated ages at death aggregated into decadal categeories in adult male skeletons from the Infirmary burial ground at Newcastle, England. The long dashed line shows the ages calculated from the morphological state of the pubic symphysis, incorporating prior probabilities of age taken from a model life table with $e_0 = 20$ years. The short dashed line shows the ages at death, calculated according to the procedure of Suchey and Brooks in which the mean age for the relevant pubic symphysis stage is assigned to each skeleton. The solid line shows the distribution of adult ages at death recorded in the Newcastle Infirmary burial registers.

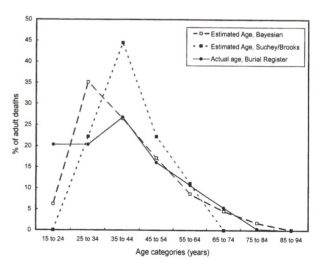

resemble that of the living population, rather than the normal mortality pattern in which the deaths of young children and older adults predominate. Furthermore, in some burial contexts there may be selective interment of particular age classes. Where there is uncertainty as to the likely age structure of the sample, it may be more appropriate to select uniform priors, as these do not commit the investigator to specific assumptions about the prior probability of age.

GENETIC PALAEODEMOGRAPHY

With continuing advances in molecular biological methods there are increasing opportunities to investigate the demographic histories of populations through genetic analysis. In studies of present-day populations the geographical variations in the frequency of classical genetic markers (mainly variants in the structural genes encoded by nuclear DNA) have been used to reconstruct large-scale prehistoric population movements.[38,39] Also useful in this regard are haploid genetic loci, including the maternally inherited mitochondrial DNA and the male-specific non-recombining parts of the Y chromosome.[40,41] These parts of the genome can be used to define distinct genetic lineages, with the divergence between the lineages being proportional to the time since the lineages shared a most recent common genetic ancestor. This allows the investigator to reconstruct the phylogenetic history of a group of related populations, and the divergence between populations may correspond to major demographic events such as large-scale migrations and colonizations.

Periods of rapid population expansion also leave a distinctive genetic signature, for example in the distribution of pairwise differences between the DNA sequences of individuals in a population and in the geometric patterns of lineage relationships.[42–44] In a population that has undergone a substantial expansion of numbers through intrinsic growth (i.e. through fertility exceeding mortality) most of the genetic mutations in the population will have occurred post-expansion, in separate genetic lineages, and each mutation will thus be present in just one or two copies in the population. A pairwise comparison between the DNA sequences of individuals will show the effects of this in a narrow distribution of differences, and a phylogeny of genetic lineages will exhibit a 'starlike' topology in which the lineages radiate from a common ancestral sequence.[41,43] In a population that is stationary or has increased only at a slow rate the proportion of shared ancestral mutations in the population will be greater and the spread of pairwise sequence differences will be broader and often multimodal.

A widely used measure of genetic diversity is F_{ST}, the proportion of total genetic variance that is attributable to differences between separate population groups. F_{ST} increases with increasing time since the initial divergence between the population groups, and increases faster when effective population sizes are small, but is decreased in proportion to the rate of migration between the groups (migration has the effect of reducing between-group genetic variance). F_{ST} is usually calculated directly from gene frequency data[39] but good proxies to F_{ST} can also be derived from the frequencies of skeletal morphological traits that have high heritabilities.[45]

Comparisons of diversity in mitochondrial DNA and Y chromosome DNA in the same populations have revealed a difference in the average transgenerational migration rate of the sexes, with the females having a history of much higher migration rates than males.[46] This finding, which has been demonstrated separately among both African and European modern population samples, has been linked to the historical predominance of patrilocality among human populations, especially since the adoption of agriculture when communities became more settled and some lineages established their tenure on land through male-line inheritance. In patrilocal societies the women, rather than the men, migrate transgenerationally and, given equivalent effective population sizes, the sex-specific between-population genetic diversity is reduced in females relative to the diversity in the males of the same population.

Studies of ancient DNA extracted from archaeological human remains (see Brown, chapter 27, in this volume) have the potential to corroborate or refute hypotheses about population history. However, the difficulty and expense of ancient DNA analysis ensures that most published projects have had very small sample sizes, limiting the extent to which inferences can be made concerning populations. An indication of the possibilities for genetic palaeodemography using ancient DNA was published by Colson et al.,[47] who examined mtDNA sequences in 3rd–9th-century AD human skeletons from a coastal settlement in the northern Netherlands. The sequences were compared with those of modern Frisian-speaking inhabitants from the mainland and from the North Frisian Islands off the north coast of The Netherlands and Germany. The distribution and diversity of the sequences in the ancient DNA samples matched that seen today in the Frisian islanders, rather than the much lower diversity of present day mainland Frisian speakers. This suggests that the archaeological population may represent a community that historically occupied a much wider geographical area, whereas today the matrilineal descendants of that population are confined to the offshore islands.

CONCLUSIONS

As emphasized above, inferring the structure and dynamics of past populations from bio-archaeological evidence is a task fraught with difficulty. The removal of systematic bias from current methods of skeletal age estimation is an urgent research priority, as it is only with unbiased methods that meaningful statements can be made about the pattern of mortality exhibited by a skeletal sample. In conjunction with appropriate population models it may then be possible to establish in particular cases whether past mortuary practices were selective (i.e. preferential deposition of particular age classes and sex) as well as allowing distinctions to be made between attritional and catastrophic mortality patterns.

The advent of procedures for extracting and characterizing ancient biomolecules in human remains provides a welcome new line of evidence for palaeodemography, in particular offering an independent source of information about past population movements. When combined with the very extensive databases of nuclear and mitochondrial DNA sequences now recorded for present day lineages the biomolecular approach has the potential to answer a range of questions about the dynamics of populations in the past.

REFERENCES

1 Binford LR. Post-Pleistocene adaptations. In: Binford LR, Binford SR (eds), *New Perspectives in Archaeology*. Chicago: Aldine, 1968: pp. 313–341.

2 Carneiro RL. A theory of the origin of the state. *Science* 1970; **169**: 733–738.

3 Renfrew C. *Before Civilisation*. London: Cape, 1973.

4 Zubrow E. The demographic modelling of Neanderthal extinction. In: Mellars P, Stringer C (eds), *The Human Revolution: Behavioural and Biological Perspectives on the Origin of Modern Humans*. Edinburgh: Edinburgh University Press, 1989: pp. 212–231.

5 Martin PS. The discovery of America. *Science* 1973; **179**: 969–974.

6 Ammerman AJ, Cavalli-Sforza LL. A population model for the diffusion of early farming in Europe. In: Renfrew C (ed.), *The Explanation of Culture Change*. London: Duckworth, 1973: pp. 343–357.

7 Anthony DW. Migration in archaeology: the baby and the bathwater. *American Anthropology* 1990; **92**: 895–914.

8 Clark GA. Migration as an explanatory concept in Paleolithic archaeology. *Journal of Archaeological Method and Theory* 1994; **1**: 305–343.

9 Härke H. Archaeologists and migrations. A problem of attitude? *Current Anthropology* 1998; **39**: 19–45.

10 Larsen CS. *Bioarchaeology: Interpreting Behavior from the Human Skeleton*. New York: Cambridge University Press, 1997.

11 Bocquet-Appel J-P, Masset C. Farewell to paleodemography. *Journal of Human Evolution* 1982; **11**: 321–333.

12 Acsádi G, Nemeskéri J. *History of Human Life Span and Mortality*. Budapest: Akadémiai Kiadó, 1970.

13 Wood JW, Milner GR, Harpending HC, Weiss KM. The osteological paradox. *Current Anthropology* 1992; **33**: 343–370.

14 Coale AJ. How the age distribution of a human population is determined. *Cold Spring Harbor Symposia on Quantitative Biology* 1957; **22**: 83–88.

15 Kirk D. Demographic transition theory. *Population Studies* 1996; **50**: 361–387.

16 Coale AJ, Demeny P. *Regional Model Life Tables and Stable Populations* (2nd edn). Princeton: Princeton University Press, 1983.

17 Milner GR, Humpf DA, Harpending HC. Pattern matching of age-at-death distributions in paleodemographic analysis. *American Journal of Physical Anthropology* 1989; **80**: 49–58.

18 Paine RR. Model life table fitting by maximum likelihood estimation: a procedure to reconstruct paleodemographic characteristics from skeletal age distributions. *American Journal of Physical Anthropology* 1989; **79**: 51–61.

19 Dawes JD, Magilton, JR. *The Cemetery of St Helen-on-the-Walls, Aldwark*. London: Council for British Archaeology, 1980.

20 White W. *The Cemetery of St Nicholas Shambles*. London: London and Middlesex Archaeological Society, 1988.

21 Ubelaker DH. *Human Skeletal Remains. Excavation, Analysis and Interpretation* (2nd edn). Washington, DC: Smithsonian Institution, 1989.

22 Klein RG, Cruz-Uribe K. *The Analysis of Animal Bones from Archaeological Sites*. Chicago: University of Chicago Press, 1984.

23 Reichs KJ.(ed.), *Forensic Osteology*. Springfield: Charles C Thomas, 1986.

24 Krogman WM, Işcan MY. *The Human Skeleton in Forensic Medicine* (2nd edn). Springfield: Charles C Thomas, 1986.

25 Jackes MK. Pubic symphysis age distributions. *American Journal of Physical Anthropology* 1985; **68**: 281–299.

26 Jackes M. Paleodemography: problems and techniques. In: Saunders SR, Katzenberg MA (eds), *Skeletal Biology of Past Peoples*. New York: Wiley, 1992: pp. 189–224.

27 Konigsberg LW, Frankenberg SR. Estimation of age structure in anthropological demography. *American Journal of Physical Anthropology* 1992; **89**: 235–256.

28   Konigsberg LW, Frankenberg SR. Paleodemography: 'not quite dead'. *Evolutionary Anthropology* 1994; **3**: 92–105.

29   Lucy D, Ackroyd RG, Pollard AM, Solheim T. A Bayesian approach to adult human age estimation from dental observations by Johanson's age changes. *Journal of Forensic Sciences* 1996; **41**: 189–194.

30   Ackroyd RG, Lucy D, Pollard AM, Roberts CA. Nasty, brutish, but not necessarily short: a reconsideration of the statistical methods used to calculate age at death from adult human skeletal and dental age indicators. *American Antiquity* 1999; **64**: 55–70.

31   Suchey JM, Wisely DV, Katz D. Evaluation of the Todd and McKern–Stewart methods for aging the male os pubis. In: Reichs KJ (ed.), *Forensic Osteology*. Springfield: Charles C Thomas, 1986: pp. 33–67.

32   Işcan MY, Loth SR. Estimation of age and determination of sex from the sternal rib. In: Reichs KJ (ed.), *Forensic Osteology*. Springfield: Charles C Thomas, 1986: pp. 68–89.

33   Hunt DR. History and demography of the Robert J. Terry anatomical collection. *American Journal of Physical Anthropology* 1999; 28 (suppl.): 156–157.

34   Molleson T, Cox M. *The Spitalfields Project*, vol. 2: *Anthropology – The Middling Sort*. Research Report 86. York: Council for British Archaeology, 1993.

35   Saunders SR, Herring DA, Boyce G. Can skeletal samples accurately represent the living population they come from? The St. Thomas' cemetery site, Belleville, Ontario. In: Grauer AL (ed.), *Bodies of Evidence: Reconstructing History through Skeletal Analysis*. New York: Liss, 1995: pp. 69–91.

36   Litton CD, Buck CE. The Bayesian approach to the interpretation of archaeological data. *Archaeometry* 1995; **37**: 1–24.

37   Brooks S, Suchey JM. Skeletal age determination based on the os pubis: a comparison of the Acsádi–Nemeskéri and Suchey–Brooks methods. *Human Evolution* 1990; **5**: 227–238.

38   Sokal RR, Oden NL, Wilson C. Genetic evidence for the spread of agriculture in Europe by demic diffusion. *Nature* 1991; **351**: 143–145.

39   Cavalli-Sforza LL, Menozzi P, Piazza A. *The History and Geography of Human Genes*. Princeton: Princeton University Press, 1994.

40   Donnelly P, Tavaré S. Coalescents and genealogical structure under neutrality. *Annual Review of Genetics* 1995; **29**: 401–421.

41   Harpending HC, Sherry ST, Rogers AR, Stoneking M. The genetic structure of ancient human populations. *Current Anthropology* 1993; **34**: 483–496.

42   Harpending HC, Batzer MA, Gurven M, Jorde LB, Rogers AR, Sherry ST. Genetic traces of ancient demography. *Proceedings of the National Academy of Sciences, USA* 1998; **95**: 1961–1967.

43   Rogers AR. Genetic evidence for a Pleistocene population explosion. *Evolution* 1995; **49**: 608–615.

44   Richards M, Côrte-Real H, Forster P, Macaulay V, Wilkinson-Herbots H, Demaine A, Papiha S, Hedges R, Bandelt HJ, Sykes B. Paleolithic and Neolithic lineages in the European mitochondrial gene pool. *American Journal of Human Genetics* 1996; **59**: 185–203.

45   Tyrrell AJ, Chamberlain AT. Non-metric trait evidence for modern human affinities and the distinctiveness of Neanderthals. *Journal of Human Evolution* 1998; **34**: 549–544.

46   Seielstad MT, Minch E, Cavalli-Sforza LL. Genetic evidence for a higher female migration rate. *Nature Genetics* 1998; **20**: 278–280.

47   Colson IB, Richards MB, Bailey JF, Sykes BC. DNA analysis of seven human skeletons excavated from the Terp at Wijnaldum. *Journal of Archaeological Science* 1997; **24**: 911–917.

8

SEX DETERMINATION IN SKELETAL REMAINS

Simon Mays and Margaret Cox

INTRODUCTION

Reliable determination of sex from human skeletal remains is clearly of fundamental importance, both for personal identification in forensic work and for studies of earlier populations using archaeological cemetery data. Sex is generally inferred using skeletal morphology, but in recent years DNA has also been used for this purpose in forensic work, and to a more limited extent in archaeological settings. This chapter concentrates on sexing using metric or non-metric recording of aspects of skeletal morphology, while sexing using DNA is covered elsewhere.[1]

From the outset it is probably useful to clarify terminology, specifically the difference between sex and gender. Sex is the biological quality that distinguishes males and females. It is fundamentally a chromosomal difference, females having two X chromosomes and males an X and a Y. In the scientific literature (e.g. [2]) the terms gender and sex are sometimes used interchangeably; however, the two are not synonymous. Gender may be defined as the social significance placed on the biological differences between males and females. It is therefore a cultural construct, linked to biological sex but not exclusively defined by it. In work on archaeological burials it is particularly useful to preserve this conceptual distinction between sex and gender, as the biological sex inferred from the skeleton can be used as a reference point from which to infer gendered differences in past societies.[3,4]

Hormone-related change is the means whereby sexual differences manifest in many tissues, including bone. It is the tissue response to these circulating levels of hormones that dictates the basics of sexual dimorphism. The development of sex differences in the skeleton reflects hormonal differences between males and females. In males, it is the hormones principally secreted by the testes that elicit the development of male physical features. In mammals, the ovaries do not appear to be necessary for the development of most female characters; the female phenotype is the one into which the foetus will develop unless redirected by male hormones.[5]

Sex determination from the skeleton relies on the existence of regular and recordable differences in skeletal morphology between males and females. The greater the degree of dimorphism, the more accurate will be the assignment of sex from skeletal remains. In the male, androgen levels vary with age; in particular they are much lower before puberty. This means that pre-pubertal sexual dimorphism in the skeleton is slight, so determination of sex in the remains of juveniles is much more difficult than it is in adults. Much of the osteological work directed at providing morphological sexing techniques for juveniles has involved attempting to extend the use of morphological indicators that work well in the adult to immature skeletons. Therefore, in this chapter we first discuss sexing techniques for the adult, and then proceed to consider immature remains. We have, unusually, devoted as much discussion to sexing infants and juveniles as to adults. This reflects the importance of understanding the difficult and contentious area of sexing immature remains and its potential importance in terms of understanding past lives and cultural practices.

SEX DETERMINATION IN THE ADULT SKELETON

When attempting to determine sex in adult skeletal remains it is essential to examine the whole skeleton, or at least as much of it as survives. The reliability of sex determination is contingent upon the completeness of the remains,[6] particularly in populations where levels of sexual dimorphism are relatively low. The two areas of the skeleton that exhibit sexual dimorphism most strongly in the adult are the pelvis and the skull, so although the whole skeleton should be assessed, indicators from these parts should be accorded the most weight.

Skeletal sex indicators

Pelvis

Sexual dimorphism in the pelvis indicates both functional modification and evolutionary adaptation. The male pelvis has evolved to ensure successful bipedality. In females, pelvic structure is modified to ensure that obstetric success is also possible.[7,8] Generally, the male pelvis is a high and narrow structure, whereas that in the female is transversely oval with a relatively wider inlet, greater pelvic diameter and outlet. Aspects of these differences provide osteological sex indicators. Phenice[9] recognized several morphological features of the pubic bone that are useful in sexing. These comprise, for females, the developed ventral arc, subpubic concavity and the ridged medial border of the inferior pubic ramus. While the shape of the greater sciatic notch is influenced by the elevation of the sacrum, a wide, shallow notch is considered to be a female feature.[10] All the above reflect the wider and more open female pelvic girdle.[11] In addition, criteria such as the morphology of the sacro-iliac joints and, in the sacrum, the relative width of the body and alae are also considered sex indicators.[12,13]

In the pelvic bones, the presence of the cortical variables pre-auricular sulci and pubic pitting have traditionally been considered indicators of female sex.[14] However, they are no longer thought to indicate this; rather they have been shown to be associated with pelvic shape and size, the large gynaecoid pelvis being associated with their presence and the android pelvis with their absence.[7,15]

For the experienced osteologist, reliability of the pelvis in sex determination in adults is generally good. Phenice's[9] criteria were tested by Sutherland and Suchey[16] with 96% accuracy on a large documented sample ($n = 1284$) aged between 11 and 99 years, although they were found to work less well by Lovell[17] who reported 83% accuracy in a smaller collection ($n = 50$). Meindl et al.,[6] using a modern sample of North American Caucasoids ($n = 100$), obtained a 96% accuracy rate using a variety of pelvic features. Some samples, however, are less dimorphic than others and may challenge even the most experienced osteologist. Variability in dimorphism between different samples has been discussed by MacLaughlin and Bruce.[18] They note that the greater sciatic notch/acetabulum index rule of thumb devised by Kelley[19] on Native American, Negroid and Caucasoid North American material was a poor discriminator of sex in a sample comprising documented British and Dutch material.

Researchers have also evaluated the use of discriminant function analysis of pelvic measurements and various indices, with differing success rates. Schulter-Ellis et al.[20] examined a sample of 100 North American Caucasoids from the Terry collection and achieved 95% accuracy using an acetabulum/pubis index and 97% accuracy when this was combined with femoral head diameter. Earlier work[21] on a sample of Negroids from the same collection produced slightly less accurate results. It is important to remember that the use of measurements in discriminant function analysis, as with diagnostic criteria in any sexing method, is most safely employed in cases or samples where the ancestry of the material under study is the same as that of the reference sample on which the method was developed.

Skull

Puberty in females occurs, on average, two years earlier than in males. Consequently, males have an extra two years of somatic growth, during which period there is acceleration in muscle mass. As a consequence, changes occur both at direct sites of muscle attachment to bone or as a response to the dissipation of forces. It is these changes that result in sexual dimorphism in the face and skull. Thus, sexual identification in adolescents depends upon the timing and duration of puberty. Multifactorial influences also have a bearing on this expression, including genetics, diet and disease.

In males, cranio-facial changes lead to an elongation of the face, an enlargement of the supra-orbital ridges and mastoid processes, and an accentuation of the chin. The upper orbital margins become thicker and blunter and the orbits become squarer. Changes in the angle of the ramus and the mandibular body also occur. Females do not undergo such changes but retain the more gracile juvenile form. Their foreheads are generally more vertical in profile with well-defined frontal eminences, while the glabellar region is smoother than in the male. Muscle markings on the nuchal crest, temporal bone, temporal crest and around the zygomatic roots, are larger and heavier in males. Various authors have advocated the use of such features as sex indicators.[13,14,22-26]

Many workers claim an accuracy for sex identification from the adult cranium alone of about 80%,[12] increasing to 90% if the mandible is included. Meindl et al.[6] found that sex could be correctly inferred in 92% of skulls from a modern collection of known sex.

Loth and Henneberg[27] have recently attempted to derive a new method for sexing the mandible. They studied a sample of 300 mandibles from documented adults (mainly Negroids) from the Dart collection. They discovered a distinct angulation on the posterior border of the mandibular ramus in adult males. The overall accuracy of sex determination using this feature, ramus flexure, was 94%. Koski,[28] however, questions the value of ramus flexure as a sex indicator. He draws attention to the subjective nature of the feature and the likely problems of inter-observer error in scoring it, as do Donnelly et al.[29] who only achieved a success rate of 62.5% using it to sex their sample.

Although sexing from the skull is potentially quite reliable, problems may arise, particularly in weakly dimorphic populations. For example, the skull may sometimes indicate one sex and the pelvis the other; in an undocumented Dutch archaeological sample ($n = 202$), the mandibles of 51% of those sexed on other criteria as female, appeared male.[30] In instances where sex indications from the pelvis and the skull are in conflict, it is possible that the former might be more reliable as dimorphism of the pelvis is directly related to function. Clearly this hypothesis needs testing on an appropriate sample of documented sex. Recently, one of the authors (MC) examined a medieval skeleton from East Anglia where the skull was characteristically male and the pelvis female. DNA analysis suggested that the individual was female, but DNA analysis is not totally reliable.

As with the pelvis, some workers have used discriminant functions for sexing the skull. In a Japanese collection, Hanihara[31] reported an accuracy of 90% using only three dimensions from the skull, while Giles[32] demonstrated that a similar approach could also be successfully applied to North American Negroid and Caucasoid samples. Sexing from the mandible alone using discriminant function analysis has also been attempted. Hanihara[31] reported 85% accuracy from four dimensions, while work conducted by Giles[33] achieved 84% from eight measurements.

High accuracy rates for sex determination have been reported when using the pelvis and skull combined. Meindl et al.[6] achieved a success rate of 97% on a modern North American sample, and Molleson and Cox[34] reported 98% correctly sexed in the documented archaeological material of the 18th–19th century from Spitalfields, London.

Other post-cranial elements

To enable fragmentary remains to be sexed, analysis of the reliability of sex determination using a wide range of bones has been conducted. Isçan et al.[35,36] report 83% accuracy for sex determination using dimensions of the sternal end of the fourth rib in a sample of 230 autopsy specimens, and Cologlu et al.[37] reported a success rate of 86–90% using discriminant function analysis. However, the problems of successfully identifying the fourth rib in fragmented material seriously reduce the usefulness of this method.

Sex differences in the appendicular skeleton have been examined extensively using discriminant function analysis. Here is not the place to review in detail this literature, but it is worth mentioning a few examples. Lui[38] examined 17 femoral dimensions, using a range of statistical approaches in a Chinese sample ($n = 141$) and concluded that femoral head diameter is the most reliable (85%). Trancho et al.'s[39] work, based on five measurements on documented Spanish femora ($n = 132$), suggests a 99% accuracy, while that of Seidemann et al.,[40] looking at the supero-inferior femoral neck diameter, achieved success rates of 87–92% for samples of different ancestral origin. It must, however, be emphasized that approaches based on metrical variation cannot be relied upon across the board; the value of each must be demonstrated for the sample under examination.

SEX DETERMINATION IN THE IMMATURE SKELETON

Bones

In the immature skeleton, much of the work that has been conducted towards establishing criteria for sex determination from bone morphology has been done on perinatal infants. The main reason for this is that reference collections of perinatal material of documented sex are more readily available than are those of older infants and children. In addition, there are theoretical reasons to expect that osteological sexual dimorphism will be more pronounced in foetal and perinatal infants than in older pre-pubescent individuals. Although always low compared with those at adolescence, testosterone levels in pre-pubertal males do vary during development. In the male foetus, testosterone levels start to rise at about 8 weeks of gestation and maintain a relatively high level until birth. Soon after birth, testosterone levels fall and remain low until puberty.[5] In theory then, although one would expect its expression to be slight compared with that in adults, sexual dimorphism in immature bones ought to be most readily detectable in perinatal and foetal age groups.

Most work on osteological sexual dimorphism in non-adults has concentrated on pelvic morphology, particularly the greater sciatic notch. It has been noted since at least the last quarter of the 19th century[41] that, as in the adult, the infant sciatic notch is narrower and deeper in males. Some more recent metric studies (generally using an index composed of notch length and breadth) support this. Boucher[42] found sexual dimorphism in British Caucasoid ($n = 107$) and North American Negroid ($n = 96$) foetal remains, males showing a deeper, narrower notch. Fazekas and Kósa,[43] obtained similar results from a study on Hungarian forensic foetal material ($n = 104$). However, other assessments (e.g. Weaver[44] on recent US foetal and infant material, and Molleson and Cox[34] on British archaeological remains of documented sex) have found no such dimorphism. Holcomb and Konigsberg,[45] working with a documented US collection ($n = 122$) of recent foetal material using an image analysis technique, also failed to find a difference in the sciatic notch depth:width ratio, although they did find that the maximum depth of the notch was more anteriorly located in the male.

Even in those studies where dimorphism in the greater sciatic notch can be demonstrated in infant and/or foetal pelves, its degree is slight compared with that seen in adults. For example, in the Fazekas and Kósa study,[43] the mean index ($100 \times$ notch depth/notch width) for males was about 32, about 4 percentage points greater than the female mean, with a large degree of overlap. Figures for adults, reported by Hager[10] give a mean of about 85 for males and 63 for females, a difference of fully 22 percentage points.

The small degree of dimorphism in greater sciatic notch morphology poses problems when one attempts to develop the observations of the existence of dimorphism in this feature into practical techniques for sex determination. The fact that sexual dimorphism varies between populations, coupled with the relatively slight sex differences in infant pelves, means that for archaeological remains, simply measuring infant pelvic bones and inferring sex by determining whether they group with male or female bones from a modern reference sample is unlikely to be a reliable method. One possible approach, if large numbers of infant bones are available from any one archaeological assemblage, is to plot the data to determine whether they fall into two separate clusters. If they do then the inference is that the two clusters correspond to male and female infants. If they do not then the degree of dimorphism in that particular population may be too low for discrete male and female clusters to appear. Another, less likely, explanation would be that all infants were of the same sex. This approach was used with perinatal remains ($n = 36$) from the mediaeval churchyard at Wharram Percy, England.[23] The width and the depth of the notch were measured using a moving stage micrometer and a binocular microscope. The results (Figure 1) showed some evidence for bimodality. There was no association between individual age at death and sciatic notch index which could have caused this, so the most likely conclusion is that the two peaks correspond to male and female infants, the males being represented by the group at the higher index value.

Some researchers have examined the value of auricular surface form for sex determination in immature remains. In the adult, an auricular surface showing elevation from the ilium is a female character[12] and can be considered a manifestation of the greater width of the female pelvis. Weaver[44] investigated dimorphism in this feature in a sample of foetal/infant skeletal material ($n = 153$). He found that a non-elevated surface characterized males (85% showed this form) and an elevated surface was associated with females (although the pattern here was less strong, with only 58% of females showing this morphology). In an indirect test of Weaver's method, Hunt[46] applied it to immature skeletons ($n = 275$), ranging up to about 6.5 years of age, of undocumented sex from archaeological sites in North America. He found an association between auricular morphology and individual age, the frequency of the non-raised form increasing markedly with age. This suggested that the auricular surface

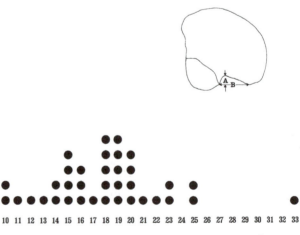

Figure 1 – Distribution of the sciatic notch index for the Wharram Percy perinatal infants. From Mays.[23]

trait was primarily a manifestation of morphological variation during the growth period rather than of sex. Mittler and Sheridan[47] evaluated Weaver's method using a juvenile archaeological sample from Sudanese Nubia ($n = 58$). The arid climate preserved soft tissue, so that sex could be determined unambiguously from preserved external genitalia. The ages ranged up to 18 years. In this study, 85% of males showed non-elevated auricular surfaces and 58% of females had the elevated form. However, there was also an age effect; the non-elevated pattern was so common in those < 9 years of age that among this subgroup a majority of both sexes showed this form. In later childhood all males showed the non-elevated form but only about two-thirds of the females displayed the elevated morphology.

A little research has also been undertaken on sex indicators in the juvenile skull. Schutkowski[48] found some evidence for sexual dimorphism in the mandible in the documented sex Spitalfields juveniles ($n = 44$). This was confirmed by Molleson et al.,[49] who investigated the form of the mentum and gonial areas, together with orbital morphology, and found that by combining these features, sex could correctly be ascertained in 78% of the Spitalfields juveniles. These morphological features of the facial skeleton were scored for a group of juveniles of undocumented sex from another archaeological site (Wharram Percy). To test the success of this technique, the sex inferred by the facial morphology was compared with permanent canine dimensions, since males tend to have larger teeth than females (see below). In the Wharram Percy sample, those inferred as male showed significantly larger permanent canine dimensions than did those inferred as female,[49] suggesting that, for this material, the sex inferred by facial morphology was generally correct.

Teeth

It has been known for some time that within a population, the dimensions of the crowns of the deciduous[50] and the permanent[51] dentition tend to be larger in males. It appears that the Y chromosome promotes growth both of tooth enamel and dentine, whereas the effect of the X chromosome seems to be confined to enamel formation. It has been suggested[52] that these differential effects of the X and Y chromosomes may underlie the sexual dimorphism in tooth size.

Tooth-crown sizes, and the degree of sexual dimorphism vary between populations.[53-55] Sex differences in crown dimensions are small. The most frequently taken measurements are bucco-lingual and mesio-distal widths. In the permanent dentition these characteristically show up to about a maximum 10% difference between the sexes; this corresponds to a difference of < 1 mm between male and female means.[56-58] The degree of dimorphism in the deciduous tooth crowns in general seems less than in the permanent teeth.[50,59,60] The small and variable degree of dimorphism means that, as with osteological metric methods, measurement standards from recent populations cannot be reliably used to determine sex in archaeological material. The best results are likely to be obtained by using as a reference sample, a subgroup of the assemblage under study that is of known sex (or at least one for which sex can reliably be inferred). To use dimensions of the deciduous dentition as a means of sex determination in this way in an archaeological assemblage we would require that a subset of the juveniles in that assemblage be of known sex. This of course is hardly ever the case, and for this reason sex determination in archaeological assemblages using dimensions of the deciduous dentition is rarely attempted. However, in adults for whom sex can reliably be determined osteologically, the permanent teeth can be used to provide a baseline from which to determine sex in those juveniles for which at least some of the permanent tooth crowns have formed (and indeed in adults for which osteological indicators are missing or damaged).

In general, the canines (particularly the lower canines) are the most dimorphic teeth,[56] so measurements from them play an important role in dental sexing. The canines erupt at about 10–11 years of age, although the crowns are complete for measurement purposes by about 6 years.[61] Consequently, if loose unerupted teeth are present they may be measured in individuals from this age. Odontometry of the permanent dentition therefore provides a potential sexing method from middle-to-late childhood.

In some instances, the degree of dental dimorphism is sufficient that measurements from a single tooth can provide an adequate means of sex determination. For example, Molleson[62] plotted mandibular canine crown widths for male and female adult skeletons from the Romano-British site at Poundbury, England, and sexed the juveniles according to whether they lay in the male or female ranges. However, for most archaeological assemblages the degree of dimorphism is insufficient for sex to be determined in juveniles in this way. In these circumstances sex determination may be achieved by discriminant function analysis, using tooth measurements of adults in the assemblage, who could be sexed osteologically, to generate the function.

Archaeological examples of sexing from dental measurements using discriminant function analysis generally report success rates of between 75 and 95%.[57,58,63–66] It is worth emphasizing though, that these are figures for the proportions of adults in the assemblage which the discriminant function sexes correctly (or at least places in the same sex group as the osteological indicators). The success with children is, strictly speaking, unknown, as there are no independent sex indicators for these individuals. In addition, despite these apparently successful applications, it should be noted that sexual dimorphism in dental dimensions sometimes proves to be too low to permit sex determination, even by discriminant function analysis (this was the case, for example, with the Spitalfields skeletons[34]).

An assumption when using dental measurements to determine sex in juveniles is that tooth dimensions in children in an archaeological assemblage are similar to those in adults of the same sex. It is possible that in some instances this assumption may be problematic. Work with animals[67–71] indicates that tooth crown size may be reduced in instances of suboptimal nutrition during development. Generational differences observed in dental size in human populations have been ascribed to nutritional factors.[72] Individuals suffering most from poor nutrition and health may tend to die early, so there is the potential for those who died in childhood to have smaller teeth than did those who survived into adult life. Some researchers claim to have identified this mortality bias in archaeological material. Guagliardo[73] found that juveniles from a North American archaeological site had smaller teeth than were seen in adults from the same assemblage. The adult sex ratio was about 1:1, suggesting that the reduced dental dimensions in the juveniles did not reflect an excess of female deaths in childhood. Guagliardo argued that the reason why juvenile teeth were smaller was because those who died in childhood were more stressed than those who survived to maturity. Simpson *et al.*[74] noted a similar discrepancy in tooth size between adults and juveniles from another North American site, and likewise ascribed it to mortality bias. At Wharram Percy, Molleson *et al.*[49] found that those juveniles sexed on the basis of the morphology of the facial skeleton showed smaller tooth size than adults of the same sex, perhaps indicating mortality bias in dental dimensions in this group also.

In the absence of archaeological assemblages with significant numbers of juveniles of documented sex, it is not possible to determine unequivocally whether this mortality bias in dental dimensions is present. However, the circumstantial evidence cited above suggests that in some assemblages it may be. When it is present, it will tend to result in males being misidentified as female, giving an erroneous impression of elevated female mortality during childhood.

CONCLUSIONS

Compared with the task of attributing sex to infant and juvenile skeletons, sexing adults is relatively straightforward and reliable. However, there are limiting factors which are all too often forgotten and which could usefully be mentioned here in order to guard against over-confidence on the part of the osteologist when sexing adult remains.

Disorders of sexual differentiation are rare but should be considered. Some are chromosomal, others gonadal, endocrine or phenotypic. They include conditions such as Klinefelter's syndrome (47XXY), Turner's syndrome (45XO) and Testicular Feminization syndrome (46XY). In such instances individual phenotypes differ from the norm to varying degrees, although little is known of the skeletal morphology in such cases.

Some disease processes may influence the morphology of the pelvis and skull. Growth conditions, such as those affected by somatotropin, can influence morphology, as can those due to disorders of the parathyroid glands.[75] Metabolic conditions such as rickets and osteomalacia can effect both pelvic and cranial morphology. The osteologist must be alert for the possibility of such changes, particularly slight or moderate cases where pathological alterations may not be immediately obvious.

Most of the sexually dimorphic features of the skull used in the estimation of sex are simply correlated with robusticity, the male being the more robust. However, dietary and other factors may influence skull robusticity. A coarse, tough diet, requiring heavy mastication, as was generally consumed by all peoples before recent times, resulted in greater skull robusticity, particularly of the facial skeleton.[76,77] Archaeological skulls may, therefore, tend to show a more 'masculine' appearance in these areas than modern reference material. Cultural practices, for example the use of the jaws in hide preparation by Eskimos,[78] can also affect skull robusticity.

Over-representation of males in some cemetery assemblages has recently been attributed to errors in sexing due to increased cranio-facial robusticity in post-menopausal females.[79]

The hypothesis of increasing cranio-facial robusticity in elderly females is not supported by evaluation of material of known sex at Spitalfields (mean age of females = 56 years) where 98% were correctly sexed;[34] however, this is still an issue which merits further investigation.

For juveniles, osteological sex determination is very difficult. Of the osteological features, greater sciatic notch morphology may be the most promising, at least as far as perinatal remains are concerned. However, one might expect the small differences that exist perinatally to be quickly blurred by the growth process, and this is supported by a radiographic study of living children.[80] Nevertheless, if only to confirm this, further work on greater sciatic notch morphology in skeletal material of older children and adolescents is still needed. Other methods, such as Weaver's auricular surface technique, have not yet provided results that would encourage their routine use on juvenile skeletal remains.

Relatively less attention has been paid to the possibility of sexual dimorphism in the juvenile skull. It may be worth testing further the features identified by Molleson et al.[49] using what few collections of juvenile skeletons of known sex exist,[81] and replacing these criteria with new ones if they are found wanting.

In general, osteological techniques for sexing juveniles suffer from the observation that sexual dimorphism is a relatively small component of the bony morphological variability seen in the juvenile cohort; the great majority of variation is due to the growth process, although other things such as mechanical factors also contribute. Multivariate statistical analyses may help us to tease out elements of osteological variation in juvenile assemblages that reflect sexual dimorphism rather than variation related to growth or other factors. However, one suspects that it will be very difficult to operationalize any insights thus gained into reliable methods that can be used routinely for sexing immature material.

Since teeth do not grow or remodel once formed, odontometric methods are perhaps likely to remain more useful as practical techniques for sex determination in juvenile remains. At present, odontometric techniques using discriminant functions generated from dimensions of the permanent dentition may be the most reliable morphological methods of sex determination in immature skeletons. However, for archaeological remains, the potential · problems associated with mortality bias, which if present will tend to give the erroneous impression of excess female mortality during childhood, should be born in mind when using these techniques.

DNA analysis is potentially a tool that could aid sex determination. However, it must be emphasized that DNA techniques have their own problems and drawbacks.[1] The difficulty and expense of conducting such analyses means that sexing using ancient DNA is unlikely to challenge the primacy of morphological techniques for routine use on archaeological remains, even for fragmentary material and immature skeletons where the techniques currently available perform poorly.

It is possible that, in future, collection of morphometric data in three dimensions using image analysis systems may provide a more sensitive method of detecting skeletal sexual dimorphism than do the use of non-metric morphological assessments or linear measurements. In addition, there is a need for the examination of further archaeological collections of documented sex, in order to provide direct information on sexual dimorphism in earlier human groups.

ACKNOWLEDGEMENTS

The authors are grateful to the referees for their valuable comments. Sue Black is particularly thanked for her input.

REFERENCES

1   Brown K. Ancient DNA applications in human osteoarchaeology: achievements, problems and potential (Chapter 27 – this volume).

2   Sutton MQ, Malik M, Ogram A. Experiments on the determination of gender from coprolites by DNA analysis. *Journal of Archaeological Science* 1996; **23**: 263–267.

3   Sofaer-Derevenski J. Age and gender at the site of Tiszapolgár-Basatanya, Hungary. *Antiquity* 1997; **71**: 875–889.

4   Lucy S. *The Early Anglo-Saxon Cemeteries of East Yorkshire*. British Archaeological Reports (British Series) No. 272. Oxford: Archaeopress, 1998.

5   Wilson JD, George FW, Griffin JE. The hormonal control of sexual development. *Science* 1981; **11**: 1278–1284.

6   Meindl RS, Lovejoy CO, Mensforth RP, Carlos LD. Accuracy and determination of error in the sexing of the skeleton. *American Journal of Physical Anthropology* 1985; **68**: 79–85.

7   Cox MJ. Evaluation of the significance of scars of parturition in the Christ Church, Spitalfields sample. Unpublished PhD thesis, University College London, 1989.

8   Tague RG. Variation in pelvic size between males and females in non-human anthropoids. *American Journal of Physical Anthropology* 1995; **97**: 213–233.

9   Phenice TW. A newly developed method of sexing the os pubis. *American Journal of Physical Anthropology* 1969; **30**: 297–302.

10 Hager L. Sex differences in the sciatic notch of great apes and modern humans. *American Journal of Physical Anthropology* 1996; **99**: 287–300.

11 Budinoff LC, Tague RG. Anatomical and developmental bases for the ventral arc of the human pelvis. *American Journal of Physical Anthropology* 1990; **82**: 73–79.

12 St Hoyme LE, Işcan MY. Determination of sex and race: accuracy and assumptions. In: Işcan MY, Kennedy KAR (eds), *Reconstruction of Life from the Skeleton*. New York: Alan Liss, 1989: pp. 53–93.

13 Bass WM. *Human Osteology. A Laboratory and Field Manual* (3rd edn). Columbia: Missouri Archaeological Society, 1987.

14 Brothwell DR. *Digging Up Bones* (3rd edn). London: British Museum (Natural History), 1981.

15 MacLaughlin SM, Cox MJ. The relationship between body size and parturition scars. *Journal of Anatomy* 1989; **164**: 258.

16 Sutherland LD, Suchey JM. Use of the ventral arc in pubic sex determination. *Journal of Forensic Sciences* 1991; **36**: 501–511.

17 Lovell NC. Test of Phenice's technique for determining sex from the os pubis. *American Journal of Physical Anthropology* 1989; **79**: 117–120.

18 MacLaughlin SM, Bruce MF. The sciatic notch/acetabulum index as a discriminator of sex in European skeletal remains. *Journal of Forensic Sciences* 1986; **31**: 1380–1390.

19 Kelley MA. Sex determination with fragmented human remains. *Journal of Forensic Sciences* 1979; **24**: 154–158.

20 Schulter-Ellis FP, Hayek LC, Schmidt DJ. Determination of sex with a discriminate analysis of new pelvic bone measurements: part II. *Journal of Forensic Sciences* 1985; **30**: 178–185.

21   Schulter-Ellis FP, Schmidt DJ, Hayek LC, Craig J. Determination of sex with a discriminate analysis of new pelvic bone measurements: part I. *Journal of Forensic Sciences* 1983; **28**: 169–180.

22   Krogman WM, Işcan MY (eds), *The Human Skeleton in Forensic Medicine* (2nd edn). Springfield: Charles C Thomas, 1986: pp. 156–162.

23   Mays S. *The Archaeology of Human Bones*. London: Routledge/English Heritage, 1998.

24   Stewart TD. *Essentials of Forensic Anthropology*. Springfield: Charles C Thomas, 1979.

25   Ubelaker D. *Human Skeletal Remains: Excavation, Analysis, Interpretation* (2nd edn). Washington, DC: Taraxacum, 1989.

26   Wienker CW. Sex determination from human skeletal remains: A case of mistaken assumption. In: TA Rathburn, JE Buikstra (eds), *Human Identification*. Springfield: Charles C Thomas, 1984: pp. 229–223.

27   Loth SR, Henneberg M. Mandibular ramus flexure: A new morphological indicator of sexual dimorphism in the human skeleton. *American Journal of Physical Anthropology* 1996; **99**: 473–485.

28   Koski K. Mandibular ramus flexure – indicator of sexual dimorphism? *American Journal of Physical Anthropology* 1996; **101**: 545–546.

29   Donnelly SM, Hens SM, Rogers NL, Schneider KL. Technical note: A blind test of mandibular ramus flexure as a morphological indicator of sexual dimorphism in the human skeleton. *American Journal of Physical Anthropology* 1998; **107**: 363–366.

30   Maat GJR, Mastwijk RW, Van der Velde EA. On the reliability of non-metrical morphological sex determination of the skull compared with that of the pelvis in the Low Countries. *International Journal of Osteoarchaeology* 1997; **7**: 575–580.

31   Hanihara K. Sexual diagnosis of Japanese long bones by means of discriminate functions. *Journal of Anthropological Society of Nippon* 1959; **67**: 21–27.

32   Giles E. Discriminate function sexing of the human skeleton. In: Stewart TD (ed.), *Personal Identification in Mass Disasters*. Washington, DC: Smithsonian Institution, 1970: pp. 99–107.

33   Giles E. Sex determination by discriminate function analysis of the mandible. *American Journal of Physical Anthropology* 1964; **22**: 129–135.

34   Molleson TI, Cox MJ. *The Spitalfields Project*, vol. 2: *The Anthropology – The Middling Sort*. Research Report 86. York: Council for British Archaeology, 1993.

35   Işcan MY, Loth SR, Wright RK. Age estimation from the rib by phase analysis: white males. *Journal of Forensic Sciences* 1984; **29**: 1094–1104.

36   Işcan MY, Loth SR, Wright RK. Age estimation from the rib by phase analysis: white females. *Journal of Forensic Sciences* 1985; **30**: 853–863.

37   Cologlu AS, Iscan MY, Yavuz MF, Sari H. Sex determination from the ribs of contemporary Turks. *Journal of Forensic Sciences* 1998; **43**: 273–276.

38   Lui W. Sex determination of Chinese femur by discriminate function. *Journal of Forensic Sciences* 1989; **34**: 1222–1227.

39   Trancho G J, Robledo B, Lopez-Bueis I, Sanchez JA. Sexual determination of the femur using discriminate functions. Analysis of a Spanish population of known sex and age. *Journal of Forensic Sciences* 1997; **42**: 181–185.

40   Seidemann RM, Stojanowski CM, Doran GH. The use of the supero-inferior femoral neck diameter as a sex assessor. *American Journal of Physical Anthropology* 1998; **107**: 305–313.

41   Schutkowski H. Geschlechtsdifferente Merkmale an kindlichen Skeletten, Kentnisstand und diagnostische Beduetung. *Zeitschrift für Morphologie und Anthropologie* 1986; **76**: 149–168.

42   Boucher BJ. Sex differences in the foetal pelvis. *American Journal of Physical Anthropology* 1957; **15**: 581–600.

43   Fazekas IG, Kósa F. *Forensic Foetal Osteology*. Budapest: Academiai Kiado, 1978.

44   Weaver DS. Sex differences in the ilia of a known sex and age sample of fetal and infant skeletons. *American Journal of Physical Anthropology* 1980; **52**: 191–195.

45   Holcomb SMC, Konigsberg LW. Statistical study of sexual dimorphism in the human fetal sciatic notch. *American Journal of Physical Anthropology* 1995; **97**: 113–125.

46   Hunt DR. Sex Determination in the subadult ilia: an indirect test of Weaver's non-metric sexing method. *Journal of Forensic Sciences* 1990; **35**: 881–885.

47   Mittler DM, Sheridan SG. Sex determination in subadults using auricular surface morphology: a forensic science perspective. *Journal of Forensic Sciences* 1992; **7**: 1068–1075.

48   Schutkowski H. Sex determination of infant and juvenile skeletons: I. Morphognostic features. *American Journal of Physical Anthropology* 1993; **90**: 199–205.

49   Molleson T, Cruse K, Mays S. Some sexually dimorphic features of the human juvenile skull and their value in sex determination in immature skeletal remains. *Journal of Archaeological Science* 1998; **25**: 719–728.

50   Black TK. Sexual dimorphism in the tooth-crown diameters of the deciduous teeth. *American Journal of Physical Anthropology* 1978; **48**: 77–82.

51   Garn SM, Lewis AB, Kerewsky RS. Sex difference in tooth size. *Journal of Dental Research* 1964; **43**: 306.

52   Alvesalo L. Sex chromosomes and human growth, a dental approach. *Human Genetics* 1997; **101**: 1–5.

53   Hanihara K. Differences in sexual dimorphism in dental morphology among several human populations. In: Butler PM, Joysey KA (eds), *Development, Function and Evolution of the Teeth*. London: Academic Press, 1978: pp. 127–133.

54   Lavelle CLB. Anglo-Saxon and modern British teeth. *Journal of Dental Research* 1968; **47**: 811–815.

55   Brace CL, Ryan AS. Sexual dimorphism and human tooth size differences. *Journal of Human Evolution* 1980; **9**: 417–435.

56   Garn SM, Lewis AB, Swindler DR, Kerewsky RS. Genetic control of sexual dimorphism in tooth size. *Journal of Dental Research* 1967; **46**: 963–972.

57   Rösing FW. Sexing immature human skeletons. *Journal of Human Evolution* 1983; **12**: 149–155.

58   Duncan C. Sex determination using tooth measurements. In: Anderson S (ed.), *Current and Recent Research in Osteoarchaeology*. Proceedings of the Third Meeting of the Osteoarchaeological Research Group. Oxford: Oxbow, 1998: pp. 51–62.

59   Moss ML, Moss-Salentijn L. Analysis of developmental processes related to human dental sexual dimorphism in permanent and deciduous canines. *American Journal of Physical Anthropology* 1977; **46**: 407–414.

60   Lysell L, Myrberg N. Mesio-distal tooth size in the deciduous and permanent dentitions. *European Journal of Orthodontics* 1982; **4**: 113–122.

61   Gustafson G, Koch G. Age estimation up to 16 years of age based on dental development. *Odontologisk Revy* 1974; **25**: 297–306.

62   Molleson T. The Human Remains. In: Farwell DE, Molleson TI (eds), *Excavations at Poundbury 1966–80*, vol. 2: *The Cemeteries*. Dorset Natural History and Archaeological Society Monograph Series No. 11. Dorchester: Dorset Natural History and Archaeological Society, 1993: pp. 142–214.

63   Langenscheidt F. Diskriminanzanalytische geschlechtsbestimmung an hand von zahnmassen – unter verwending von verfahren zur angenähert unverzerrten schätzung der trennstärke. *Homo* 1983; **34**: 22–27.

64   Scott GT, Parham KR. Multivariate dental sexing: discrimination of the sexes within an East Tennessee Mississippian skeletal sample. *Tennessee Anthropologist* 1979; **4**: 189–198.

65   Mays S. The human skeletal remains. In: Timby JR (ed.), *The Anglo-Saxon Cemetery at Empingham II, Rutland*. Monograph 70. Oxford: Oxbow, 1996: pp. 21–33.

66   Ditch LE, Rose JC. A multivariate dental sexing technique. *American Journal of Physical Anthropology* 1972; **37**: 61–64.

67   Searle AG. Genetical studies on the skeleton of the mouse XI. The influence of diet on the variation within pure lines. *Journal of Genetics* 1954; **52**: 413–424.

68   Holloway PJ, Shaw JH, Sweeney EA. Effects of various sucrose:casein ratios in purified diets on the teeth and supporting structures of rats. *Archives of Oral Biology* 1961; **3**: 185–200.

69   Tonge CH, McCance RA. Severe under-nutrition in growing and adult animals. 15. The mouth, jaws and teeth of pigs. *British Journal of Nutrition* 1965; **19**: 361–372.

70   Bunyard MW. Effects of high sucrose cariogenic diets with varied protein-calorie levels on the bones and teeth of the rat. *Calcified Tissue Research* 1972; **8**: 217–227.

71 Paynter KJ, Grainger RM. The relation of nutrition to the morphology and size of rat molar teeth. *Journal of the Canadian Dental Association* 1956; **22**: 519–531.

72 Suzuki N. Generational differences in size and morphology of tooth crowns in the young modern Japanese. *Anthropological Science* 1993; **101**: 405–429.

73 Guagliardo MF. Tooth crown size differences between age groups: a possible new indicator of stress in skeletal samples. *American Journal of Physical Anthropology* 1982; **58**: 383–389.

74 Simpson SW, Hutchinson DL, Larsen CS. Coping with stress: tooth size, dental defects and age at death. In: Larsen CS (ed.), *The Archaeology of the Mission Santa Catalina de Guale: 2. Biocultural Interpretations of a Population in Transition*. Anthropological Paper No. 68. New York: American Museum of Natural History, 1990: pp. 66–77.

75 Aufderheide AC, Rodriguez-Martin C. *The Cambridge Encyclopedia of Human Palaeopathology*. Cambridge: Cambridge University Press, 1998.

76 Goose DH. Reduction of palate size in modern populations. *Archives of Oral Biology* 1962; **7**: 343–350.

77 Moore WJ, Lavelle CLB, Spence TF. Changes in the size and shape of the human mandible in Britain. *British Dental Journal* 1968; **125**: 163–169.

78 Tomenchuk J, Mayhall JT. A correlation of tooth wear and age among modern Igloolik Eskimos. *American Journal of Physical Anthropology* 1979; **51**: 67–78.

79 Walker PL. Problems of preservation and sexism in sexing: some lessons from historical collections for palaeodemographers. In: Saunders SR, Herring A (eds), *Grave Reflections: Portraying the Past through Cemetery Studies*. Toronto: Canadian Scholars, 1995: pp. 31–46.

80 Reynolds EL. The bony pelvis in pre-pubertal childhood. *American Journal of Physical Anthropology* 1947; **5**: 165–200.

81 Saunders SR, DeVito C. Subadult skeletons in the Raymond Dart anatomical collection: research potential. *Human Evolution* 1991; **6**: 421–434.

9

ASSESSMENT OF PARTURITION

Margaret Cox

'The Queen of Scots is but this day leichter [*sic.*] of a fair son, and I am but of a barren stock.'

Elizabeth I (1533–1603)

INTRODUCTION

Were UK biological anthropologists to be presented with the skeletal remains of the two early post-medieval women noted above, it is likely that most would not even stop to consider the issue of whether either had borne children. If we use the literature as a guide, having been a subject of much concern in the 1970s and 1980s, the issue of assessment of parturition in human skeletal samples seems not to be significant to today's *biological* anthropologist. Indeed, many modern textbooks on skeletal biology do not even mention parity assessment.[1,2] It is perhaps paradoxical that, reflecting the paramount importance of childbearing, and consequently fertility to individuals and social groups across the world, the *cultural* anthropologist would devote considerable energy to this subject.

DEFINITIONS AND RESEARCH BACKGROUND

It is prudent to open this discussion with the definition of terms, some of which are used arbitrarily in the literature. *Fecundity* is the ability to produce live offspring; hence, the period from puberty to menopause in females and from puberty to death in males. *Gravid* is the state of pregnancy and the number of pregnancies, where known, is denoted by the prefix of a Roman numeral. *Parturition* is the process of childbirth; so assessment of parturition or parity status is the determination of whether a woman has given birth and is parous, or has not and is nulliparous. A woman who has undergone several pregnancies is referred to as multiparous. *Fertility* is the number of live births delivered to a female during her fecund period and one that excludes miscarriages or stillbirths.

This chapter is concerned with the assessment of parturition in the female skeleton. It is not going to include discussion of population fertility, which is covered elsewhere[1] and based upon the use of palaeodemographic data, particularly mortality profiles.

Parity assessment

There are three areas of research relevant to this field of inquiry. They comprise so-called 'scars of parturition' (i.e. areas of cortical resorption on the anterio-inferior ilium adjacent to the sacro-iliac joints and postero-superior pubic symphysis), extension of the pubic tubercle, and finally changes to bone micromorphology and cortical dynamics.

Scars of parturition

As would be expected, concern with attempting to assess parturition in skeletal material has concentrated on the bony pelvis. Particularly on the antero-inferior ilium adjacent to the sacro-iliac joints, where interosseous ligaments connect ilium to sacrum, and the postero-superior symphysis pubis where ligaments are important in strengthening the articulation (both are secondary cartilaginous joints and the sacro-iliac joint has a synovial component). Neither joint facilitates much movement and the primary function of both is in relation to the stability of the pelvic girdle, an important structure in the transfer of weight from the trunk to the lower limbs.

Research, producing equivocal results, has concentrated upon the distribution of cortical resorption and remodelling adjacent to the ventral pre-auricular margins of the ilium and sacrum and on the dorsal aspect of the pubic body, both of which are strongly sexually dimorphic. The morphology and dynamics of muscle/ligament/tendon to bone interface is extremely complex[3] and not entirely understood. However, in the context of providing a background to this area of research, understanding was that hormonally mediated relaxation of the joints takes place during pregnancy. This involves the hormone relaxin, possibly acting synergistically with oestrogen, which is produced during pregnancy by the corpus luteum.[4] This was followed by a 'hyperaemia of the joint capsules and ligaments as well as by minor haemorrhages at the bone/cartilage interfaces during parturition … ventral ligaments are heavily stretched and in part lacerate, and the periosteum may be lifted … disintegrated masses injected into the ligaments … lead to pea sized bulges in the joint capsule … there forming debris cysts which cause lacunar bone resorption … ' (p. 25).[5] Simplified, this means that as a consequence of pregnancy and childbirth, ligaments involved in pelvic articulation, which are known to be affected by endocrine changes[4] and their attachment sites, are under stress and possibly incur trauma, after which processes of cortical reorganization, repair and resorption take place. It was believed that macroscopic skeletal manifestations of this process of recovery and repair to bone following parturition were apparent on female pelves. Research focused on the pre-auricular sulcus and pitting of the postero-superior pubis.

The deep and 'scooped' pre-auricular sulcus (Figure 1) was first described in 1866 by Zaaiger.[6] It was, and still is, noted almost exclusively in females.[6–15] Less clearly marked and shallower areas of resorption (Figure 2) at the pre-auricular margins were, and are occasionally seen in males.[14–17] The same is true for pitting of the dorsal pubis (Figure 3), which was first described by Luschka in 1854[5] as a dimorphic feature, and by Putschar in 1931[7] as an indicator of parturition.

Following hypotheses postulated by such researchers as Angel,[18] Stewart,[19] Houghton,[20,21] and Ullrich 1975,[5] this dimorphism resulted in the pre-auricular sulcus and pubic pitting

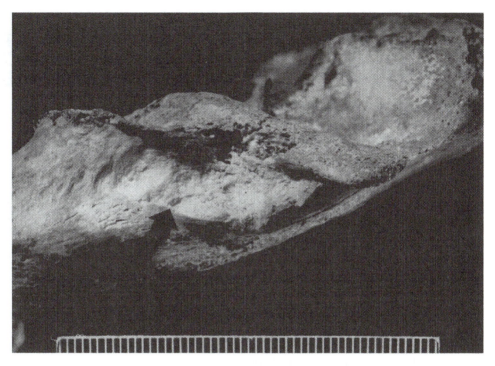

Figure 1 – Deep and rugged pre-auricular sulcus in a female of unknown parity status from Christ Church, Spitalfields, London.

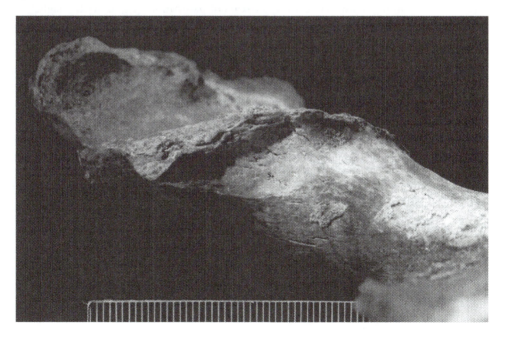

Figure 2 – Pre-auricular sulcus with less marked and shallower features than that shown in Figure 1. Observed on the same female of unknown parity status from Christ Church, Spitalfields.

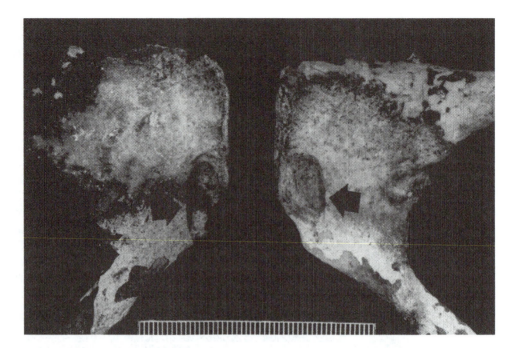

Figure 3 – Cortical resorption on the dorsal aspect of the pubic body. Observed in a female with five recorded births from Christ Church, Spitalfields.

becoming known collectively as 'scars of parturition' (e.g. Ullrich,[5] Tague[17]). It should be noted that in all cases, methods and diagnostic criteria were devised using skeletal samples of unknown parity status.

Meaningful evaluation of the obstetric significance of pre-auricular sulci and dorsal pubic pitting was impaired by the lack of reliably documented skeletal samples where the obstetric history of females was known. Affirmative evaluation of these methods was undertaken on such material as the Hamann-Todd[22,23] and Terry collections. With these samples parity assessment was largely determined by soft tissue analysis. Depending upon the soft tissue criterion employed, this method is not necessarily considered reliable (i.e. where abdominal stretch marks were used as an indicator of pregnancy). Contrary to earlier work, Anderson[24] found no significant relationship between scars of parturition and obstetric histories in the Hamann-Todd collection.

From the 1980s, small samples of reliably documented autopsy/willed body material became increasingly available. Obstetric histories were derived from medical histories and families. While this method may not be 100% reliable it is probably the best that can be achieved. The same decade also saw the recovery of a documented archaeological sample, the skeletons excavated from the vaults beneath Christ Church, Spitalfields, London, in 1984–86.[25,26]

Of studies undertaken on these more reliably documented autopsy/willed body samples, Suchey *et al.*[16] found only a weak correlation between full-term pregnancies and pubic pitting in an autopsy sample of known parity status. Bergfelder and Herrmann[27] also found no unequivocal relationship between pubic pitting and pregnancy and parturition. Dunlap[12] concluded that no accurate prediction of obstetric events was possible but that a deep and grooved pre-auricular sulcus was associated with parturition. Conversely, using a radiographic sample, Spring et al.[13] found no relationship between the two.

The opportunity to assess obstetric histories in archaeological material is rare. Defining obstetric histories in the Christ Church, Spitalfields sample (died 1729–1852) relied upon the association of legible coffin plates in secure archaeological association with a skeleton and the availability of relevant and reliable historical documentation. Clearly, this sample and method has limitations and identified problems (i.e. live births which were not baptized or registered and stillbirths which, in the UK, are historically invisible) which could cast doubt on the reliable identification of nulliparous females. However, a sample of 94 females with obstetric histories was identified with reasonable confidence. In this sample, there was no statistically significant association between the absence, presence, severity, type or size of the pre-auricular sulcus with parity status; the same proved to be the case with pubic pitting.[14,15]

A more recent study on material from a Coroner's Office[28] concludes that pubic pitting increases in relation to the number of births, but notes that such pitting can also be associated with stature. MacLaughlin and Cox[29] also observed a correlation between the presence of sulci and pits with body size in modern Dutch and archaeological British material. Anderson[24] observed that pitting and sulci relate to pelvic flexibility in females and Cox[14] observed that the presence or absence of pubic pitting, and pre-auricular sulci, were positively associated with a wide range of pelvic dimensions. Such work suggests that the presence of pre-auricular sulci and pubic pitting may relate to biomechanics not parturition.

Recent research by Tague,[30] examining pre-auricular and pubic morphology of macaques in relation to parturition and age, suggests that in humans there might be different aetiologies for resorption of the pubic and pre-auricular areas. He considers that pubic pitting in reproductively active human females reflects oestrogen-induced resorption, which, in macaques, inhibits synostosis of the inter-pubic joint. But, that as both males and nulliparous females in both species can also present such resorption, reproduction is not the single aetiology and probably not the primary one.

In light of the literature reviewed above, it must be concluded that if parturition is one aetiology associated with either pubic pitting or pre-auricular sulci, it is unequivocally not the only etiological factor involved and certainly not the most important.

Pubic tubercle extension

A largely ignored breakthrough in this field occurred when Bergfelder and Hermann[27] examined the pubic tubercle (Figure 4) as a possible indicator of parity status. The rationale underlying this investigation was that the tubercle is part of the attachment site of *rectus abdominis*. *Rectus abdominis* is a superficial muscle of the abdomen, that is one of a group of muscles which is responsible for (among other things) anterior containment and compression of the abdominal viscera, a task which is particularly important during the later months

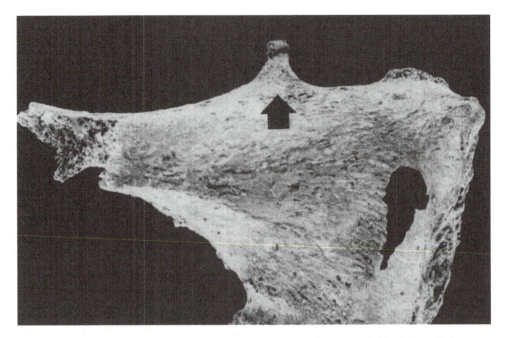

Figure 4 – Extended pubic tubercle (dorsal view) seen on a female with one recorded birth from Christ Church, Spitalfields.

of pregnancy. The superficial abdominal musculature has a further role in childbirth in that it assists in expelling the foetus from the uterus.

Abdominus rectus is a long flat muscle that extends along the whole length of the front of the abdomen. It is attached to the pubis by two tendons, the larger of which is attached to the crest of the os pubis and the pubic tubercle. The smaller tendon attaches to the other pubic crest where it also connects to the ligamentous tissue covering the anterior pubic symphysis. The muscle is attached superiorly to the cartilage of the fifth, sixth and seventh ribs. Some fibres attach to the anterior extremity (largely to the costal cartilage) of the fifth rib and the xiphoid. No work has been published looking at associated cortical remodelling at these attachment sites. The pubic tubercle is also the attachment site of the inguinal ligament, which also attaches to the supero-anterior iliac spine. This is also under stress during the latter months of pregnancy.

Hirschberg *et al.*[3] consider that the complexity and morphology of ligamentous/tendon interfaces with bone, whether convexities or concavities, are related to the precise form and angle of attachment of ligaments/tendons and stresses that are applied. Consequently, observation of such characteristics on the skeletal pelvis suggests that sulci and pitting appear to relate to lateral tension, and tubercles seem to relate to longitudinal stress. In light of this theory, it seems unlikely that stress to the tubercle relating to the inguinal ligament during later pregnancy would result in the form of tubercle extension under discussion.

Considering the implications of distension of abdominus rectus during pregnancy, the subsequent stress on the attachment sites at the pubic crest, and stretching of the inguinal ligament, Bergfelder and Hermann[27] evaluated the relationship between the degree of extension of the pubic tubercle and obstetric events. They found no unequivocal relationship between the extension of tubercle and parity status (i.e. either nulliparous or parous). However, despite this, the extended tubercle was usually associated with females known to have experienced more than three births. Evaluating this relationship in females with known obstetric histories at Christ Church[14,15] it was found that unlike Bergfelder and Hermann's sample, the pubic tubercle was statistically significantly associated with parity status. Results showed a concordance with the earlier study in that this sample also demonstrated a significant statistical relationship between tubercle extension and the number of births. Unfortunately, the results of Galloway et al.'s[28] work on modern autopsy material are not yet available in any detail.

Bone micromorphology and cortical bone dynamics

Little attention has been paid to evaluating the possibility that there might be a relationship between pregnancy and lactation and bone micromorphology, including cortical bone dynamics and involution, in samples with documented obstetric histories or otherwise. Bone loss in healthy adults affects both sexes. Beginning in the fourth decade it becomes more pronounced with increasing age.[31] Cortical bone dynamics have been examined in relation to lactation and pregnancy by Mensforth and Lovejoy[32] in the Libben sample which is of unknown parity status and whose ages have been determined by multifactorial methods. They note a reduction of mid-shaft femoral cortex in females presumed to have died in their third decade, with a higher level being restored in females by the middle of the fourth decade, before decreasing thereafter (reflecting menopausal hormonal influences). A similar trend has been noted elsewhere.[33–36] It is suggested that this age-specific bone loss, one forming an inverse curve with Weiss's[37] modal fertility curve, may represent calcium stress imposed by the increased nutritional demands of pregnancy and lactation.

Although, in theory, the potential of such studies is clear, this is an extremely complex area of research. It is known from clinical studies that pregnancy tends to increase bone mass, with nulliparity increasing a female's risk of developing osteoporosis, and that the greater the number of births, the lower the risk of hip fracture.[38] (It should be noted that Wyshak's[38] clinical study was based on a sample of 827 females (90% Caucasoid) aged over 65 years, with obstetric histories. The study did not consider race, weight, or any other relevant variables.) However, prolonged lactation can deplete bone mass.[34,36] A controlled clinical trial by Kent et al.[39] ($n = 80$) suggests that the deficit is compensated for by an elevated bone formation rate following weaning in those lactating for 6 months. Consideration of these variables complicates matters and it has to be further remembered that in archaeological samples we rarely have any real understanding of the status of other variables known to influence bone involution (e.g. race, weight, activity levels, diet, smoking) in clinical trials.

Mensforth and Lovejoy[32] also noted an increase in the prevalence of unremodelled porotic hyperostosis (i.e. cribra orbitalia and cranii) in females of the same age range. Following others,[35,40–42] the authors consider that this might reflect iron deficiency anaemia resulting from pregnancy and lactation. It is postulated that this might represent the increased nutritional demands of pregnancy and lactation in parous females dying during their fertile period. Both the reduction of cortex and porotic hyperostosis reflecting higher than normal demands for calcium and iron associated with pregnancy and lactation.

PRESENT STATUS OF METHODOLOGY

The methods discussed above fall into three research areas. The first, examining the deep pre-auricular sulcus and dorsal pubic pitting, suggest that they reflect biomechanical influences associated with the role of the pelvic girdle in transmitting weight from the trunk to the lower limbs, overall body and pelvic size, and locomotion. There are little, if any, convincing data to suggest that either is significantly associated with obstetric events.

The second, pubic tubercle extension is considered unequivocally to reflect increased stress on abdominal musculature, and its attachment sites to the pubic crest and tubercle, via ligamentous tissue, during the later stages of pregnancy. Consequently, research to date suggests that the extended tubercle in females does relate to parturition and seems to increase with the number of obstetric events. Data from Christ Church[14,15] show that the relationship between parity status and an extended tubercle is statistically significant at $p < 0.01$ ($n = 33$). A relationship between extension and the number of births is also apparent ($p < 0.05$). However, as mentioned above, concern must be raised with this sample that nulliparous females may be over-represented. Of those believed to be nulliparous, 33.3% had an extended tubercle. Nevertheless, the similarity between these results and the earlier work of Bergfelder and Hermann,[27] where medical histories were available for a dissecting room sample lends credibility to the results obtained on the archaeological material. What these results indicate is that this method provides a reliable indication of parity status in both archaeological skeletons and modern autopsy material. This suggests that the underlying biological processes are not modified by extraneous variables. However, extreme caution should be applied when considering its application to *individual* forensic cases. In such cases it should also be considered that Galloway *et al.*'s work[28] suggests that tubercle extension can relate to arcuate angle, while that from Christ Church produced no convincing correlations between tubercle extension and either stature or pelvimetry.[14]

Changes to bone microstructure as a consequence of pregnancy and lactation have been little explored in the anthropological literature. While its utility might be largely confined to assessment of fertility of those dying within their fecund period, analysis of cortical bone maintenance might merit further work. Unfortunately, Mensforth and Lovejoy's work[32] appears not to have been followed through by others. This is undoubtedly a difficult area to pursue. The clinical literature makes it clear that while multiple pregnancies tend to increase bone mass, nulliparity generally has the opposite effect. Combine this with the fact that prolonged lactation can deplete bone mass and the picture becomes very complex.

FUTURE RESEARCH

The present trend apparent in the literature is that while much energy is being applied to resolving the significance and aetiology of pre-auricular sulci and dorsal pubic pitting,[28,30] less is being expended in determining parturition in skeletal material. This is perhaps unfortunate and can, in part, be explained by a shortage of reliably documented material to evaluate. Perhaps it also reflects a lack of current interest in assessment of parturition. It is an interesting reflection of research priorities, where focus appears to dwell on minute cortical variables rather than on larger issues which were fundamentally important to the peoples whose lives we profess to seek to understand, and engage with, on their terms.

How should we progress in this subject area? Clearly, if there is no interest within biological anthropology we cannot. However, this situation if it exists now will not – indeed cannot – persist. Unless we practice an anthropology that has public and social, and consequently some funding relevance, we will lose public support. This could be critical if the UK and other countries ever have to face the reburial movement, resulting in not only the reburial of collections, but also a climate where the excavation of cemetery assemblages is either reduced or forbidden.

Areas that clearly merit further research are bone histomorphology and extension of the pubic tubercle. Examination of the xiphoid in older females, to which *abdominus rectus* also attaches, might also yield useful data. Childbearing and lactation place a considerable physiological cost upon the mother; demands that might be reflected in anomalous bone micromorphology, involution and cortical dynamics. Further work is required to assess the extent of such changes to individuals during their childbearing years. This could utilize a wide range of material from autopsy samples to radiographic data and material from documented archaeological contexts. As tests for bone density are now frequently taken on living samples, such data might also be fruitfully applied to this area of research.

Clearly, the issue of the reliability of the extension of the pubic tubercle needs further investigation on large samples of material with known obstetric histories. These can be procured through autopsy/willed body samples in some countries (e.g. USA, Italy) or through archaeological material from the 18th and 19th centuries where skeletons are recovered in a secure context with legible coffin plates. Given the extent and nature of ecclesiastic and civic registration at this time, the reconstruction of reliable obstetric histories is possible. Though as stated above, confidence placed upon those who were apparently nulliparous needs to be cautious.

If further research verifies the significance of the extended pubic tubercle, another issue needs to be considered. It is a matter of concern that the excavation of human remains is often undertaken by those with limited or no relevant experience.[43] Morphological characteristics such as the pubic tubercle are extremely fragile projections on an anterior aspect of the skeleton prone to post-mortem decay and damage. As McKinley and Roberts[44] observe, while all archaeologists have a skeleton, it does not follow that they have any real understanding of the form or components of the same. Unfortunately, it is an indisputable fact that many field archaeologists have no real understanding of pelvic morphology and it is within the realms of possibility, indeed almost a probability, that the pubic tubercle will be damaged during excavation and post-excavation processing. To prevent this from occurring, it is essential that archaeology undergraduates should be taught human skeletal morphology as an essential component of their education. The field archaeologist who is never required to excavate a human skeleton is a rarity, and it is the excavators and finds processors who facilitate the analysis of the remains by the biological anthropologist.

Ultimately, our analyses and interpretation of the past are in the hands of the field archaeologist. The realization of the potential of human remains from archaeological deposits is at the mercy of their level of skill and their excavation strategies. It behoves us to work more closely with them ensuring that they share our aims and understand the requirements of our methods.

ACKNOWLEDGMENTS

Sue Black and Simon Mays kindly acted as referees for this chapter and are thanked for their useful and thought provoking comments. The figures are reproduced with kind permission of The Natural History Museum, London. Photographs were taken by Phillip Crabbe.

REFERENCES

1   Larsen CS. *Bioarchaeology: Interpreting Behavior from the Human Skeleton.* Cambridge: Cambridge University Press, 1997.

2   Mays S. *The Archaeology of Human Bones.* London: Routledge, 1998.

3   Hirschberg J, Milne N, Oxnard CE. The interface between muscle and bone: biomechanical implications. *American Journal of Physical Anthropology* 1998; 26 (suppl.): 96.

4   Casey ML, Macdonald PC. The endocrinology of human parturition. *American Academy of Sciences* 1997; **26**: 273–284.

5   Ullrich H. Estimation of fertility by means of pregnancy and childbirth alterations at the pubis, the ilium and the sacrum. *Ossa* 1975; **2**: 23–39.

6   Derry DE. Note on the innominate bone as a factor in the determination of sex. *Journal of Anatomical Physiology* 1909; **43**: 266–276.

7   Putschar WGJ. *Entwicklung, wachstum und pathologie der beckenverbindungen des menschen, mit besonderer berücksichtigung von schwangerschaft, geburt und ihren Folgen.* Jena: Gustav Fischer, 1931.

8   Cornwall IW. *Bones for the Archaeologist.* New York: Macmillan, 1956.

9   Krogman WM. *The Human Skeleton in Forensic Medicine.* Springfield: Charles C Thomas, 1962.

10 Bass WM. *Human Osteology: A Laboratory and Field Manual.* Columbia: Missouri Archaeological Society, 1971.

11 Putschar WGJ. The structure of the human symphysis pubis with special consideration of parturition and its sequelae. *American Journal of Physical Anthropology* 1976; **45**: 589–594.

12 Dunlap SS. A study of preauricular sulci in a cadaver population. Unpublished PhD thesis, Michigan State University, 1981.

13 Spring DB, Lovejoy CO, Bender GN, Duerr M. The radiographic preauricular groove of pregnancy: its non-relationship to past parity. *American Journal of Physical Anthropology* 1989; **79**: 247–252.

14 Cox MJ. An evaluation of the significance of 'scars of parturition' in the Christ Church, Spitalfields sample. Unpublished PhD thesis, University College London, 1989.

15 Cox MJ, Scott A. Evaluation of the obstetric significance of some pelvic characters in an 18th century British sample of known parity status. *American Journal of Physical Anthropology* 1992; **89**: 431–440.

16   Suchey JM, Wisely DV, Green RF, Noguchi TT. Analysis of dorsal pitting in the os pubis in an extensive sample of modern American females. *American Journal of Physical Anthropology* 1979; **51**: 517–540.

17   Tague RG. Bone resorption of the pubis and preauricular area in humans and non-human mammals. *American Journal of Physical Anthropology* 1988; **76**: 251–267.

18   Angel JL. The bases of palaeodemography. *American Journal of Physical Anthropology* 1969; **30**: 427–437.

19   Stewart TD. Identification of scars of parturition in the skeletal remains of females. In: Stewart TD (ed.), *Personal Identification in Mass Disasters.* Washington, DC: National Museum of Natural History, 1970: pp. 127–135.

20   Houghton P. The relationship of the preauricular groove of the ilium to pregnancy. *American Journal of Physical Anthropology* 1974; **41**: 381–390.

21   Houghton P. The bony imprint of pregnancy. *New York Academy of Medicine* 1975; **51**: 655–661.

22   Holt CA. The relationship of the preauricular scars on the female pelvis. *American Journal of Physical Anthropology* 1978; **49**: 381–390.

23   Kelley MA. Parturition and pelvic changes. *American Journal of Physical Anthropology* 1979; **51**: 541–546.

24   Anderson BC. Pelvic scarring analysis: parturition or excess motion. *American Journal of Physical Anthropology* 1987; **75**: 181.

25   Molleson TI, Cox MJ. *The Spitalfields Project*, vol. 2: *The Anthropology – The Middling Sort.* Research Report 86. York: Council for British Archaeology, 1993.

26   Cox MJ. *Life and Death in Spitalfields: 1700–1850.* York: Council for British Archaeology, 1996.

27   Bergfelder T, Herrmann B. Estimating fertility on the basis of birth traumatic changes in the pubic bone. *Journal of Human Evolution* 1980; **9**: 611–613.

28   Galloway A, Snodgrass JJ, Suchey J. Markers of childbirth? Effect of body size and pubic morphological change. *American Journal of Physical Anthropology* 1998; 26 (suppl.): 102.

29   MacLaughlin SM, Cox MJ. The relationship between body size and parturition scars. *Journal of Anatomy* 1989; **164**, 258.

30   Tague RG. Morphology of the pubis and preauricular area in relation to parity and age at death in Macaca mulatta. *American Journal of Physical Anthropology* 1990; **82**: 517–525.

31   Gallager and Riggs, 1978, cited in 32.

32   Mensforth RP, Lovejoy CO. Anatomical, physiological and epidemiological correlates of the ageing process: a confirmation of the multifactorial age determination in the Libben population. *American Journal of Physical Anthropology* 1985; **68**: 87–106.

33   Sorenson JA, Cameron JR. A reliable *in vivo* measurement of bone mineral content. *Journal of Bone and Joint Surgery* 1967; **49A**: 481–97.

34   Atkinson PJ, West RR. Loss of skeletal calcium in lactating women. *Journal of Obstetrics and Gynaecology* 1970; **75**: 555–560.

35   Armelagos GJ. Disease in ancient Nubia. *Science* 1969; **163**: 167–259.

36   Goldsmith NF, Johnston JO. Bone mineral: effects of oral contraceptives, pregnancy and lactation. *Journal of Bone and Joint Surgery* 1975; **57A**: 657–68.

37   Weiss KM. *Demographic models for anthropology.* Memoir 27. Washington, DC: Society for American Archaeology, 1973.

38   Wyshak G. Hip fracture in elderly women with reproductive history. *Journal of Gerontology* 1981; **36**: 424–427.

39   Kent GN, Price RI, Gutteridge DH, *et al.* Human lactation: forearm trabecular bone loss, increased bone turnover, and renal conservation of calcium and inorganic phosphate with recovery of bone mass following weaning. *Journal of Bone and Mineral Research* 1990; **5**: 361–369.

40   Dewey JR, Armelagos GJ, Bartley MH. Femoral cortical bone loss in three Nubian populations. *Human Biology* 1969; **41**: 13–28.

41   Martin DL, Armelagos GJ. Morphometrics of compact bone: an example from Sudanese Nubia. *American Journal of Physical Anthropology* 1979; **51**: 571–578.

42 Stout S, Simmons DJ. Use of histology in ancient bone research. *Yearbook of Physical Anthropology* 1979; **22**: 228–49.

43 Bashford L, Pollard T. 'In the burying place': the excavation of a Quaker burial ground. In: Cox M (ed.), *Grave Concerns: Death and Burial in Post-Medieval England.* Research Report 113. York: Council for British Archaeology, 1998.

44 McKinley JI, Roberts CA. *Excavation and Post-excavation Treatment of Human Remains.* Technical Paper 13. Birmingham: Institute of Field Archaeology, 1993.

Section III

Disease in the past

That this section is the longest in this volume reflects the pre-eminence of palaeopathology in human osteology in Britain in recent decades. The medical backgrounds of many British osteologists working in the 1970s and 1980s meant that most palaeopathological work was directed at medico-historical questions. This situation is now changing as more have come to the discipline from an archaeological background, with the result that there has been a shift to the use of palaeopathology to address broader questions of health and lifestyle in earlier populations.

This section opens with an assessment of infectious disease by Charlotte Roberts. She surveys evidence for non-specific infections, and for tuberculosis, leprosy and treponemal disease, with a particular emphasis on the rich skeletal record for these conditions in Britain. She emphasizes the value of a biocultural perspective in which population-level data for patterns of disease are fully integrated with cultural evidence. Juliet Rogers provides a discussion of joint diseases, covering erosive arthropathies, hypertrophic joint disease, sero-negative spondyloarthropathies and some other joint disorders. The palaeopathology of the metabolic diseases is discussed by Megan Brickley, who focuses on scurvy, rickets, osteomalacia and osteoporosis, with an emphasis on diagnostic techniques. Trevor Anderson considers the evidence for congenital disorders and neoplastic disease in earlier British populations. Providing immensely useful tables of published cases, he goes on to discuss the likely prevalence of these conditions in archaeological material. Chrissie Freeth covers approaches to the study of dental health. In particular, she considers the methodological approaches to the recording of dental pathology in skeletal assemblages.

Specific methodological approaches to the diagnosis of disease are dealt with in the last two chapters. That by Angela Gernaey and David Minnikin reflects on the development of biomolecular techniques in palaeopathology. A variety of possible biomarkers for diagnosing disease in ancient bones is discussed, including DNA and protein residues from infecting microorganisms. This work has the potential to extend palaeopathological work beyond those diseases which cause skeletal lesions to those which do not. In the final chapter, Lynne Bell and Kim Piper examine the benefits of making greater use of bone histology in differential diagnosis of disease in ancient bones.

10

INFECTIOUS DISEASE IN BIOCULTURAL PERSPECTIVE: PAST, PRESENT AND FUTURE WORK IN BRITAIN

Charlotte Roberts

INTRODUCTION

The aims of this chapter are to review the types of information which are potentially retrievable from a study of infectious disease in antiquity, and the range of published research already extant worldwide on infectious disease, to document the range and quality of work already completed on British material, and to recommend the way forward and best practice. In such a short chapter it will not be possible to include all aspects of infectious disease in past populations but the more common approaches will be considered. It is of necessity that a biocultural approach needs to be considered. The term refers to the biological evidence for disease within its cultural context, e.g. did the living environment of populations predispose them to infectious disease? While some British researchers in palaeobiological anthropology do follow this biocultural approach to studying palaeopathology, others find it inappropriate for British material.

The infectious diseases cover a wide range of conditions affecting both soft tissue (e.g. plague, cholera, malaria) and the skeleton. While those infections which involve soft tissue will not be observed in the skeletal record (even though they may be studied in other ways, e.g. a palaeodemographic study of a plague cemetery,[1] and identification of the plague bacillus using ancient DNA[2]), in many infectious diseases only a small percentage of people will have skeletal involvement (e.g. 3–5% in tuberculosis[3]), and some people may have died before bone changes occurred, i.e. in the acute phase of the disease. It should also be noted that healed lesions represent chronicity and a healthy immune system that prevented the individual succumbing from the disease in the acute stage.[4] In many respects the study of infections in antiquity potentially provides a window on how humans have evolved and adapted to, or changed, their environment. As suggested,[5] 'infectious diseases have played a major role in the evolution of the human species . . . a prime mover in cultural transformation, as societies have responded to the social, economic, political, and psychological disruption engendered by acute epidemics . . . and chronic debilitating infectious diseases'

(p. 31). They are, therefore, a fascinating area of research in anthropology as a whole and need considering from a multidisciplinary perspective.

A range of pathogenic organisms consisting mainly of viruses, bacteria, fungi and parasites cause infections. Of course, whether a person is vulnerable to an infectious disease depends on many intrinsic and extrinsic factors. Pathogenicity of the agent, route of transmission, nature and strength of host response,[5] age, sex, genetic predisposition, nutritional status (there is a relationship between quality of diet and infection), occupation, trade and contact, climate, population density, economy, sanitation, quality of housing, and many more factors must be considered when interpreting the evidence for infectious disease in the past. However, much of the information needed to complete this jigsaw will not be available to the biological anthropologist because of the fragmentary nature of the data we deal with. Today, infectious disease remains *the* major cause of death worldwide and causes much ill health and misery in human populations.[6] Thus, it deems itself an important area of study in anthropology as a whole. By studying how infectious diseases have evolved, and the factors inherent in their appearance, transmission and maintenance in a population, they may help shed light on the epidemiology of infectious disease today.

This chapter will concentrate on those infections that affect the bones of the skeleton and have been recorded most commonly in skeletal material worldwide. These infections may be classified as specific (known causative organism) and non-specific (could be caused by a variety of organisms). Infections are usually associated with inflammation, or a cellular reaction to the invading organism, manifested as pain, swelling, tenderness and raised temperature.[7] In antiquity the infections evident in the skeletal record were more often caused by bacteria rather than viruses, as the latter would have been more rapidly overcome (or proved fatal), leaving no bone change. However, there are potential avenues for identifying viral infections that have been noted in the published literature. For example, smallpox can leave osteomyelitic and arthritic variolosa lesions, usually in the elbow joint,[8] and a possible example of these changes has been reported in the archaeological record.[9] Furthermore, poliomyelitis may be identified in the skeleton in the form of atrophy and osteoporosis of limb bones as a result of paralysis.[7] Finally, Paget's disease of bone, despite being of unknown specific aetiology, is suspected to be the result of a slow viral infection.[8] Although the bone changes of formation and/or destruction, *per se*, of non-specific and specific infections are the same, it is their distribution pattern which is characteristic in diagnosing the specific infections.

Many books, chapters, and major review articles have been published on the infectious diseases in antiquity.[7–18] These range in content from historical documentation, through diagnostic texts, to interpretative bioculturally focused discussions of data.

The infections most commonly reported and analysed in the palaeopathological literature are the non-specific infections affecting the periosteum (periostitis), cortex (osteitis) and medullary cavity (osteomyelitis) of bone. These changes, however, can also be seen as manifestations of a specific infection (but in a specific distribution pattern), or be focused on a particular part of the body. Leprosy, tuberculosis and treponemal disease are those specific infections reported most frequently (the fungal infections, seen in North

America have not yet been reported in British material and therefore are not considered here). However, focal non-specific infections in the sinuses (maxillary sinusitis), meninges (meningitis), ears (mastoiditis, otitis media), and lungs (affecting ribs) have seen increasing interest in biological anthropology in recent years, particularly in Britain. Non-specific periostitis, osteitis and osteomyelitis, however, may occur anywhere on the body, and periostitis (especially of the tibial shafts) has been the focus of much work in the palaeopathology of indicators of stress.[19]

Studies of infectious disease in past human skeletal populations have focused on a number of areas, all of which have, and still can, contribute in different ways to the palaeoepidemiology of infections. Much work has been undertaken on developing diagnostic criteria (particularly for the specific infections) which, in itself, is essential and the starting point for identification of infections in skeletal remains. Moreover, it has highlighted some problems in the clinically based diagnostic approach where diagnostic criteria from clinical sources may not always be appropriate for archaeological material. Case studies of specified infectious diseases, while not contributing to the advocated 'biocultural population approach' *per se*, do (when collated) add to the picture, i.e. without them there would be less data. However, the population-based biocultural approach is the one currently advocated. This enables the biological data to be linked meaningfully with cultural data and the data produced to have a more significant role in the reconstruction of past human evolution and adaptation. This approach inevitably considers ecological factors in the appearance and maintenance of infections in a population,[20] for example the impact of urban and rural environments on infectious disease and the change in frequency in infectious disease in hunter-gatherer as opposed to agricultural communities. The origin, evolution and spread of infectious disease worldwide, as a study in its own right, has been enabled by the production of data, while hypotheses about infectious disease have been raised on the basis of evidence reported. All these approaches are valid in the British context, although some areas have not been tackled using British data.

NON-SPECIFIC INFECTION

Non-specific infection appears to consistently increase in frequency with the transition to agriculture in many populations around the world.[21] The increase in population size and density, settled and permanent housing, poor sanitation, changes in nutrition, and increase in trade and contact are believed to have lead to an increase in susceptibility to infection. In addition, the development of urbanization and industrialization worldwide has contributed to increased rates of infectious disease. In British contexts it has not been possible to assess health at the transition to agriculture due to the lack of skeletal material available for study from pre-agricultural contexts. However, much skeletal material exists from specific contexts, which could be used for looking generally at infectious disease prevalence. Although a population study of sex differences in infectious disease (maxillary sinusitis) in urban and rural contexts has recently been undertaken,[22,23] urban infections, particularly in British medieval contexts, have rarely been a focus of interest (with some exceptions[24–26]). This is particularly surprising considering the wealth of contemporary historical data available for study and interpretation. Non-specific infection is recorded as case studies[27,28] and is routinely reported in the archaeological literature in British contexts in the form of periostitis, usually on the tibiae and fibulae, and osteitis and osteomyelitis (although the latter two tend to merge and are often both classed as osteomyelitis). Of course, other areas of the skeleton can also be involved especially when the changes are the result of a specific infection. However, periostitis can also be an indicator of other conditions that must all be considered in a differential diagnosis, e.g. trauma. The differential diagnosis of the infectious diseases has also been discussed from a British perspective.[29]

Data in Britain are generally presented as individuals affected rather than actual prevalence rates (both should be given). Few people have taken the data further than this, with some exceptions where non-specific infection has been considered along with other 'indicators of stress'. For example, in one study[30] nearly 60% of subadult individuals suffered long bone periostitis in both urban and rural populations. In North America this information is routinely recorded for archaeologically derived skeletal material (for examples, see [21]), and the way forward is to acquire prevalence rates for this condition for British material. In addition, recording of the nature of the bone formed as a response to inflammation (i.e. woven or lamellar, denoting active or healed), its distribution pattern and prevalence rate, may help in some way to assess its aetiology. Of course, periostitis may be the result of trauma and, more specifically, has been reported as an indicator of child abuse,[31] and could be part of injury patterning in torture victims.[32] Whatever its aetiology, it does tend to occur more frequently on the tibiae, which, because of their extensive vascularity and physiologically inactive surfaces, slower blood circulation, and lack of soft tissue covering, are most vulnerable to develop bone changes of infection from colonization of the area with bacteria.[15] A point to note, although it is problematic to distinguish, is that in very young individuals, periosteal new bone formation should not be mistaken for new bone as a result of normal growth. In addition, there have been several instances where normal porosity on certain bone elements (e.g. the brow ridges and zygomatic bones of the skull) have been mistaken for periostitis.

A survey of published and unpublished data from British contexts reveals some problems. The first point to make is that, as there is no standard format for skeletal reports, non-specific infection tends to be assigned either to the infectious disease category or nutritional/metabolic disease, the former being preferred. Second, a common trend noted is the reporting of prevalence rates for non-specific infection by individuals affected and not as an absolute rate of bones affected compared with bones present,[33,34] with some exceptions.[35-39] No non-specific infection is reported for the post-medieval sample from Christ Church, Spitalfields, London,[40] which is surprising considering the historical evidence suggesting environmental factors predisposing to infection. In some instances specific individual skeletons are described in detail but no specific prevalence rates given.[41] While *individual* prevalence rates are essential for interpretation, this assumes that all bones for all individuals were present for observation (not the case for archaeological material). For example, if many skeletons are missing their lower leg bones then the most frequently affected bones in non-specific infection cannot be recorded and therefore the *actual* prevalence rate may be incorrect. *Actual* bone prevalence rates are also required to enable any meaningful interpretations and/or comparisons with populations both geographically and temporally. Valid and useful recommendations on the study of non-specific infection have been made,[19] which included narrowing down age ranges for individuals affected (which, for adults, is problematic considering the inaccuracy of ageing methods), distinguishing degree of severity, exact location and evidence of healing, considering factors associated with infection, nutrition and culture, age and sex differences, and integrating the data with other stress indicators.

When dealing with specific parts of the body with respect to non-specific infection (rib involvement is reserved for the section on tuberculosis), involvement of the maxillary sinuses is sometimes mentioned,[37,42,43] and infection of the ears,[43,44] but on an individual basis and not as a true prevalence rate. Population studies of these conditions are rare. In addition, there is increasing work considering changes on the endocranial surface of the skull which may be consistent with meningitis, or inflammation of the meninges.[45] In fact, a case of pituitary dwarfism in a 4th-century AD British context showing bone formation endocranially was suggested to be the result of tuberculous meningitis, a common cause of damage to the pituitary gland.[46] There is debate, however, about whether a person in the past could have survived long enough with meningitis for bone change to occur; changes in virulence of the causative organism (i.e. an increase in virulence through time) may be one explanation. Recent work on ear infection[47,48] has indicated respectively that of 136 ear bones examined from 471 temporal bones, 51% had erosive lesions indicating infection, and of 1244 temporal bones representing 688 individuals from seven Roman to late medieval cemeteries, there were similar infection rates to modern figures. In addition, preliminary studies on the evidence for maxillary sinusitis, although previously higher in Anglo-Saxon individuals (6.8% of individuals examined[49]) compared with earlier and later groups, have shown higher rates in urban compared with rural populations (55%:39% respectively[22]), and high frequencies in individuals from a medieval leprosy hospital.[50] As these conditions are common in modern populations (e.g. middle ear infection[51]), it would be recommended that they are recorded for archaeological material using protocols already developed,[48,50] and considered with respect to age and sex differences. It should be noted, however, that elsewhere in the world it is periostitis/osteomyelitis of long bones, which are usually recorded, and not infections of the ears or sinuses, save for a few exceptions.[52–57]

SPECIFIC INFECTIONS

The most common specific infections reported in the palaeopathological literature[7,17,18] are leprosy, tuberculosis and treponemal disease which all have bone changes which overlap in nature with each other (e.g. facial changes).[58] It is therefore particularly important to consider the characteristics and distribution pattern of lesions in the skeleton to ensure an attempt at an accurate diagnosis. All these infectious diseases have increased through time until factors such as developments in chemotherapy and improvement in living conditions decreased their frequency (e.g. tuberculosis[59]); however, in some areas of the world these infections are still prevalent and are increasing. They have a fascinating history, which has been revealed both by historical and skeletal evidence worldwide. In Britain and the rest of Europe, along with the skeletal evidence we are also fortunate to be furnished with a wealth of contemporary historical documentation, especially in the medieval and later periods. However, the trend in palaeopathology has been on case studies, and theoretical approaches to the origin, development and transmission of these infections, with very little attention paid to looking at real prevalence rates in populations through time and throughout the world, especially in Britain. In British contexts, however, some researchers have figured very prominently in developing diagnostic criteria for identification of these infections in skeletal remains.

Leprosy

An infection cause by *Mycobacterium leprae*, leprosy is contracted via the pulmonary route through droplet infection, and possibly via skin to skin contact.[8] It is predominantly found today in the southern hemisphere, but in the past the northern hemisphere appears to have harboured the majority of cases, particularly in northern Europe, and leprosy was not introduced into the New World until European contact in the 15th century AD.[15] The clinical expression of leprosy is very much determined by the individual's immune response and, for palaeopathological purposes, if the person is highly resistant to the infection he or she may not develop any bony involvement, thus precluding diagnosis in an archaeological context. Britain figures very prominently in the history of this disease, which makes its study in skeletal remains particularly important. Although much of the history of leprosy is documented (not always reliably) in written texts[60] and illustrated in iconography,[61] the primary evidence for the infection can only be considered from skeletal remains.

Although the first written evidence of leprosy comes from India and is dated to about 600 BC,[7] the first evidence from human remains is dated to the 2nd century BC,[62] and in Britain to the 4th century AD,[63] although there is some dispute about the diagnosis of this case.[34] However, and this is mirrored in many other European countries, from AD 1000 to 1600 over 200 leprosy hospitals were founded in Britain, mainly in England,[64] suggesting that the disease was prevalent (although this cannot be taken *per se* as an indication of the disease frequency). Increasing population density, poverty, increase in trade and contact, and nutritional stress may all have contributed to its rise in prevalence. Historical sources indicate that people with leprosy were stigmatized and, once diagnosed, banished into the local leprosy hospital, an event not infrequent today in many parts of the world.[65] However, it is very probable that many were not diagnosed and others were misdiagnosed,[66] which probably explains why leprous skeletons are found not only in leprosy hospital cemeteries, but also in non-leprosy hospital graveyards, something to remember when considering the skeletal evidence.

The key figure in highlighting the bone changes of leprosy in archaeological contexts was Moller-Christensen when he excavated and analysed the Danish leprosy hospital cemeteries,[67–68] but British research, in particular, has refined the diagnostic criteria for leprosy by developing these initial findings.[70–74] Diagnosed cases of leprosy have mainly come from Denmark[67–69] and England,[75–81] although evidence for leprosy in Western Micronesia,[82] Israel,[83] Hungary[84] and France[85] has been reported. Apart from the Danish, and English work (on the medieval leprosy hospital from Chichester, Sussex), no collective studies anywhere in the world have been undertaken charting the development and frequency of the disease (incorporating unpublished work), the age and sex distribution of leprous sufferers, and their status. Considering the wealth of historical documentation available on the antiquity of leprosy, including its social aspects and how it was diagnosed and treated, and the confidence in diagnosing this infection in skeletal remains, it is surprising that this has not yet been attempted, especially in Britain.

Tuberculosis

Tuberculosis in humans is caused by the two organisms, *Mycobacterium tuberculosis* (via droplet infection from human to human) and *M. bovis* (via ingested meat and milk from animals, particularly cattle, or via droplet infection). It is becoming an increasing problem today worldwide,[86] especially drug-resistant disease in people of low socio-economic status with HIV and AIDS, and it has been termed a disease of poverty. Only a few per cent of people with tuberculosis will develop skeletal changes and therefore its identification in skeletal material may be expected to be rare. Primarily the spine, hip and knee joints are those parts of the body most affected,[18] but work suggesting that periostitis on visceral rib surfaces (Figure 1) may indicate pulmonary infection (most likely tuberculosis) is gaining more support.[87,88] The study of tuberculosis in human populations is particularly important because of its strong link with tuberculosis in animals,[89] particularly cattle, and the suggestion that it developed in humans with the advent of domestication. Not only is more work needed in tracing the appearance, development and prevalence of this infection in antiquity in humans, but also in non-humans in the past, something which, until recently,[90] has been neglected in archaeozoological studies worldwide. Interestingly, it is tuberculosis upon which most diagnosis of disease using ancient DNA[91,92] and mycolic acids[93] has been focused.

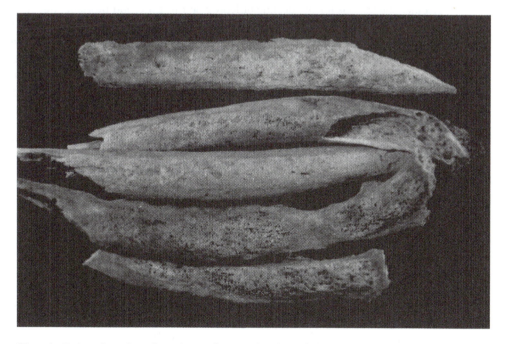

Figure 1 – Periosteal new bone formation on the visceral surfaces of ribs (Romano-British).

Written and artistic representation of tuberculosis is somewhat problematic to interpret as the signs and symptoms of pulmonary tuberculosis are similar to a whole range of other lung complaints. Also, the hunchback deformity depicted in many paintings, sculptures and reliefs could be purely artistic license and/or represent other diseases affecting the spine. Palaeopathological evidence of tuberculosis is found worldwide; in the Old World, cases are reported as early as the 4th millennium BC from Italy,[94,95] and in the pre-Columbian New World as early as AD 700 in South America.[96,97] Tuberculosis is a population density dependent disease and with increasing urbanization, poverty and malnutrition, and close contact with animals and their products, its prevalence in the past would have been affected by these contributory factors. Again, Britain was witness to large numbers of tuberculosis sufferers, particularly in the later medieval and post-medieval periods. For example, 'Touching for the King's Evil' (tuberculosis) was practised on thousands of victims as a cure, and in the 17th century in London 20% of all deaths were reported to be due to tuberculosis.[7] Of course, like leprosy, historical documentation of the disease cannot, *per se*, be taken as indicative of the actual prevalence of tuberculosis, but may be regarded as an indication of the problem at the time.

Diagnosed cases of tuberculosis have come from a variety of countries in the Old and New Worlds, e.g. Japan[98], Egypt[99] and Jordan[100] but remain basic case reports with no collation of data looking at the frequency of tuberculosis. In Britain the first evidence for tuberculosis is dated to the 4th century AD,[33,101] but cases have been reported through into the post-medieval period[102] and increase particularly in the later medieval period, as seen in both skeletal[102] and historical evidence.[103,104] The decline in leprosy around the 14th century AD may reflect the cross immunity between leprosy and tuberculosis.[105] There are, however, other suggestions for the decline of leprosy at this time, and mortality due to the plague is highlighted.[106] The idea that sufferers of leprosy were not resistant to the plague bacillus and could not escape its ravages is not as compelling an argument as tuberculosis cross immunity causing the decline. It has been suggested that the leprous were no more vulnerable than the poor in general.[60] Other suggestions for leprosy disappearing include a drop in mean annual temperature, eating fish and drinking goat's milk, and segregation of the affected.[64]

Because the numbers of tuberculous individuals diagnosed in British contexts have been low,[102] it has been suggested that the criteria being used may not be wholly adequate.[7] In addition, there are many individuals in the British skeletal record with occurrence of periostitis on ribs,[102] and evidence to support the theory that tuberculosis induces these changes is increasing.[107] If these lesions are accepted as tuberculous induced, then the clinical diagnostic criteria for tuberculosis may be deemed, for biological anthropologists, partially inadequate. Based on the currently accepted diagnostic criteria described[7] what is now needed is collation of data on the actual prevalence of skeletal tuberculosis through time in Britain, and a correlation of these data with culturally relevant information. In addition, a consideration of the frequency of periostitis on rib surfaces as a possible indicator of pulmonary tuberculosis must be made to enable more realistic figures for tuberculosis to be produced. Finally, studying the relationship between human and non-human tuberculosis in archaeological contexts would help clarify information on the appearance, development and maintenance of tuberculosis throughout the world over long periods.

Treponemal disease

The bacterial infection treponemal disease covers four syndromes that can potentially affect humans, although one (pinta) does not affect the skeleton and is therefore invisible with respect to palaeopathological studies. Endemic syphilis (or treponarid/bejel), yaws and venereal syphilis all affect bone and are caused by spirochetes of the genus *Treponema*. All these syndromes are associated with specific regions, climates, and socio-cultural factors,[108] i.e. pinta: tropical regions of America, yaws: hot tropical humid areas, bejel: temperate and subtropical arid regions, especially the Middle East, and venereal syphilis: ubiquitous around the world in urban environments today. They are transmitted via skin to skin contact through open lesions, and venereally in the case of venereal syphilis. It is believed that 'every human population has the kind of treponematosis that is adapted to its physical environment and socio-cultural status' (p. 155).[8] The current (and long-standing) historical question which is still being debated is where did venereal syphilis originate, in the Old or New World.[109–113] The current answer, based on the evidence to date, is that it was present in both the Old and New Worlds before Columbus made his journey to the New World. However, the abundant evidence in the New World does tend to overshadow the more limited data from Europe. This was recently reviewed in a symposium at the Annual Meeting of the American Association of Physical Anthropologists, which considered a series of systematic critical evaluations of treponemal disease in ten regions of North America.[114]

All the syndromes affecting the skeleton produce similar bone changes, which consist of periostitis, osteitis and osteomyelitis. In yaws the tibia is most affected but the nasal area of the skull may be destroyed. In endemic syphilis the cranium is rarely involved (as in yaws) but the naso-palatal area can be, Again, the tibia is the most affected bone, resulting in the sabre shin shape due to new bone apposition anteriorly.[7] In venereal syphilis the frontal bone of the skull (caries sicca lesions) and nasal area, plus long bones (particularly tibia), are the most frequently observed bones affected. In addition the joints may be destroyed in the tertiary phase (Charcot joint). Venereal syphilis can, of course, pass to an unborn child from an infected mother via the placenta and give rise to congenital syphilis, manifest mainly in the tibiae and dentition (mulberry and moon molars and Hutchinson's incisors occur in 30% of children with congenital syphilis[15]).

Based on diagnostic criteria developed by Hackett,[115] palaeopathological evidence of published treponemal disease is found worldwide in the form of collective works,[109,111] but also as case studies,[116,117] In Britain the (scarce) evidence for treponematosis dates from the late medieval period and has been summarized.[118] However, it is the author's opinion that some of the cases diagnosed in New World contexts on the basis of periostitis/osteomyelitis may benefit from being re-evaluated (e.g. [109]). Recording these changes as indicative of treponemal disease may be a diagnosis for another disease causing the same changes, and therefore only recording cranial and facial involvement as treponemally induced may be the most accurate way of recording true prevalence rates (there has been a tendency in Old World contexts to do the latter).

The treponematoses clearly need specific environmental (often rural) conditions, poor sanitation, and lack of clothing for survival and maintenance, but for venereal syphilis to make an impact on a population there are usually higher levels of sanitation and the infection increases rapidly in urban situations[15] where trade and contact between people occurs more readily. Although few cases so far have been reported in British contexts, biological anthropologists should make accurate identification of cases one of the highest priorities because of the numerous hypotheses and questions which have been raised over the years about the treponematoses. Britain plays a large part in the debate and could contribute more.

CONCLUSION

This review of infectious disease in British palaeopathology has, necessarily, been summarized. It is clear that there is still a lot to achieve, but achievements are possible with the skeletal material available. Basic training in identification of these conditions and then following the recommendations outlined below should, even minimally, provide some sound data from which to develop ideas about the infections in Britain. However, there is a need to isolate the gaps we have in knowledge by reviewing the work already undertaken on skeletal material from British contexts. When those gaps (which are many) have been identified, it will then be possible to raise hypotheses about infectious disease. In addition, these gaps should be discussed with the archaeological community so that current issues in our discipline are known, and future cemetery excavations may help to test these hypotheses. However, before those hypotheses can be tested, accurate, detailed descriptions of pathological lesions using standard terminology, stating whether lesions are active or healed are needed (Figures 2–4). It is inevitable that macroscopic and radiographic methods of examination will be used primarily for analysis and could be limited in some respects, but physical, biological, and chemical analytical techniques may help in disease diagnosis in problematic circumstances, or when a specific question cannot be answered using basic analytical methods. Clinically based diagnostic criteria, with consideration of differential diagnoses, are the pre-requisite for any work in the infectious diseases (and in palaeopathology as a whole). Particular problems to note with reference to recording of infections are, in leprosy, survival of the hand and foot bones, which is a problem as they are often missing from the archaeological record and are affected in leprosy. In addition, in leprosy, tuberculosis, and treponemal disease, the facial damage (Figures 5 and 6) can be very similar and potentially confusing, which emphasizes the need to consider accurate description and the distribution pattern of pathological alteration of the skeleton. In tuberculosis there are many differential diagnoses for the spinal changes, and the periostitis of ribs at this stage can only be considered as a non-specific response to infection. Finally, in treponemal disease and leprosy, the non-specific infective changes of the lower legs may be part of both those disease processes but could occur in other conditions.

It is recommended that both prevalence rates for individuals in a population, and prevalence rates for numbers of elements observed, should be presented, and by sex and age at death. All data should also be considered within its cultural context e.g. is it a rural or urban site, and what might the impact of these environments be on infection? In addition, period of site, geographic region, and funerary context are important, as is a consideration of sample representativeness. Probably one of the most interesting outcomes of any palaeopathological study is the interpretation of the evidence in relation to lifestyle, which may include stigma

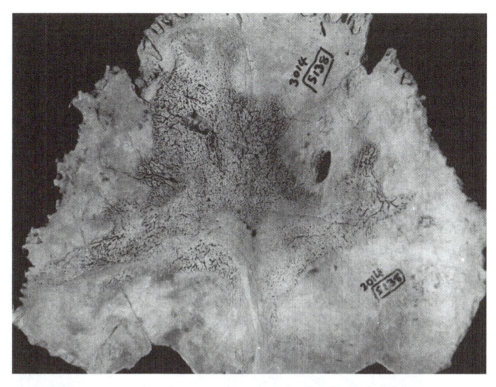

Figure 2 – Woven (active) new bone formation on the endocranial surface of the occipital bone (Anglo-Saxon).

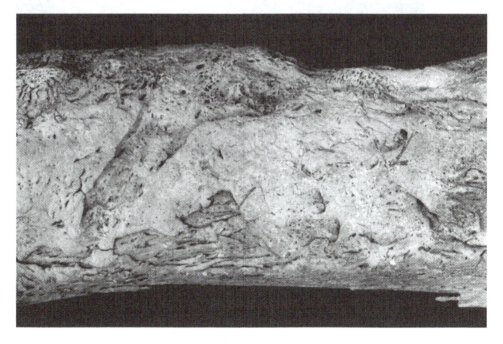

Figure 3 – New bone formation (lamellar) on a long bone (healed).

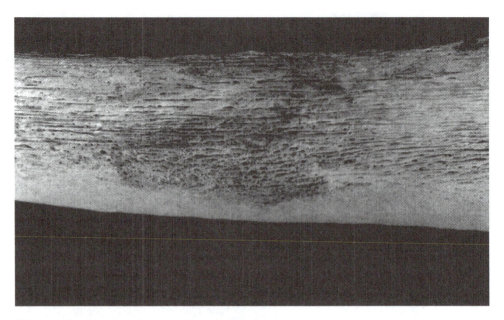

Figure 4 – New bone formation on long bone (mixed woven and lamellar bone).

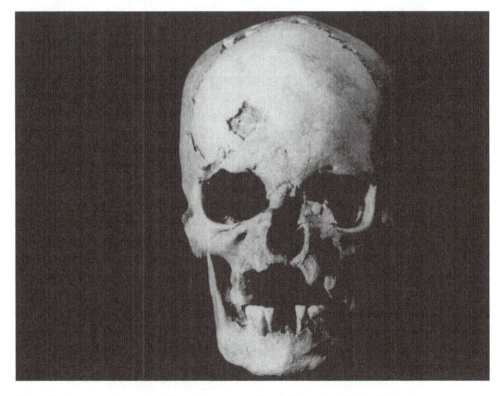

Figure 5 – Damage to the nasal and frontal bone areas of the skull in an individual suffering from treponematosis (later medieval).

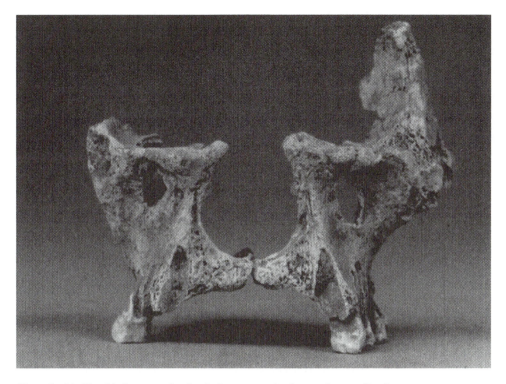

Figure 6 – Maxilla with damage to the alveolar bone suggesting leprosy (later medieval).

and disability in leprosy, for example. As previously outlined, the lack of published, population-based studies in Britain means that there is little data to work with at present but, in addition to advocating further population studies, the collation and review of reported case studies of infectious disease would be extremely useful. Once data has been collected and analysed in the manner suggested we can then start to compare our data with that of other countries to gain a population based assessment of the development and spread of the infections in antiquity, and how humans have (successfully or unsuccessfully) adapted to them.

ACKNOWLEDGEMENTS

Don Ortner is thanked for the production of Figure 5 as a slide. Jean Brown, Department of Archaeological Sciences, University of Bradford, produced the other photographs for this chapter. I also thank two referees for constructively reviewing the text.

REFERENCES

1   Margerison B. A comparison of the palaeodemography of catastrophic and attritional cemeteries. Unpublished PhD dissertation, University of Bradford, 1997.

2   Drancourt M, Aboudharam G, Signoli M, Dutour O, Raoult D. Detection of 400 year old *Yersinia pestis* DNA in human dental pulp: an approach to the diagnosis of ancient septicemia. *Proceedings of the National Academy of Sciences, USA* 1998; **91(21)**: 12637–12640.

3   Resnick D, Niwayama G (eds), *Diagnosis of Bone and Joint Disorders*. Edinburgh: WB Saunders, 1988.

4   Wood JW, Milner GR, Harpending HC, Weiss KM. The osteological paradox. Problems of inferring prehistoric health from skeletal samples. *Current Anthropology* 1992; **33**: 343–370

5   Inhorn MC, Brown PJ. The anthropology of infectious disease. In: Inhorn MC, Brown, PJ (eds), *The Anthropology of Infectious Disease. International Health Perspectives*. Gordon & Breach, 1997; pp. 31–67.

6   Inhorn MC, Brown PJ. Introduction. In: Inhorn MC, Brown PJ (eds), *The Anthropology of Infectious Disease. International Health Perspectives*. Gordon & Breach, 1997; pp. 3–29.

7   Roberts CA, Manchester K. *The Archaeology of Disease*. Stroud: Sutton, 1995.

8   Aufderheide AC, Rodriguez-Martin C. *The Cambridge Encyclopedia of Human Paleopathology*. Cambridge: Cambridge University Press, 1998.

9   Jackes M. Osteological evidence for smallpox. A possible case from 17th century Ontario. *American Journal of Physical Anthropology* 1983; **60**: 75–81.

10 Brothwell DR, Sandison AT (eds), *Diseases in Antiquity. A Survey of the Diseases, Injuries and Surgery of Early Populations*. Springfield: Charles C Thomas, 1967.

11 Birkett DA. Non-specific infections. In: Hart GD (ed.), *Disease in Ancient Man*. Toronto: Clarke Unwin, 1983; pp. 99–105.

12 Cockburn A, Cockburn E. *The Evolution and Eradication of Infectious Disease*. Baltimore: Johns Hopkins Press, 1963.

13 Kelley MA. Infectious disease. In: Isçan MY, Kennedy KAR (eds), *Reconstruction of Life from the Skeleton*. New York: Alan Liss, 1989; pp. 191–199.

14 Kiple KF (ed.), *The Cambridge World History of Human Disease*. Cambridge: Cambridge University Press, 1993.

15 Larsen CS. *Bioarchaeology. Interpreting Behavior from the Human Skeleton*. Cambridge: Cambridge University Press, 1997.

16 Merbs CF. A new world of infectious disease. *Yearbook of Physical Anthropology* 1992; **35**: 3–42.

17 Ortner D, Putschar W. *Identification of Pathological Conditions in Human Skeletal Remains*. Washington, DC: Smithsonian Institution Press, 1981.

18 Steinbock RT. *Paleopathological Diagnosis and Interpretation*. Springfield: Charles C Thomas, 1976.

19 Goodman AH, Brooke Thomas R, Swedlund AC, Armelagos GJ. Biocultural perspectives on stress in prehistoric, historical and contemporary population research. *Yearbook of Physical Anthropology* 1988; **31**: 169–202.

20 Learmonth A. *Disease Ecology*. Oxford: Basil Blackwell, 1988.

21 Cohen MN, Armelagos GJ (eds), *Paleopathology at the Origins of Agriculture*. London: Academic Press, 1984.

22 Lewis ME, Roberts CA, Manchester K. A comparative study of the prevalence of maxillary sinusitis in medieval urban and rural populations in northern England. *American Journal of Physical Anthropology* 1995; **98(4)**: 497–506

23 Roberts CA, Lewis ME, Boocock P. Infectious disease, sex and gender: the complexity of it all. In: Grauer AL, Stuart-Macadam P (eds), *Sex and Gender in Palaeopathological Perspective*. Cambridge: Cambridge University Press, 1998: pp. 93–113.

24 Brothwell DR. On the possibility of urban–rural contrasts in human populations palaeobiology. In: Hall AR, Kenward HK (eds), *Urban–Rural Connexions: Perspectives from Environmental Archaeology*. Monograph 47. Oxford: Oxbow 1994; 129–136.

25 Manchester K. The palaeopathology of urban infections. In: Bassett S (ed.), *Death in Towns*. Leicester: Leicester University Press, 1992; pp. 8–14.

26 Waldron T. The effect of urbanisation on human health: the evidence from skeletal remains. In: Serjeantson D, Waldron T (eds), *Diet and Crafts in Towns. The Evidence from the Roman to the Post-Medieval Periods*. Oxford: British Archaeological Reports, British Series 1989; **199**: 55–73.

27 Anderson T, Carter AR. Periosteal reaction in a newborn child from Sheppey, Kent. *International Journal of Osteoarchaeology* 1994; **4**: 47–48.

28 Anderson T, Carter AR. An unusual osteitic reaction in a young medieval child. *International Journal of Osteoarchaeology* 1995; **5**: 192–195.

29 Rogers J, Waldron T. Infections in palaeopathology: the basis of classification according to most probable cause. *Journal of Archaeological Science* 1989; **16**: 611–625.

30 Ribot I, Roberts C. A study of non-specific indicators and skeletal growth in two medieval subadult populations. *Journal of Archaeological Science* 1996; **23**: 67–79.

31 Walker PL, Cook DC, Lambert PL. Skeletal evidence for child abuse: a physical anthropological perspective. *Journal of Forensic Science* 1997; **42(2)**: 196–207.

32 Petersen HD, Wandall JH. Evidence of physical torture in a series of children. *Forensic Science International* 1995; **75**: 45–55.

33 Wells C. The human burials. In: McWhirr A, Viner L, Wells C. *Romano-British Cemeteries at Cirencester*. Cirencester: Excavation Committee, 1982; pp. 135–202.

34 Molleson T. The human remains. In: Farwell DE, Molleson TI. *Poundbury*, vol. 2: *The Cemeteries*. Dorchester: Dorset Natural History and Archaeological Society. Monograph Series, 1993.

35 Boghi F, Boylston A. The medieval cemetery of Pennell Street, Lincoln, Lincolnshire. Unpublished skeletal report, Bradford, 1997.

36 Boocock P, Manchester K, Roberts C. The human remains from Eccles, Kent. Unpublished skeletal report, Bradford, 1995.

37 Stroud G, Kemp, RL. *Cemeteries of St Andrew, Fishergate. The archaeology of York. The Medieval Cemeteries* 12/2. York: Council for British Archaeology for York Archaeological Trust, 1993.

38 Wiggins R, Boylston A, Roberts C. Castledyke, Barton on Humber. Human skeletal report. Unpublished skeletal report, Bradford, 1992.

39 Wiggins R, Boylston A, Roberts C. Report on the human remains from Blackfriars, Gloucester (19/91). Unpublished skeletal report, Bradford, 1993.

40 Waldron T. The health of the adults. In: T. Molleson and M. Cox (eds), *The Spitalfields Project*, vol. **2**: *The Anthropology. The Middling Sort*. Research Report 86 York: Council for British Archaeology 1993: 67–89.

41 Miles AEW. *An Early Christian Chapel and Burial Ground on the Isle of Ensay, Outer Hebrides, Scotland with a Study of the Skeletal Remains*. Oxford: British Archaeological Reports British Series 1989; 212.

42 Brothwell DR, Browne S. Pathology. In: Lilley JM, Stroud G, Brothwell DR, Williamson MH (eds), *The Jewish burial ground at Jewbury. The Archaeology of York. The Medieval Cemeteries* 12/3. York: Council for British Archaeology for York Archaeological Trust, 1994: pp. 457–494.

43 Cross JF, Bruce MF. The skeletal remains. In: Stones JA (ed.), *Three Scottish Carmelite Friaries: Aberdeen, Linlithgow, and Perth*. Edinburgh: Society of Antiquaries of Scotland. Monograph Series 1989; **6**: 119–141.

44 Mann GE. The identification of chronic ear disease in the dried skull. *International Journal of Osteoarchaeology* 1992; **2**: 19–22.

45 Teschler-Nicola M. Differential diagnosis of tuberculosis: the diagnostic value of endocranial features. *Paper presented at the International Congress on 'The Evolution and Palaeoepidemiology of Tuberculosis', Hungary* (1997).

46 Roberts CA. A rare case of dwarfism from the Roman period. *Journal of Paleopathology* 1988; **2(1)**: 9–21.

47 Bruintjes TJ. The auditory ossicles in human skeletal remains from a leper cemetery in Chichester. *Journal of Archaeological Science* 1990; **17**: 627–633

48 Dalby G. Middle ear disease in antiquity. PhD Dissertation, University of Bradford, 1994.

49 Wells C. Disease of the maxillary sinus in antiquity. *Medical and Biological Illustration* 1977; **27**: 173–178.

50 Boocock P, Roberts CA, Manchester K. Maxillary sinusitis in Medieval Chichester. *American Journal of Physical Anthropology* 1995; **98**: 483–495.

51 Daniel HJ, Schmidt RT, Fulghum RS, Ruckriegal L. Otitis media: a problem for the physical anthropologist. *Yearbook of Physical Anthropology* 1988; **31**: 143–167.

52 Gregg JB, Gregg PS. *Dry Bones: Dakota Territory Reflected. An Illustrated Descriptive Analysis of Health and Well Being of Previous Peoples and Culture as Mirrored in their Remains*. Sioux Falls: Sioux Printing Co., 1987.

53 Loveland CJ, Pierce LC, Gregg JB. Ancient temporal bone osteopathology. *Annals of Otology, Rhinology and Laryngology* 1990; **99**: 146–154.

54   Mann RW, Owsley DW, Reinhard KJ. Otitis media, mastoiditis and infracranial lesions in two Plains Indian children. In: Owsley DW, Jantz RL (eds), *Skeletal Biology in the Great Plains. Migration, Health, Warfare and Subsistence*. Washington, DC: Smithsonian Institution Press, 1994; pp. 131–146.

55   McKenzie W, Brothwell DR. Diseases in the ear region. In: Brothwell DR, Sandison AT (eds), *Diseases in Antiquity. A Survey of the Diseases, Injuries and Surgery of Early Populations*. Springfield: Charles C Thomas, 1967; pp. 464–473.

56   Rathbun TA, Mallin R. Middle ear disease in a prehistoric Iranian population. *Bulletin New York Academy of Medicine* 1977; **53(10)**: 901–905.

57   Wells C. Three cases of aural pathology of Anglo-Saxon date. *Journal of Laryngology and Otology* 1962; **76**: 931–933.

58   Manchester K. Rhinomaxillary lesions in syphilis: differential diagnosis. In: Dutour O, Palfi G, Berato J, Brun J-P (eds), *L'origine de la syphilis en Europe: avant ou apres 1493?* Toulon: Centre Archeologique du Var, Editions Errance, 1994; pp. 79–80.

59   Barkham TMS, Drury A, Pearson AD, Dybowski R, Atkinson H. Tuberculosis in Inner London: evidence for an increase in young adults and immigrants. *Epidemiology and Infection* 1995; **115**: 133–137.

60   Richards P. *The Medieval Leper and his Northern Heirs*. Cambridge: D.S. Brewer 1978.

61   Manchester K, Knusel C. A Medieval sculpture of leprosy in the Cistercian Abbaye de Cadouin. *Medical History* 1994; **38(2)**: 204–206.

62   Dzierzykray-Rogalski T. Palaeopathology of the Ptolemaic inhabitants of Dakhleh Oasis (Egypt). *Journal of Human Evolution* 1980; **9**: 71–74.

63   Reader R. New evidence for the antiquity of leprosy in early Britain. *Journal of Archaeological Science* 1974; **1**: 205–207.

64   Roberts CA. Leprosy and leprosaria in Medieval Britain. *M.A.S.C.A. Journal* 1986; **4(1)**: 15–21.

65   Jopling W. Leprosy stigma. *Leprosy Review* 1991; **62**: 1–12.

66   Roberts CA. Leprosy and tuberculosis in Britain: diagnosis and treatment in antiquity. *Museum Applied Science Center for Archaeology (MASCA) Journal* 1987; **4(4)**: 166–171.

67   Moller-Christensen V. *Bone Changes of Leprosy*. Copenhagen: Munksgaard, 1961.

68   Moller-Christensen V. Evidence of leprosy in earlier peoples. In: Brothwell DR, Sandison AT (eds), *Diseases in Antiquity. A Survey of the Diseases, Injuries and Surgery of Early Populations*. Springfield: Charles C Thomas, 1967: pp. 295–306.

69   Moller-Christensen V. *Leprosy Changes of the Skull*. Odense: Odense University Press, 1978.

70   Anderson J, Manchester K. Grooving of the proximal phalanx in leprosy: a palaeopathological and radiological study. *Journal of Archaeological Science* 1987; **14**: 77–82.

71   Anderson J, Manchester K. Dorsal tarsal exostoses in leprosy: a palaeopathological and radiological study. *Journal of Archaeological Science* 1988; **15**: 51–56.

72   Anderson J, Manchester K. The rhinomaxillary syndrome in leprosy: a clinical, radiological and palaeopathological study. *International Journal of Osteoarchaeology* 1992; **2**: 121–129.

73   Anderson J, Manchester K, Ali RS. Diaphyseal remodelling in leprosy: a radiological and palaeopathological study. *International Journal of Osteoarchaeology* 1992; **2**: 211–219.

74   Anderson J, Manchester K, Roberts CA. Septic bone changes in leprosy: a clinical, radiological and palaeopathological review. *International Journal of Osteoarchaeology* 1994; **4**: 21–30.

75   Bishop M. Burials from the cemetery of the hospital of St. Leonard, Newark, Nottinghamshire. *Transactions of the Thoroton Society of Nottinghamshire* 1983; **87**: 23–35.

76   Magilton J, Lee F. Leper hospital of St James and St Mary Magdalene, Chichester. In: Roberts CA, Lee F, Bintlif JL (eds), *Burial Archaeology. Current Research, Methods and Developments*. Oxford: British Archaeological Reports British Series 1989; **211**: 249–265.

77   Farley M, Manchester K. The cemetery of the leper hospital of St. Margaret, High Wycombe, Buckinghamshire. *Medieval Archaeology* 1989; **33**: 82–89.

78   Manchester K. A leprous skeleton of the 7th century from Eccles, Kent, and the present evidence of leprosy in early Britain. *Journal of Archaeological Science* 1981; **8**: 205–209.

79   Wells C. A possible case of leprosy from a Saxon cemetery at Beckford. *Medical History* 1962b; **6**: 383–386.

80   Wells C. A leper cemetery at South Acre, Norfolk. *Medieval Archaeology* 1967; **11**: 242–248.

81   Anderson A. Leprosy in a medieval churchyard in Norwich. In: Anderson S, Boyle A (eds), *Proceedings of the 3rd Meeting of the Osteoarchaeology Research Group. Current and Recent Research in Osteoarchaeology.* Oxford: Oxbow, 1998: pp. 31–37.

82   Trembly D. On the antiquity of leprosy in Western Micronesia. *International Journal of Osteoarchaeology* 1995; **5(4)**: 377.

83   Zias J. Leprosy in the Byzantine monasteries of the Judaean Desert. *Koroth* 1985; 9(1–2): 242–248.

84   Palfi G. The first osteoarchaeological evidence of leprosy in Hungary. *International Journal of Osteoarchaeology* 1991; **1**: 99–102.

85   Blondiaux J, Duvette J-F, Vatteon S, Eisenberg L. Microradiographs of leprosy from osteoarchaeological contexts. *International Journal of Osteoarchaeology* 1994; **4**: 13–20.

86   Raviglione MC, Snider DE, Kochi A. Global epidemiology of tuberculosis. Morbidity and mortality of a worldwide epidemic. *Journal of the American Medical Association* 1995; 273(3): 220–226.

87   Eyler WR, Monsoin LH, Beute GH, Tilley B, Schultz LR, Schmitt, WGH. Rib enlargement in patients with chronic pleural disease. *American Journal of Radiology* 1996; **67**: 921–926.

88   Roberts CA, Lucy D, Manchester K. Inflammatory lesions of ribs: an analysis of the Terry Collection. *American Journal of Physical Anthropology* 1994; **95(2)**: 169–182.

89   O'Reilly LM, Daborn CJ. The epidemiology of Mycobacterium bovis in animals and man: a review. *Tubercle and Lung Disease* 1995; **76** (suppl. 1): 1–46.

90   Lignereux Y, Peters J. Elements for the Retrospective Diagnosis of Tuberculosis on Animal bones from Archaeological sites. In: Pálfi G, Dutour O, Déak J, Hutás I (eds), *Tuberculosis Past and Present.* Golden Books/Tuberculosis Foundation, Budapest, pp. 339–348.

91   Arriaza B, Salo W, Aufderheide AC, Holcomb TA. Pre-Columbian tuberculosis in Northern Chile: molecular and skeletal evidence. *American Journal of Physical Anthropology* 1995; **98**: 37–45

92   Salo WL, Aufderheide AC, Buikstra JE, Holcomb TA. Identification of Mycobacterium tuberculosis DNA in a pre-Columbian Peruvian mummy. *Proceedings of the National Acacdemy of Sciences, USA* 1994; **91**: 2091–2094.

93   Gernaey AM, Minnikin DE, Copley MS, Ahmed AMS. Correlation of the occurrence of mycolic acids with tuberculosis in an archaeological population. In: Pálfi G, Dutour O, Déak J. Hutás I (eds), *Tuberculosis Past and Present.* Golden Books/Tuberculosis Foundation, Budapest, pp. 275–282.

94   Canci A, Minozzi S, Borgognini S. New evidence of tuberculous spondylitis from Neolithic Liguria (Italy). *International Journal of Osteoarchaeology* 1996; **6**: 498–502.

95   Formicola V, Milanesi Q, Scarsini C. Evidence of spinal tuberculosis at the beginning of the 4th millenium BC from Arene Candide cave (Liguria, Italy). *American Journal of Physical Anthropology* 1987; **72**: 1–6.

96   Buikstra JE (ed.), *Prehistoric tuberculosis in the Americas.* Evanston: Northwestern University Archeology Program, 1981.

97   Buikstra JE. Palaeoepidemiology of tuberculosis in the Americas. In: Pálfi G, Dutour O, Déak J, Hutás I (eds), Tuberculosis Past and Present. Golden Books/Tuberculosis Foundation, Budapest, pp. 479–494.

98   Suzuki T. Palaeopathological diagnosis of bone tuberculosis in the lumbosacral region. *Journal of the Anthropological Society of Nippon* 1985; **93**: 381–390.

99   Strouhal E. Vertebral tuberculosis in ancient Egypt and Nubia. In: Ortner DJ, Aufderheide AC (eds), *Human Paleopathology. Current Syntheses and Future Options.* Washington, DC: Smithsonian Institution Press, 1991: pp. 181–194.

100 Ortner D. Disease and mortality in the Early Bronze Age people of Bab edh-Dhra, Jordan. *American Journal of Physical Anthropology* 1979; **51**: 589–598.

101 Stirland A, Waldron T. The earliest cases of tuberculosis in Britain. *Journal of Archaeological Science* 1990; **17**: 221–230.

102   Roberts CA. The modern scourge: reflections on tuberculosis old and new. In: Pollard A, Downes J (eds), *The Loved Body's Corruption*. Leicester: Leicester University Press, 1999: pp. 159–174.

103   Crawfurd R. *Touching for the King's Evil*. Oxford: Clarendon, 1911.

104   Clarkson L. *Death, Disease and Famine in Pre-Industrial England*. Dublin: Gill and Macmillan, 1975.

105   Manchester K. Tuberculosis and leprosy: evidence for interaction of disease. In: Ortner DJ, Aufderheide AC (eds), *Human Paleopathology. Current Syntheses and Future Options*. Washington, DC: Smithsonian Institution Press, 1991: pp. 23–35.

106   Gottfrieder RS. *Epidemic Disease in 15th Century England. The Medical Response and the Demographic Consequences*. Leicester: Leicester University Press, 1978.

107   Roberts CA, Boylston A, Buckley L, Chamberlain A, Murphy E. Rib lesions and tuberculosis: the palaeopathological evidence. *Tubercle and Lung Disease* 1998; **79(1)**: 55–60.

108   Powell ML. *Status and Health in Prehistory. A Case Study of the Moundville Chiefdom*. Washington, DC: Smithsonian Institution Press, 1988.

109   Baker B, Armelagos GJ. Origin and antiquity of syphilis: a paleopathological diagnosis and interpretation. *Current Anthropology* 1988; **29(5)**: 703–737.

110   Brothwell DR. Microevolutionary change in human pathogenic treponemes, an alternative hypothesis. *International Journal of Systematic Bacteriology* 1981; **31(1)**: 82–87.

111   Dutour O, Palfi G, Berato J, Brun J-P. *L'origine de la syphilis en Europe: avant ou apres 1493?* Toulon: Centre Archeologique du Var, Editions Errance, 1994.

112   Hackett C. The human treponematoses. In: Brothwell DR, Sandison AT (eds), *Diseases in Antiquity. A Survey of the Diseases, Injuries and Surgery of Early Populations*. Springfield: Charles C Thomas, 1967: pp. 152–169.

113   Hudson EH. Christopher Columbus and the history of syphilis. *Acta Tropica* 1968; **25**: 1–16.

114   Powell M.L, Cook DC. Palaeopathology IV: North American treponematoses: a natural history. *American Journal of Physical Anthropology*, 1998; **26** (suppl.): 32–33.

115   Hackett C. *Diagnostic Criteria of Syphilis, Yaws and Treponarid (Treponematoses) and of Some Other Diseases in Dry Bone*. New York: Springer, 1976.

116   Jacobi K, Cook D, Corruccini R, Handler J. Congenital syphilis in the past: slaves at Newton Plantation, Barbados, West Indies. *American Journal of Physical Anthropology* 1992; **89**: 145–158.

117   Trembly D. Treponematosis in Pre-Spanish Western Micronesia. *Journal of Human Evolution* 1996; **6**: 397–402.

118   Roberts CA. Treponematosis in Gloucester, England: a theoretical and practical approach to the pre-Columbian theory. In: Dutour O, Palfi G, Berato J, Brun J-P (eds), *L'origine de la syphilis en Europe: avant ou apres 1493?* Toulon: Centre Archeologique du Var, Editions Errance, 1994: pp. 101–108.

11

THE PALAEOPATHOLOGY OF JOINT DISEASE

Juliet Rogers

INTRODUCTION

Joint disease is the most frequent type of post-cranial pathology to be found in both skeletal material and in modern populations. The diseases occurring in joints are responsible for a great deal of pain and disability and are an increasing burden for modern ageing populations.[1] The potential hardships caused by joint diseases in past populations make them a very important part of palaeopathological studies. Furthermore, changes in and around the joints may represent modifications due to biomechanical factors such as activity or trauma, which may have implications in the interpretation of the lifestyle of earlier populations.

Joints, which are the organs surrounding the junctions of two bones, enable free movement (in the case of synovial joints) or a relatively stable conjunction (in fibrous or cartilagenous joints). Joint disease may be defined as any disease afflicting any or all of the structures, such as ligaments, joint capsule, synovium, cartilage and bone, which comprise the various tissues found in a joint. Naturally, in skeletal palaeopathology, the pathological changes undergone by the various tissue components of the joint are only recognized if manifest on bone. It is the interpretation of the various changes and their location within the joint and around the skeleton that enables the skeletal osteologist to diagnose a particular joint disease.

The recognition, classification and nomenclature of the various types of joint disease have undergone considerable changes over the centuries. The classification of most disease has depended upon the appreciation of groups of clinical signs and symptoms, which, of course, are not applicable for the diagnosis of disease in dry bone. It was only with the introduction of X-rays in the later years of the 19th century that the appearance of the bone pathology played any part in disease classification. It was common to divide the joint diseases into 'acute' or 'chronic' depending on the time course run by the various forms of arthritis. It was after the introduction of X-rays that Garrod,[2] for example, categorized the joint diseases as *hypertrophic* or *atrophic* depending on either the amount of new bone or destructive lesions around the joints. What we now call osteoarthritis (OA) was in the former group and rheumatoid arthritis (RA) was in the latter. The further investigation, use of new tests, such as the identification of biochemical markers, and increased knowledge of disease processes and clinical progress has led to further refinement of disease definitions and introduction of new disease categories. It is against this background that the dry bone appearance of the various joint diseases has to be placed as well as earlier accounts of palaeopathological investigations.[3] These latter can be difficult to interpret because of the use of unfamiliar and archaic terminology and the application of contemporary descriptions of disease.

The interpretation of the morphological changes depends to a great extent on the recognized radiological appearances, but often these are only manifest in the later stages of a disease. Much that can be seen on dry bone is not seen on X-ray[4] and this can complicate the palaeopathological recognition. The various arthropathies typically display characteristic changes, such as marginal new bone (osteophyte) or erosion of a joint, which in a particular disease will present a characteristic configuration both around the joint (Figure 1) and around the skeleton (Figure 2). If the whole skeleton is present and the case typifies the

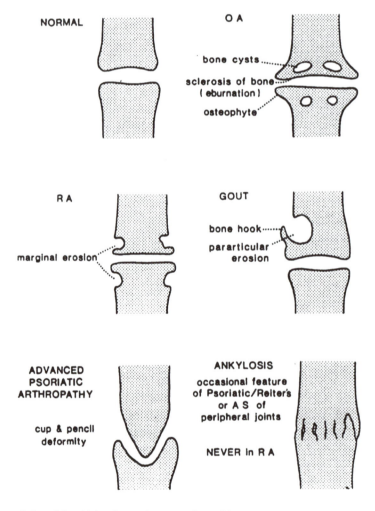

Figure 1 – Characteristic peripheral joint changes in some arthropathies.

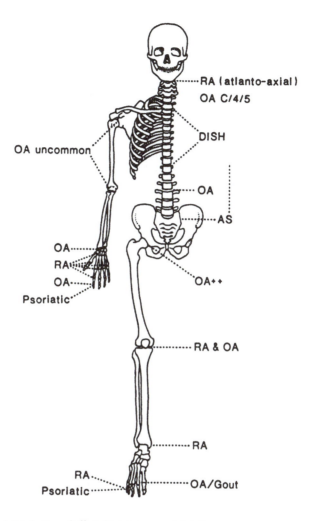

Figure 2 – Typical distribution of affected joints in some joint diseases.

classic presentation of the disease diagnosis should be possible,[5] but in many examples detailed classification will not be feasible. For the purposes here, joint diseases are discussed under four main headings: hypertrophic diseases, erosive arthropathies, seronegative spondyloarthropathies and other joint diseases.

HYPERTROPHIC DISEASES

Osteoarthritis

OA is the commonest of all the joint diseases in both modern and ancient populations. It is found in animals,[6] in fossil humans[7] and in all types of more modern skeletal assemblages from all over the world.[8–15] Osteoarthritis affects synovial joints and its frequency increases with age.[16] It is somewhat more common in females and, although any synovial joint can be affected, it most frequently affects facet joints of vertebrae, hands, hips, knees, the acromio-clavicular joint and the first metatarsophalangeal (MTP) joint.

OA involves damage to the cartilage, which can degrade to such an extent that the under-lying bone is exposed, and other changes such as the formation of marginal osteophytes or thickening of the joint capsule. Because of the focal loss of cartilage, OA has always been considered as a degenerative disease but a more recent understanding suggests that there are more complex processes going on than simple wear and tear. The changes apparent on and around the joint are manifestations of reaction to and attempts to repair joint failure.[17] There are many elements that may lead to a predisposition to this failure including age, systemic and genetic predisposition as well as biomechanical alteration. The latter may be a consequence of major changes to joint geometry such as that resulting from fracture or other disease (this used to be known as secondary OA) or more subtle alterations due to the inherent shape of the joint[18] or unusual use. Indeed Hutton[19] hypothesized that during the course of evolution the alteration of range of movement of some joints, such as, for example, the thumb base with the acquisition of opposition of the thumb, and the patellofemoral joint with attainment of bipedal gait, would predispose these joints to OA. Work by Lim et al.[20] and Mair et al.[21] supported this hypothesis by finding that primates had almost no OA of the thumb base or patellofemoral (PFJ) knee joints, whereas equivalent human skeletal material had a high frequency of thumb base and PFJ OA.

The features of OA that are used for clinical or radiological diagnosis such as pain or swelling, or joint space narrowing are obviously unavailable to the palaeopathologist so that morphological changes have to be used. The most frequent change to be seen around the joint margins is osteophytes. They also very frequently occur on both margins of the verte-bral bodies. Around joint margins osteophytes may take several forms: a thin rim, a large florid and irregular bone fringe or a flat ribbon. They can be situated around the whole joint margin or around only a portion. The joint surface itself can also be the location for patches of new bone, so called surface osteophytes, in the form of 'buttons' or 'pancakes' of bone (Figure 3). Other changes that can be seen on the joint surface in OA include areas of porosity or pitting, with the openings sometimes visibly connecting with subchondral cysts. Frequently, the bony contour of the joint may be altered, especially if the most diagnostic joint change, eburnation, is present (Figure 4).

Eburnation is an area of polishing on the joint surface caused by the total degradation of cartilage and the friction upon each other of the two opposing bone surfaces. It is an unequivocal marker of the presence of OA.[22] On X-ray the presence of joint space narrowing and osteophyte is a definite marker for the diagnosis of OA, but palaeopatholog-ically the joint space does not exist and osteophyte presence on its own can mislead as to the real prevalence of OA.[4] Osteophytes are very easily observed in dry bone, and although common in OA can also occur in other conditions and indeed may be a 'normal' part of age-related change.[23] The inclusion of osteophyte by itself as an indicator of OA may explain the wide variation of OA frequency reported in the palaeopathological literature.

Table 1 displays the prevalence of OA for various archaeological populations. The data displayed were extracted from published sources.[9,12,14,24–27] Many differences in the

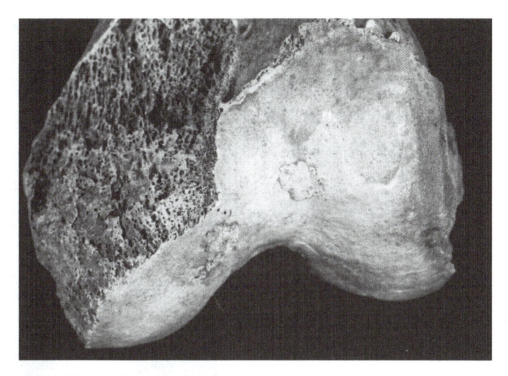

Figure 3 – Distal end of a femur showing both surface and marginal osteophytes.

Table 1 – Osteoarthritis of different joints in various skeletal samples.

Archaeological site	Joints (% skeletons affected)						
	Spine	Shoulder	Elbow	Wrist	Hip	Knee	Ankle
South Eastern USA[9]	–	35.0	40.0	15.0	3.0	27.0	8.0
Fishergate, York, North Yorkshire[14]	–	12.5	17.0	15.0	18.2	15.2	4.0
Dordrecht, Holland[12]	36.8	14.3	5.6	–	12.0	5.2	–
Trowbridge, Wiltshire[25]	–	2.9	1.9	1.4	3.4	1.4	0.4
Castledyke, N. Lincolnshire[24]	–	7.6	1.8	5.2	2.3	3.8	0.0
England:[26]							
Pre-medieval	31.9	31.9	2.1	8.5	12.8	2.1	0.0
Medieval	31.7	33.5	2.1	3.6	5.7	5.0	0.0
Post-medieval	24.0	27.7	2.6	1.9	2.9	4.4	0.0
St Oswald's Priory, Gloucestershire[27]							
Early medieval	18.6	0.0	0.9	5.7	1.9	0.0	0.0
Medieval	22.5	0.9	0.0	2.7	4.6	0.9	0.0
Post-medieval	25.9	0.0	4.6	8.0	3.4	5.7	0.0

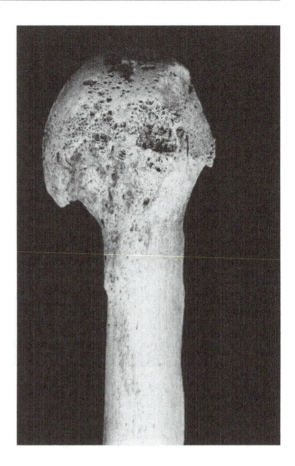

Figure 4 – Proximal end of a humerus
showing extensive changes due to OA:
eburnation, osteophyte formation, pitting
and contour change of the joint surface.

prevalence of OA at different joints and different archaeological sites are apparent. If these are real they might be of significance in the interpretation of the potential causes of the disease and its implications for the various populations. However, many of the variations may be spurious because of the different diagnostic criteria for OA adopted. For example, Bridges[9] uses the presence of osteophytes alone or in conjunction with other changes for inclusion, whereas many of the other researchers use eburnation. Care also needs to be taken that the definitions of the joints are always comparable. Rogers[25,27] for instance, in the example in Table 1, defines the shoulder joint as the glenohumeral joint whereas Waldron[26] includes both the gleno-humeral joint and the acromio clavicular joint. As the latter is one of the most frequently affected by OA[28] this probably explains the very high frequency of OA found by Waldron in his sample. There is often still incomplete agreement between osteologists as to whether particular pathological changes are present and the degree of their severity.[29]

If an agreed set of diagnostic criteria are used then comparisons may be made between archaeological and modern populations which may allow some inferences to be drawn about the effect OA would have had on the former.

Table 2 presents evidence for the frequency of OA at various joints from four archaeological sites.[13,24,27,30] They all used the same diagnostic criteria for OA, i.e. the presence of

Table 2 – Prevalence of osteoarthritis (%) in four archaeological samples.

	Shoulder	Elbow	Wrist	Hip	Knee	Ankle
St Oswald's Priory Glos.[27]						
early medieval	0	0.9	5.7	1.9	0	0
post medieval	0	4.6	8.0	3.4	5.7	0
Lund, Sweden 10th-15th Century AD[13]0.5	1.9	2.0	2.6	2.2	0.3	
Castledyke, Barton-on-Humber[24]	7.6	1.8	5.2	2.3	3.8	0
St Peter's, Barton-on-Humber[30]						
10th-11th century AD	1.1	2.6	0	2.4	3.3	0.4
12th-13th century AD	0	2.8	4.4	6.4	4.6	0
14th-15th century AD	2.8	3.4	2.6	2.2	2.3	1.0
16th-17th century AD	0	4.0	2.2	5.0	3.2	0
18th-19th century AD	0.6	12.2	5.0	7.1	11.8	0.9

eburnation or the combined presence of joint surface pitting, bony contour change and osteophytes. It can be seen that in many cases there is remarkable conformity. Ankle joint OA, for example, is rare; this is still true today, usually only occurring as an aftermath of trauma or some other pathological change. The shoulder is another joint at which there is generally little OA; the fact that there is an unusually high prevalence at Castledyke, Barton on Humber, in the 6th and 7th centuries AD would suggest some unusual environmental factor, activity or genetic predisposition. It is also obvious from these figures that the prevalence of OA of most joints shows a marked increase in the post-medieval phases. This is likely to be because of a higher prevalence of older individuals in these groups. Over the age of 65, most individuals have some OA.[31] These figures also partly support the previous findings of Rogers and Dieppe[32] who found a change in the frequency of hip and knee OA over time.

Because of the part played by biomechanics in the aetiology of OA, the pattern of OA distribution has always been thought by anthropologists to be a good marker for occupation and activity.[33] There is mixed evidence from the clinical literature about the association of particular activities with specific OA locations,[31] and a varying amount of evidence for the association of OA with occupation in the anthropological literature.[34,35]

Spondylosis

Spondylosis, or degenerative disc disease, is a separate entity from the OA, which occurs at the apophyseal joints (facet joints) of the vertebrae. These are synovial joints, and are very often affected in the same spines where there are signs of disc degeneration. Spondylosis is very common,[28] one of the most obvious manifestations being marginal osteophytes of the vertebral bodies. There is usually also coarse pitting, sometimes associated with new bone growth, on the superior and inferior surfaces of the vertebral bodies (this is called intervertebral osteochondrosis) (Figure 5). It is most frequently found in mid- and lower cervical, upper thoracic and lower lumbar regions of the spine. Schmorl's nodes are frequently associated with the other changes and are recognized as indentations on the upper or lower surfaces of the vertebral bodies. They represent the site of herniation of intervertebral disc

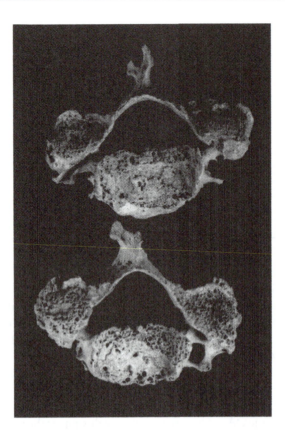

Figure 5 – Two cervical vertebrae showing changes characteristic of spondylosis, marginal osteophytes and coarse pitting of the vertebral body surface. The facet joints are also affected with changes associated with OA.

material through the end plates. They are most common in the lower thoracic and lumbar regions and can occur on both surfaces of the vertebral bodies.

Diffuse idiopathic skeletal hyperostosis

The spines of many older individuals, as mentioned above, frequently have osteophytes around the margins of the vertebral bodies. A quite different phenomenon is what appears to be an over-growth of osteophyte from one vertebral body to another, frequently fusing them together. At one time this was thought to be a version of OA or spondylosis but it is now recognized as a syndrome in its own right. Forestier and Rotes-Querol[36] described a disease of the spine in older individuals in which a fusion distinct from that of ankylosing spondylitis (discussed below) occurred. The condition, which usually affected the thoracic vertebrae with fusion of the anterior longitudinal ligament and which resembled dripping candle wax down the right hand side of the spine, was called Forestier's disease or senile ankylosing hyperostosis. Resnick *et al.*,[37] in further studies of patients with Forestier's disease, noted that most had ossification and new bone formation of peripheral ligament and tendon insertion sites (entheses) as well as the spinal changes previously described. They suggested that the condition be called diffuse idiopathic skeletal hyperostosis (DISH). They defined DISH as a condition with fusion of four adjacent vertebrae and the presence of enthesophytes. Fusion is often present in more than four thoracic vertebrae and can occur in other spinal segments. In the examination of skeletal material, fusion of less than four vertebrae may be seen which is representative of an earlier stage of the disease. The facet joints are not usually involved and the disc spaces are generally maintained. DISH occurs more frequently in males and increases in prevalence with age. It is found in between 3 and 5% of the population, rising to > 10% in those over the age of 65 years.[38] The symptoms are generally insignificant and there is a measurable association with obesity and diabetes.[28]

The extra spinal ossifications or enthesophyte formation is widespread in DISH cases but can occur in individuals who have not developed the conventional spinal involvement. It has been found that individuals with DISH and enthesophyte formation are likely to have more osteophyte formation around the joints and other sites;[39] this subset of the population have been termed 'boneformers'. They form about 20–30% of British skeletal samples but this phenomenon is not present in all populations. DISH and its extra-spinal manifestation are rare in some American Indian and South East Asian populations. In Northern Europe, DISH and boneforming individuals have been found in much greater frequency at monastic or other high status burial sites than in the general population (e.g. Merton Priory,[40] Wells Cathedral[41] and St Servaas Cathedral, Maastricht[42]). The known association of DISH with obesity may be reflecting the better nutrition of the individuals in these graveyards. On the other hand it could be caused by the higher frequency of older age groups within the high status sites. DISH, osteophyte, and enthesophyte all increase with age. However, a study at Wells Cathedral revealed that there were two separate chapels, which contained higher status burials than the rest of the cemetery and which contained all the burials with DISH and the majority of boneformers. Linear regression analysis determined that 'status', i.e. the location in one of the chapels, was more important than age in the distribution of DISH and at this site.[41]

Caution is needed in interpreting these results, however; not all individuals who have DISH or who are boneformers are necessarily of high status or vice versa, but the phenomenon of boneforming may affect the interpretation of enthesophyte formation as a marker of activity. If there is a section of the population who react by forming bone very readily, the amount of reaction to activity may be modified, which may make interpretation of activity related to enthesophytes confusing.

Despite the fact that DISH is one of the most easily recognized of all the joint diseases it has sometimes been misdiagnosed[3] but it is reported widely in the literature. The earliest case so far recognized is that of DISH in a Neanderthal skeleton,[42] and it occurs from many other sites[12,14] for all periods.

EROSIVE ARTHROPATHIES

Another group of joint diseases to be recognized in skeletal material are the erosive arthropathies. Clinically some of these diseases, such as gout, are not related and might be classified as metabolic diseases, but in palaeopathological material it may be difficult to differentiate them on visual grounds alone. The presentation of a skeleton with erosions around one or more joints can cause problems even to the most experienced osteologist. The erosions, which can occur in any area of the joint, are caused by pathological changes in the various soft tissues of the joints that can impinge upon and destroy bone tissue. The possibility of distinguishing and identifying the disease causing the erosions in skeletal material depends very greatly on having sufficient skeletal material present for examination, as well as observing and describing in detail the distribution of pathological change around the joint and the distribution around the skeleton of joints affected. Erosions may be distributed marginally around the joint, away from the articular surface or on the joint surface itself. The edges of an erosion may have new bone proliferating around them or there may be no new bone. They may have smooth or sharp margins. The distribution of lesions may be symmetrical or asymmetrical and affect differing joint groups. If the disease in a particular skeleton is characteristic for its type, these features will help distinguish it from the other conditions. However, diseases are dynamic processes and the course of a disease in a particular individual is not static; the bony pathology will vary according to the stage the disease had reached at the time of death and also according to the individual's bony response. People with DISH or who are boneformers, for example, may modify the expression of their disease making the bony changes atypical.

Erosive osteoarthritis

In some cases of OA erosions are found in the interphalangeal joints. The lesions are unlike typical erosions in other erosive arthropathies as they are articular rather than marginal.[43] On X-ray they produce a characteristic gull-wing appearance. Erosive osteoarthritis (EOA) is considered to be a severe form of interphalangeal OA with an inflammatory component.

Gout

Gout is a clinical syndrome caused by an inflammatory response to urate crystals, which may form in people with hyperuricaemia. In archaeological material the morphological appearance of the erosions caused in bone by deposits of crystals or tophi are the only signs present and have to be differentiated from other causes of joint erosion.

Clinically, gout most commonly affects middle-aged males and in the past was much less frequent in females. It has recently become more common in females over the age of 60 because of diuretic treatment. It is found worldwide but there are regional differences. It is associated with obesity, heavy alcohol intake, renal impairment and hypertension. There is an increased frequency of gout in individuals with DISH. Gout can occur in an acute or chronic form with the first metatarsophalangeal joint being affected in 90% of individuals. In the majority of attacks of acute gout only one joint is affected, but other areas that are targeted are the tarsus, heels, ankles and knees. It is the chronic form of gout that is associated with tophus formation and bone and joint destruction. This, and the deposition of crystals, make gout a very painful condition.[44]

The X-ray appearance displays well-preserved joint spaces and no juxta articular osteopaenia. The erosions characteristically have a 'punched out' appearance with overhanging edges and, on X-ray, sclerotic margins. The erosions are frequently situated in a juxta articular location (i.e. away from the joint margins) and are sometimes eccentrically placed on one side of the digit only (Figure 6).

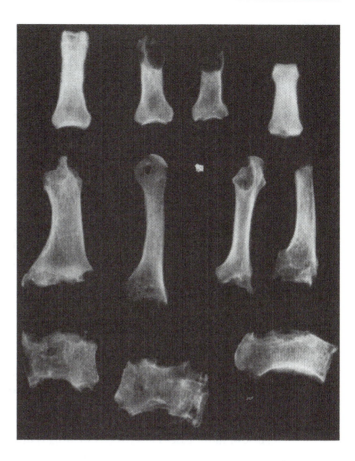

Figure 6 – Example of the X-ray appearance of gout in a male skeleton from St Peters Church, Barton on Humber. Sharp edged undercut marginal erosions on metatarsophalangeal, intertarsal, metacarpophalangeal and interphalangeal joints can be seen.

Recognizable descriptions of gout appear in the early medical literature, such as that of the Hippocratic School, but reports of cases are rather rare in the palaeopathological literature. One case was reported in an Egyptian Mummy,[45] with findings confirmed by the identification of urate crystals. Normally in skeletal material this cannot be done and the X-ray appearance of the erosions has to suffice. Calvin Wells[8] described three cases of gout from the assemblage of Romano-British skeletons he examined from Cirencester. One of these does not have lesions of a typical appearance and may have been an inflammatory arthropathy. However, the two others fulfil all the radiological criteria for gout.

From the site of St Peters Church, Barton on Humber, 12 individuals displayed signs of gout (five males, three females, four unsexed). The overall prevalence was 1.19% with very little variation through the phases from the 10th century AD to the post-medieval period. This is well within the modern prevalence rate of between 0.1 and 3%. For females at Barton, the prevalence was 0.8%, and for males 1.2%. There are, however, wide variations in the occurrence of gout reported from archaeological sites. No cases were reported from a recent detailed study of > 5000 skeletons from medieval Lund in Sweden.[13] However, in other studies it is difficult to be sure whether gout was not present, or whether it appears absent because the population was too small, there was poor survival of pathological bones or there was non-recognition of the disease.

Hallux valgus

Another condition in which the site of erosions may mimic gout is hallux valgus of the first tarsometatarsophalangeal joint. The erosions, like those found in gout, may be single or multiple but they usually have smooth, rounded margins, not sharp or undercut edges as is typical in gout. In gout, lesions may occur elsewhere in the skeleton, but by definition in hallux valgus the lesions are restricted to the first metatarsophalangeal joint.[28]

Rheumatoid arthritis

RA is a common severe inflammatory disorder affecting men and women of all ages, with a peak incidence in young adult and pre-menopausal females. It is an autoimmune disease but there are other etiological factors including a genetic predisposition and hormonal and reproductive factors influencing susceptibility to the disease. In the light of these it is not surprising that females are affected more frequently than males. A prevalence of between 0.5 and 1% has been reported, with a higher frequency in certain American Indian groups and a lower frequency or absence in parts of rural Africa.[46]

RA affects the synovial membrane, with the inflammation of this tissue causing increased vascularity and thickening. The inflammation can become chronic and then the thickened synovium is called 'pannus'. This can destroy first the articular cartilage and then the bone, erosions appearing at the joint margins. Joints can become deformed and patients are frequently very disabled. Typically RA involves the small joints of the hands and feet with the proximal interphalangeal joints, the metacarpophalangeal and metatarsophalangeal joints being most frequently affected. The distal interphalangeal joints in RA are less often affected. Other joints, such as the knee, elbow or shoulder may become involved later in the course of the disease. The erosions are usually distributed symmetrically on the margins of the joints without any proliferative new bone around their margins (Figure 7). In severe cases eburnation can be present as a by-product of the alteration of the joint morphology. Many rheumatoid patients have antibodies called rheumatoid factor IgG molecules (an immunoglobulin) in their blood, which is one way in which this disease can be clinically distinguished from other erosive polyarthropathies.

Historically this disease was first reported by Landre Beauvais in 1800.[47] There have been suggestions that RA is a new disease,[48] so the palaeopathology of RA is of particular interest both to clinicians and palaeopathologists. Many earlier reported cases[49] are not clear-cut and could be other forms of inflammatory arthritis. As in gout there may be under-reporting of cases because of non-survival of lesions or non-recognition of lesions. There has also been some disagreement and difficulty over the precise diagnosis of some cases[50] but it is clear that likely instances of RA have been reported from, among other places, the USA.[51-56] Examples have also been published from Japan[57] and from ancient Scythian material.[58] Cases have been reported from the past two millennia. The skeletons from St Peters, Barton on Humber, yielded three cases dating from the medieval period with an overall prevalence of 0.2%; this is much less frequent than gout or the seronegative spondyloarthropathies. The frequency of RA found in the group at Barton is similar to that found currently in rural Africa.[46] Undoubtedly RA is present in many different past populations but on present evidence it seems to have been rarer in the past than it is currently.

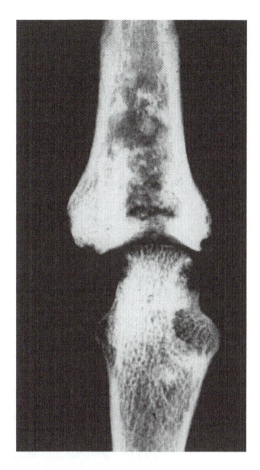

Figure 7 –X-ray of a metacarpophalangeal joint from a possible case of RA. The skeleton dates from the 10th to 11th centuries AD and is from Trowbridge, Wiltshire. The joint has symmetrical marginal erosions with no proliferation.

SERONEGATIVE SPONDYLOARTHROPATHIES

The seronegative spondyloarthropathies are a group of erosive, inflammatory polyarthropathies like RA, but they also affect the ligament and tendon insertions or entheses. They were originally considered to be variants of RA but it was found that the patients lacked the rheumatoid factor in their blood; hence they are seronegative, and have other clinical differences. The conditions in this group all have overlapping clinical features, which include sacroiliitis, spondylitis and peripheral arthropathy. They include ankylosing spondylitis, psoriatic arthritis and Reiter's disease or reactive arthritis. Although Reiter's disease and psoriatic arthropathy can usually be separated clinically, especially some time after disease onset, skeletally some cases show overlapping features. However, there are some characteristic morphological changes and distribution of lesions, which, if enough of the skeleton survives, should allow a palaeopathological diagnosis to be attempted.

Ankylosing spondylitis (AS)

AS is a chronic inflammatory disorder mainly affecting the axial skeleton. Clinically, it presents with low back pain and gradual stiffening of the spine; involvement of hips and shoulders and enthesopathies are also common. In Caucasians it occurs with a prevalence of between 0.5 and 1.0% with a male to female ratio of 5:1. It presents typically in the third decade of life.[59]

There is a very strong genetic predisposition associated with the HLA-B27 tissue type. The disease usually commences in the sacro-iliac joints and in the lumbar spine, with spinal fusion progressing steadily upwards (the so-called Bamboo Spine). Ribs can become fused to the vertebrae and the sacro-iliac joints are affected symmetrically (Figure 8).

The spinal and sacro-iliac fusion seen in DISH is usually easily distinguished from the changes characteristic of AS. In DISH the syndesmophytes are usually much more irregular and are restricted to the right-hand side of the thoracic spine. In AS the sacro iliac joint fusion involves the whole surface of the joint, not just the superior margin as in DISH.

There are many cases of AS reported in the palaeopathological literature[60,61] although there have undoubtedly been some misdiagnosed examples reported, especially before DISH and Forestier's disease were described.[3]

Reiter's disease (reactive arthritis)

This condition was first described in 1916 by Hans Reiter when he described an army officer with a dysenteric illness who also had arthritis, urethritis and conjunctivitis,

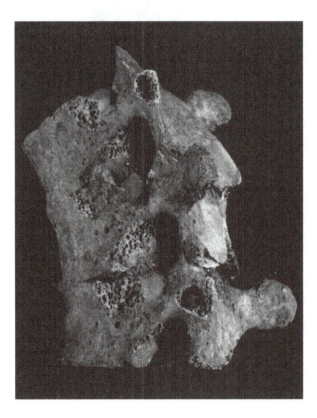

Figure 8 – Block of vertebrae from a spine affected with ankylosing spondylitis with fusion of vertebral bodies and facet joints.

although even in the 16th and 17th centuries physicians had recognized arthritis as a complication of urethitis. The disease most commonly affects young adults between the ages of 20 and 40 years. It occurs worldwide, and 1–4% of people with enteric infections such as salmonella, shigella or campylobacter may develop this condition. As in AS there are genetic associations with a strong relationship with HLA-B27. It occurs more often in males than in females. The clinical onset occurs in the form of joint discomfort from a few days to 2 weeks after an enteric or urogenital infection.[62] It is a systemic disease with varying joint symptoms from mild joint pain to a disabling polyarthritis. It can occur in one joint only or a few weight-bearing joints can be affected but others, especially the feet, can become involved as well. Enthesopathy and tendon inflammation are also present in a high percentage of cases, and this can lead to entheseal proliferation or 'whiskering', which is especially prominent around the calcaneum. Periosteal reaction on the metatarsals and tibiae and fibulae can also occur together with asymmetrical involvement of the sacro-iliac joint and spondylitis with 'skip' lesions, i.e. blocks of vertebrae alternating between affected or non-affected.[5]

Psoriatic arthropathy

Alibert first made an association between arthritis and psoriasis in the 1850s. However, until the first half of the 20th century this type of arthropathy was thought to be RA affecting patients who also had psoriasis. The discovery of rheumatoid factor helped to differentiate the two. Psoriatic arthritis (PsA) was recognized as a distinct clinical entity in the 1960s.[63]

Psoriasis affects about 1% of the population but only about 5–8% of patients with this condition go on to develop the arthropathy. Males and females are affected equally with the most common age of onset between 20 and 40 years. Spinal involvement tends to be more common in males and peripheral arthritis in females. The prevalence rate is between 0.2 and 1.0 per 1000. It is uncommon in Asians. The arthropathy is usually asymmetrically distributed with erosions affecting the distal interphalangeal, proximal interphalangeal and metatarsophalangeal joints. Changes are often mild, but in a few patients 'arthritis mutilans' can develop. The interphalangeal joints are destroyed leading to bony ankylosis and shortening of the digits (Figure 9). The proximal end of the distal phalanx is often enlarged while the distal end of the middle phalanx becomes pointed to produce the 'cup and pencil' deformity sometimes seen on X-ray. This appearance can lead to confusion with possible cases of leprosy. A skeleton from the Romano-British site of Poundbury diagnosed as a case of PsA was first classified as that of a leper; there is still some doubt about the correct diagnosis of this and other possible cases of PsA from this site.[64]

As in the other arthropathies in this group there is involvement of the sacro-iliac joints, which in this arthropathy may occur bilaterally but asymmetrically. The spine is also affected, sometimes displaying bulky asymmetrical para-vertebral ossification.

Palaeopathologically it is often very difficult to differentiate psoriatic arthropathy from reactive arthritis, especially if the skeleton is incomplete. In both arthropathies the erosions are asymmetrically distributed with marginal proliferative new bone. However, in PsA the small joints of both hands and feet can be affected whereas in reactive arthritis the feet are

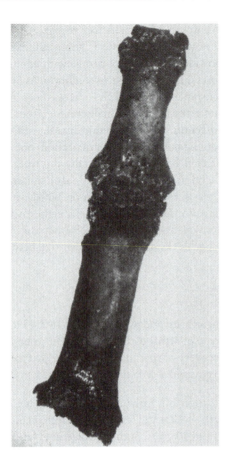

Figure 9 – Phalanges fused and shortened from a probable case of psoriatic arthropathy from St Peters, Barton on Humber (medieval).

more often affected, often with periosteal new bone on the metatarsals. Bony ankylosis can occur in both types but arthritis mutilans only occurs in PsA. In psoriatic arthropathy the cervical spine is more commonly affected and in reactive arthritis there may be skip lesions. Also in reactive arthritis the enthesis on the plantar surface of the calcaneum may show marked spurring. There are few cases of psoriatic arthropathy or reactive arthritis in the literature. One case of PsA has been is described[64] and other possible cases have been seen[50] but many may have been misdiagnosed as other erosive arthropathies. At St Peters, Barton on Humber, eight skeletons were identified as having seronegative type erosive arthropathy; one was definitely AS and two were likely to be PsA. The others could not be differentiated, although most were probably reactive arthropathies. A diagnosis of erosive arthropathy or seronegative type arthropathy usually has to suffice.

OTHER JOINT DISEASES

There are many other conditions which can affect joints and which may be recognized in skeletal material, such as trauma or infection. It is unlikely that traumatic change such as an old dislocation or a fracture through a joint will cause confusion with other sorts of joint disease but the changes caused by infection in a joint may at first be difficult to differentiate from perhaps some of the erosive arthropathies. Septic arthritis is usually mono-articular, and it generates a lot of proliferative new bone that may be very irregular in form. This new bone can occur on the articular surface as well as the margins of the joints. The proliferation may be so great that bony ankylosis may occur; this is particularly so in infection subsequent to trauma. Erosions can also occur which need to be distinguished from erosions in inflammatory arthropathies. For joints affected by specific infections such as tuberculosis or leprosy see Roberts, chapter 10, in this volume.

Osteochondritis dissecans

Osteochondritis dissecans is a lesion resulting from an area of micro-trauma and consequent necrosis of bone on the convex articular surface of a joint.[28] It most frequently occurs on the medial condyle of the femur in the knee but also occurs on the radiohumeral joint of the elbow and on the talar side of the ankle joint among others. The effect in the subchondral bone can appear as an oval but circumscribed area of bone. Some lesions appear hollow because the central area of dead bone has completely separated from the joint surface. Osteochondritis dissecans is more common in males than females, it commences between the ages of 15 and 20 years and is usually unilateral.

CONCLUSIONS

Joint disease is of fundamental importance in palaeopathological and osteological studies. It is the most frequently occurring type of post-cranial bony abnormality and can encompass many different types of disease. They can have a major influence on the life of an individual.

The palaeopathology of joint disease has developed a great deal in the last few years fulfilling the need, expressed by Bourke[65] in his review of the palaeopathology of arthritis, for much more detailed observation and description to be carried out. Diagnostic criteria have been developed for many of the joint diseases, enabling comparisons to be made between populations in a more standardized manner. More examples of the rarer erosive arthropathies have been recognized, presented and discussed which enables palaeopathology to address both the development and natural history of these diseases and the role they may have played in the biocultural history of human populations.

It is essential that the diagnostic criteria be applied in an agreed manner, as without some standardization, comparisons with other populations, modern or archaeological, cannot be made. It is only by investigating these diseases in the context of population studies that accurate conclusions may be drawn about the impact of this group of diseases on individuals and ancient populations and whether they reflect in any way aspects of activity or lifestyle.

REFERENCES

1   Dieppe P, Kirwan J, Billingham M (eds), Report of an international symposium held in Bristol, November 1996. *Annals of the Rheumatic Diseases* 1997; **56**: 444.

2   Garrod AE. Rheumatoid arthritis, osteoarthritis and arthritis deformans. In: Albitt TC, Rolleston HD (eds), *A System of Medicine*. London: Macmillan, 1907: pp. 3–43.

3 Rogers J, Watt I, Dieppe P. The palaeopathology of spinal osteophytosis, vertebral ankylosis, ankylosing spondylitis and vertebral hyperostosis. *Annals of the Rheumatic Diseases* 1985; **44**: 118–120.

4 Rogers J, Watt I, Dieppe P. Comparison of visual and radiographic detection of bony changes at the knee joint. *British Medical Journal* 1990; **300**: 367–368.

5 Rogers J, Waldron T, Dieppe P, Watt I. Arthropathies in palaeopathology: The basis of classification according to most probable cause. *Journal of Archaeological Science* 1987; **14**: 179–193.

6 Baker J, Brothwell D. *Animal Diseases in Archaeology*. London: Academic Press, 1980.

7 Trinkaus E. Pathology and posture of the La Chapelle-aux-Saints Neanderthal. *American Journal of Physical Anthropology* 1985; **61**: 19–41.

8 Wells C. The Human Burials. In: McWhirr A, Viner L, Wells C (eds), *Romano-British Cemeteries at Cirencester*. Cirencester: Cirencester Excavation Committee, 1982: pp. 134–202.

9 Bridges P. Degenerative joint disease in hunter gatherers and agriculturalists from the South Eastern United States. *American Journal of Physical Anthropology* 1991; **85**: 379–391.

10 Rogers J. The human skeletal material. In: A Saville (ed.), *Hazelton North, Gloucestershire, 1979–82: The Excavation of a Neolithic Long Cairn of the Cotswold-Severn Group*. London: English Heritage, 1990: pp. 182–198.

11 Waldron HA. Prevalence and distribution of osteoarthritis in a population from Georgian and early Victorian London. *Annals of the Rheumatic Diseases* 1991; **50**: 301–307.

12 Maat G, Mastwijk RW, van der Velde EA. Skeletal distributions of degenerative changes in vertebral osteo-phytosis, vetebral osteoarthritis and DISH. *International Journal of Osteoarchaeology* 1995; **5**: 289–298.

13 Arcini C. Health and disease in early Lund. Unpublished PhD thesis, Medical Faculty, Lund University, 1999.

14 Stroud G, Kemp RL (eds), *Cemeteries of the Church and Priory of St Andrew, Fishergate*. The Archaeology of York, vol. 12, *The Medieval Cemeteries*. London: Council for British Archaeology for York Archaeological Trust, 1993.

15 Jurmain R, Kilgore L. Skeletal evidence of osteoarthritis, a palaeopathological perspective. *Annals of the Rheumatic Diseases* 1995; **54**: 443–450.

16 Van Saase J, Romunde L, Cats A, Vandenbroucke J, Valkenberg H. Epidemiology of osteoarthritis. Zoetermeer survey. Comparison of radiological osteoarthritis in a Dutch population with that in ten other populations. *Annals of the Rheumatic Diseases* 1989; **48**: 271–280.

17 Dieppe P, Lim K. Osteoarthritis and related disorders; clinical features and diagnostic problems. In: Klippel J, Dieppe P (eds), *Rheumatology* (2nd edn). London: Mosby, 1998: 8.3.1–8.3.16.

18 Shepstone L, Rogers J, Kirwan J, Silverman B. The shape of the distal femur: a palaeopathological compar-ison of eburnated and non-eburnated femora. *Annals of the Rheumatic Diseases* 1999; **58**: 22–28.

19 Hutton C. Generalized osteoarthritis, an evolutionary problem. *Lancet* 1987; **8548**: 1436–1465.

20 Lim K, Rogers J, Shepstone L, Dieppe P. The evolutionary origins of osteoarthritis: A comparative skeletal study of hand disease in two primates. *Journal of Rheumatology*, 1995; **22**: 2132–2134.

21 Mair F, Rogers J, Lim K, Dieppe P. Patterns of joint involvement in osteoarthritis. Support for the evolu-tionary hypothesis. *British Journal of Rheumatology*, 1998; **37**(suppl. 1): 155.

22 Rogers J, Waldron T. *A Field Guide to Joint Disease in Archaeology*. Chichester: Wiley, 1994.

23 Ahlbach S. Osteoarthrosis of the knee. A radiographic investigation. *Acta Radiologica* 1968; **277**(suppl. 1).

24 Boyleston A, Wiggins R, Roberts C. The human skeletons. In: Drinkall G, Foreman M (eds), *The Anglo Saxon Cemetery at Castledyke South, Barton on Humber*. Excavation Report 6. Sheffield: Sheffield Academic Press, 1998: pp. 221–236.

25 Rogers J. The palaeopathology. In: Graham AH, Davis SM (eds), *Excavations in the Town Centre of Trowbridge, Wiltshire, 1977 and 1986–1988*. Archeological Report 2. Old Sarum: Trust for Wessex Archaeology, 1993: pp. 122–127.

26 Waldron T. Changes in the distribution of osteoarthritis over historical time. *International Journal of Osteoarchaeology* 1975; **5**: 385–389.

27 Rogers J. Burials: the human skeletons. In: Heighway C, Bryant R (eds), *The Golden Minster: The Anglo-Saxon and Later Medieval Priory St Oswald at Gloucester*. Research Report 117. London: Council for British Archaeology, 1999: pp. 229–246.

28 Resnick D, Niwayama G. *Diagnosis of Bone and Joint Diseases* (3rd edn). Philadelphia: WB Saunders, 1995.

29 Waldron T, Rogers J. Inter-observer variation in coding osteoarthritis in human skeletal remains. *International Journal of Osteoarchaeology* 1991; **1**: 49–56.

30 Rogers J, Barber G, Waldron T, Rodwell W. *A Parish and its Community – St Peter's Church, Barton on Humber*, vol. 1 (in preparation)

31 Cooper C. The epidemiology of osteoarthritis. In: Klippel J, Dieppe P (eds), *Rheumatology* (2nd edn). London: Mosby, 1998: 8.2.1–8.2.8.

32 Rogers J, Dieppe P. Is tibiofemoral osteoarthritis in the knee joint a new disease? *Annals of the Rheumatic Diseases* 1994; **53**: 612–613.

33 Merbs CF. *Patterns of Activity Induced Pathology in a Canadian Inuit Population*. Ottawa: National Museums of Canada, 1983.

34 Waldron T, Cox M. Occupational arthropathy: evidence from the past. *British Journal of Industrial Medicine* 1989; **46**: 420–422.

35 Roberts C, Manchester K. *The Archaeology of Disease* (2nd edn). Stroud: Sutton, 1997.

36 Forestier J, Rotes-Querol I. Senile ankylosing hyperostosis of the spine. *Annals of the Rheumatic Diseases* 1950; **9**: 321–330.

37 Resnick D, Shaul SR, Robins JM. Diffuse Idiopathic Skeletal Hyperostosis, DISH: Forestier's disease with extra spinal manifestations. *Radiology* 1975; **115**: 513–524.

38 Julkunen H, Heinonen OP, Pyörälä K. Hyperostosis of the spine in an adult population. *Annals of the Rheumatic Diseases* 1971; **30**: 605–612.

39 Rogers J, Shepstone L, Dieppe P. Boneformers; osteophyte and enthesophyte formation are positively associated. *Annals of the Rheumatic Diseases* 1997; **56**: 85–90.

40 Waldron T. DISH at Merton Priory: evidence for a 'new' occupational disease. *British Medical Journal* 1985; **291**: 1762–1763.

41 Rogers J, Young P, Dieppe P. 'Boneformers' – positive correlations between osteophyte and enthesophyte formation. *British Journal of Rheumatology* 1993; **32**(suppl. 2): 51.

42 Crubezy E, Trinkaus E. Shanidar I: a case of hyperostotic disease (DISH) in the Middle Palaeolithic. *American Journal of Physical Anthropology* 1992; **89**: 411–420.

43 Rogers J, Waldron T, Watt I. Erosive osteoarthritis in a mediaeval skeleton. *International Journal of Osteoarchaeology* 1991; **1**: 151–153.

44 Cohen MG, Emmerson B. Gout. In: Klippel J, Dieppe P (eds), *Rheumatology* (2nd edn). London: Mosby, 1998: 8.14.1–8.14.4.

45 Elliot-Smith G, Dawson W. *Egyptian Mummies*. New York: Dial, 1924.

46 MacGregor AJ, Silman AJ. Rheumatoid arthritis, classification and epidemiology. In: Klippel J, Dieppe P (eds), *Rheumatology* (2nd edn). London: Mosby, 1998: 5.2.1–5.2.6.

47 Snorrason E. Landre-Beauvais and his goute asthenique primitive. *Acta Medica Scandinavica* 1952; **142**(suppl. 266): 115.

48 Short CL. The antiquity of rheumatoid arthritis. *Arthritis and Rheumatism* 1974; **17**: 193.

49 Ortner DJ, Utermohle CJ. Polyarticular inflammatory arthritis in a pre-Columbian skeleton from Kodiak Island, Alaska, USA. *American Journal of Physical Anthropology* 1981; **56**: 23–31.

50 Dieppe P, Rogers J. *The antiquity of the erosive arthropathies*. Arthritis and Rheumatism Council for Research Conference Proceedings No. 5, 1988.

51 Rothschild BH, Turner KR, De Luca MA. Symmetrical erosive peripheral polyarthritis in the late archaic period of Alabama. *Science* 1988; **241**: 1948–1501.

52 Waldron T, Rogers J, Watt I. Rheumatoid arthritis in an English Mediaeval skeleton. *International Journal of Osteoarchaeology* 1994; **4**: 165–167.

53 Hacking P, Allen T, Rogers J. Rheumatoid arthritis in a mediaeval skeleton. *International Journal of Osteoarchaeology* 1994; **4**: 251–255.

54   Rogers J, Watt I, Dieppe P. Arthritis in Saxon and medieval skeletons. *British Medical Journal* 1981; **283**: 1668.

55   Blondiaux J, Cotten A, Fontaine C, Hanni C, Bera A, Flipo R-M. Two Roman and medieval cases of symmetrical erosive polyarthropathy from Normandy. *International Journal of Osteoarchaeology* 1997; **7**: 451–466.

56   Arcini C. Rheumatoid arthritis – rare reality as recovered among Sariian skeletal remains from Viking and mediaeval times. In: *Lectures in Medical History from the 24th Scandinavian Congress of Rheumatology in Malmö*. Lund: Sydsvenska Medicinhistoriska Sällskapets, 1992: pp. 11–21.

57   Inoue K, Hukuda S, Nakjai M, Katayama K, Huang J. Erosive peripheral polyarthritis in ancient Japanese skeletons: a possible case of rheumatoid arthritis. *International Journal of Osteoarchaeology* 1999; **9**: 1–7.

58   Murphy EM. An osteological and palaeopathological study of the Scythian and Hunno-Sarmatian period populations from the cemetery complex of Aymyrlyg, Tuva, South Siberia. Unpublished PhD thesis, Queens University, Belfast, 1998.

59   Grau JT, Husby G. Ankylosing spondylitis: prevalence and demography. In: Klippel J, Dieppe P (eds), *Rheumatology* (2nd edn). London: Mosby, 1998: 6.15.1–6.15.6.

60   Ortner D, Putschar WG. *Identification of pathological conditions in human skeletal remains*. Washington, DC: Smithsonian Institution, 1981.

61   Steinbock RT. *Palaeopathological diagnosis and interpretation*. Springfield: Charles C Thomas, 1976.

62   Lipsky PE, 1998. Reactive arthritis and Reiter's syndrome: aetiology and pathogenesis. In: Klippel J, Dieppe P (eds), *Rheumatology* (2nd edn). London: Mosby, 1998: 6.12.1–6.12.8.

63   Helliwell PS, Wright V, 1998. Psoriatic arthritis: clinical features in rheumatology. In: Klippel J, Dieppe P (eds), *Rheumatology* (2nd edn). London: Mosby, 1998: 6.22.1–6.22.8.

64   Farwell DW, Molleson TL. *Excavations at Poundbury, Dorchester, Dorset 1966–1980*, vol. 2: *The Cemeteries*. Monograph No. 11. Dorchester: Dorset Natural History and Archaeology Society, 1993.

65   Bourke JB. A review of the palaeopathology of the arthritic diseases. In: Brothwell D, Sandison A (eds), *Disease in Antiquity*. Springfield: Charles C Thomas, 1967: pp. 352–370.

12

THE DIAGNOSIS OF METABOLIC DISEASE IN ARCHAEOLOGICAL BONE

Megan Brickley

INTRODUCTION

There are many metabolic diseases that are detectable in archaeological skeletal material. This chapter will cover those that, for a variety of reasons, are likely to be of most value in studies of the lifestyle, health, and mortality of past populations. The metabolic bone diseases covered here are scurvy, rickets/osteomalacia and osteoporosis. Descriptions of a wider range of metabolic conditions in archaeological bone can be found in palaeopathology textbooks.[1,2]

Advances in the development of techniques applied to the study of such conditions have not occurred at the same rate. For each disease covered by this chapter, the range of techniques currently available and the ways in which our understanding of these conditions may be advanced in the future are examined. The possible implications of the presence of the condition for the understanding of past populations are also considered.

BONE BIOLOGY

The term metabolic bone disease was first used in 1948 to describe those diseases caused by a disruption of bone formation, remodelling, mineralization, or a combination of these.[3] To understand metabolic bone disease, some knowledge of the mechanisms involved in the formation and growth of bone, and changes within it throughout life is required. The main features of bone, which are important for the study of these diseases, are briefly covered here.

An important feature of bone is that, despite its hardness, it is not a static tissue. Throughout the growth period in childhood and early adulthood, there are extensive changes as bones increase in size. Bone growth takes place in two main ways, namely endochondral and intramembranous ossification. Endochondral ossification involves bone growth at the cartilage plate between the diaphysis and the epiphysis. This type of growth ceases once epiphyses have fused. Intramembranous ossification occurs at the surface of the bone below the periosteum and allows a growth in the diameter of bones. Clearly, evidence for metabolic bone diseases will be most apparent in areas of greatest bone activity, and it is therefore necessary to be aware of the pattern of bone development across the skeleton at different ages. Such an understanding will also give an appreciation of what is normal, i.e. where within the skeleton sites of new bone formation might be expected in a healthy individual.

Bone, like most tissues of the body, is constantly renewed even after achieving full growth. Continual remodelling, involving bone formation and resorption, takes place in both trabecular and cortical bone. Trabecular bone makes up about 20% of the skeletal mass,[4] forming the main component of the vertebral bodies and the epiphyses of the long bones. There are also small amounts at other sites within the skeleton such as the iliac crest. Within these bones, trabeculae form a semi-rigid framework of bony struts with a high surface area, arranged to provide support to the structure of the bone in relation to the forces placed upon it. The areas of trabecular bone are enclosed within a thin layer of more compact cortical bone, which comprises about 80% of the mass of the skeleton. Cortical bone is formed from Haversian systems, consisting of a central Haversian canal surrounded by a concentric arrangement of bone tissue.[5] Such bone is found throughout the skeleton, for example in the diaphyses of the long bones.

The two major cell types involved in bone remodelling are osteoblasts (bone forming cells) and osteoclasts (bone resorbing cells). Osteoblasts secrete the organic components of bone matrix, which are subsequently mineralized over months. Newly laid-down bone enters a 'resting' phase during which it is covered by bone-lining cells (resting osteoblasts). At a later date, osteoclasts may resorb this bone. Osteoclasts are cells that have the ability to resorb all mineralized tissues by bonding onto them and secreting proteolytic enzymes.[6] Areas of bone where resorption has taken place exhibit characteristic resorption pits or Howship's lacunae. Both bone formation and resorption are continually in operation and, under normal circumstances, in mature adults a dynamic equilibrium exists between them. Turnover rate is widely quoted as being about 25% per annum in trabecular bone and 2–3% in cortical bone.[7] Trabecular bone is generally assumed to be more metabolically active.[8] This continuous turnover of bone prevents structural damage due to fatigue and is important in maintaining calcium homeostasis.[9]

With metabolic bone disease any of the stages of bone formation, remodelling and mineralization can either be increased or decreased, but the predominant disturbance will affect the gross, radiographic and histological appearance of bone. The three main changes produced are:

- An increased in the amount of tissue present.
- A reduction in the amount of tissue present.
- Poorly mineralized bone.

SCURVY

Scurvy is caused by a lack of vitamin C (ascorbic acid). There are a wide range of foods that contain vitamin C, for example fruits (in particular citrus fruits) and many vegetables.

However, there are many circumstances, particularly in past populations, which may have resulted in a deficiency of vitamin C in the diet. Although many of the above food types can be stored, levels of vitamin C will decrease rapidly. Scurvy is more prevalent in regions with cooler climates, and is generally associated with times of hardship or famine. Stuart-Macadam gives clear descriptions of the clinical manifestations of scurvy and some examples of early historical references to the condition.[10]

All these factors mean that potentially scurvy could be of great value in aiding interpretations of past populations. As today, there will have been variations in the amount of vitamin C consumed both within and between different societies. Any interpretation of what varying levels of scurvy mean will of course be difficult, but could be used to infer information on environmental conditions, past economies, lifestyle, cooking methods, and occupation. Differential access to vitamin C between males and females may also aid interpretation of the above points in the context of what is known about the society in question. For example, scurvy has been more common in men than women, as men were more often involved in wars and long voyages, situations in which there would have been a lack of fresh produce.[10] However, due to the nature of skeletal markers of the condition and problems of interpretation, work undertaken on scurvy in archaeological bone has been limited.

Many of the skeletal changes related to scurvy are the result of an absence or reduction in the amount of bone matrix formation, as vitamin C is essential for the formation of collagen, the main organic component of bone. In long-standing cases, there may be a net loss of bone due to impaired bone formation. Bone changes will therefore be clearer where rapid bone formation is taking place, and are consequently far more marked in infants than adults. However, many changes primarily affect soft tissues and so will be absent from the archaeological record.

In infantile scurvy (Möller–Barlow's disease) the main sites in which primary bone changes are manifest is in the region of the growth plate of bones. Alteration of the mechanical structures around these areas often leads to fracture at the metaphysis, which may re-unite with the epiphysis in an abnormal position. While the condition is active the metaphyseal end of affected long bones may be sclerotic and dense, while the region behind is of diminished density. This pattern of bone change is known as the 'scurvy line' and may be visible on radiographs.[11] Scurvy is often fatal, but if the individual survives, remodelling of the damaged metaphysis tends to be slow. New bone formation associated with growth will gradually leave an isolated area of damaged bone below the growth plate which, when radiographed, can appear as a band of 'coarsely structured bone'.[1] Subperiosteal haematomas, particularly on the long bones, are common in infantile scurvy, although the likelihood of discovering 'pumice-bone' related to such an event are limited as a result of its fragile nature. Haemorrhage and related dislocation at the costochondral junction of the ribs may lead to the development of a 'rosary' appearance due to new bone formation.[1] Scurvy may also cause porotic and, occasionally, hypertrophic changes in the skull. A recent study[12] identified areas of the skull in which such changes commonly occur. The pattern of possible bone changes is complex, but was related to scorbutic soft tissue changes. Care must be taken when considering a differential diagnosis of scurvy, as some changes are similar to those produced by infections and anaemias. It was also noted that more than one pathology may be present in such infants. However, 'bilateral, porous lesions of the external surface of the greater wing of the sphenoid' (p. 214).[12] appeared to be pathognomic of scurvy.

In adults, the skeletal manifestations of the condition are difficult to identify. Although subperiosteal haematomas do occur, they are often not as severe as in younger individuals, and the possibility of recognizing resulting periosteal new-bone formation caused by scurvy is limited.

Another change that can occur in both infantile and adult scurvy, is new-bone formation in the roof of the orbits[13] (Figure 1) due to bleeding into this area. Care should be taken not to confuse these changes with those associated with anaemia, such as cribra orbitalia. This difficulty is illustrated by Larsen[14] where changes in the orbital region in a American Guale skeleton described as cribra orbitalia resemble changes characteristic of scurvy. After contact with Europeans the nutritional quality of the diet of these individuals decreased, with a heavy dependency on maize.[15] Such a diet is known to predispose individuals to scurvy.[13] The possibility that a misdiagnosis may have occurred in an otherwise excellent text serves to illustrate the lack of knowledge about the appearance of scurvy in archaeological bone material. This suggestion is merely conjecture, as detailed examination of the entire skeleton would be required to produce a more accurate differential diagnosis.

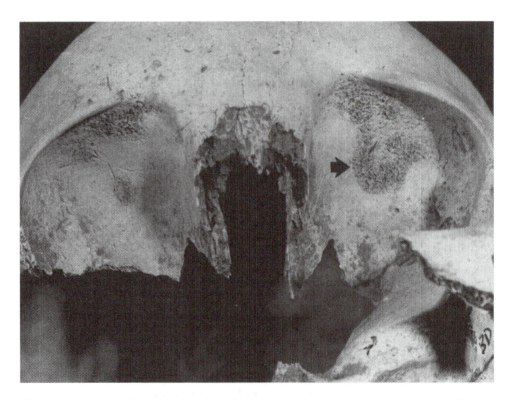

Figure 1 – The arrow indicates orbital new bone formation representing scurvy, from the 1st century BC, Beckford, Worcestershire. Photo: courtesy Department of Archaeological Sciences, University of Bradford.

One region of the skeleton in which soft tissue changes may be apparent in both adults and children is the jaw. Swollen and bleeding gums are a classic sign of scurvy. Clearly, these will not be apparent in the skeleton, but associated defects of the periosteum and ligaments holding the teeth in their sockets can lead to tooth loss and periodontal disease. In isolation, such changes are not diagnostic of scurvy, but such features have been used in conjunction with other skeletal changes to produce a more reliable diagnosis.[13] The occurrence of periosteal new-bone formation and tooth loss has been used to argue for high levels of the condition in medieval European populations.[16] However, care should be taken as, it is known that both lesions can be caused by a wide range of pathological conditions. Although some of the cases discussed[16] may be scurvy, this is not certain due to the diagnostic criteria used. In future studies, a far wider range of features, of the type discussed here, should be identified before scurvy is suggested as the pathology involved. One clear description of scurvy in archaeological bone, is a study of the skeletons of Dutch sailors who died of the disease.[17] This study provides a clear account of the osseous lesions caused by scurvy.

The ambiguity of skeletal markers of scurvy, and the obvious necessity of having relatively complete and well preserved skeletal material, go some way to explaining the paucity of reported cases of the condition in the archaeological literature. There are other papers that deal with the condition,[18–23] but the fact that most references to findings of scurvy can be included here probably reflects the difficulties in diagnosing the condition. It is also likely that scurvy has often not been considered in differential diagnoses of pathological conditions. Clearly, with the difficulties associated with identification of skeletal changes related to scurvy, particularly in adults, new ways of detecting the disease should be investigated. An alternative approach to the study of scurvy in adult skeletal material might be through the analysis of bone density. As mentioned previously, scurvy may cause bone loss. If the condition persisted for any length of time, classic features of osteoporosis may develop. In past populations, as scurvy was often fatal, few individuals with scurvy would have lived sufficiently long for features, such as fractures commonly associated with age-related osteoporosis, to be manifest. However, it is possible, although unlikely, that scurvy could have led to fracture and therefore some care with diagnosis may be required. In such cases the classic features associated with age-related osteoporosis should also be carefully considered (see below).

A more likely result of scurvy would be osteopenia, a lower than expected bone density of an individual for a particular age. It is possible that techniques developed to assess bone density could be used to help identify individuals with scurvy. However, such an approach would only be viable in juveniles and younger adults (less than 25 years). This approach would only be feasible if there was a large enough sample, from the same site, with which the results obtained could be compared. Most importantly, other skeletal indicators associated with scurvy should be present before a differential diagnosis of scurvy is suggested.

RICKETS

In contrast to scurvy, rickets has been widely reported in archaeological material. However, this condition will only be dealt with briefly, as Lewis (chapter 4, in this volume) discusses it further. Rickets is caused by a failure (in sub-adults) to obtain adequate levels of vitamin D from diet and/or exposure to sunlight. Lack of exposure to sunlight is often the main factor in the development of rickets, as 90% of the body's requirements can be obtained through exposure to sunlight.[24]

Vitamin D is essential for normal mineralization of bone and inadequate amounts can lead to a failure in this stage of the bone formation process. The classic sign of the condition is a bowing of the long bones due to poor mineralization. However, the manifestation of such signs depends on weight being placed upon these bones. The region of the skeleton where such features are present will depend upon the age of the affected child. For example, before walking occurs the long bones of the arms may be deformed from weight placed upon them during crawling, while in infants who have started to walk, the leg bones may become bowed.[1]

Other skeletal features of the condition include 'flaring' of the ends of long bones due to the presence of large amounts of unmineralized osteoid. If the condition persists for some time these changes at the metaphysis can become very marked and the end of the bone may have a 'frayed' appearance.[25] Deformation of the spine resulting in either kyphosis or scoliosis may also occur. Other attributes that can be related to rickets, visible on dry bone, have recently been described in the Wharram Percy skeletal collection.[26] The features attributed to rickets were, among others, cranial vault porosity (Figure 2), flared costo-chondral ends of ribs (Figure 3) and deformation of the mandibular ramus. This study found that many affected individuals did not exhibit all of the features of the condition, and, in isolation, many of these features may not be diagnostic. This is certainly the case with those such as the porotic changes described on the skull. As in many pathological conditions, ideally examination of the complete skeleton is necessary to add credence to any diagnosis made. Any metabolic disease that occurs during childhood may disrupt enamel development causing enamel hypoplasia.[27] However, such changes are not in themselves diagnostic, as they may reflect numerous conditions.[28]

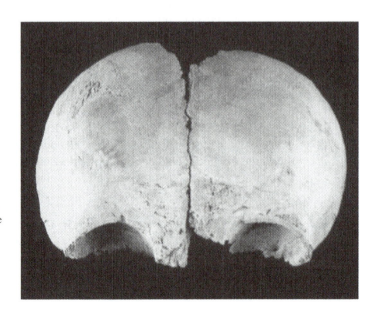

Figure 2 – Areas of porous new bone formation on the frontal bone, 10th–16th centuries AD, Wharram Percy, North Yorkshire. Photo: courtesy Ancient Monuments Laboratory, English Heritage.

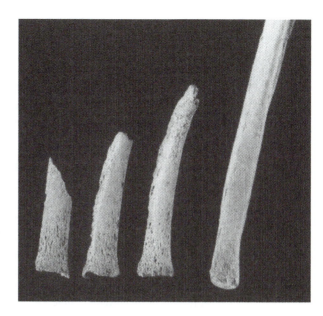

Figure 3 – Three rib fragments from Wharram Percy that display pitting of their cortices and flaring of their sternal ends. A normal rib is included for comparison (far right). Photo: courtesy Ancient Monuments Laboratory, English Heritage.

As rickets is not fatal, signs of its presence can persist into adulthood. One of the most serious changes that can remain in adulthood is the abnormal angulation of the sacrum and deforming of the ischium, creating a narrow and constricted pelvic girdle, which, if severe, can cause difficulties in parturition for females. As the aetiology of rickets is the same as that for osteomalacia, the implications of these conditions, for an understanding of past populations, will be considered together below.

OSTEOMALACIA

Osteomalacia has the same aetiology as rickets, although there are rare diseases that may also produce the condition, such as steatorrhoea and renal glomerular failure.[29]

As a result of their identical aetiology and the possibility of persistence of rachitic features in the adult skeleton, often in the form of bowing of the long bones, it could be unclear if the condition observed should be classified as osteomalacia or rickets. If bowing of the long bones is significantly greater than normal for the collection in question, but there is doubt as to whether osteomalacia or rickets is the cause, the safest option is to classify the condition as vitamin D deficiency. In general, changes such as bowing of the long bones will be less marked in osteomalacia. This is because in mature individuals, increases in the percentage of osteoid and poorly mineralized bones occur at a slower rate than in younger individuals. As the aetiology of rickets and osteomalacia is identical, it might be expected that there would be a similar spatial and temporal distribution of the two conditions. However, there are virtually no conclusive reported cases of osteomalacia in archaeological bone. One possible example is an isolated angulated sacrum from a Twelfth dynasty tomb, Lisht, Upper Egypt.[1] Individuals with angulated sacra have also been reported for the post-medieval population from Spitalfields, London.[30] Lack of reported cases is probably partly due to the fact that as yet no pathognomic features have been identified.

Skeletal deformation due to osteomalacia may occur across the skeleton. In particular the spine is susceptible to changes and, as with sub-adults, scoliosis or kyphosis may develop. Another change that can affect the spine in adults, is the development of depressed centres in the vertebral bodies due to ballooning of the intervertebral discs. Skeletal deformities may also occur in the rib cage and pelvis[27,31] due to weight and stresses at these sites. However, all such deformities will only be apparent in severe and long standing cases of the condition.

Ideally, some of the features discussed above would be detectable from visual analysis of the skeleton, as individually the types of skeletal changes outlined above are not in themselves pathognomic of osteomalacia. This can make diagnosing osteomalacia through gross examination of dry bone difficult, especially where the condition is not severe or long-standing. Radiological examination of bones may be of assistance in some instances. There are radiological features produced by the condition, such as Looser's zones, but these are rare and are not apparent in the early stages of the condition. Looser's zones, which can resemble fractures, appear as poorly mineralized zones perpendicular to the bone surface. They are 2–3 mm thick and surrounded by denser bone. Characteristic areas where these may be observed are the proximal femur, humeral neck, pubic rami, ribs, metatarsals, and the axiliary border of the scapula.[25,31] In cases where the condition is of very long standing, fractures may occur in Looser's zones. More general radiological features of the condition are a generalized loss of opacity affecting both cortical and trabecular bone, in particular trabecular bone may be less sharply defined than expected.[25] Clearly radiographic interpretation of archaeological bone may be made more difficult by diagenetic change and ingress of soil into bones.

There will no doubt be cases where, even after visual and radiological examination, uncertainty remains regarding the diagnosis of pathology in a skeleton. In such cases, if time and money are available, histological analysis may assist in producing a diagnosis. Either thin sections or embedded blocks of bone could be prepared for analysis. However, due to the fragile nature of archaeological bone, preparing embedded blocks may be more successful. Such blocks can be analysed using scanning electron microscopy (SEM). SEM backscattered imaging allows investigation of the arrangement of bone tissue and levels of mineralization, although care must be taken that diagenesis has not altered mineralization levels. Characteristic features include areas of poorly organized bone with low levels of mineralization. There may also be a thinning of micro-architectural elements due to areas of unmineralized osteoid at the time of death. Care must be taken, as a reduction in bone caused by osteomalacia could be mistaken for osteoporosis. However, although bone is lost with osteoporosis, mineralization of remodelled bone is normal, unlike with osteomalacia.

Today both osteomalacia and rickets are rarely observed in developed countries. In Britain, the rare cases of osteomalacia are most commonly observed in Asian women.[32] Osteomalacia is more prevalent in areas where, for cultural reasons, individuals have little exposure to sunlight, for example, Bedouin women and Islamic groups in Saudi Arabia and Pakistan.[33] Such modern patterns of occurrence should help in making interpretations about past societies in whom the condition is found. For example, both are often prevalent where levels of vitamin D in an individual may be low due to poor diet and limited exposure to sunlight. Rickets can, in extreme cases, produce severe deformity, but the extent to which an individual could participate in society, and societies view of that individual, may vary widely through time and across cultures.

OSTEOPOROSIS

'Osteoporosis is a disease characterized by abnormalities in the amount and architectural arrangement of bone tissue that lead to impaired skeletal strength and an undue susceptibility to fracture'.[34] The condition is divided into two main groups, primary and secondary, depending upon the causative factors involved. Primary osteoporosis includes Type I postmenopausal, related to hormonal changes, and Type II senile.[35] Secondary osteoporosis is defined as being attributed to one known cause, such as disease or reaction to drugs. The term osteoporosis should only be used in cases of extreme osteopenia where natural bone loss has been exaggerated and the individual is liable to suffer from one of the associated fractures.[36] These are hip fracture (proximal femur), Colles' fracture (distal radius) and vertebral crush fracture.

The imbalance in the remodelling processes, which results in a net loss of bone, occurs with advancing age and as a consequence of certain medical conditions, such as scurvy. This may lead to the clinical condition of osteoporosis. There is still considerable debate as to the exact role each cell type plays in producing an imbalance in the bone remodelling process. However, senile osteoporosis may be due to a reduction in activity of osteoblasts.[7] In postmenopausal osteoporosis, a brief phase of rapid loss is seen after the menopause[37], apparently caused by a rapid turnover rate of bone with increased osteoclastic activity.[38,39] Many factors such as exercise and nutrition have been linked to the development of an imbalance in bone remodelling, but ageing is one of the most important.

As discussed here on bone biology, bone turnover and therefore potential bone loss is greater in trabecular than cortical bone. This is reflected in the pattern of osteoporosis-related fractures observed clinically. Regions of the skeleton with a high proportion of trabecular bone are more susceptible to osteoporosis-related fracture.[40] Imbalance between bone formation and resorption results in the thinning of the cortex, from its inner (endosteal) surface, through its replacement by trabecular bone (trabecularization). Such bone is, of course, eventually impossible to tell apart from the original area of trabecular bone. The porosity of the cortex also increases.[7] These changes in the bone structure lead to micro-architectural deterioration of trabecular support structures and a reduction in density.

The simplest approach to the study of osteoporosis in archaeological material is to examine the bone for evidence of fracture. In considering a diagnosis of osteoporosis a number of factors should be taken into account, for example location of the fracture and estimated age and sex of the individual. Owing to the range of diagenetic changes that can occur, feeling the weight of bones is not an acceptable way of diagnosing the condition. With growing awareness of the condition some osteoporosis-related fractures, mostly crush fractures of the spine, have been reported.[41–45] Few cases of fracture of the femoral neck have been reported in the archaeological literature. This is probably because such fractures produce problems in healing, and can lead to premature death.[46] Distinguishing fractures that occurred close to death from post-mortem damage can be very problematic. However, as it is known that density and structural alteration may occur within bone before a fracture,[47] some studies have investigated ways of detecting these changes.[48,49]

Density

As might be expected with the variety seen in adult size and build, there is a large and continuous range in the amount of bone present in normal individuals.[34] Consequently it is impossible to give a specific figure for peak bone density expected in any one adult. However, clinically, calculations of bone mineral density or content are frequently used to aid diagnosis, and density criteria have been produced by the World Health Organisation.[50] The WHO defined osteoporosis and osteopenia relative to young adult reference means. Individuals who have density values reduced by 1 SD of the young adult reference mean have 'low bone mass (osteopenia)', and those < 2.5 SD have 'osteoporosis'. There are, however, a wide range of figures for bone mass at which osteoporotic fractures occur.[51] Research indicates that the link between osteoporotic fracture and density is poor.[51–54] There is a significant body of opinion that considers the trabecular structure of the bone more important in the occurrence of osteoporosis-related fractures.[47,55–58] However, for practical reasons, the most common clinical techniques for assessing bone loss are non-invasive, and measure whole bone mass or density.

Dual energy X-ray absorptiometry (DEXA) is a commonly used clinical tool designed to measure bone mineral density and content. Such equipment has been used on archaeological bone in some studies.[47,55,56] Although these studies have produced interesting results, there are problems with applying this technique to archaeological bone. In particular, DEXA cannot detect diagenetic changes[59,60] and the use of soft tissue replication when examining archaeological bone can be problematic.

In contrast Energy Dispersive Low Angle X-ray Scattering (EDLAXS), an energy-dispersive diffraction technique, has produced excellent results on archaeological material. This technique has the advantage that it is not designed for clinical use and consequently no soft tissue replication is required. The mineral spectrum produced for each bone also enables the type as well as the quantity of minerals present to be determined.[60] This enables altered samples to be excluded from study. Unfortunately this technique has very limited availability and the equipment required is very expensive.

Optical densitometry is a technique that allows an equivalent 'optical density' to be calculated from radiographs of bone taken with an aluminium step-wedge, as shown in Figure 4 (or other calibration standard). A light densitometer is required for analysis of radiographs. The technique produces good results, and the equipment needed is available in many universities. However, it is not always possible to detect diagenetic changes from examination of radiographs[49] and care must be taken with the interpretation of results.

Trabecular structure

Some studies have examined changes in the structure of trabecular bone in relation to ageing and osteoporosis in vertebral bodies.[48,61] A depletion of the number of vertical plates

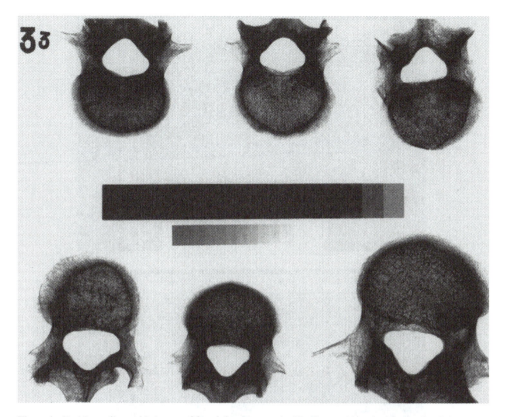

Figure 4 – Positive radiographic image of fourth lumbar vertebral bodies, positioned with two aluminium step wedges to allow analysis of density.

was observed, resulting in an apparent increase in the length of horizontal trabeculae (Figure 5). A thinning of horizontal trabeculae was also noticed, with some trabeculae having free ends (Figure 6). All these processes will predispose an individual to fracture. Close range photogrammetry enables the measurement of structures in three dimensions, and such a technique is ideal for gaining an objective measure of micro-architectural trabecular structures. It has been found that measurable length of horizontal trabeculae is closely related to age and sex. Although a study by the author[49] found this to be the best technique for the detection of age- and sex-related bone loss, there are drawbacks. The technique requires that a slice is removed from bones for analysis and, although not as expensive and limited in availability as EDLAX, equipment is not widely available and is relatively expensive.

The Singh Index,[62] which is used to assess bone loss and osteoporosis from examination of radiographs of the femoral head and neck region, should, in theory, provide a quick and easy way of analysing bone for osteoporosis. A score is given which relates to changes in the pattern of trabecular bone. However, a pilot study carried out by the author[49] found the technique to be of limited use in predicting bone loss. It was also found that there was great difficulty in obtaining repeatable results. Although this was only a pilot study, the author would not recommend the use of this technique.

(a)

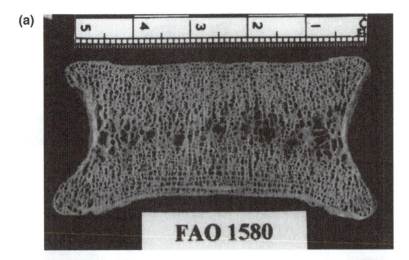

FAO 1580

(b)

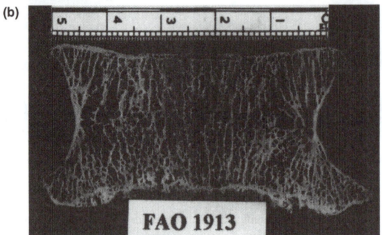

FAO 1913

Figure 5 – (a) Coronal section through the fourth lumbar vertebral body of a young adult (15–25 years). The trabecular bone is densely packed and evenly distributed. (b) Coronal section through the fourth lumbar vertebral body of an older adult (46+ years). There has been a loss of trabecular bone resulting in a more open structure.

Considerable research has been undertaken on adapting techniques for the study of archaeological bone, and successful studies have been mentioned. To understand fully the history and development of osteoporosis, results of studies undertaken across geographical regions and periods need to be compared. Consequently, the author is working in collaboration with Dr Farquharson of City University, London to develop a 'standard' that can be used with optical densitometry or DEXA. Although it has many limitations, DEXA is available in over 90 hospitals in the UK and so is widely accessible. Use of a 'standard' with optical densitometry or DEXA will not overcome the problems of diagenetic change and this will have to be tested for using other methods. However, it will allow calibration of results and direct comparison between future studies. Such an approach will allow a fuller understanding of the condition to be gained. Where bones can be sectioned and funds are available trabecular structure should also be studied.[61] This would enable a clearer picture of the relationship between density and structure to be gained.

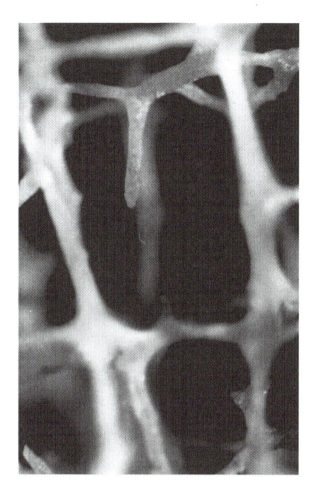

Figure 6 – Typical free-ending trabecula (centre field). Length of free-ending element about 1.5 mm.

In theory, levels of age-related bone loss and osteoporosis across different societies could be used to examine changes in factors such as levels of nutrition and exercize in different populations. At present, the data to undertake such a study do not exist. What may be found is that osteoporosis is so multifactoral that determining which lifestyle factors are responsible for variations observed is difficult. However, it may be possible to discern broad trends, and the results of such a study would potentially be of interest to epidemiologists and palaeopathologists. The impact of the condition upon societies would have been the same as that from any other type of fracture, although it has been noted that femoral fractures can result in premature death.

CONCLUSIONS

Although in recent years interest in metabolic bone disease has increased, apart from rickets, very little attention has been paid to the conditions discussed in this chapter in past studies of archaeological bone. One possible reason why these pathologies have not been widely studied in skeletal remains, is the difficulty of diagnosing such conditions in dry bone material; the limited number of ways in which bone can respond to such conditions makes diagnosis difficult.

There is now a better understanding of many metabolic bone diseases among the public and archaeological community, and it is appreciated that these conditions have a valuable contribution to make to our understanding of past populations. The variety of useful techniques that could be developed to aid the study of metabolic bone disease in archaeological bone is illustrated by the range of techniques developed to investigate osteoporosis.

Although analysis of archaeological material at a gross level will undoubtedly remain the primary means of investigation, newer techniques are still extremely valuable. Investigation of material using such techniques can give an indication of the number of cases that may be missed using visual examination. Hopefully, continued interest in this important group of conditions will lead to the development of alternative ways of detecting conditions such as scurvy and osteomalacia. This in turn will provide a fuller picture of the everyday lives of past populations.

REFERENCES

1   Ortner DJ, Putschar WGJ. *Identification of Pathological Conditions in Human Skeletal Remains.* Washington, DC: Smithsonian Institution Press, 1985.

2   Aufderheide AC, Rodriguez-Martin C. *The Cambridge Encyclopaedia of Human Paleopathology.* Cambridge: Cambridge University Press, 1998.

3   Albright F, Riefenstein E. *The Parathyroid Glands and Metabolic Bone Disease.* Baltimore: Williams & Wilkins, 1948.

4   Woolf AD, St John Dixon A. *Osteoporosis a Clinical Guide.* London: M Dunitz, 1988.

5   Sambrook P, Kelly P, Eisman J. *Bone Mass and Ageing.* Ballieres Clinical Rheumatology 7. London: Balliere Tindal, 1993: pp. 445–457.

6   Arnett TR. Physiology of the skeleton: In Stevenson JC (ed.), *Osteoporosis.* Guildford: Reed Healthcare, 1991: pp. 10–14.

7   Dempster DW, Lindsay R. Pathogenesis of osteoporosis. *Lancet* 1993; **341**: 797–801.

8   Dargent P, Breart G. Epidemiology and risk factors of osteoporosis. *Current Opinion in Rheumatology* 1993; **5**: 339–345.

9   Peel N, Eastell R. ABC of rheumatology: Osteoporosis. *British Medical Journal* 1995; **15(310)**: 989–992.

10 Stuart-Macadam PL. Nutritional deficiency diseases: a survey of scurvy, rickets, and iron-deficiency anemia. In: Isçan MY, Kennedy KAR (eds), *Reconstructing Life from the Skeleton.* New York: Wiley, 1989: pp. 210–222.

11 Resnick D, Niwayama G. *Diagnosis of Bone and Joint Disorders*, vol. 5 (2nd edn). Philidelphia: WB Saunders, 1988.

12 Ortner DJ, Erickson MF. Bone changes in the human skull probably resulting from scurvy in infancy and childhood. *International Journal of Osteoarchaeology* 1997; **7**: 212–220.

13 Roberts C, Manchester K. *The Archaeology of Disease* (2nd edn). New York: Sutton, 1997.

14 Larsen CS. *Bioarchaeology: Interpreting Behavior from the Human Skeleton.* Cambridge: Cambridge University Press, 1997.

15 Larsen CS. Telltale bones. *Archaeology* 1992; **45(2)**: 43–46.

16 Wells C. *Bones Bodies and Disease.* London: Thames & Hudson, 1964.

17 Maat GJR. Scurvy in Dutch whalers buried at Spitzbergen. In: *Proceedings of the IVth European Members Meeting of the Paleopathology Association at Middleberg/Antwerp on 16–19 September 1982.* Utrecht, 1982: pp. 82–93.

18 Ortner DJ. Bone lesions in a probable case of scurvy from Metlatavik, Alaska. *Museum Applied Science Center for Archaeology (MASCA) Journal* 1984; **3**: 79–81.

19 Roberts CA. Case Report **9**: Scurvy. *Paleopathology Society Newsletter* 1987; **57**: 14–15.

20 Saul F. The human skeletal remains of Altar de Sacrificios. *Papers of the Peabody Museum of Archaeology and Ethnology* 1972; **63**: 3–75.

21 Wells C. Prehistoric and historical changes in nutritional disease and associated conditions. *Progress in Food and Nutrition Science* 1975; **1**: 729–79.

22 Holk P. Scurvy as a paleopathological problem. *Paleopathology Society Newsletter* 1984; **47** (suppl. 5): Abstract.

23 Janssens PA, Marcsik A, Meyere C.de, Roy G. de. Qualitative and quantitative aspects of scurvy in ancient bones. *Journal of Paleopathology* 1993; **5**: 25–36. .

24 Passmore R, Eastwood MA. *Human Nutrition and Dietetics*. London: Churchill Livingstone, 1986.

25 Grech P, Martin TJ, Barrington NA, Ell PJ. *Diagnosis of Metabolic Bone Disease*. London: Chapman & Hall Medical, 1985.

26 Ortner DJ, Mays S. Dry-bone manifestations of rickets in infancy and early childhood. *International Journal of Osteoarchaeology* 1998; **8**: 45–55.

27 Parsons V. *A Colour Atlas of Bone Diseases*. Amsterdam: Wolfe, 1980.

28 Hillson S. *Dental Anthropology*. Cambridge: Cambridge University Press, 1996.

29 Pitt MJ. Rachitic and osteomalacic syndromes. *Radiologic Clinics of North America* 1981; **19**: 580–99.

30 Molleson T, Cox M. *The Spitalfields Project*, vol. **2**: *The Anthropology. The Middling Sort*. Research Report 86. York: Council for British Archaeology, 1993.

31 Francis RM, Selby PL. *Osteomalacia*. Ballieres Clinical Endocrinology and Metabolism. International Practice and Research. Metabolic Bone Disease 11. Balliere Tindall: London, 1997: pp. 145–163.

32 Fitch PJ, Ang L, Eastwood JB. Maxwell JD. Clinical and histological spectrum of osteomalacia among Asians in south London. *Quarterly Journal of Medicine* 1992; **83**: 439–48.

33 Lowenthal MN, Shany S. Osteomalacia in Bedouin women of the Negev. *Israel Journal of Medical Science* 1994; **30**: 520–3.

34 Melton JL, III, Chrischilles EA, Cooper C, Lane AW, Riggs LB. Perspective, how many women have osteoporosis. *Journal of Bone and Mineral Research* 1992; **7**: 1005–1010.

35 Riggs BL, Melton LJ. Evidence for two distinct syndromes of involutional osteoporosis. *American Journal of Medicine* 1983; **75**: 899–901.

36 Gallagher JC. The pathogenesis of osteoporosis. *Bone and Mineral* 1990; **9**: 215–227.

37 Riggs BL, Melton LJ. Involutional osteoporosis. *New England Journal of Medicine* 1986; **314**: 1676–86.

38 Heaney RP, Yates AJ, Santora AC (II). Bisphosphonate effects and the bone remodelling transient. *Journal of Bone and Mineral Research* 1987; **12**: 1143–1151.

39 Eriksen EF, Mosekilde L, Melsen F. Trabecular bone resorption depth decreases with age: Differences between normal males and females. *Bone* 1985; **6**: 141–6.

40 Barlow DH (ed.), *Report By the Advisory Group on Osteoporosis*. London: Department of Health, 1994.

41 Dequeker J, Ortner DJ, Stix AI, Cheng X, Brys P, Boonen S. Hip fracture and osteoporosis in a XIIth dynasty female skeleton from Lisht, Upper Egypt. *Journal of Bone and Mineral Research* 1997; **12**: 881–888.

42 Foldes AJ, Moscovici A, Popovtzer MM, Mogle P, Urman D, Zias J. Extreme osteoporosis in a sixth century skeleton from the Negev desert. *International Journal of Osteoarchaeology* 1995; **5**: 157–162.

43 Frigo P, Lang C. Osteoporosis in a woman of the Early Bronze Age. *New England Journal of Medicine* 1995; **333**: 1468.

44 Mays SA. Age-dependent cortical bone loss in a medieval population. *International Journal of Osteoarchaeology* 1996; **6**: 144–154.

45 Roberts C, Wakely J. Microscopical findings associated with the diagnosis of osteoporosis in palaeopathology. *International Journal of Osteoarchaeology* 1992; **2**: 23–30.

46 Spector TD. The epidemiology of osteoporosis. In: Stevenson JC (ed.), *Osteoporosis*. Guildford: Reed Healthcare, 1991: pp. 7–9.

47   Beck TJ, Ruff CR, Bissessur K. Age-related changes in female femoral neck geometry: Implications for bone strength. *Calcified Tissue International* 1993; **53** (suppl. 1): S41–S46.

48   Jayasinghe JAP. A study of change in human trabecular bone structure with age and during osteoporosis. Unpublished PhD thesis, University of London, 1991.

49   Brickley M. Age-related bone loss and osteoporosis in archaeological bone: a study of two London populations Redcross Way and Farringdon Street. Unpublished PhD thesis, University of London, 1998.

50   World Health Organisation. *Assessment of Fracture Risk and its Application to Screening for Postmenopausal Osteoporosis.* Report of a WHO Study Group; Technical Report Series 843. Geneva: WHO, 1994.

51   Ross PD, Davis JW, Vogel JM, Wasnich RD. A critical review of bone mass and the risk of fractures in osteoporosis. *Calcified Tissue International* 1990; **46**: 149–161.

52   Chappard D, Alexandre C, Riffat G. Spatial distribution of trabeculae in iliac bone from 145 osteoporotic females. *Acta Anatomica (Basel)* 1988; **132**: 137–42.

53   Cummings SR. Epidemiology of hip fractures. In: Christiansen C, Johansen JS, Riis BJ (eds), *Osteoporosis 1987.* Viborg: Nohaven A/S, 1987: pp. 40–44.

54   Pødenphant J, Herss Nielsen VA, Riis BJ, Gotfredsen A, Christiansen C. Bone mass, bone structure and vertebral fractures in osteoporotic patients. *Bone* 1987; **8**: 127–130.

55   Jensen KS, Mosekilde L, Mosekilde L. A model of vertebral trabecular bone architecture and its mechanical properties. *Bone* 1990; **11**: 411–415.

56   Mosekilde LI, Mosekilde LE, Danielson CC. Biomechanical competence of vertebral trabecular bone in relation to density and age in normal individuals. *Bone* 1987; **8**: 79–85.

57   Lees B, Molleson T, Arnett TR, Stevenson JC. Differences in proximal femur bone density over two centuries. *Lancet* 1993; **341**: 673–675.

58   Mays, S. Lees, B. Stevenson, J. Age-dependent bone loss in the femur in a medieval population. *International Journal of Osteoarchaeology* 1998; **8**: 97–106.

59   Farquharson MJ, Brickley M. Determination of mineral composition of archaeological bone using energy-dispersive low-angle X-ray scattering. *International Journal of Osteoarchaeology* 1997; **7**: 95–99.

60   Farquharson MJ, Brickley M, Speller RD. Measuring bone mineral density in archaeological bone using energy dispersive low angle X-ray scattering techniques. *Journal of Archaeological Science* 1997; **24**: 765–772. .

61   Brickley M, Howell PGT. Measurement of changes in trabecular structure with age in an archaeological population. *Journal of Archaeological Science* 1999; **24**: 765–772.

62   Singh M, Nagrath AR, Maini PS. Changes in the trabecular pattern of the upper end of the femur as an index of osteoporosis. *Journal of Bone and Joint Surgery* 1970; **52**: 457–467.

13

CONGENITAL CONDITIONS AND NEOPLASTIC DISEASE IN BRITISH PALAEOPATHOLOGY

Trevor Anderson

INTRODUCTION

Congenital conditions and neoplastic diseases are both well-known problems in modern medicine. In the past 3 years there have been 9883 papers devoted to congenital conditions and 57 583 referring to cancer (source: MEDLINE). Based on skeletal material, both congenital and neoplastic diseases *appear* to be less frequent in archaeological populations.

It is true that modern radiation hazards[1] and excessive alcohol intake during pregnancy can damage the foetus.[2] Modern pollutants, synthetic dyes, modern chemicals as well as tobacco and alcohol have all been implicated as causative factors in various forms of cancer.[3–6] In addition, metastatic carcinoma is a disease of the elderly; in earlier urban societies, it was not unusual for 25–30% of the population to die during childhood,[7] and only a small percentage of the adults reached old age.

However, direct comparison between modern and archaeological data is handicapped by various factors. Modern figures are based on clinical data with individuals presenting symptoms, and it is possible to calculate the incidence of any disease, whether affecting skeletal or soft tissue. Biopsy and histological examination can achieve definitive diagnosis. Archaeological information is by and large based on skeletal material. Not only are the recovered remains often incomplete and damaged, but also they invariably represent only a small proportion of the community from which they were derived.[8] Also, skeletons without externally visible lesions are not normally examined radiographically for internal pathology. Interpretation is handicapped by the fact that, in comparison with modern day populations the number of skeletal remains is extremely small. The larger cemetery samples probably span a wide period. As such it is impossible to gauge the incidence of specific disease.

All these factors must be considered when examining the apparent rarity of congenital and neoplastic disease in the archaeological record. The following sections outline our current state of knowledge, and consider the problems of the data, its limitations and interpretation. Thought is also given to the question of future developments.

PRESENT STATE OF KNOWLEDGE

Major congenital anomalies and neoplastic disease are not unknown from earlier British skeletal samples. The earliest examples date to the prehistoric period.[9–11] Compared with many other pathological conditions that may involve the skeleton, both are rare findings. A search of the literature has revealed 31 cases of congenital anomalies and 43 examples of neoplastic disease (Tables 1–5). This excludes osteoma of the cranial vault and solitary osteochondroma. The former typically develop on the cranial vault as small, circular dense bone overgrowths.[12] The latter develop at the growing end of long bones, especially the knee region, and present as a smooth pedunculated or sessile bone overgrowth.[13] Both occur frequently but current data do not permit calculation of their prevalence rates.

Congenital conditions

The most frequently reported archaeological example of a major congenital condition is congenital dislocation of the hip (CDH). The earliest British example is dated to the Bronze Age, and, apart from one Anglo-Saxon case, the rest are all medieval (Figure 1). The well-known female bias is evident.[14] Hydrocephaly, enlargement of the skull due to an abnormal increase in cerebrospinal fluid, has been recorded from four sites.[15–18] Hydrocephaly need not be congenital, it can occur as a consequence of meningitis, trauma or infection. Congenital hydrocephaly is often associated with spina bifida, cleft lip and club foot.[19]

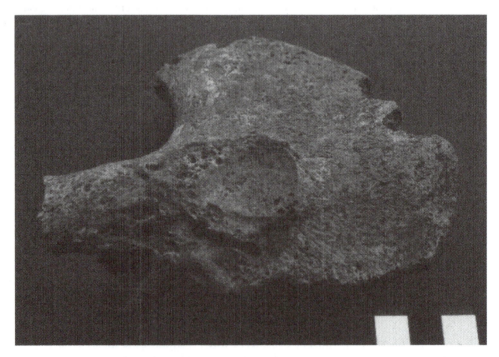

Figure 1 – Right pelvis of a 20–25-year-old medieval female, St Gregory's Priory, Canterbury. Complete remodelling of the original acetabulum and formation of a new, shallow, false joint. Evidence for congenital dislocation of the hip. Note the eburnation, indicating that, despite the instability, movement and use of the joint was still possible. Scale: cm.

Table 1 – Skeletal evidence: congenital conditions.

Sex	Age (years)	Location	Date	Source
ARTHROGRYPOSIS MULTIPLEX CONGENITA				
M	35–45	St Gregory's Priory, Canterbury, Kent	Medieval	74
CONGENITAL DISLOCATION OF THE HIP				
M	?	Thixendale, North Yorkshire	Bronze Age	9, 15
?	?	Guildown, Surrey	Anglo-Saxon	9, 15
F	20–25	St Gregory's Priory, Canterbury, Kent	Medieval	7
F	45–55	Shouldham, Norfolk	Medieval	134
F	Adult	Jewbury, York, North Yorkshire,	Medieval	77
F	21–23	Abingdon, Oxfordshire	Medieval	135
CLEFT PALATE				
?	Child	Burwell, Cambridgeshire	Anglo-Saxon	21
?	8–9	Raunds Furnells, Northamptonshire	Anglo-Saxon	20
M	40–50	St Gregory's Priory, Canterbury, Kent	Medieval	22
CLUB FOOT				
?	?	Nether Swell, Gloucester	Neolithic	15
DOWN'S SYNDROME (MONGOLISM)				
?	about 9?	Breedon-on-the-Hill, Leicestershire	Anglo-Saxon	15, 76
?	25	Nazeingbury, Essex	Anglo-Saxon	16
HEMIVERTEBRAE				
?	?	Crichel Down, Dorset	Bronze Age	15
HYDROCEPHALY				
M?	Young adult	Norton, North Yorkshire	Roman	15
?	14–16	Eccles, Kent	Anglo-Saxon	17
M	25	Nazeingbury, Essex	Anglo-Saxon	16
?	6–7	Doonbought Fort, Co. Antrim, N. Ireland	Medieval	18
MICROCEPHALY				
?	?	Hythe, Kent	Medieval	15
OSTEOCHONDROMATOSIS (DIAPHYSEAL ACLASIA)				
F	Adult	Poundbury, Dorset	Roman	67
?	Child	Winchester, Hampshire	Anglo-Saxon	96
M	Young adult	St Nicholas Shambles, London	Medieval	136
OSTEOGENESIS IMPERFECTA				
?	17–18	Burgh Castle, Suffolk	Anglo-Saxon	137
OSTEO-ONYCHODYSPLASIA (FONG'S SYNDROME/NAIL-PATELLA SYNDROME)				
?	?	Eccles, Kent	Anglo-Saxon	24, 138
?	?	Eccles, Kent		
?	?	Eccles, Kent		
PARTIAL APLASIA: BASI-OCCIPUT				
M	Young adult	York, North Yorkshire	Roman	15, 75
PARTIAL APLASIA: SPINOUS PROCESS				
F	30–35	St Gregory's Priory, Canterbury, Kent	Medieval	73
PARTIAL APLASIA: FIBULAE				
?	?	Dunstable, Bedfordshire	Anglo-Saxon	15, 139
PARTIAL APLASIA: PECTORAL GIRDLE				
M	28–30	Worthy Park, Hampshire	Anglo-Saxon	140
SPONDYLO-EPIPHYSEAL DYSPLASIA				
M	45+	Abingdon, Oxfordshire	Medieval	141

Table 2 – Neoplastic disease: primary malignant tumours.

Sex	Age (years)	Location	Date	Source
OSTEOSARCOMA				
M	20–30	Standlake, Oxfordshire	Anglo-Saxon	10
M	30–40	St Andrew, Fishergate, York, North Yorkshire	Medieval	59
MULTIPLE MYELOMA				
F?	45+	Abingdon, Oxfordshire	Medieval	61

Table 3 – Neoplastic disease: primary benign tumours.

Sex	Age (years)	Location	Date	Source
ENCHONDROMA				
F	28–33	Brackmills, Northampton, Northamptonshire	Anglo-Saxon	48
M	35–45	St Gregory's Priory, Canterbury, Kent	Medieval	66
GIANT CELL TUMOUR				
SK	44	Finglesham, Kent	Anglo-Saxon	10
OSTEOID OSTEOMA				
F	20–30	Caister-on-Sea, Norfolk	Anglo-Saxon	65
M	Adult	Sedgeford, Norfolk	Anglo-Saxon	9, 10
F	Elderly	West Heslerton, North Yorkshire	Anglo-Saxon	64
OSTEOMA (EXCLUDING CRANIAL VAULT IVORY OSTEOMATA)				
M	30–40	Brackmills, Northampton, Northamptonshire	Anglo-Saxon	62
?	?	Petersfinger, Cambridgeshire	Anglo-Saxon	82
M	40–50	St Gregory's Priory, Canterbury, Kent	Medieval	78
M	40–50	St Gregory's Priory, Canterbury, Kent	Medieval	63
F	45–50	Timberhill, Norwich, Norfolk	Medieval	142
M	45+	St Andrew, Fishergate, York, North Yorkshire	Medieval	59
F	Adult	Jewbury, York, North Yorkshire	Medieval	77

Three cases of cleft palate are known, two in Anglo-Saxon children[20,21] and one in an elderly medieval male[22] (Figure 2). Interestingly, cleft palate was one of the few problems for which the Anglo-Saxon medical texts advocated a medical procedure, perhaps suggesting that it was not an uncommon condition.[23] Three cases of the hereditary condition osteochondromatosis, also known as diaphyseal aclasia, have been published (Table 1). In clinical medicine, this condition predisposes to malignant degeneration.[2] Three individuals with iliac horns may be suffering from Fong's syndrome.[24] Other congenital conditions are represented by single examples (Table 1).

Minor congenital anomalies

A wide range of minor skeletal anomalies occurs in the hands and feet, including fusions, bipartitions and accessory bones.[25,26] There is some evidence that certain variations may be familial.[27–37] Symphalangism (fusion of the phalanges), often associated with tarsal coalitions, is known to be hereditary.[38–41] Indeed, it has been traced through 14 generations of the Talbot family from an ancestor who died in 1453.[42]

Table 4 – Neoplastic disease: secondary tumours (metastases).

Sex	Age (years)	Location	Date	Source
OSTEOLYTIC				
M	35	Poundbury, Dorset	Roman	67
?	?	Winchester, Hampshire	Anglo-Saxon	10
M	30–50	Barrington, Cambridgeshire	Anglo-Saxon	80
F	40+	Eccles, Kent	Anglo-Saxon	52
F	75	Spitalfields, London	Post-medieval	143
MIXED				
M	about 50	Chichester, West Sussex	Medieval	54
OSTEOBLASTIC				
M	45–55	St Gregory's Priory, Canterbury, Kent	Medieval	51
M	60+	St Gregory's Priory, Canterbury, Kent	Medieval	55
M	30–50	Wharram Percy, North Yorkshire	Medieval	53
M	59	St Bride's, London	Post-medieval	81
MULTIPLE MYELOMA/METASTATIC CARCINOMA				
?	?	Stonar, Kent	Medieval	60
?	?	St James, Ipswich, Suffolk	Medieval	60

Table 5 – Neoplastic disease: soft tissue neoplasia eliciting bone response

Sex	Age (years)	Location	Date	Source
ADENOMA				
M	Mature	Abingdon, Oxfordshire	Medieval	144
HAEMANGIOMA				
M	Adult	Masham, North Yorkshire	Bronze Age	145
MENINGIOMA				
F	Adult	Burton Fleming, East Yorkshire	Iron Age	69
F?	Adult	Deal, Kent	Iron Age	112
F	Adult	Radley, Oxfordshire	Roman	10
F	35–50	Rochester, Kent	Medieval	56, 57, 58
M	50+	St Andrew, Fishergate, York, North Yorkshire	Medieval	59
M	Adult	Hertfordshire	Medieval/post-medieval	70
F	45+	Hertfordshire	Medieval/post-medieval	70
M	Adult	Hertfordshire	Medieval/post-medieval	70
NASOPHARYNGEAL				
?	?	East Yorkshire	Anglo-Saxon	9, 10
NEUROFIBROMA				
M	Adult	Dunstable, Bedfordshire	Anglo-Saxon	9, 10
UNCERTAIN: BENIGN				
M	Adult	Maiden Castle, Dorset	Iron Age	9
F	Adult	Maiden Castle, Dorset	Iron Age	9
UNCERTAIN: MALIGNANT				
?	?	All Saints Church, York, North Yorkshire	Medieval	79

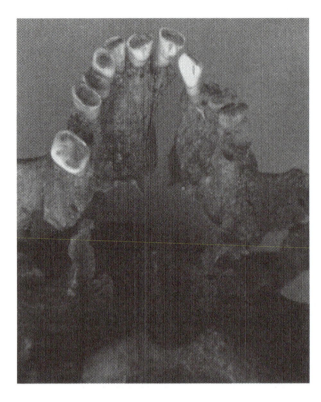

Figure 2 – Cranium of a 40–50-year-old medieval male from St Gregory's Priory, Canterbury, displaying cleft lip and palate.

At Apple Down, Chichester, Sussex, it was suggested that five Anglo-Saxons with additional vertebrae and sagittal ossicles were possibly related.[43] However, identifying genetic links by examining patterns of minor congenital anomalies in archaeological samples has generally been overlooked. Indeed, several congenital anomalies may not be recognized as such. For instance, seven cases of what appears to be a facet for an accessory bone known as *os tibiale*[44,26] have been published as being of possible traumatic aetiology.[45] Anatomical studies suggest that the incidence of *os tibiale* is 10–11.5%,[26] and that it may give rise to painful flat feet.[46]

Two examples of a rare variant, hypoplastic hamulus (reduced size of the hook of the hamate)[47] were discovered on a site at Brackmills, Northamptonshire, with only 24 burials. Based on these two bones, it has been suggested that a small inbreeding community may have been farming the land at Brackmills from the Iron Age through to the Anglo-Saxon period, with minimal disturbance from the Roman invasions.[48,49]

Neoplastic diseases

Neoplastic diseases have been subdivided into three broad categories:

i   *Primary bone tumours:* those that develop initially in bone. They are subdivided into (a) *benign* such as osteoma and (b) *malignant* and life threatening, such as osteosarcoma.

ii *Secondary bone tumours:* those that develop in soft tissue and then metastasize to bone. Such deposits favour areas of red marrow, namely the axial skeleton and also long bone metaphyses.[50] The sex of the individual, the morphology of the lesions, whether they are predominantly bone forming (osteoblastic) or bone reducing (osteoclastic) or a mixed response, may permit diagnosis of the likely original site of the soft-tissue lesion.[51–55]

iii *Soft tissue tumours eliciting a bone response:* soft tissue involvement causing bone alteration although the tumour has not metastasized, e.g. hyperostosis secondary to cranial meningioma.[10,56–58]

Primary malignant bone tumours are extremely rare in archaeological material (Table 2). The best known British example is from Standlake, Oxfordshire, where a young Anglo-Saxon man was suffering from a large malignant overgrowth at his knee joint.[10] A tentative diagnosis of osteosarcoma has been made for a porous swelling of a sphenoid bone from medieval York[59] (although the age of the individual, 30–40 years, is rather old for a primary osteosarcoma and too young to represent Pagetic osteosarcoma). Osteolytic lesions on two medieval crania may be multiple myeloma or metastatic carcinoma.[60] A case of multiple myeloma has been identified from Abingdon, Oxfordshire.[61]

With the exception of cranial vault osteomata and isolated osteochondroma of the limb bones, primary benign tumours of bone have been reported infrequently (Table 3). Osteomata of unusual sites, such as the mandible[59,62] and the frontal sinus[63] are known. Osteoid osteoma[9–10,64,65] and enchondroma[48,66] are probably under-represented since they require radiography for diagnosis. Benign tumours without external changes, such as lipoma and osteoblastoma, have not been recognized in British material. Also, early stage central chondrosarcoma is restricted to internal bone destruction and is unknown in the archaeological record.

Ten cases of secondary bone tumours (metastatic lesions) are known, the earliest dating to the Roman period[67] (Table 4). All presented external osseous alteration. Osteoblastic metastases, all in males, are confined to the medieval and post-medieval periods (Figure 3 and Table 4). This may suggest that prostatic carcinoma may not have existed before the medieval period. However, we must bear in mind that routine radiography of outwardly normal spines, femora and pelves would almost certainly increase the detection of both primary and secondary bone cancers.[68] It should be noted that in archaeological dry bone material, the definition of the radiograph is improved by (1) a lack of soft tissue which could mask subtle osseous involvement and (2) the ability to use high definition radiography which would not be possible on bones of living patients due to the danger of an overdose of radiation.

The most common type of tumour is that in which soft tissue involvement has lead to an alteration in skeletal remains (Table 5). Bone response to an underlying benign brain tumour, a meningioma, is the most frequently encountered lesion in this group[10,56–59,69,70] (Figures 4 and 5).

Limitations

It must be stressed that other examples of congenital conditions and neoplasia do undoubtedly exist. This search of the literature is based mainly on reported case studies, review

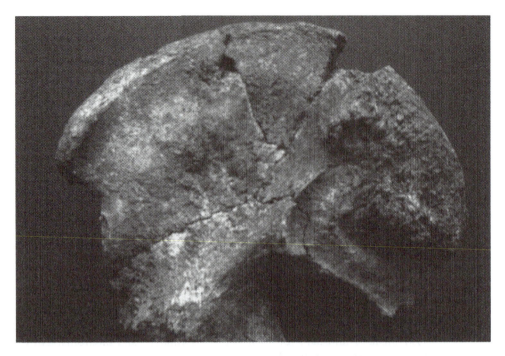

Figure 3 – Right innominate of a 45–55-year-old medieval male, St Gregory's Priory, Canterbury. New woven bone on the internal surface of the ilium. Similar deposits were located on the pleural surface of the ribs and the internal surface of the mandibular rami. Internal osteoblastic changes were noted radiographically in the pelvis; spine; proximal femorae. The form and distribution of the lesions, combined with the sex of the individual, are indicative of metastases from carcinoma of the prostate.

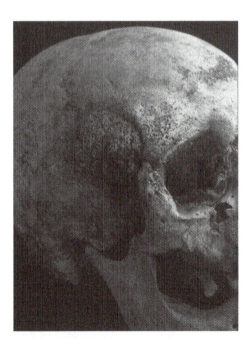

Figure 4 – Cranium of a 35–45-year-old medieval female from Rochester. Hyperostosis secondary to an intracranial meningioma.

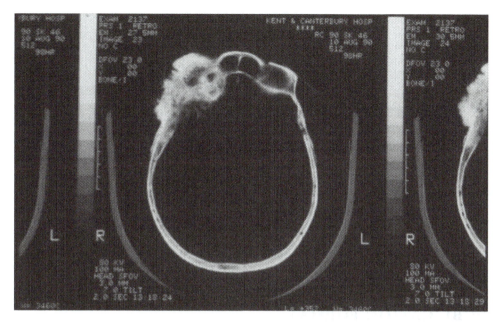

Figure 5 – CT scan of the cranium in Figure 4. Displaying the internal destruction typical of an intracranial meningioma.

articles and cemetery excavations which have been published as monographs. However, other examples may not be readily accessible, as they are contained in unpublished reports or hidden away in local archaeological journals.

A lack of funding may mean that certain cemetery samples have not been analysed, or only examined in a very cursory fashion. Also earlier workers may not have recognized examples of congenital conditions and neoplastic disease. This is especially true of forms of diseases that lead to overall reduction in bone quantity or replacement by non-osseous tissue. After hundreds of years in the ground, with the pathological bone compromised by post-mortem damage, its final appearance may not be identifiable as neoplastic. This will particularly affect expansive, lytic lesions in which bone quantity is reduced, including giant cell tumour, angiosarcoma, lymphoma and desmoplastic fibroma.[71] In addition, the presentation of archaeological tumours may be at variance with clinical specimens that have received extensive medical treatment.[72]

Almost half the congenital conditions that are mentioned here were reviewed by Brothwell several years ago or are cases published by the author, mainly from his work in Kent.[7,9,15,21,22,24,73–77] Over a third of reports referring to British examples of neoplastic disease have been published by the same two authors,[9,10,51,56–58,62,63,66,67,77–79] which seems to suggest that many other cases remain unpublished. The fact that other syndromes have been recognized from medieval documents and illustrations indicates that the skeletal evidence is far from complete (Table 6). The following sections suggest avenues that could be pursued to gain a better understanding of congenital conditions and neoplastic disease in earlier British societies.

Table 6 – Documentary and illustrative evidence: congenital conditions.

Sex	Age (years)	Location	Date	Source
CLEFT LIP				
M	New born	Maidstone, Kent	1568	22, 44, 119, 121, 122
CONJOINED TWINS				
FF	New born	Biddenden, Kent	about 1100	146, 147
FF	New born	Herne, Kent	1565	148
FF	New born	Stony Stratford, Northamptonshire	1565	148
MF	New born	Swanburne, Buckinghamshire	1566	149
PACHYDERMIA				
F	New born	Mitcham, Surrey	1566	149
SPINA BIFIDA CYSTICA				
M	New born	Maidstone, Kent	1568	22, 44, 119, 121, 122
TETRADYSMELIA				
M	New born	Much Horkesley, Colchester, Essex	1562	44, 120

PUBLICATION FORMAT

Many examples have been published as case studies, which generally discuss the aetiology of the condition and often review the existing literature.[22,53,55–58,70,80,81] Other cases are included as part of a bone report.[16,20,56,64,67,69,77,82] Recently, work on neoplastic diseases in British populations has been extended by Eugen Strouhal who has been funded to identify British examples.[53,61,80]

Ideally, a database should be created. Only then will we identify possible geographical, chronological or environmental variation for these conditions. However, osteologists would need to be aware of factors that are known to influence modern day congenital conditions and neoplastic disease. For example, a medieval skeleton was found with both a cleft lip and palate and an odontome.[22] Based on clinical studies, facial clefting and odontome formation may be related to avitaminosis.[83,84] Odontome formation in laboratory rats has been related to a diet deficient in vitamin A.[83] It is therefore possible that this medieval individual was suffering from a shortage of vitamin A as well as facial clefting and abnormal dental formation.[22]

In the case of neoplastic diseases, we may indicate that variation in earlier societies is related to any of the following:

- Urban and rural samples.
- Geographical location (related to blood group type?).
- Social status.
- Environment/occupation.
- Diet and vitamin intake.
- Sexual activity.
- Familial.
- Stature.

In clinical studies, all of the above have been implicated in the development of neoplastic disease. Based on death rates, breast and rectal cancer are more frequent in higher social classes in urban contexts,[85] whereas there is evidence that lower socio-economic classes may be at greater risk of carcinoma of liver, oral cavity, scrotum and uterus.[86] Meningiomas are also slightly more frequent in lower social classes.[87]

Many cancers, including gastric and prostatic, display a predilection for blood group A.[5,85,88] This may explain the high incidence of prostatic carcinoma in modern day Scandinavia, a region with a high frequency of blood group A. There may be a direct relationship between blood group A and a weak immunological system, in which the body fails to destroy the cancer cells. The fact that there is a link between individuals with an overactive immune system (who may develop autoimmune disease) and blood group O supports this hypothesis.[88]

Soot was implicated in scrotal carcinoma (chimney sweeper's cancer) as early as 1775.[6] Inhalation of lead dust may lead to laryngeal carcinoma.[6] Coal miners may be susceptible to gastric carcinoma[5] and workers in the dye industry are reported to be prone to urinary bladder cancer.[6] Occupational exposure to leather and wood dust appears to predispose to carcinoma of the nasal sinus.[86] In archaeological material, a case of bronchogenetic carcinoma has been tentatively linked to occupation.[89]

Pulmonary carcinoma appears to be inhibited by a diet rich in vitamin A.[6] Certain cancers develop more rapidly if the patient is lacking vitamin A.[6] Colon and rectal carcinoma are closely related to the Western civilized diet, i.e. a lack of fibre combined with excess fat and animal protein.[6] There is evidence from migrant studies that gastric carcinoma and cancer of the bowel are, in part, related to diet.[85]

The development of prostatic carcinoma appears to be directly linked to the level of the male hormone, testosterone.[90] It appears that it may be related to coital frequency, number of partners, and age of first sexual intercourse.[5] Although recent work in America has suggested that a high fat intake may predispose to prostatic carcinoma,[91] other researchers have not replicated these results.[92] It has also been suggested that there may be a weak familial tendency.[86]

Cancer of the breast is known to be familial; daughters with affected mothers have a risk factor 15 times greater than the general population.[86] Also, nulliparous women are more prone to develop mammary carcinoma.[86] As such, it would be most interesting to examine radiologically skeletons from medieval nunneries, although it has to be remembered that these frequently housed widows.

There is some evidence that taller, rapidly growing individuals are more prone to primary bone neoplasms.[93,94] It would be interesting to see if there is a relationship between stature attainment and primary tumour formation in the archaeological record.

If a database were to be set up we would need to consider what information should be included in addition to a description of the pathology and details of the individual(s) involved. Areas that seem to be profitable include:

- Prevalence rate by both individual and by bone element. In diseases that affect specific bones, such as congenital dislocation of the hip, we need to know how many acetabula were available for study, subdivided by sex and age.
- Size of sample and chronological period.
- Demographic profile of the sample. In the case of secondary tumours, which develop in old age, it is essential to known how many individuals in the sample were old enough to be at risk.
- Archaeological information, such as anything atypical about the burial. Were the individual(s) with congenital conditions or neoplastic disease treated differently in death?
- Environmental evidence from the grave. There may be the possibility of identifying plant remains indicative of diet or medical treatment.

EXAMINATION OF THE REMAINS AND DIAGNOSIS

For variations in the axial skeleton, an excellent text has been published by Barnes.[95] Standard monographs on palaeopathology make reference to the more frequently encountered disease processes.[96,97] Many osteologists base their diagnoses on the latter books. Perhaps some may even try to fit their diagnosis into something that is included within these books. However, a very wide range of congenital conditions and numerous forms of neoplasia may directly or indirectly involve the skeleton. Ideally, one should consult the specialist clinical literature. The latter will provide detailed information, including classification, typical presentations, sex and age biases, typical bone sites and aetiology[2,71,98–100] (Tables 7a, b and 8). In addition, the older clinical texts provide a valuable insight into the end result of tumours that have received limited treatment[101,102] and will equate more closely with the appearance of untreated archaeological cases.

Something that has rarely been considered in palaeopathology is the fact that various skeletal anomalies that appear to be totally unrelated may equate with a well-known clinical syndrome (Table 9). Only by being aware of the major syndromes will it be possible to realise that external changes to certain bones may be associated with internal alteration (Table 10). It is more likely that we are dealing with a disease, or an atypical manifestation of a known condition, than to argue the skeletal changes represent a totally unknown condition.[24]

Fusion of the cervical spine may be congenital Klippel–Feil syndrome, rather than the result of underlying disease.[100] Bilateral bowing of long bones, particularly the legs, is known to be a congenital condition and need not be evidence for metabolic disease.[2] Also, the classic 'sabre-shin' although present in syphilis is the major finding in Weismann–Netter–Stuhl syndrome, possibly in association with short stature and spinal deformity.[2]

Clinical texts show that a wide range of neoplastic conditions may affect the skeleton.[71,99] However, archaeological skeletal remains are frequently weakened by the pathology, lack the soft tissue component of a tumour, and may be compromised by post-mortem damage, as well as being atypical in appearance to modern day post-chemotherapy radiographic presentation. As osteoarchaeologists we must therefore be aware of the limitations and precision of diagnoses based on dry bone material.

Table 7a – Clinical evidence for the sex, age and osseous distribution of selected benign neoplastic diseases.

Neoplasia	Sex M:F	Age (yrs)	Skull	Spine	Distribution Humerus	Radius	Hand	Pelvis	Femur	Tibia	Foot
Bone-forming											
OSTEOID OSTEOMA (n214){n57}	2:1	> 50% 11–20							(26.6%){40.4%}	(25.2%){26.3%}	
OSTEOBLASTOMA (n51){n0}	3:1	90% < 30 years		(21.6%)					(11.8%)	(9.8%)	
Cartilage-forming											
ENCHONDROMA (n466){n99}	1:1	81% > 20 years					(62.4%){56.6%}		(6.9%){12.1%}		(8.2%){6.1%}
OSTEOCHONDROMA (n783){n272}	1.5:1	69% > 20 years			(16.1%)[a]{19.1%}				(26.4%)[b]{29.0%}	(21.5%)[c]{13.6%}	
CHONDROBLASTOMA (n115){n17}	1.7:1	Most 10–20 years			(17.4%)[d]{17.6%}			(0.0%){23.5%}	(28.7%)[e]{41.2%}	(19.1%)[f]{0.0%}	
CHONDROMYXOID FIBROMA (n44){n13}	1:1	68% 5–25 years								(50.0%)[g]{46.2%}	
Vascular											
HAEMANGIOMA (n36){n13}	1:1	Adult	(44.4%){69.2%}	(13.9%){15.4%}							
Connective tissue											
DESMOPLASTIC FIBROMA (very rare){n35}	1:1	Most > 30 years			{8.6%}				{34.3%}	{40.0%}	

For Table 7a and b, osteoma is classed as hamartoma rather than true neoplasms and is omitted here.

Source: figures in (parentheses) are based on Schwajowicz[71]; those in {curly brackets} are based on Dahlin[98].

For Table 7a: osteochondroma: [a]humerus 95.2% proximal; [b]femur 83.1% distal; [c]tibia 66.7% proximal; chondroblastoma: [d]humerus 90.0% proximal; [e]femur 54.5% distal; [f]tibia 90.9% proximal; chondromyxoid fibroma: [g]tibia 63.6% proximal metaphysis.

211

Table 7b – Clinical evidence for the sex, age and osseous distribution of selected malignant neoplastic diseases.

Neoplasia	Sex M:F	Age (yrs)	Skull	Spine	Distribution Humerus	Radius	Hand	Pelvis	Femur	Tibia	Foot
Bone-forming											
OSTEOSARCOMA (n512){n490}	3:2	> 60% 11–20			(10.2%}{7.8%}			{8.2%}	(48.2%}{43.7%}	(24.0%}{19.2%}	
Cartilage-forming											
CHONDROSARCOMA[a] (n287){n137}	3:2	> 60% 11–20			(10.2%}{5.8%}			{18.2%}	(48.2%}{24.8%}	(24.0%}{21.2%}	
Marrow tumour											
EWING'S SARCOMA (n210){n141}	1.1:1	Most 5–15			(11.0%}{7.1%}			{18.2%}	(29.0%}{26.2%}	(15.2%}{10.6%}	
RETICULOSARCOMA (n102){n0}	1:1.4	20–70		(4.5%)	(3.8%)			(7.7%)	(9.0%)	(4.5%)	
MYELOMA (n404){n140}	3:2	Peak 40–60	{12.1%}	{39.3%}				{14.3%}			
Connective tissue											
FIBROSARCOMA (n142){n106}	1:1	Most 20–60			(10.6%}{5.7%}			{6.6%}	(33.8%}{39.6%}	(20.4%}{24.5%}	
Other											
GIANT CELL TUMOUR (36){13}	1:1.5	20–40			(9.7%)[b]{5.5%}	(9.9%)[c]{8.3%}		{10.1%}[f]	(24.9%)[d] {33.9%}	(28.2%)[e] {22.9%}	
CHORDOMA (n23){n80}	1.1:1	20–40			{27.5%}	{72.5%}[g]					
ADAMANTINOMA (n11){n5}	7:5	11–50[h]								{100.0%}[i]	

Chondrosarcoma: [a]central type, which accounts for 91.7% of chondrosarcoma in the series. Juxta articular type (3.5% of the series) is largely found on the femoral shaft; the mesenchymal from is also rare (4.8%) and may affect a wide range of bones but has a predilection for ribs and mandible.[71]

Giant cell tumour: [b]humerus 88.6% proximal; [c]radius 97.2% distal; [d]femur 85.6% distal; [e]tibia 87.3% proximal; [f]confined to the sacrum.

Chordoma: [g]spinal division: 53.8% sacral.

Adamantinoma: [h]male age range 31–50 years; female age range 11–30 years; [i]practically all cases in the tibia, but very rarely examples are found in ulna; femur; humerus; capitate; and first cuneiform.[71]

Table 8 – Factors influencing selected congenital conditions.

Congenital condition	Influencing factors	References
Congenital dislocation of the hip	Female bias; shallow acetabula; left side; joint laxity; first borns; breech delivery; winter births	14, 150
Cleft palate	Avitaminosis; mother subject to long periods on feet?; cranial morphology of parents; genetic influence	83, 84, 151, 152
Club foot	Genetic influence; seasonality (June conception) related to enterovirus	153, 154
Down's syndrome	Increased maternal age: early 20s: 1:1500; early 40s: 1:70; > 45: 1:25	155
Microcephaly	Malnutrition?	156
Osteogenesis imperfecta	Genetic influence: both dominant and recessive forms known	157
Osteo-onychodysplasia	Genetic influence	2

Table 9 – Clinical conditions with outwardly visible skeletal manifestations.

Condition	Skeletal manifestations	Source
Cleidocranial dysplasia	Imperfect cranial ossification; hypoplastic clavicles; slight stunting of growth; minor hand and feet anomalies	100, 2 (PAL)★
Congenital bowing	Bowing of long bones, especially the lower limbs	2
Dyschondrosteosis	Madelung deformity and mesomelic★★ dwarfism	158
Foetal alcohol syndrome	Microcephaly, hypoplastic maxilla, radio-ulnar synostosis	2
Frontometaphyseal dysplasia	Prominent supraorbital ridge; hypoplastic mandible; dysplasia of vertebral bodies and femoral heads; deformity of pelvis	2
Mesomelic dwarfism (Robinow's type)	Mesomelic dwarfism; hemivertebrae; costal fusion; bifid distal phalanges	2
Mesomelic dwarfism (Werner's type)	Mesomelic dwarfism; polydactyly; absence of thumbs	2
Osteo-onychodysplasia	Iliac horns; hypoplastic patellae (abnormal nails)	2, 24 (PAL)
Metachondromatosis	Exostoses of digits; metaphyseal and iliac enchondromata	2
Roberts' syndrome	Cleft palate and limb deficiencies	159
Schwarz-Lélek syndrome	Cranial hyperostosis; lateral bowing and metaphyseal widening of the femora	2
Spondyloepiphyseal dysplasia (SED)	Kyphoscoliosis; platyspondyly; dysplastic hip joints	2
Upington bone disease	Perthes disease of femoral heads; multiple enchondromata	2
Weismann-Netter-Stuhl syndrome	Anterior bowing of tibia and fibula 'sabre shin'; some cases: stunted stature and spinal deformities	2

★(PAL) palaeopathological reference.
★★Mesomelic: shortened lower arm and lower leg bones (rhizomelic: shortened upper arm and upper leg bones).

Table 10 – Clinical conditions with outwardly visible skeletal and internal radiological manifestations.

Condition	Skeletal manifestations	Source
Congenital syphilis	Bone infection: especially tibiae, cranium, and facial bones; dental defects (Turner teeth; mulberry molars); *Wimberger's Sign*, proximal tibiae	160, 161
Craniodiaphyseal dysplasia	Hyperostosis and *sclerosis* of skull and mandible; ribs and clavicles abnormally wide; *undermodelling* of tubular bones	2
Diaphyseal dysplasia	Thickened diaphyses; *narrowing of the medullary canal*	2
Endosteal hyperostosis	*Sclerosis of the calvarium; cranial base; mandible; endosteal thickening of the tubular bones*	2
Larsen syndrome	Dislocations; abnormal hand phalanges; supernumerary bones; *calcanei with secondary ossification centre*	162
Ollier's disease	Multiple enchondroma of digits; *radiological lucencies in metaphyses (especially the tibia)*	2
OS-CS	*Osteopathia striata; cranial sclerosis; scoliosis; fibulae aplasia*	163
Pycnodysostosis	Short stature; hypoplastic clavicles and distal phalanges; persistence of anterior fontanelle; misplaced teeth; *generalized sclerosis*	2
Pyle's disease (metaphyseal dysplasia)	Widening of the metaphyses especially distal femur and proximal humerus; *thinning of cortices*	2

Internal variation requiring radiography in *italics*.

The morphology of the borders of a tumour should permit differentiation between fast-growing malignant forms and slow-growing indolent and benign lesions. However, the situation may be confused when a benign lesion develops malignant tendencies.[56] The morphology and location of the lesions are of fundamental importance in reaching a reliable diagnosis.[103–105] Ideally, histological examination of neoplastic bone should be undertaken. However, problems of bone degradation, the cost and difficulty of obtaining access to the equipment mean that, at the moment, it is an unattainable luxury for most osteoarchaeologists.

It is essential to define the criteria on which a diagnosis is being made. The study of meningioma illustrates this point. In clinical practise, meningioma affects 20 people per million, making it the second most common brain tumour[70,87] (glioma being the most common). In British archaeological material, until recently, only two cases of meningioma had been reported.[10,56] Based on an estimated sample of 20 000 archaeological crania, this is an incidence of 100 per million, five times greater than the present-day figure. Both archaeological cases involved external hyperostosis, which is reported to occur in only 20–25% of modern day intracranial meningiomas.[106–108] As such, the true incidence of archaeological meningiomas, including those without external alteration, may be in the region of 400–500 per million: 200–250 times greater than modern-day figures.

Based solely on internal changes, enlarged vascular channels and smooth cystic cavitation, Campillo recorded five cases of suspected meningiomata from 3000 Spanish archaeological crania, an incidence some 85 times greater than found in clinical practise.[109] Again based on endocranial alterations, Waldron has published three cases from a medieval/post-medieval site in Hertfordshire,[70] which equates with a figure 900 times greater than found in modern material.

What is causing this variation? Is there some exogenous factor in earlier Hertfordshire causing this cluster of brain tumours? It is more likely that we are dealing with variation in data collection and presentation. When post-mortem figures are taken into account, meningiomata are the most common modern day brain tumour.[110,111] In other words the true incidence of meningiomas in modern populations is under-represented, as many are asymptomatic. Possibly the minor vascular variations reported by Campillo[109] and Waldron[70] represent asymptomatic meningiomas. This may solve the discrepancy in figures but it leaves us with an intriguing problem. If the individuals concerned were unaffected by the meningiomatous changes and carried on their daily lives as normal how meaningful is it to say they were *suffering* from a brain tumour? This is certainly an area that requires further consideration. The author believes it may be better to record the endocranial findings as vascular abnormalities and indicate that they *may* represent asymptomatic meningiomata. Similar vascular variation in the greater wing of a sphenoid bone has been published as a possible but uncertain meningioma.[112]

It would be possible to record sites in which endocranial vascular variation occurred. Only crania that were incomplete, damaged or broken could be examined internally. Therefore, it would be necessary to record the lesions as a percentage of available observations (number of damaged crania). A cluster may be related to those sites in which there are a large number of broken crania. That is to say, any cluster may be directly related to:

- High density of burials, with intercutting and damaged crania, i.e. medieval and post-medieval urban sites.
- Geology: heavy clay soil making it difficult to lift crania intact.
- Level of funding and speed at which site is excavated: stripping sites with machine may lead to damage of the upper levels of the cemetery, i.e. a tendency for large-scale medieval and post-medieval urban cemeteries to be involved.
- Sites in which there has been a great deal of disturbance, with foundations and service trenches cutting into deposits, i.e. urban cemeteries.

VARIATION BETWEEN ARCHAEOLOGICAL AND MODERN DAY FREQUENCIES OF CONGENITAL CONDITIONS AND NEOPLASTIC DISEASE

We must consider if the level of congenital conditions and neoplastic disease has changed significantly between archaeological samples and modern day Britain. Furthermore, can we identify significant variations between earlier British societies?

One problem is that archaeological and clinical data are not directly comparable. The archaeological data will identify cases in which there are external bone changes, and generally diseases without osseous involvement or only internal alteration will not be recognized. For example, there are no known British archaeological cases of osteopathia striata or osteopoikilosis, both of which present only internal bone changes.[2] In the clinical data, with the exception of incidental findings, only cases that give rise to symptoms will be identified.

In the absence of a database with information on numbers of individual skeletal elements, divided by period as well as by age and sex, it is not possible to provide any precise archaeological disease frequencies. However, based on various unpublished sources, it appears that about 50 000 inhumations have been excavated in living memory. Not all of these have been examined, only a small percentage are written up and even fewer are published. Also, not all of these skeletons would be complete.

At the moment, therefore, it is rather premature to compare archaeological and modern day frequencies. However, as an experiment, it is suggested that we base our approximate figures on an archaeological population sample of between 25 000 and 50 000. From this, we can present archaeological disease frequencies as number of individuals affected per million. It appears that congenital conditions are much more frequent in the modern population, although an exception to this is diaphyseal aclasia (Table 11).

It *appears* that neoplastic disease was much less frequent in earlier societies (Tables 2–5). However, the situation is complicated by various factors. Primary bone tumours are extremely rare, accounting for only 0.04% of all deaths in England and Wales in 1993.[113] If we assume that about 20% of the available skeletal sample died before adolescence, we have a 'population' of about 40 000 at risk from primary tumours. If the archaeological frequency of deaths from primary bone tumours is identical to the modern (1993) rate we should expect 16 cases. Admittedly, this is slightly higher than our figures. However, many cases may remain unpublished or unidentified. As such, it appears that the frequency of primary bone tumours has not altered greatly over the centuries.

Table 11 – Frequency of archaeological and modern day congenital conditions.

Congenital condition	Archaeological (frequency per million)	Modern (frequency per million)	Modern source
Arthrogryposis multiplex congenita	20–40	18	164
Congenital dislocation of the hip	120–240	1000	14
Cleft palate	60–120	765	84
Club foot	20–40	1000	100
Down's syndrome (mongolism)	40–80	670*	165
Hemivertebrae	40–80	?	
Hydrocephaly	80–160	400	166
Microcephaly	20–40	?	
Osteochondromatosis (diaphyseal aclasia)	60–120	20	167
Osteogenesis imperfecta	20–40	25	100
Osteo-onychodysplasia (Fong's syndrome)	60–120	100	2
Spondylo-epiphyseal dysplasia	20–40	?	

*There is a clear link between Down's syndrome and maternal age. As such, the lower archaeological frequency is not surprising.

Metastatic lesions present in the older age groups, i.e. those > 45 years. In urban archaeo-logical samples, the majority of individuals (perhaps 90%) were dying younger than this. If this is correct, only about 2000 individuals were at risk from secondary carcinoma. Also, based on skeletal material, we can only identify tumours that metastasize to bone.[114] The highest frequencies of metastatic bone involvement occur in prostatic (33–85%) and mammary (47–85%) carcinoma.[115] Other primary foci are much less likely to metastasize to bone.[50,115] In archaeological material the frequencies of bone involvement were probably lower due to the lack of surgical treatment, radiotherapy and chemotherapy that permit modern day patients to live longer.

Data from the late Victorian period indicate that death rate from cancer was 758 per million.[113] Based on a sample of about 50 000 skeletons, if the death rates had remained unchanged, we should expect 38 cases of fatal cancer in the archaeological record. We have located 15 malignant tumours (Tables 2 and 4). However, several examples may still remain unpublished or undiscovered. Also, if 50–70% of the cases did not involve bone metastases they would not be diagnosed, leaving us with 11–19 cases available for recognition in skeletal remains. It appears that the frequency of neoplastic disease and malignant tumours may not be so different to that found in modern populations. The apparent rarity is based on the fact that, in population terms, we are dealing with small samples.

About 80% of congenital conditions and 65% of neoplastic diseases occur during the Anglo-Saxon and medieval periods (Tables 1–5). This apparent bias may be related to the fact that about two-thirds of securely dated skeletal material comes from these two periods.

ARCHAEOLOGICAL AND DOCUMENTARY EVIDENCE

One area that appears to be largely overlooked is how contemporaries regarded the deceased person. We may recognize from the skeleton that a person was suffering from a congenital condition or a form of neoplasia, but how did this affect his/her relationship with society, friends and relatives? The burial environment is the only direct link between ourselves and the individuals that were responsible for the interment of the deceased. We may glean clues to how a person was regarded during life by the way that they were treated in death.

Today, congenital diseases are feared but are generally understood. In earlier societies the situation was quite different. Ambroise Paré, a French surgeon, writing in 1570, thought that monsters, including congenital deformities of human beings, could be caused by:

God's Glory or His Wrath

Too much or insufficient seed

Imagination

Narrowness of the womb

Indecent posture of the mother during pregnancy

Injury to the womb, a fall or by blows

Hereditary or accidental illness

Rotten or corrupt seed

Mixture or mingling of the seed

Artifice of wicked spital beggars

Through Demons and Devils.[116]

A condition which today would be recognized as anencephaly, a severe neural tube defect, in part related to diet, was formerly described by outward appearance as a human with a frog's face.[116] Up to this century, the mother's imagination, maternal impressions, was considered to affect the form of a newborn child. It was suggested that Mrs Merrick had been knocked over and scared by a circus elephant while pregnant with her son, Joseph and this resulted in his terrible deformities, which earned him the epithet 'the elephant man'.[117]

Based on British 16th-century documentary and illustrative material, we know that congenital conditions were regarded as the work of God.[118] Recent work has identified several individuals with congenital conditions that have not previously been recognized in British skeletal material[44,119–122] (Figure 6). Of course, it is possible that these and similar cases, regarded as the wrath of God, were denied burial in consecrated ground, and as such may well be lost to the archaeological record (see, for example, Pliny's comments on infants

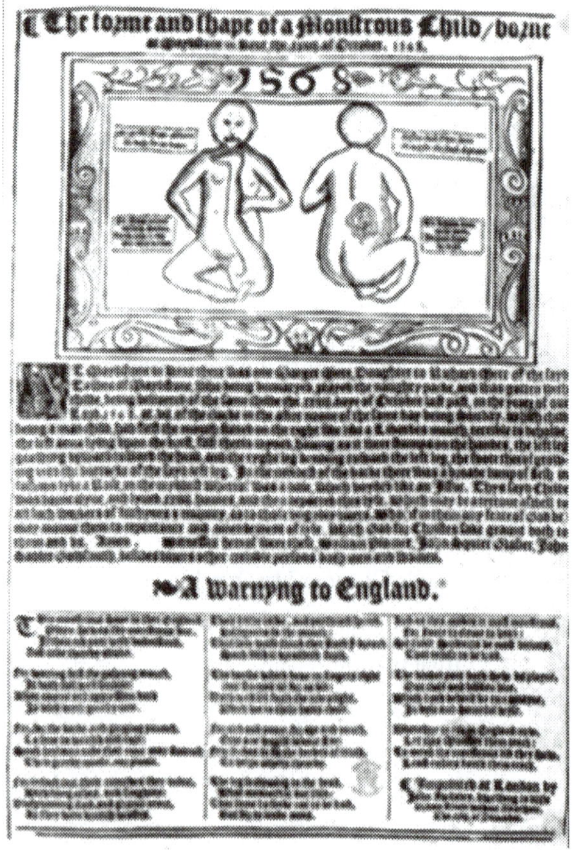

Figure 6 – Documentary and illustrative evidence for cleft lip and spina bifida cystica, possible clubfoot and congenital dislocation of the knee from Maidstone, Kent (1568). '*A Warnyng to England*' indicates that the 'monstrous childe' was a punishment for the immorality of the unmarried mother. The fact that these congenital conditions were thought to be the work of God suggests that similar cases would not receive burial within a cemetery and may be missing from the archaeological record. Huth Collection 50(38) by permission of the British Library.

with congenital deformities[123]). In addition, extreme poverty may have persuaded parents to bury neonates within their own homes to avoid cemetery fees.[124]

There is no evidence that those suffering from neoplastic diseases were excluded from cemetery burial. Old English texts contain the word *cancer* but it appears to refer to any form of ulceration, perhaps translating better as canker.[125] However, the '*ulcus cancri*', which debilitates and finally kills a nun may be a malignancy.[125] If so, it would be tempting to consider mammary carcinoma, the most common fatal cancer in females today.[86]

There is documentary evidence concerning herbs and plants that were believed beneficial in the treatment of various conditions.[126–129] For instance, Discorides, writing in the first century AD, advocated the use of squirting cucumber (*Ecballium elaterium*). The latter was used up until 1958 to treat sarcoma.[128] However, very little environmental work has been carried out to prove which medicinal plants were being used to treat patients.[130–133] As yet, we have not combined osteological evidence (specific disease in an individual) with environmental evidence from the grave (pollen/seeds/plant remains) to investigate if treatment was provided.

Osteologist and archaeologist may not be working in the same office. However, it should be possible for them to communicate and to exchange ideas and suggestions, ideally before the excavation or *at least* long before the final report is written. Factors which osteologists might consider for a particular burial in order to decide if it has received any atypical treatment, include:

The grave:
- Location: outside a cemetery; peripheral to the cemetery.
- Orientation.
- Size: depth; width; length.
- Coffin/uncoffined; coffin type.
- Grave fill: large stones over body to stop body rising?, quicklime?

The body:
- Position: prone/supine; extended; flexed; crouched.
- Treatment: embalming?
- Grave goods: consider the position of the finds as well as the inventory of artefacts.

Environmental evidence:
- Diet.
- Treatment: medicinal herbs.

CONCLUSION

The current evidence and its presentation only permits us to say that certain congenital conditions and neoplastic diseases have been identified from various sites and periods. Ideally, we should create a database of congenital conditions and neoplastic disease. Only then will we assess prevalence by skeleton and individual bone, as well as identify possible geographical, chronological or environmental variation for these conditions.

It is important for osteologists to be aware of clinical studies, since they provide information on classification, incidence, typical presentations and aetiologies. Future work should address the fact that various skeletal anomalies, which appear to be unrelated, may equate with well-known clinical syndromes. It is more likely that we are dealing with a disease or an atypical manifestation of a known condition than to argue that the skeletal changes represent a totally unknown condition.

It is essential to define the criteria on which a diagnosis is being made. However, when based on dry bone material, which can be weakened by the pathology and possibly compromised by post-mortem damage, we must be aware of the limitations and precision of our diagnoses. As such, the publication of *Problematica* is to be welcomed.

We should consider whether the level of congenital conditions and neoplastic disease has altered significantly between archaeological samples and modern day Britain. Also, is it possible to identify significant variations between earlier British societies? Examination of our admittedly incomplete data suggests that congenital conditions (with the exception of diaphyseal aclasia) are more frequent in modern Britain. Also, neoplastic diseases are rarely encountered in archaeological material. However, archaeological samples are relatively small as the majority of secondary tumours occur in the elderly and only those that lead to bone involvement will be recognized. Our preliminary work suggests the possibility that there may not be great variation between modern and archaeological frequencies of neoplasia.

The study of the burial environment in which pathological bones have been found is an area that has been largely overlooked by osteologists. Is there any evidence for an atypical treatment of the deceased that might provide clues for how they were regarded by their contemporaries? Also, a wide range of minor skeletal anomalies, some of which are known to be hereditary, may provide clues for genetic links either spatially or chronologically.

Although congenital abnormalities and neoplastic disease account for a small percentage of palaeopathological conditions, careful study of all British cases has the potential to reveal a great deal about how our ancestors lived and died.

ACKNOWLEDGEMENTS

I thank the Canterbury Archaeological Society for £400 towards costs and expenses in the preparation of this chapter. Photographs were provided by Andrew Savage, Canterbury Archaeological Trust, and the original CT scan (Figure 5) was provided by Kent and Canterbury Hospital. I also thank Mrs Sue Cover and staff at the Postgraduate Medical Centre Library for obtaining numerous inter-library loans with marked efficiency.

REFERENCES

1   James DK, Steer PJ, Weiner CP, Gonik B. *High Risk Pregnancy Management Options*. London: WB Saunders, 1994.

2   Beighton P. *Inherited Disorders of the Skeleton* (2nd edn). Edinburgh: Churchill Livingstone, 1988.

3   Ahsan H, Neugut AI, Gammon MD. Association of adenocarcinoma and squamous cell carcinoma of the oesophagus with tobacco-related malignancies. *Cancer, Epidemiology, Biomarkers and Prevention* 1998; **6**: 779–782.

4   Kjaerheim K, Gaard M, Andersen A. The role of alcohol, tobacco and dietary factors in upper aerogastric cancers: a prospective study of 1099 Norwegian men. *Cancer Causes and Control* 1998; **9**: 99–108 .

5   Raffle PAB, Lee WR, McCallum RI, Murray R. *Hunter's Diseases of the Occupations* (6th edn). London: Hodder & Stoughton, 1978.

6   Raven RW. *The Theory and Practice of Oncology.* Carnforth: Parthenon, 1990.

7   Anderson T, Andrews J. The human skeletons. In: Hicks M, Hicks A. *The Priory of St Gregory's Priory, Canterbury* (in press).

8   Waldron T. *Counting the Dead: The Epidemiology of Skeletal Populations.* Chichester: John Wiley, 1994.

9   Brothwell D. The palaeopathology of early British man: an essay of the problems and diagnosis and analysis. *Journal of the Royal Anthropological Institute* 1961; **91**: 318–344.

10 Brothwell D. The evidence for neoplasms. In: Brothwell D, Sandison AT (eds), *Diseases in Antiquity.* Springfield: Charles C Thomas, 1967: pp. 320–345.

11 Chamberlain AT, Rogers S, Romanowski CA. Osteochondroma in a British Neolithic skeleton. *British Journal of Hospital Medicine* 1992; **47**: 51–53.

12 Capasso L. Osteoma: palaeopathology and phylogeny. *International Journal of Osteoarchaeology* 1997; **7**: 615–620.

13 Birkett D. Osteochondroma (cartilaginous exostosis). In: Bellard FG, Sanchez JA (eds), *Proceedings of the 6th European Meeting of the Paleopathological Association.* Madrid, 1986: pp. 321–323.

14 Kelsey JL. *Epidemiology of Muscoskeletal Disorders.* Oxford: Oxford University Press, 1982.

15 Brothwell D. Major congenital anomalies of the skeleton. In: Brothwell D, Sandison AT (eds), *Diseases in Antiquity.* Springfield: Charles C Thomas, 1967: pp. 423–443.

16 Huggins PJ. Excavations of Belgic and Romano-British farm with middle Saxon cemetery and churches at Nazeingbury, Essex. *Essex Archaeology and History* 1978; **10**: 29–117.

17 Manchester K. Hydrocephalus in an Anglo-Saxon child from Eccles. *Archaeologia Cantiana* 1980; **96**: 77–82.

18 Murphy E. A possible case of hydrocephalus in a medieval child from Doonbought Fort, Co. Antrim, Northern Ireland. *International Journal of Osteoarchaeology* 1996; **6**: 435–442.

19 Bamforth SJ, Baird PA. Spina bifida and hydrocephalus: a population study over a 35 year period. *American Journal of Human Genetics* 1989; **44**: 225–232.

20 Boddington A. *Raunds Furnells The Anglo-Saxon Church and Churchyard.* Archaeological Report 7. London: English Heritage, 1996.

21 Brothwell DR. *Digging Up Bones* (2nd edn). London: British Museum Natural History, 1972.

22 Anderson T. An archaeological example of cleft lip and palate from medieval Canterbury, Kent, England. *The Cleft Palate-Craniofacial Journal* 1994; **31**: 466–472.

23 Vrebos J. Cleft lip surgery in Anglo-Saxon Britain: The *Leech Book* (circa AD 920). *Plastic and Reconstructive Surgery* 1986; **77**: 850–853.

24 Anderson T. Bars of bone on hip bones in antiquity. A differential diagnosis: osteo-onychodysplasia (Fong's Syndrome). *Human Evolution* 1993; **8**: 291–292.

25 O'Rahilly R. A survey of carpal and tarsal anomalies. *Journal of Bone and Joint Surgery* 1953; **35A**: 626–642.

26 Sarrafian SK. *Anatomy of the Foot and Ankle.* Philadelphia: JB Lipincott, 1983.

27 Barnes CL, Frazier GT, Hixson ML. Bilateral congenital fusion of the scaphoid and trapezium in identical twins. *Orthopedics* 1992; **15**: 739–741.

28 Boyd HB. Congenital talonavicular synostosis. *Journal of Bone and Joint Surgery* 1944; **26**: 682–686.

29 Case DT, Ossenberg NS, Burnett SE. Os intermetatarseum: a heritable accessory bone of the human foot. *American Journal of Physical Anthropology* 1998; **107**: 199–209.

30 Challis J. Hereditary transmission of talonavicular coalition in association with anomaly of the little finger. *Journal of Bone and Joint Surgery* 1974; **56A**: 1273–1276.

31 Glessner JR, Davis GL. Bilateral calcaneonavicular coalition occurring in twin boys. *Clinical Orthopaedics and Related Research* 1966; **47**: 173–176.

32 Leonard MA. The inheritance of tarsal coalition and its relationship to spastic flat foot. *Journal of Bone and Joint Surgery* 1974; **56B**: 520–526.

33   Regan MH, Case DT, Brundige JC. Articular surface defects in the third metatarsal and third cuneiform: nonosseous tarsal coalition. *American Journal of Physical Anthropology* 1999; **109**: 53–65 .

34   Rothberg AS, Feldman JW, Schuster OF. Congenital fusion of astragalus and scaphoid: bilateral; inherited. *New York State Journal of Medicine* 1935; **35**: 29–31.

35   Webster FS, Roberts WM. Tarsal anomalies and peroneal spastic flat foot. *Journal of the American Medical Association* 1951; **146**: 1099–1104.

36   Wray JB, Herndon CN. Hereditary transmission of congenital coalition of the calcaneus to the navicular. *Journal of Bone and Joint Surgery* 1963; **45A**: 365–372.

37   Zeide MS, Weisel SW, Terry RL. Talo navicular coalition. *Clinical Orthopaedics and Related Research* 1977; **126**: 225–227.

38   Austin FH. Symphalangism and related fusions of the tarsal bones. *Radiology* 1951; **56**: 882–885.

39   Castle JE, Bass S, Kanat IO. Hereditary symphalangism with associated tarsal synostosis and hypophalangism. *Journal of the American Podiatric Medical Association* 1993; **83**: 1–9.

40   Geelhoed GW, Neel JV, Davidson RT. Symphalangism and tarsal coalitions: a hereditary syndrome. *Journal of Bone and Joint Surgery* 1969; **51B**: 278–289.

41   Harle TS, Stevenson JR. Hereditary symphalangism associated with carpal and tarsal fusions. *Radiology* 1967; **89**: 91–94.

42   Drinkwater H. Phalangeal enarthrosis (synostosis, ankylosis) transmitted through fourteen generations. *Proceedings of the Royal Society of Medicine* 1917; **10**: 60–68.

43   Harman M. The human remains. In: Down A, Welch M. *Chichester Excavations VII. Apple Down and the Mardens.* Chichester: Chichester District Council, 1990: pp. 183–213.

44   Anderson T. Palaeopathology: more than just dry bones. *Proceedings of the Royal College of Physicians of Edinburgh* 1994; **24**: 554–580.

45   Cardy A. The human bones. In: Hill P. *Whithorn and St Ninian The Excavation of a Monastic Town 1984–1991.* Stroud: Sutton, 1998: pp. 519–562.

46   Lepore L, Pagliuca S, Francobandiera C. Os tibiale externum: etiopathogenesis, cases, clinical aspect and treatment. *La Chirurgia Degli Organi do Movimento* 1990; **75**: 307–310.

47   Pierre-Jerome C, Bekkelund SI, Husby G, Mellgren SI, Osteaux M, Nordstrom R. MRI Anatomical variants of the wrist in women. *Surgical and Radiologic Anatomy* 1996; **18**: 37–41.

48   Anderson T. The human skeletal material. In: Chapman A. *Excavations at Brackmills, Northampton.* Northampton: Northampton Archaeological Unit (forthcoming).

49   Chapman A. Brackmills, Northampton. *Current Archaeology* 1998; **159**: 92–95.

50   Willis RA. *The Spread of Tumours in the Human Body* (3rd edn). London: Butterworths, 1973.

51   Anderson T, Wakely J, Carter A. Medieval example of metastatic carcinoma: A dry bone, radiological and SEM study. *American Journal of Physical Anthropology* 1992; **89**: 309–323.

52   Manchester K. Secondary cancer in an Anglo-Saxon female. *Journal of Archaeological Science* 1983; **10**: 475–482.

53   Mays S. Strouhal E, Vyhnánek L, Němečková A. A case of metastatic carcinoma of medieval date from Wharram Percy, England. *Journal of Paleopathology* 1996; **8**: 33–42.

54   Ortner DJ, Manchester K, Lee F. Metastatic carcinoma in a leper skeleton from a medieval cemetery in Chichester, England. *International Journal of Osteoarchaeology* 1991; **1**: 91–98.

55   Wakely, J, Anderson T, Carter A. A multidisciplinary case study of prostatic(?) carcinoma from medieval Canterbury. *Journal of Archaeological Science* 1995; **22**: 469–77.

56   Anderson T. A medieval example of meningiomatous hyperostosis. *British Journal of Neurosurgery* 1991; **1**: 499–504.

57   Anderson T. An example of meningiomatous hyperostosis from medieval Rochester. *Medical History* 1992; **36**: 207–213.

58   Anderson T. A medieval example of meningiomatous hyperostosis. *Journal of Paleopathology* 1993; **4**: 141–154.

59   Stroud G, Kemp RL. *Cemeteries of the Church and Priory of St Andrew, Fishergate.* York: York Archaeological Trust 12/2, 1993.

60   Wells C. Two medieval cases of malignant disease. *British Medical Journal* 1964; **1**: 1611–1612.

61   Wakely J, Strouhal E, Vyhnánek L, Němečková A. Case of a malignant tumour from Abingdon, Oxfordshire, England. *Journal of Archaeological Science* 1998; **25**: 949–956.

62   Anderson T. A probable example of osteoma of the mandible from Northamptonshire, Great Britain. *Journal of Paleopathology* 1997; **9**: 69–72.

63   Anderson T, Carter A. The first archaeological evidence for Madelung deformity?. *International Journal of Osteoarchaeology* 1995; **5**: 168–173.

64   Cox M. *The Human Bones from West Heslerton North Yorkshire*. English Heritage Ancient Monuments Laboratory Report 112/90, 1990.

65   Wells C. Pathological Anglo-Saxon femur. *British Journal of Radiology* 1965; **38**: 393–394.

66   Carter AR, Anderson T. An archaeological example of enchondroma. *International Journal of Osteoarchaeology* 1996; **6**: 411–413.

67   Farwell DE, Molleson TI. *Excavations at Poundbury 1966–1980*, vol. **2**: *The Cemeteries*. Monograph Series No. 11. Dorset: Dorset Natural History and Archaeological Society, 1993.

68   Rothschild BM, Rothschild C. Comparison of radiologic and gross examination for detection of cancer in defleshed skeletons. *American Journal of Physical Anthropology* 1995; **96**: 357–363 .

69   Stead S.The human bones. In: Stead IM. *The Iron Age Cemeteries in East Yorkshire*. London: English Heritage, 1991.

70   Waldron T. An unusual cluster of meningiomas? *International Journal of Osteoarchaeology* 1998; **8**: 213–217.

71   Schajowicz F. *Tumors and Tumorlike Lesions of Bone and Joints*. New York: Springer, 1981.

72   Ragsdale BD. The irrelevance of contemporary orthopedic pathology to specimens from antiquity (continued). *Paleopathology Society Newsletter* 1997; **97**: 8–12.

73   Anderson T. Cleft neural arch and spinous process aplasia in the lower thoracic spine of a medieval skeleton. *Journal of Paleopathology* 1996; **8**: 57–59.

74   Anderson T, Thomas GT. Arthrogryposis multiplex congenita from medieval Canterbury. *International Journal of Osteoarchaeology* 1997; **7**: 181–185.

75   Brothwell DR. Congenital absence of the basi-occipital in a Romano-Briton. *Man* 1958; **58**: 73–74.

76   Brothwell DR. A possible case of mongolism in a Saxon population. *Annals of Human Genetics* 1960; **24**: 141–150.

77   Brothwell DR, Browne S. Pathology. In: Lilley JM, Stroud G, Brothwell DR, Williamson MH (eds), *The Jewish Burial Ground at Jewbury*. York: York Archaeological Trust 12/3, 1994: pp. 457–494.

78   Anderson T. Computerised tomographic investigation of a medieval frontal osteoma. *Journal of Paleopathology* (under review).

79   Brothwell D. Problematica I. Possible evidence of soft tissue neoplasm from All Saints Church, York. *Journal of Paleopathology* 1996; **8**: 121–123.

80   Duhig C, Strouhal E, Němečková A. Case of a secondary carcinoma of Anglo-Saxon period from Edix Hill, Barrington, Cambridgeshire, England. *Journal of Paleopathology* 1996; **8**: 25–31.

81   Waldron T. A nineteenth century case of carcinoma of the prostate, with a note on the early history of the disease. *International Journal of Osteoarchaeology* 1997; **1**: 241–247.

82   Leeds ET, Shortt H de S. *An Anglo-Saxon Cemetery at Petersfinger near Salisbury Wiltshire*. Salisbury: South Wiltshire and Blackmore Museum, 1953.

83   Hitchin AD. The aetiology of calcified composite odontomes. *British Dental Journal* 1971; **130**: 475–482.

84   Tolarovà M. Genetic findings in cleft lip and palate. In: Bardach J, Morris HL (eds), *Multidisciplinary Management of Cleft Lip and Palate*. Philadelphia: WB Saunders, 1990: pp. 113–121.

85   Glücksmann A. *Sexual Dimorphism in Human and Mammalian Biology and Pathology*. London: Academic Press, 1981.

86   Mould RF. *Cancer Statistics*. Bristol: Adam Hilger, 1983.

87   Preston-Martin S. Descriptive epidemiology of primary tumours of the brain, cranial nerves and cranial meninges in Los Angeles County. *Neuroepidemilogy* 1989; **8**: 283–295.

88   Mourant AE. *Blood Relations and Blood Groups and Anthropology*. Oxford: Oxford University Press, 1985.

89   Grupe G. Metastasizing carcinoma in a medieval skeleton: differential diagnosis and etiology. *American Journal of Physical Anthropology* 1988; **75**: 369–374.

90   Vesey MP, Gray M (eds), *Cancer Risks and Prevention*. Oxford: Oxford University Press 1985.

91   Fair WR, Fleshner NE, Heston W. Cancer of the prostate: a nutritional disease? *Urology* 1997; **50**: 840–848 .

92   Veierod MB, Laake P, Thelle DS. Dietary fat intake and risk of prostate cancer: a prospective study of 25,708 Norwegian men. *International Journal of Cancer* 1997; **73**: 634–638.

93   Gelberg KH, Fitzgerald EF, Hwang S, Dubrow R. Growth and development and other risk factors for osteosarcoma in children and young adults. *International Journal of Epidemiology* 1997; **26**: 272–278.

94   Lane JM, Hurson B, Boland PJ, Glasser DB. Osteogenic sarcoma. *Clinical Orthopaedics and Related Research* 1986; **204**: 93–110.

95   Barnes E. *Developmental Defects of the Axial Skeleton in Paleopthaology*. Niwot: University Press of Colorado, 1994.

96   Ortner DJ, Putschar WGJ. *Identification of Pathological Conditions in Human Skeletal Remains*. Washington, DC: Smithsonian Institution Press, 1985.

97   Steinbock RT. *Paleopathological Diagnosis and Interpretation. Bone Diseases in Ancient Human Populations*. Springfield: Charles C Thomas, 1976.

98   Dahlin DC. *Bone Tumors General Aspects and an Analysis of 2,276 Cases*. Springfield: Charles C Thomas, 1957.

99   Resnick D, Niwayama Gen. *Diagnosis of Bone and Joint Disorders*. Philadelphia: WB Saunders, 1981.

100 Tachdjian MO. *Pediatric Orthopedics*. Philadelphia: WB Saunders, 1972.

101 Coley BL. *Neoplasms of Bone*. New York: PB Hoeber, 1930.

102 Geschickter CF, Copeland MM. *Tumors of Bone* (3rd edn). Philadelphia: JB Lipincott, 1949.

103 Jacobsen HG, Popppel MH, Shapiro JH Grossberger S. The vertebral pedicle sign: a roentgen finding to differentiate metastatic carcinoma from multiple myeloma. *American Journal of Roentgenology* 1958; **80**: 817–821.

104 Ragsdale BD. Morphologic analysis of skeletal lesions: correlation of imaging studies and pathologic findings. *Advances in Pathology and Laboratory Medicine* 1993; **6**: 445–490.

105 Strouhal E. Myeloma multiplex versus osteolytic carcinoma: differential diagnosis in dry bones. *International Journal of Osteoarchaeology* 1991; **1**: 219–224.

106 Cushing H. The meningiomas (dural endotheliomas): their source, and favoured seats of origin. *Brain* 1922; **45**: 282–316.

107 Rowbotham GF. The hyperostoses in relation with the meningiomas. *British Journal of Surgery* 1939; **26**: 593–623.

108 Walton J (ed.), *Brain's Disease of the Nervous System*. Oxford: Oxford University Press, 1985.

109 Campillo D. The possibility of diagnosing meningiomas in palaeopathology. *International Journal of Osteoarchaeology* 1991; **1**: 225–230.

110 Nakasu S, Hirano A, Shimura T, Llena JF. Incidental meningiomas in autopsy study. *Surgical Neurology* 1987; **7**: 19–22.

111 Robbins SL, Cotran RS, Kumar V. *Pathological Basis of Disease* (3rd edn). Philadelphia: WB Saunders, 1984.

112 Anderson T. The human bones. In: Parfitt K (ed.), *The Iron Age Burials from Mill Hill, Deal, Kent*. London: British Museum Press, 1995: pp. 114–144.

113 Waldron T. What was the prevalence of malignant disease in the past? *International Journal of Osteoarchaeology* 1996; **6**: 463–470.

114 Tofe, AJ, Francis MD, Harvey, WJ. Correlation of neoplasms with incidence and localization of skeletal metastases. An analysis of 1355 diphosphonate bone scans. *Journal of Nuclear Medicine* 1975; **16**: 986–989.

115 Galasko CSB. *Skeletal Metastases*. London: Butterworths, 1986.

116 Pallister JL. *Ambroise Paré on Monsters and Marvels*. Chicago: Chicago University Press, 1982.

117 Howell M, Ford P. *The True History of the Elephant Man*. Harmondsworth: Penguin, 1980.

118   Wilson D. *Signs and Portents Monstrous Births from the Middle Ages to the Enlightenment*. London: Routledge, 1993.

119   Anderson T. Evidence of birth deformities in 16th century Kent. *British Medical Journal* 1994; **308**(6970): 1748.

120   Anderson T. Artistic and documentary evidence for tetradysmelia from sixteenth century England. *American Journal of Medical Genetics* 1994; **52**: 475–477.

121   Anderson T. The earliest evidence for arthrogryposis multiplex congenita or Larsen's syndrome. *American Journal of Medical Genetics* 1997; **71**: 127–129.

122   Anderson T. Documentary and artistic evidence for congenital conditions from sixteenth century England. *International Journal of Osteoarchaeology* 1997; **7**: 625–627.

123   Pliny, the Elder. *Natural History* [*Historia Naturalis*], 10 vols, with an English translation by WHS Jones. London: Heineman, 1963.

124   Anderson T, Parfitt K. Two unusual burials from medieval Dover. *International Journal of Osteoarchaeology* 1998; **8**: 123–124.

125   Thompson P. The disease that we call cancer. In: Campell S, Hall B, Klausner D (eds), *Health, Disease and Healing in Medieval Culture*. London: Macmillan, 1992: pp. 1–11.

126   Getz FM. *Healing and Society in Medieval England*. Madison: Wisconsin University Press, 1991.

127   Hunt T. *Popular Medicine in Thirteenth Century England*. Woodbridge: DS Brewer, 1990.

128   Riddle J. Ancient and medieval chemotherapy for cancer. *Isis* 1985; **76**: 319–330.

129   Voigts LE. Anglo-Saxon plant remedies and the Anglo-Saxons. *Isis* 1979; **70**: 250–268.

130   Moffat B. Investigations into medieval medical practise: the remnants of some herbal treatments on archaeological sites and archives. In: Deegan M, Scragg DG (eds), *Medicine in Early Medieval England*. Manchester: Manchester forum of Anglo Saxon Studies, 1979: pp. 33–40.

131   Moffat B (ed.), *The First Report on Researches into the Medieval Hospital at Soutra, Lothian Region*. SHARP, 1986.

132   Moffat B, Fulton J (eds), *The Second Report on Researches into the Medieval Hospital at Soutra, Lothian Region*. SHARP, 1988.

133   Moffat B, Thompson BS, Fulton J (eds), *The Third Report on Researches into the Medieval Hospital at Soutra, Lothian/Borders Region*. SHARP, 1989.

134   Wells C. Hip disease in ancient man. Report of three cases. *Journal of Bone and Joint Surgery* 1963; **45B**: 790–791.

135   Wakely J. Bilateral congenital dislocation of the hip, spina bifida occulta and spondylolysis in a female skeleton from the medieval cemetery at Abingdon, England. *Journal of Paleopathology* 1993; **5**: 37–45.

136   White WJ. *Skeletal Remains from the Cemetery of St Nicholas Shambles, City of London*. London: London and Middlesex Archaeological Society, 1988.

137   Wells C. Osteogenesis imperfecta from an Anglo-Saxon burial ground at Burgh Castle, Suffolk. *Medical History* 1965; **9**: 88–89.

138   Roberts C. Bars of bone on hip bones in antiquity: pathological, occupational or genetic?. *Human Evolution* 1987; **2**: 539–545.

139   Dingwall D. A barrow at Dunstable, Bedfordshire. Part II. The skeletal material. *The Archaeological Journal* 1932; **88**: 210–217.

140   Hawkes SC, Wells C. Absence of the left upper limb and pectoral girdle in an unique Anglo-Saxon burial. *Bulletin of the New York Academy of Medicine* 1976; **52**: 1229–1235.

141   Wakely J. Spondylo-epiphyseal dysplasia in a medieval skeleton from Oxfordshire. *Clinical Anatomy* (in press).

142   Anderson S. *Human Skeletal remains from Timberhill, Castle Mall, Norwich (excavated 1989–91)*. English Heritage Ancient Monuments Laboratory Report 73/96, 1996.

143   Molleson T, Cox M. *The Spitalfields Project*, vol. 2: *The Anthropology The Middling Sort*. Research Report 86. York: Council for British Archaeology, 1993.

144   Hacking P. A pituitary tumour in a medieval skull. *International Journal of Osteoarchaeology* 1995; **5**: 390–393.

145   Manchester K. Jugular vein occlusion in the Bronze Age. *Yorkshire Archaeological Journal* 1980; **52**: 167–169.

146   Ballantyne JW. The Biddenden Maids: the medieval pygopagus. *Teratologia* 1895; **2**: 268–274.

147   Bondeson J. The Biddenden Maids: a curious chapter in the history of conjoined twins. *Journal of the Royal Society of Medicine* 1992; **85**: 217–221.

148   Collman HL (ed.), *Ballads and Broadsides chiefly of the Elizabethan Period and printed in Black Letter Most of which were formerly in the Heber Collection and are now in the Library at Britwell Court Buckinghamshire.* Oxford: Roxburghe Club, 1872.

149   Huth H. *Ancient Ballads and Broadsides Published in England in the Sixteenth Century Chiefly in the Earlier Years of the Reign of Queen Elizabeth.* London: Whittingham & Wilkins, 1867.

150   Holck P. The occurrence of hip dislocation in early Lappic populations of Norway. *International Journal of Osteoarchaeology* 1991; **1**: 199–202.

151   Lin S, Gensburg L, Marshall EG, Roth GB, Dlugosz L. Effects of maternal work activity during pregnancy on infant malformations. *Journal of Occupational and Environmental Medicine* 1998; **40**: 829–34 .

152   Mossey PA, McColl J, O'Hara M. Cephalometric features in the parents of children with orofacial clefting. *British Journal of Oral and Maxillofacial Surgery* 1998; **36**: 202–212.

153   Lochmiller C, Johnston D, Scott A, Risman M, Hecht JT. Genetic epidemiology study of idiopathic talipes equinovarus. *American Journal of Medical Genetics* 1998; **79**: 90–96.

154   Robertson WW, Corbett D. Congenital club foot. Month of conception. *Clinical Orthopaedics and Related Research* 1997; **338**: 14–18.

155   Winchester AM, Mertens TR. *Human Genetics (*4th edn). Columbus: Charles E Merrill, 1983.

156   Skull SA, Ruben AR, Darwin, NT. Malnutrition and microcephaly in Australian aboriginal children. *Medical Journal of Australia* 1997; **166**: 412–414.

157   Smith R, Francis MJO, Houghton GR. *The Brittle Bone Syndrome Osteogenesis Imperfecta.* London: Butterworths, 1983.

158   Carter AR, Currey HLF. Dyschondrosteosis (mesomelic dwarfism) – a family study. *British Journal of Radiology* 1974; **47**: 634–640.

159   Roberts JB. A child with double cleft lip and palate, protrusion of the intermaxillary portion of the upper jaw and imperfect development of the bones of the four extremities. *Annals of Surgery* 1919; **70**: 252.

160   Hackett CJ. *Diagnostic Criteria of Syphilis, Yaws and Treponarid (Treponematoses) and of some other Diseases in Dry Bones.* Berlin: Springer, 1976.

161   Hillson S, Grigson C, Bond S. Dental defects of congenital syphilis. *American Journal of Physical Anthropology* 1998; **107**: 25–40.

162   Larsen LJ, Schottstaedt ER, Bost FD. Multiple congenital dislocations associated with a characteristic facial abnormality. *Journal of Pediatrics* 1950; **37**: 574–581.

163   Pellegrino JE, McDonald-McGinn DM, Schneider A, Markowitz RI, Zackai EH. Further clinical delineation and increased morbidity in males with osteopathia striata with cranial sclerosis: an X-linked disorder? *American Journal of Medical Genetics* 1997; **70**: 159–65 .

164   Wynne-Davis R, Lloyd-Roberts GL. Arthrogryposis multiplex congenital search for prenatal factors in 66 sporadic cases. *Archives of Disease in Childhood* 1976; **51**: 618–623.

165   Steele J, Stratford B. The United Kingdom population with Down syndrome: present and future projections. *American Journal of Mental Retardation* 1995; **99**: 664–682.

166   Schrander-Stumpel C, Fryns JP. Congenital hydrocephalus: nosology and guidelines for clinical approach and genetic counselling. *European Journal of Pediatrics* 1998; **157**: 355–362.

167   Schmale GA, Conrad EU, Raskind WH. The natural history of hereditary multiple exostoses. *Journal of Bone and Joint Surgery* 1994; **76A**: 986–992.

14

DENTAL HEALTH IN BRITISH ANTIQUITY

Chrissie Freeth

INTRODUCTION

The aim of this chapter is to highlight recent areas of research concerning dental disease in archaeology. Dental diseases are among the most commonly seen pathological conditions in archaeological remains and can potentially provide a great deal of information. For example, they can tell us about subsistence strategy and about the content, texture and preparation of diet. They may provide information about oral hygiene and dentistry practises, or the lack of them, the use of teeth as a third hand or as a tool, and therefore occupation, and also about the general health and stress of a population under study.

The dental diseases are a complex, interrelated, multifactorial series of conditions that affect the teeth and surrounding tissues. The manifestations of these disorders are limited, the most commonly seen archaeologically being dental calculus, periodontal disease, caries, abscess, ante-mortem tooth loss and enamel hypoplasia. Although wear is due to a mechanical rather than disease process, it is included in this review as it is a commonly observed and reported condition and may affect the prevalence of the diseases.

This overview of the study of dental health in antiquity aims to illustrate the types of dental problems that may be seen in human remains and to consider how such evidence has been interpreted and used to contribute to the archaeology of the people of the past. Following this review, some of the problems faced by researchers of dental diseases will be discussed and ways forward for future research proposed.

ARCHAEOLOGICAL EVIDENCE FOR DENTAL DISEASE

Calculus

Dental plaque, a matrix that adheres to teeth and houses microorganisms, may, if mineralized, form calculus deposits (Figure 1). Calculus may occur on any surface of the tooth, including the roots should they become exposed. Two forms can be identified: supragingival calculus, which forms above the gum, and subgingival calculus, which forms below it. These two forms can be distinguished by the amount of the deposit (subgingival calculus is

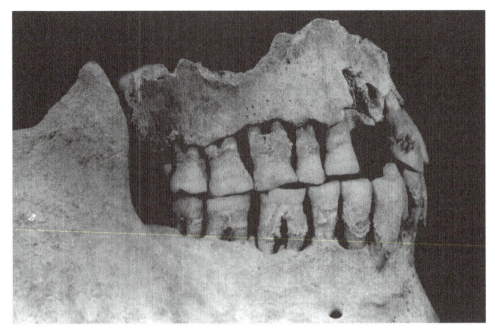

Figure 1 – Mandible and maxilla with periodontal disease and calculus deposits.

thinner) and colour (subgingival calculus is green or black whereas supragingival deposits are grey or brown).[1] Unfortunately calculus deposits are very fragile and can be easily broken off during excavation and subsequent processing. This has obvious consequences when trying to record its presence.

Periodontal disease

Periodontal disease can be recognized as exposure of the roots caused by the resorption of the alveolar bone (Figure 1). The form of such bone loss may be seen as trenches, dehiscences and fenestrations and it is important to record which form is being observed.[2] However, periodontal disease is not the only cause of root exposure. Continuing eruption (super-eruption) allows the occlusal surface to remain at a particular height during life as teeth wear down,[3] the result of which is exposure of the roots. Another factor to take into account is the phenomenon of hypercementosis caused by the deposition of excessive cement at the root tip.[2] Because of these additional factors, it is probable that periodontal disease is over-reported in archaeological publications. A further problem in the study of periodontal disease is that its diagnosis is hampered by damage to the bone around the teeth, which may prevent it from being recorded and even be mistaken for periodontal disease by inexperienced workers.

Continuing eruption

The phenomenon of continuing eruption has been reported by Whittaker *et al.*[4,5] who examined remains from a Romano-British cemetery at Poundbury Camp in Dorset.

Although they found it to be associated with occlusal wear, a later study by Whittaker *et al.*[6] of the skeletal remains retrieved from the crypt of Christ Church, Spitalfields, London, showed that continuing eruption will occur even if no wear is present and that during life, facial height may increase by as much as 5 mm. Evidence of wear-induced continuing eruption has also been reported in pre-industrial Irish remains.[7] Kerr and Ringrose[8] argued that continuing eruption was a major and underestimated factor in ante-mortem tooth loss before the 17th century AD, when levels of tooth wear decreased. Kerr[9] then argued that because of continuing eruption and the subsequent lack of bony support and exposure of the fork of the molar roots, the use of instruments (such as the 'Key' and 'Pelican') to extract teeth would have been quite effective. However, this procedure would have been more painful when the rate of continuing eruption decreased and this, he argues, was the trigger for an improvement of techniques, and the transformation of dentistry from a trade to a profession.

Caries

Dental caries (Figure 2) is one of the most common oral pathological conditions seen clinically[10] and is one of the most commonly seen and reported in archaeological remains.[1] Caries is caused by the acids secreted by microorganisms after digesting carbohydrates such as sugar and starch. These microorganisms are housed in plaque, so wherever plaque accumulates caries may develop.

An example of the value of caries in archaeological investigations is its use as an indicator of a change in diet and subsistence strategy. Larsen[11] found an increase in caries when a North

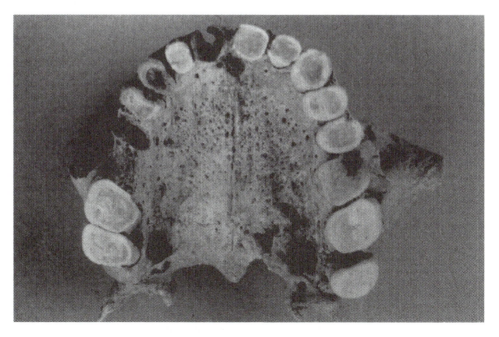

Figure 2 – Maxillary dentition with caries and pulp exposure, tooth wear, ante-mortem loss of the right first molar and post-mortem loss of right central incisor and second premolar.

American population moved from a hunter-gathering and fishing economy, to one with a greater dependency on maize agriculture. Lukacs[12] also found an increase in caries in a population from Bronze Age Pakistan as they increased their dependence in agriculture. A study of two populations in Nubia by Beckett and Lovell[13] showed that, although both populations practised a mixed subsistence strategy, an increase in caries in the later period could be interpreted as evidence of a greater dependency on agricultural produce. A decrease in caries was found by Walker and Erlandson[14] as a population from Santa Rosa Island, California, became less dependent on plant foods and more dependent on fish as the staple in the diet.

In the 1970s Moore and Corbett produced a series of four papers[15–18] that traced the prevalence of dental caries in British remains from the Iron Age to the 19th century AD. They found that there was little statistically significant change in the prevalence and location of caries during the Iron Age to medieval periods. Investigations of dentition from medieval Scotland have shown a similar pattern in the location of caries, but a lower prevalence rate than in England.[19–21] They found that in the 17th century AD the prevalence increased and the occlusal surface and contact points between neighbouring teeth became the most common location for caries to develop.[17] Before the 17th century the cemento-enamel junction (CEJ), was the most common area attacked. The increase in prevalence was attributed to the increased availability of cane sugar.[17] The change in location was attributed to the introduction of refined flour that softened the diet, caused less tooth wear and allowed plaque to accumulate between the teeth and in the fissures of the occlusal surfaces. The decrease in wear, and therefore continuing eruption, would also prevent the CEJ from becoming as exposed as in previous centuries; this may also help to explain why the CEJ became a less common location for carious lesions as well as changes in the prevalence of root exposure caused by periodontal disease.

Caries is best observed macroscopically, with good lighting and supplemented as necessary with some form of magnification. Rudney et al.[22] suggested that visual examination is a more reliable method than the use of X-rays and had a lower rate of inter-observer error. Caries that has not yet broken down the enamel may appear as white opaque spots, and arrested caries as brown spots due to staining. However, in archaeological remains only those caries that have produced a cavity are usually recorded; therefore, the true prevalence of caries is probably underestimated. This is compounded by the fact that teeth lost ante-mortem may well have been lost because of carious destruction. Various attempts have been made to correct for this and Lukacs'[23] caries correction factor is an example. However, it assumes that caries and wear induced pulp exposure were the main causes of tooth loss. If Kerr and Ringrose's[8] theories on continuing eruption as a major culprit are correct then the use of the correction factor is a less valid approach to determine the true prevalence of carious teeth. However, as caries may infect adjacent tooth surfaces, teeth lost due to caries may be indicated by adjacent incipient caries that have become arrested due to the loss of the adjacent tooth and subsequent exposure to saliva and plaque removal. Work is needed to determine if this approach is feasible for helping to estimate the caries frequencies.

Periapical lesions

Some defence mechanisms can be initiated in the dentine to protect the pulp cavity from excess wear and caries. However, these barriers, such as the development of secondary dentine, may eventually be overcome by wear or microorganisms and, once the pulp is exposed, it may become infected. A consequence of such an infection is its spread through the root canal and subsequent inflammation of the periapical area.

The result of such inflammation can be seen as a cavity in the alveolar bone, which is commonly reported in the archaeological literature as an abscess. However, Dias and Tayles[24] have recently proposed that these cavities were more likely to be ultimately formed and occupied by peri-apical granuloma or apical periodontal cysts rather than the build up of pus associated with acute infections and true abscesses. It is important to try to distinguish these lesions as they have different implications regarding the health of the individual in life as the former two lesions are relatively benign while a true abscess can ultimately result in death. However, this may be difficult as an abscess may form in a cavity previously created by a granuloma or cyst. Factors such as size of the lesion (granulomas are usually < 3 mm and cysts greater), shape of the margins of the perforation (usually circumscribed in granulomas and ragged in abscesses) and characteristics of the wall of the cavity (smooth in granulomas and roughed in abscesses) should be taken into account.[24]

It can be difficult for inexperienced workers to distinguish sinuses from pseudo-sinuses caused by post-mortem damage, as well as distinguish the differences between true ante-mortem lesions. Features that may help exclude pseudo-sinuses from true ones include the tooth involved; maxillary canines are the most prone to post-mortem damage as the bone over their roots is very thin. The shape and proximity of the hole to the root may also help in diagnosis. If the post-mortem damage was caused post-excavation, the colour of the edges of the 'sinus' may be different to the surrounding bone; the edges of a true sinus are normally smooth and rounded. Presence of pulp exposure due to caries or wear may also support the diagnosis of infection, as may the presence of porosity or new bone formation around the aperture. A further complication in the analysis of periapical lesions is that they may be visible radiographically before they are seen macroscopically, and as it is only the latter that are routinely recorded, the true prevalence of these lesions is likely to be under-estimated.

Tooth loss

The loss of a tooth (Figure 2) may be for many reasons such as periodontal disease, continuing eruption and intentional extraction for cosmetic, therapeutic or ritual purpose. Unlikely as it may seem, Silverstone et al.[10] stated that in the early 1970s 37% of the modern English and Welsh population over the age of 16 had no natural teeth remaining. Teeth may also be absent congenitally. For inexperienced workers, unless a crypt is remodelling or has remodelled following the loss of a tooth during life, distinguishing it from a post-mortem loss may be difficult. When trying to distinguish ante-mortem tooth loss from congenital absence a number of factors should be taken into consideration. Such factors include the presence or absence of wear on the opposing tooth, the presence of contact facets on adjacent teeth and the space available for the tooth.

Tooth wear

Tooth wear is seen as a wearing away of enamel and an exposure of dentine and is almost always present in early British populations (Figure 2). However, it is now becoming a clinical problem because improved dental hygiene and increased lifespan means people are keeping their own teeth longer.[26] Because of this, tooth wear has attracted much attention in the clinical literature. In addition, because tooth wear is used as an age estimation method (although a problematic one) for adults in biological anthropology, and is easily recognizable and scoreable, its presence in various populations is also widely reported in the archaeological literature. Potentially, the study of tooth wear can give an indication of diet content and food preparation methods, activity and of non-dental pathology.

There are three types of tooth wear: attrition, abrasion and erosion. Dental attrition is caused by contact of tooth on tooth.[27] This may occur during normal mastication or through bruxism, a stress-related grinding of teeth. Attrition can also occur through normal occlusal rest, and is seen on both the biting surface and at contact points between neighbouring teeth.

Dental abrasion is caused by contact between teeth and a foreign object.[27] This type of wear may be caused by abrasive elements in the diet, for example grit in flour, or by chewing tobacco. Dental abrasion may also be intentionally induced for cosmetic or ritual purposes. This type of wear may also be seen to be 'activity induced' and is related to the use of the teeth either as a tool or a third hand. There are numerous published studies that describe lesions associated with various activities. Examples have been published from Pakistan,[28] North America[29,30] and Australia,[31] although the Australian findings have been contested by Frayer[32] who argued the lesions were caused by the use of toothpicks.

Attack by chemicals, especially those that are acidic may cause dental erosion. In the clinical literature it is associated with regurgitative conditions such as the eating disorders, gastrointestinal disorders and alcoholism.[33] It is also associated with diets containing sugary acidic carbonated drinks and citrus fruits, as well as with some industrial working conditions. Robb et al.[34] discussed its presence in British archaeological dental remains and argued that it was detected on 20 of the 151 individuals studied. Robb et al.[35] also argued that regurgitative erosion may be the cause of lingual surface attrition of maxillary anterior teeth (LSAMAT), a condition argued to be due to a type of abrasion caused by using the teeth to remove the outer layer of manioc.[36–39] This outer layer has to be removed as it is acidic and, therefore, may be caused by a combination of both abrasion and non-regurgitative erosion. Cox et al.[40] discuss buccolabial erosion resulting from the use of acidic dental treatments designed to remove plaque and whiten teeth.

RECOMMENDATIONS FOR FUTURE RESEARCH

As this review has sought to illustrate the data derived from dental disease, once integrated with the archaeological record, can contribute to various debates in archaeology. There are ways in which research in the archaeology of British dental disease may progress.

Much of the published work describes the dental health of a single population instead of comparing it with others. This is, in part, due to the lack of a standard recording system, the absence of which precludes the comparison of data between workers using different methods. Furthermore, unpublished bone reports usually provide an inventory of diseases present rather than the results of an integration of this data with the other archaeological evidence, for example regarding diet and subsistence, thus preventing the broader questions regarding dental disease in antiquity being addressed.

It is only by comparing populations dependent on different resources, and living in different environments etc. that differences can be identified and investigated. Geographical areas need to be compared; is there a difference between the north and south of England, for example? Although dental health is considered in all skeletal reports, additional detailed research appears biased towards particular sites, for example Poundbury,[4,5,41–43] and areas, for example Scotland[19–21,44–48].

Different subsistence strategies need to be compared. Examples looking at the transition to, and intensification of, agriculture have already been given. Obviously, this is difficult in the British Isles where the osteological evidence is lacking from the Mesolithic period. However, difference between later British urban and rural populations is one example of work that could be pursued in this area. Comparisons also need to be made between different types of site. For example comparisons of lay cemeteries to monastic sites and hospitals may provide an opportunity to compare different socio-economic groups.

As well as these geographic and socio-economic comparisons, temporal comparisons also need to be developed. There is a bias towards Roman, Anglo-Saxon and later medieval periods, although this may reflect availability or preservation of remains. Nevertheless, early work in this area[49,50] did look at prehistoric remains.

The most commonly researched (as opposed to reported) dental conditions are caries, enamel hypoplasia and wear. Although work into other dental pathologies is needed, a reassessment of periodontal disease in the light of recent publications on continuing eruption is necessary. An assessment of the potential of investigating pre-cavity caries and arrested caries, and the relationship of dental diseases to non-dental diseases needs to be investigated. What is the relationship of the dental diseases to one another? Does this balance change through time, by geographic region, by sex, or by environment?

The prevalence of dental disease in different sex and age groups should also be considered. Is any particular group more likely to be affected by a particular dental disease? Does this change through time? However, for such comparisons to be made standardization of age groups used to report the prevalence of diseases is necessary as well as standardized sex and age estimation methodology and diagnostic criteria. Larsen's study,[11] looking at the caries frequency in a sample at its transition to agriculture, found that the increase in caries frequency in females was higher than in males. This he attributes to the men having access to more protein when hunting and the females more carbohydrate from gathering. However, problems can occur when investigating age groups and dental disease, as it is not possible to know when a disease occurred in relation to the age at death of the individual. If it is possible to determine that a tooth was lost ante-mortem due to caries it may be possible to determine if the absence of that tooth was long-standing. Factors such as 'drifting' of adjacent teeth and dentine exposure on the opposing tooth, which may be expected to be at a lesser stage than the rest of the dentition, may be of use. Dental calculus, which is prone to post-mortem damage and hygienic removal during life, may be a less reliable indicator of long-term loss of the opposing tooth. Again, further research is needed to investigate the feasibility of these approaches.

RECORDING DENTAL DISEASE

As already mentioned, one of the fundamental problems regarding the research of dental disease in the past is the absence of a standard recording methodology. As no universal recording system exists, workers are forced to develop their own individual systems from a menu of different published and newly devised techniques. This results in inventories of data that are not directly comparable. Buikstra and Ubelaker[51] have attempted to provide a universal recording method, although some conditions are omitted (e.g. peri-apical lesions) and the ability to record some conditions in detail lacking (e.g. caries size). By far the most useful and comprehensive recommendations can be found in Lukacs.[52]

From the battery of recording techniques for the individual diseases available to the worker, the most commonly used methods are listed below. As well as considering what diseases to record and which methods to use, it is important to consider the format in which this data is stored; this should be a format which will enable an analysis of different zones (e.g. anterior and posterior) to be conducted.

Data recorded regarding carious lesions should include the location on the tooth (e.g. crown or root), and surface affected (e.g. buccal or mesial) as well as the size of the lesion. Definitions of the latter can be found in Lukacs.[51] When recording peri-apical lesions, their size[52] should be recorded as well as the location (e.g. buccal or lingual) of the aperture. The most popular methods of recording tooth wear are those recommended by Buikstra and Ubelaker;[51] namely, Smith,[53] which is a modified version of Murphy's[54] system for the anterior teeth and premolars and Scott's[55] system for the molars. Brothwell's[56] visual standard for recording calculus deposits is commonly used, although more detailed methods are available.[57] A review of methods of recording periodontal disease can be found in Hildebolt and Molnar.[58] Methods of recording its severity often rely on the amount of root exposure, which is of course difficult if the tooth is missing or if other causes such as continuing eruption are responsible for the exposure.

CONCLUSION

In a summary of Kerr and Ringrose's[8] work on continuing eruption, Newman[59] said that 'the history of dentitions available from the past has much to teach us about the dental problems of the present.' However, he also stated 'dental opinions on archaeological material are best left to the dental experts'. If, by this latter, he means clinical experts, it should be retorted that the vast clinical literature is just as available to palaeopathologists and should be made use of. It must also be stated that if dental disease in the past is to be understood (whether done so to investigate dental diseases today or to answer archaeological questions), and because dental diseases are a multifactorial manifestation, we must integrate the clinical and archaeological data. Only then can the potential of dental disease to tell us about diet, subsistence, hygiene, occupation, general health, and stress of British archaeological populations be realised.

REFERENCES

1 Roberts CA, Manchester K. *The Archaeology of Disease*. Stroud: Sutton, 1995.

2 Hillson S. *Dental Anthropology*. Cambridge: Cambridge University Press, 1996.

3 Levers BGH, Darling AI. Continuous eruption of some adult human teeth of ancient populations. *Archives of Oral Biology* 1983; **28**: 401–408.

4 Whittaker DK, Parker JH, Jenkins C. Tooth attrition and continuing eruption in a Romano-British population. *Archives of Oral Biology* 1982; **27**: 405–409.

5 Whittaker DK, Molleson T, Daniel AT, Williams JT, Rose P, Resteghini R. Quantitative assessment of tooth wear, alveolar-crest height and continuing eruption in a Romano-British population. *Archives of Oral Biology* 1985; **30**: 493–501.

6 Whittaker DK, Griffiths S, Robson A, Roger-Davies P, Thomas G, Molleson T. Continuing tooth eruption and alveolar crest height in an eighteenth-century population from Spitalfields, East London. *Archives of Oral Biology* 1990; **35**: 81–85.

7 Glass G. Continuous eruption and periodontal status in pre-industrial dentitions. *International Journal of Osteoarchaeology* 1991; **1**: 265–271.

8 Kerr NW, Ringrose TJ. Factors affecting the life span of the human dentition in Britain prior to the seventeenth century. *British Dental Journal* 1998; **184**: 242–246.

9 Kerr NW. Dental pain and suffering prior to the advent of modern dentistry. *British Dental Journal* 1998; **184**: 397–399.

10 Silverstone L, Johnston N, Hardie J, Williams R. *Dental Caries. Aetiology, Pathology and Prevention*. London: Macmillan, 1981.

11 Larsen C. Behavioural implications of temporal change in cariogenesis. *Journal of Archaeological Science* 1983; **10**: 1–8.

12 Lukacs J. Dental palaeopathology and agricultural intensification in South Asia: new evidence from Bronze Age Harappa. *American Journal of Physical Anthropology* 1992; **87**: 133–150.

13 Beckett S, Lovell N. Dental disease evidence for agricultural intensification in the Nubian C-group. *International Journal of Osteoarchaeology* 1994; **4**: 223–240.

14 Walker P, Erlandson J. Dental evidence for prehistoric dietary change on the northern Channel Islands, California. *American Antiquity* 1986; **51**: 375–383.

15 Moore W, Corbett E. Distribution of dental caries in ancient British populations I: Anglo-Saxon Period. *Caries Research* 1971; **5**: 151–68.

16 Moore W, Corbett E. Distribution of dental caries in ancient British populations II: Iron Age, Romano-British and medieval periods. *Caries Research* 1973; **7**: 139–53.

17 Moore W, Corbett E. Distribution of dental caries in ancient British populations III: 17th century. *Caries Research* 1975; **9**: 163–175.

18 Corbett M, Moore W. Distribution of dental caries in ancient British populations. IV. The 19th century. *Caries Research* 1976; **10**: 401–414.

19 Watt ME, Lunt DA, Gilmour WH. Caries prevalence in the permanent dentition of a medieval population from the south west of Scotland *Archives of Oral Biology* 1997; **42**: 601–620.

20 Kerr N, Bruce M, Cross J. Caries experience in the permanent dentition of late medieval Scots (1300–1600AD). *Archives of Oral Biology* 1988; **33**: 143–148.

21 Kerr N, Bruce M, Cross J. Caries experience in medieval Scots. *American Journal of Physical Anthropology* 1990; **83**: 69–70.

22 Rudney J, Katz RV, Brand JW. Interobservor error reliability of methods for palaeopathological diagnosis of dental caries. *American Journal of Physical Anthropology* 1983; **62**: 243–8.

23 Lukacs J. The 'caries correction factor' a new method of calibrating dental caries rate to compensate for antemortem loss of teeth. *International Journal of Osteoarchaeology* 1995; **5**: 151–6.

24 Dias G, Tayles N. Abscess cavity: a misnomer. *International Journal of Osteoarchaeology* 1997; **7**: 548–554.

25 Gray PG, Todd JE, Slack GL, Bulman JS. *Adult Dental Health in England and Wales 1968*. London: HMSO, 1970.

26 Smith BGN, Knight JK. An index for measuring the wear of teeth. *British Dental Journal* 1984; **156**: 435–440.

27 Powell ML. The analysis of dental wear and caries for dietary reconstruction. In: Gilbert RI, Mielke JH (eds), *The Analysis of Prehistoric Diets*. New York: Academic Press, 1985; pp. 307–338.

28 Lukacs JR, Pastor RF. Activity-induced patterns of dental abrasion in prehistoric Pakistan: Evidence from Mehrgarh and Harappa. *American Journal of Physical Anthropology* 1988; **76**: 377–398.

29 Schulz PD. Task activity and anterior tooth grooving in prehistoric Californian Indians. *American Journal of Physical Anthropology* 1977; **46**: 87–92.

30 Merbs C. *Patterns of Activity Induced Pathology in a Canadian Inuit Population*. Ottawa: National Museums of Canada, 1983.

31 Brown T, Molnar S. Interproximal grooving and task activity in Australia. *American Journal of Physical Anthropology* 1990; **81**: 545–553.

32 Frayer DW. On the aetiology of interproximal grooves. *American Journal of Physical Anthropology* 1991; **85**: 299–304.

33 Smith BGN, Knight JK. A comparison of patterns of tooth wear with aetiological factors. *British Dental Journal* 1984; **157**: 16–19.

34 Robb ND, Cruwys E, Smith BGN. Regurgitation erosion as a possible cause of tooth wear in ancient British populations. *Archives of Oral Biology* 1991; **36**: 595–602.

35 Robb N, Cruwys E, Smith B. Is lingual surface attrition of the maxillary teeth (LSAMAT) caused by dental erosion? *American Journal of Physical Anthropology* 1991; **85**: 345–347.

36 Turner CH, Machado LMC. A new dental wear pattern and evidence for high carbohydrate consumption in a Brazilian archaic skeletal population. *American Journal of Physical Anthropology* 1983; **61**: 125–130.

37 Irish JD, Turner CG. More lingual surface attrition of the maxillary anterior teeth in American Indians: prehistoric Panamanians. *American Journal of Physical Anthropology* 1987; **73**: 209–213.

38 Turner C, Irish J, Machado L. Reply to Robb, Cruwys, and Smith, with additional remarks on LSAMAT. *American Journal of Physical Anthropology* 1991; **85**: 348–351.

39 Irish JP. First evidence of LSAMAT in non native Americans – historic Senegalese from West Africa. *American Journal of Physical Anthropology* 1997; **102**: 141–146.

40 Cox M, Chandler J, Kneller P, Haslam R. Nineteenth century dental restoration, treatment and consequences in an English nobleman. *British Dental Journal* (in progress).

41 Whittaker DK, Ryan S, Weeks K, Murphy WM. Patterns of approximal wear in cheek teeth of a Romano-British population. *American Journal of Physical Anthropology* 1987; **73**: 389–396.

42 Whittaker DK, Molleson T, Bennet RB, Edwards I, Jenkins PR, Llewelyn JH. The prevalence and distribution of dental caries in a Romano-British population. *Archives of Oral Biology* 1981; **26**: 237–245.

43 Whittaker DK, Davies G, Brown M. Tooth loss, attrition and temporo-mandibular joint changes in a Romano-British population. *Journal of Oral Rehabilitation* 1985; **12**: 407–419.

44 Lunt DA. The dentition in a group of medieval Scottish children. *British Dental Journal* 1972; **132**: 443–446.

45 Lunt D. The prevalence of dental caries in the permanent dentition of Scottish prehistoric and medieval Danes. *Archives of Oral Biology* 1974; **19**: 431–437.

46 Kerr N. The prevalence and pattern of distribution of root caries in a Scottish medieval population. *Journal of Dental Research* 1990; **69**: 857–860.

47 Kerr N. Prevalence and natural history of periodontal disease in Scotland: the medieval period. *Journal of Periodontal Research* 1991; **26**: 346–354.

48 Watt M, Lunt DA, Gilmour WH. Caries prevalence in the deciduous dentition of a medieval population from the south west of Scotland. *Archives of Oral Biology* 1997; **42**: 811–820.

49 Brothwell DR. Teeth in earlier human populations. *Proceedings of the Nutrition Society* 1959; **18**: 59–65.

50 Brothwell DR. The macroscopic dental pathology of some earlier human populations. In: Brothwell DR (ed.), *Dental Anthropology*. London: Pergamon, 1963: 179–277.

51 Buikstra JE, Ubelaker DH (eds), *Standards for Data Collection from Human Skeletal Remains: Proceedings of a Seminar at the Field Museum of Natural History*. Fayetteville: Arkansas Archaeological Survey Research Series 44, 1994.

52 Lukacs J. Dental Palaeopathology: methods for reconstructing dietary patterns. In: Isçan M, Kennedy K (eds), *Reconstruction of Life from the Skeleton*. New York: Alan Liss, 1989; pp. 261–286.

53 Smith BH. Patterns of molar wear in hunter-gatherers and agriculturists. *American Journal of Anthropology* 1984; **63**: 39–56.

54 Murphy T. Gradients of dentine exposure in human molar attrition. *American Journal of Physical Anthropology* 1959; **17**: 179–166.

55 Scott EC. Dental wear scoring technique. *American Journal of Physical Anthropology* 1979; **51**: 213–218.

56 Brothwell DR. *Digging Up Bones* (3rd edn). London: British Museum, 1981.

57 Dobney K, Brothwell D. A method for evaluating the amount of dental calculus on teeth from archaeological sites. *Journal of Archaeological Science* 1987; **14**: 343–351.

58 Hildebolt C, Molnar S. Measurement and description of periodontal disease in anthropological studies. In: Kelley M, Larsen C (eds), *Advances in Dental Anthropology*. New York: Wiley-Liss, 1991; pp. 225–240.

59 Newman H. Do not confuse the bone loss of periodontitis with root exposure due to supereruption. *British Dental Journal* 1998; **184**: 229.

15

CHEMICAL METHODS IN PALAEOPATHOLOGY

Angela Gernaey and David Minnikin

INTRODUCTION

Currently, osteological study uses visual examination, with additional X-radiographic and microscopical examination of selected bones. These methods are designed to detect abnormalities, which must not be the result of post-mortem change (taphonomy). In the early 1990s, the novel application of molecular biological methods to detect specific DNA sequences opened up the field producing much discussion. Since then, biochemical methods have successfully been applied to detect specific proteins that indicate disease.[1] This paper introduces yet another new field, 'chemical palaeopathology', and discusses its potential.

The application of chemical methods to archaeologically derived human material for disease diagnosis alone, chemical palaeopathology, is concerned with the detection of specific molecules (biomarkers) characteristic/diagnostic for a disease. It is hoped that chemical detection will prove to be more sensitive, and therefore more successful, than visual, radiological and microscopical examination of archaeologically derived human remains.

WHAT ARE BIOMARKERS?

Biomarkers are specific, characteristic molecules that resist taphonomic change; if change occurs, the resulting molecule must be diagnostic for its native precursor. Biomarkers have been used in the medical,[2,3] geological[4] and archaeological[5] sciences for a number of years. The molecular classes are nucleic acids, proteins, carbohydrates, lipids and combinations of these (e.g. glycoproteins). Methods of detection depend on molecular character. This chapter will investigate the possibility of palaeopathological diagnosis using chemical methods of detection (e.g. chromatography, spectrometry).

EFFECTS OF THE BURIAL ENVIRONMENT

The environmental conditions of burial will affect the survival of human remains[6,7] and, therefore, the survival of biomarkers for palaeopathology (see below), but there are other considerations.

Equivocal results

A range of microorganisms causes infectious diseases. In certain cases, these organisms, and/or their close relatives, may be present in the natural (burial) environment. In the case of laboratory diagnosis, the demonstration of biomarkers for environmental (but pathogenic) microorganisms in archaeological materials cannot be taken as diagnostic of disease. This must be so, regardless of any supporting pathology, because soil contamination can never be excluded. Biomarker concentration may help towards an interpretation, but taphonomy must also be considered (see below).

Effects of cause of death

The cause of death may also have a significant effect on bone survival. Infections that cause soft tissue necrosis, and diseases that alter the integrity of bone collagen (e.g. Marfan's syndrome), will affect the rate of soft and hard tissue degradation, possibly to the extent that the skeleton will not survive archaeological time spans.

Biomarker overprinting

It is possible that a disease biomarker could be overprinted by non-specific compounds of a similar molecular character deriving from sediment contamination. To understand how this may be so, an appreciation of the composition of bone is required. Specifically, the importance of the highly reactive mineral surface, with which infiltrating molecules will react, must be appreciated. In bone, the interactive surfaces are the crystal lattice faces of calcium hydroxyapatite ($Ca_{10}(PO_4)_6(OH)_2$); these react strongly with the free amide and carboxyl groups on proteins (e.g. the bone protein, osteocalcin[8,9]) and perhaps with carboxyl groups on fatty acids. Accumulation of soil-derived molecules (e.g. proteins, humic and fulvic acids) may occur in a bone, obliterating the signal of interest. The activity of this mineral surface is explained more fully in the chapter on the chemical degradation of the protein and mineral phases of bone.[7]

BIOMARKER STABILITY

The value to osteological examination of the so-called 'molecular markers' (i.e. the nucleic acids) is discussed elsewhere,[10] as are bone proteins.[7] A brief overview of their stability is presented here, for comparative purposes. While taphonomy covers all post-mortem changes, diagenesis refers only to those changes that occur in the burial environment.

Nucleic acids

Fingerprint sequences of DNA are used as standard diagnostic targets in modern laboratory confirmation of disease.[11] Considerable academic interest has been sparked by the demonstration of DNA preserved in archaeological materials, including ancient bones[12] and mummified individuals.[13] DNA studies have obvious value for palaeopathology,[10] but, to date, palaeopathological applications appear to be confined to studies using microbial (e.g. *Mycobacterium tuberculosis*)[14] or protozoal (e.g. *Plasmodium falciparum*)[15] DNA.

Since DNA is subject to degradation in the burial environment, is it reasonable to expect that DNA will survive sufficiently to address osteological questions? Studies comparing the preservation of DNA in mummified soft tissue and bone show that, where degradation is severe, DNA preservation is better in bone than in soft tissue.[16] In aqueous environments, DNA is subject to depurination and subsequent chain cleavage. Chain cleavage will produce shorter fragments, which can no longer be amplified with certainty.[17] Target sequences in DNA will probably be relatively short, since long sequences are unlikely to survive for prolonged periods. In consequence, the preservational potential for DNA (vertebrate or microbial) is compromised in most burial environments where water is available for these diagenetic processes.

Microbial DNA may survive for prolonged periods if protected from hydration and oxidation damage. Certain microorganisms (e.g. *Mycobacterium* spp., *Cryptococcus neoformans*) have cell envelopes that contain unusually hydrophobic lipids or glycolipids, and still others produce resistant bodies (spores); these microorganisms might be expected to have a high preservation potential for their cell contents.

Below, molecular techniques are suggested as a possible means of detecting disease in archaeological bones, but caution must be exercized. Target regions must not only be specific, but also success is more likely if multiple copies are present, as in mitochondrial DNA. Human genomic DNA may not be an appropriate target. Bacteria are unusual in that they do contain a DNA target in multiple copy within their genome: the 16S ribosomal RNA (rRNA) gene.

rRNA genes are characterized by highly conserved sequences[18] but, as with other DNA targets, there are concerns about the demonstration of these sequences in archaeological materials. Routine amplification and cloning of 16S rRNA genes from bacteria within environmental soil samples have resulted in the generation of chimeric sequences, leading to errors of interpretation.[19,20]

Proteins

Many proteins are used as biomarkers of disease in modern populations.[21,22] Archaeological proteins may be subject to chain shortening (i.e. peptide bond hydrolysis) and other diagenetic changes (e.g. racemization of component amino acids) which result in short peptide formation. Since archaeological peptides are usually detected by immunochemical means, and the target region (epitope) for the monoclonal antibody reaction (six-to-eight amino acids) is much smaller than the PCR target for DNA (> 100 bp), epitope recognition may not be compromised for considerable periods compared with the loss of DNA amplification.[17] Prolonged epitope survival has been demonstrated in diagenesis experiments by targeting a particular part (the γ-carboxyglutamic acid α-helix) of a small bone protein, osteocalcin.[23]

Peptide bond hydrolysis is more likely between some amino acids than others.[24,25] Peptides that contain no proline or serine residues, high numbers of acidic amino acids and a helical conformation that aligns these residues in one plane, have a high chance of survival if bound to a mineral surface. Studies on bone specific proteins show that survival requires strong mineral reaction,[23] but it is also possible that protein fragments that are strongly bound to the mineral surface may degrade faster, since the attraction may distort them, and perhaps over-stress the peptide bonds. Certainly, adsorption onto mineral surfaces will change the configuration of proteins.[26]

Carbohydrates

It is perhaps counter-intuitive to expect that saccharides would survive in sediments and archaeological materials, since they are rapidly assimilated by microorganisms, and their contribution to organic matter could be assumed to be negligible.[27] Carbohydrates, as hydrolysable saccharides, comprise 2–20% while lipids are only 10% of the organic matter of sediments.[4,28,29] The saccharides survive as part of condensation complexes (Maillard reaction products) with other organic molecules present.[30] The sources of these recalcitrant saccharides are suggested to be plant (for glucose and xylose) and microbial (for amino sugars, fucose, ribose, mannose and galactose),[31] rather than animal. The potential for animal (including human) carbohydrates to survive in sediments would appear to be slight.

Lipids

Lipids are hydrophobic and more resistant to hydrolytic change than carbohydrates and proteins. The more common degradation pathways for lipids are oxidative, and can involve bacterial/enzymic degradation pathways. Lipids have been demonstrated in such wide ranging archaeological materials as ancient ceramics,[32] coprolites,[5] bog bodies,[33] and bone.[34] Lipids are well known to survive for prolonged (geological) time spans,[27] but could they be useful biomarkers for disease in ancient populations? Methods that demonstrate microbial fatty acids have both a modern diagnostic and an epidemiological application.[35,36] It is this epidemiological application that has most relevance to palaeopathology since, if microbial lipids are so characteristic that they are used as the basis of epidemiological studies, then that same specificity can be harnessed to distinguish between environmental microbial contamination and pathogenic microorganisms in an archaeological sample. To date, there has only been one palaeopathological application using archaeological microbial lipids[37,38] for the demonstration of mycobacterial disease in ancient bone.

Summary

Biomarkers are specific, environmentally stable molecules that include nucleic acids, proteins, carbohydrates and lipids. Many proteins are useful as disease markers in modern medicine. Studies on archaeological proteins have shown that certain characteristic parts of protein molecules may survive, if protected from hydrolysis and enzyme degradation by interaction with mineral surfaces. Although the concentration of lipids in sediments is usually less than that of carbohydrates, nonetheless, carbohydrates have a reduced potential as biomarkers, since their hydrophilicity facilitates enzymic degradation and their exact origin is often unclear. Hydrophobic lipids are the most stable of the biomarkers and certain microbial lipids have a modern diagnostic and epidemiological function.

BIOMARKERS FOR ANCIENT METABOLIC DISEASE

The current increase in our understanding of the extracellular matrix is changing our concepts regarding the mechanisms of pathological connective tissue diseases. This has been, in major part, a result of the increase in molecular biological studies, and it is to this field that palaeopathologists must turn for metabolic disease biomarkers. The spectrum of genetic matrix disorders is much broader than previously thought and now also includes diseases of organs such as the kidney, eye and muscle. The phenotypes of genetic matrix disorders are determined by the basic biological characteristics of the extracellular matrix, so that diseases of these reflect a cascade of pathological events. These result in such conditions as abnormal protein synthesis, which in certain conditions leads to malformation of bone (e.g. Bruck syndrome, osteogenesis imperfecta).

A perusal of the literature shows that there are as yet very few single, non nucleic acid biomarkers for metabolic disease, but myeloma is one exception.[1] For example, diagnosis of bone remodelling (Paget's disease, osteoporosis, primary hyperparathyroidism and renal osteodystrophy) currently relies on assaying several indicators of bone formation (e.g. osteocalcin, osteonectin, procollagen type 1 and bone alkaline phosphatase) and several for bone resorption (e.g. urinary hydroxyproline and hydroxylysine glycosides, and urinary hydroxy-pyridinium cross-links of collagen). All of these markers are normally present, it is variations from their normal serum concentrations that indicate a disease state.[39]

There are very few lipids or abnormal amino acids, the biomarkers best suited for chemical detection, that are diagnostic for metabolic diseases. Plant sterols are found in the plasma in a rare lipid storage condition, sitosterolaemia.[40] A genetic disorder, it is characterized by high plasma cholesterol and the presence of excessive amounts of plant sterols (e.g. campesterol and sitosterol). Other metabolic diseases are characterized by abnormal concentrations of normal lipid constituents, and this picture is seen almost universally with all biomarkers for the diagnosis of metabolic disease.

This leaves the chemical palaeopathology of metabolic diseases with an apparently insurmountable problem. Given the uncertainties of diagenetic loss, it would be optimistic to measure concentrations of a biomarker (e.g. sitosterol) within individuals in a population under study, in the hope of finding high concentrations in a few individuals, so that extrapolations concerning metabolic disorders within that population could be made. This is because the concentration in ancient tissues will depend on two factors. The first, and least important, will be the initial concentration of the compound in the tissue at death; the overriding factor will be the diagenetic alterations of the molecule.

BIOMARKERS FOR ANCIENT INFECTIOUS DISEASES

As with modern medicine, it will be easier for palaeopathological diagnosis to demonstrate a factor not normally present, than measure a variation in concentration of normal components. For biomarkers of ancient infectious disease, however, there will still be problems of interpretation for archaeological samples. Contamination by soil microbes may occur leading to confusion, if not obliteration, of any pathological signal.

Before we can identify target molecules, we need to outline the characteristics of some of the types of organisms involved in the infectious diseases of human and other animals. Although some of the information below has not been derived using chemical methods, it is included for completeness.

Rickettsial, chlamydial, fungal and parasitical diseases

These diseases will be considered together, since the current likelihood of appropriate biomarkers being identified is slight. Almost all, perhaps, could be identified using molecular techniques, but how valid would these data be? To understand the problems inherent in identifying components of microbial origin, very brief descriptions of the different groups and their environmental niches and characteristics are required.

Rickettsia and chlamydia

Rickettsia and chlamydia are of similar dimensions to viruses, but they contain both DNA and RNA and, like the bacteria, are susceptible to antibiotics. Unfortunately for chemical palaeopathology, to date, only nucleic acid biomarkers have been identified.

Fungal diseases

The problem inherent with a demonstration of fungal biomarkers in archaeological materials is that most fungi that are pathogenic to humans are present in the environment. This gives rise to a significant problem with interpretation, so much so that even the demonstration of coiled fungal hyphae, associated with microconidia, penetrating surviving archaeological skin *must* be regarded as taphonomic change, rather than ringworm. Only one yeast, *Candida albicans*, does not appear to have an environmental reservoir, yet the organism contains no obvious biomarker component, other than DNA. There is a qualification, however. *C. albicans* is often present in individuals with no disease so, even if methods could be refined, the validity of a palaeopathological survey must be questionable.

Parasitical diseases

Much evidence has been accumulated that shows that enteric (and visceral) infestations by nematodes and helminths were common in members of past societies.[41,42] More recently, molecular techniques have been applied to the detection of the malarial parasite, *Plasmodium falciparum,* in an ancient individual.[15] As with the other types of organism here, it is unlikely that there will be practical chemical biomarkers for these diseases, but there is value in continuing to be vigilant in this area.

Viral diseases

Viruses are very small, intracellular agents; only the poxviruses are large enough to be seen by light microscopy. Viruses comprise an outer protein coat surrounding a nucleic acid centre (either DNA or RNA, but never both). Certain viruses (e.g. influenza) have a lipid bilayer membrane (envelope) surrounding the outer protein coat (capsid); envelope components derive from the host cell. If the virus is released by budding through the host cell membrane, the virus is enveloped. If virus release follows rupture of the cell, the virus has no envelope. The poxviruses of humans, including smallpox and vaccinia virus (but not chicken pox), are the only viruses that contain lipids of non-human origin. In modern viral disease diagnosis, immunochemical methods coupled with tissue culture and molecular biological techniques provide laboratory confirmation.

An RNA-enveloped virus causes influenza. The pandemic of 1917–19 was responsible for at least an estimated 20 million deaths,[43] although in the UK this was also aggravated because of public health mis-management.[44] The production of vaccines to protect individuals at risk depends upon using a virus with appropriate surface proteins (haemagglutinin (H) and neuraminidase (N)) and these are usually predictive. Past influenza pandemics may hold the key to accurate future predictions. Work is underway to look at victims of the 1917–18 episode, using tissue from individuals buried in permafrost regions.[45] The aim is to determine the character of the surface proteins (H1:N1) using molecular biological methods to look at the viral RNA.

Bacterial diseases

Bacteria contain a variety of proteins, lipids and polysaccharides, some of which are species-specific. There are two major divisions within the eubacteria, based upon the chemical composition of their cell envelope, which is tested by the Gram reaction (see below). Systematic analysis of the chemical components of bacterial envelopes has led to the development of chemotaxonomy.[46,47] Recent advances in this field have meant that chemical palaeopathology is now an attractive possibility.

The bacterial cell envelope is usually based on a cell wall and a plasma membrane permeability barrier. The cell wall usually contains peptidoglycan, in which glycan strands are cross-linked by small peptides. Peptidoglycan may function as a covalent anchorage for wall polymers, such as teichoic acids and mycolylarabino-galactan in certain Gram-positive bacteria. In general, Gram-negative bacteria have an external membrane that may incorporate highly complex lipopolysaccharides in their outer leaflet. Certain Gram-positive actinomycetes, the so-called mycolata, also have a characteristic outer membrane, based in covalently bound long-chain mycolic acids.[48,49]

A series of experimental studies involving host-bacterium interactions supports the suggestion that dormant bacteria are involved in latent infections. It is probable that most bacteria, exposed to the deleterious environment within a host, can change form. For example, in certain streptococcal and nocardial infections, wall-defective forms can be induced, which can survive and persist within the host, causing pathological responses compatible with disease.[50] The persistence of some of the mycobacteria in the infected host is a well-known phenomenon, but the mechanisms of persistence within the host are an active area for study. An *in vitro* model suggests that once in a granuloma (i.e. surrounded by efficient macrophages) their metabolism changes to allow them to survive in the altered environment.[51] Since these organisms remain latent within the host, it may be possible to devise strategies to detect some of their remaining components in archaeological individuals, however, detection methods will need to be highly sensitive.

It is not the function of a review such as this to list all the different bacteria and their components that are currently used as markers of clinical disease. It is better, perhaps, to consider some diseases representative of palaeopathological and/or archaeological interest, and look at the potential of chemical methods for diagnosis.

Gram-negative bacteria

Yersinia pestis, causative organism of plague

Plague has two forms, bubonic and pneumonic. Which disease type develops is governed by the source/route of infection. During both forms of the disease, a bacteraemia disseminates the organism throughout the body, and no bone changes occur. Because of the archaeological and historic importance of the disease, the archaeological difficulties of excavating 'plague pits' and the difficulties of diagnosing death due to Y. pestis in past populations, any biomarker, chemical or otherwise, would be an advantage.

Modern diagnosis relies on culture of the organism, but immunochemical[52] and molecular techniques[53] are being investigated. Members of the bacterial genus Yersinia share many common proteins, lipids and sugars, so there is a problem in identifying species-specific molecules. However, there are two possible biochemical markers and a DNA sequence.

- Vaccination with the Fraction 1 (F1) protein of the capsule of Y. pestis protects against both the pneumonic and bubonic forms of the disease.[54,55] This protein is 17 kDa in size, and is a major virulence factor, bound to the surface of the bacterium.
- The V antigen is a 37 kDa secreted protein, which does not contain many acidic amino acid residues. All pathogenic members of the genus produce V antigens, and two evolutionary distinct groups are described.[56] Antibodies for their detection and differentiation are widely available.
- The nucleotide sequences that encode for both the Y. pestis V antigen (lcrV) and the mature form of F1 antigen (caf1) are well described.[57,58] it may be possible to detect these sequences.

Any demonstration of either of these targets in archaeologically derived human material must consider the numbers of bacteria present at death. In the bubonic form, the numbers of bacteria in the buboes are high initially, but upon necrosis, bacterial numbers will fall. In the pneumonic form, bacterial numbers remain high in the sputum, bloodstream and spleen until death.[59]

Treponema pallidum, causative organism of syphilis

Venereal syphilis is a chronic multistage infection caused by the non-cultivatable spirochaete, *Treponema pallidum,* that has both an inner cytoplasmic (CM) and outer (OM) membrane. In the tertiary stages of syphilis when bone change occurs, the numbers of bacteria present in the host fall to almost undetectable levels. Diagnosis relies on the demonstration of the host response to the bacterium, rather than on the direct detection of the bacteria or their contents. Modern diagnosis is additionally hampered by the fact that most of the antigenic material (lipoprotein) is on the CM and, in its native form, immunologically inaccessible.

Unfortunately, the accessible OM contains only a few antigens, having a low protein/lipid ratio, and these lipids are non-specific. It is the OM proteins that have the best chance of reacting with bone mineral; there are three: 28, 31 and 65 kDa,[60] and all are species-specific. If there is to be a biomarker for syphilis, it is probable that it will be components of the acidic 65 kDa OM protein, but this has not yet been fully characterized[60,61] and the low numbers of bacteria present in the host probably preclude its demonstration in archaeological populations.

Gram-positive bacteria

Streptococcus pyogenes, causative organism of scarlet fever
Before the introduction of antibiotics, serious infections (e.g. scarlet fever) with *Streptococcus pyogenes* were commonplace, as were the sequelae, rheumatic fever and kidney disorders (streptococcal glomerulonephritis). These infections appear to be on the increase.[62] Manifestations include toxic shock syndrome, septicaemia from a deep-seated bone infection and scarlet fever. The organism produces a range of distinguishing, species-specific molecules (e.g. streptolysin O, exotoxin A, B and C, DNases A, B, C and D) but unfortunately for chemical palaeopathology, there are no species-specific lipids. There are two protein groups that may be of value for biochemical detection, however.

- M proteins are expressed on the surface of the bacterial cell. The majority of the molecule is α-helical, and the N-terminus (distal from the bacterial surface) is highly negatively charged to react with Ca^{2+} on the bone mineral surface.[63,64]
- Exotoxin A (the scarlet fever toxin) is released from the bacterium into the bloodstream and surrounding tissues. The molecule is 29kDa in size, but no relationship has been noted between toxin concentration and severity of the disease.[62]

Both of these are detected using immunochemical methods in modern populations. Given the possibility for interaction with the bone mineral surface, it is possible that these markers may survive in archaeological individuals, but the total bacterial number present at death must also be considered. The organisms are present in large numbers in the throat and larynx, but numbers are not so high in the regional lymph glands. The streptococcal toxins have the potency to stimulate massive T-cell proliferation and subsequent release of large amounts of cytokines – the toxic-shock syndrome.[65] This suggests that the exotoxins themselves may not be present in high enough concentration to survive archaeological periods sufficiently to allow detection.

Corynebacterium diphtheriae, causative organism of diptheria
Diphtheria is an upper respiratory tract infection which, in severe cases, induces the extension of the naso-pharynx to the larynx and trachea, obstructing breathing. The organism rarely, if ever, induces a bacteraemia. Corynebacteria produce mycolic acids with chain lengths between C_{28} and C_{36}, which are saturated, and mono- and di-unsaturated with, predominantly, saturated C_{12} and C_{16} side chains.[66] These mycolic acids will have limited applications for skeletal chemical palaeopathology, since the bacteria are unlikely to enter the bones, but their presence in surviving mummified soft tissue is a distinct possibility.

C. diphtheriae produces an exotoxin, however, which enters the bloodstream and inhibits cellular protein synthesis, although the concentration is very low. The toxin is a protein of two fragments, A (M_r = 21 kDa) and B (38 kDa). Fragment B has an intermediate hydrophobic region that is [alpha]-helical, and commercial antibodies are available. Apart from DNA, to date, this is the most likely candidate biochemical biomarker for diphtheria, but again, concentration must be considered.

Mycobacterium leprae, causative organism of leprosy

Leprosy is a systemic infection which shows two poles of manifestation, tuberculoid and lepromatous, and many intermediate states. It is the immune status of the individual that dictates which form will develop. This is governed both by human genetic considerations (i.e. the HLA type[67]) and the *Mycobacterium* sp. that constitutes 'original mycobacterial sin'.[68] The tuberculoid form is 'self-limiting', the numbers of bacteria in the tissues are low and the immune response competent. The lepromatous form can descend to death, with many bacteria present in the tissues, skin damage, blindness, nerve and tissue (including bone) loss and a necrosing immune response.[69]

Surviving records show that in Europe, leprosy was a major scourge between the 12th and 14th centuries AD,[70] and osteological studies support this. Many skeletons excavated from leprosy hospital cemeteries show lepromatous changes. This suggests that diagnosis of the lepromatous stage in past times was reasonably accurate, although there is evidence to show that there were exceptions to correct diagnosis.[71] In the mid–14th century AD the prevalence fell, leprosy hospitals could not be filled and their function changed.[72]

M. leprae produces several species-specific lipids: mycolic acids, phthiocerol dimycocerosates (PDIM) and phenolic glycolipids (PGL). *M. leprae* has distinct mycolic acids, comprising only α-mycolic acids (no oxygen substitutions) and ketomycolic acids.[73] In lepromatous leprosy, whether there is bone change, all individuals will have very high numbers of bacteria within all their tissues,[74] and preliminary studies have demonstrated the presence of the lipids of *M. leprae* in the altered left navicular bone from an individual in a medieval leprosy cemetery (unpublished data). Based on studies with *Mycobacterium tuberculosis* (see below), the lipids of *M. leprae* could perhaps be used to detect lepromatous leprosy in individuals who died before bone change occurred.

Mycobacterium tuberculosis *and* M. bovis *(MTB complex)*

Tuberculosis (TB) is hypothesized to be a systemic disease, since no other explanation suffices for the speed with which, in some individuals, many organs are involved. Infection with members of the MTB complex does not always result in disease formation, and this will depend on infecting dose and immune status of the individual. There is the suggestion that the prevalence of leprosy in Britain fell in the 14th century AD because TB prevalence rose,[75] since *M. tuberculosis* is more pathogenic[69] than *M. leprae* and may also act as an effective vaccine against the development of leprosy.[76]

Classically, the disease affected individuals from overcrowded, insanitary homes, usually with a poor diet, and the concomitant stress brought about by these conditions.[77] Perhaps studies of TB prevalence in archaeological populations will help us to understand the current TB pandemic.

Members of the MTB complex share identical mycolic acids, having α-mycolates, methoxy-mycolates and ketomycolates. Studies have already shown that mycolic acids are informative biomarkers for TB in archaeological populations.[37,38,78] The former Newcastle Infirmary (18th–19th centuries AD) burial ground yielded 210 articulated individuals. In a pilot study, 10% of the population was examined and 24% was had mycolic acids specific for MTB complex in mid-shaft rib samples with no lesions. This correlated well with the recorded 27% deaths with tuberculosis for the site.[38,79] Mycolic acids have been shown to be an effective chemical biomarker for tuberculosis.

THE FUTURE OF CHEMICAL PALAEOPATHOLOGY

Recent studies have shown that chemical palaeopathology is a robust and reliable approach for investigating the a prevalence of TB for an archaeological population, and there are preliminary indications that leprosy can also be diagnosed in post-cranial bones with lepromatous change.

The initial outlay for equipment to carry out these studies is significant, but techniques can be automated, unlike osteological examination. It is possible that costs could be reduced sufficiently to allow for the routine examination of entire archaeological populations, if rapid screening techniques could be introduced. There are several new methods for the rapid, sensitive detection of biomarkers,[80] so it may be possible to introduce new procedures that are both more sensitive and easier to operate. For the moment, available chemical methods should be aimed at the testing of hypotheses. Given the rapid advances in the medical and geochemical sciences, perhaps a routine screening service for a number of diseases that do not cause gross alteration to the bone may become available.

REFERENCES

1   Cattaneo C, Gelsthorp K, Phillips P, Waldron T, Booth JR, Sokol RJ. Immunological diagnosis of multiple myeloma in a medieval bone. *International Journal of Osteoarchaeology* 1994; **4**: 1–2.

2   Lohmander LS. What is the current status of biochemical markers in the diagnosis, prognosis and monitoring of osteoarthritis? *Baillières Clinical Rheumatology* 1997; **11**: 711–726.

3   Belisle JT, Brandt ME, Radolf JD, Norgard MV. Fatty acids of *Treponema pallidum* and *Borrelia burgdorferi* lipoproteins. *Journal of Bacteriology* 1994; **176**: 2151–2157.

4   Hamilton SE, Hedges JL. The comparative geochemistries of lignins and carbohydrates in an anoxic fjord. *Geochimica et Cosmochimica Acta* 1988; **52**: 129–142.

5   Evershed RP, Bethall PH. Application of multimolecular biomarker techniques to the identification of fecal material in archaeological soils and sediments. *ACS Symposium Series* 1996; **625**: 157–172.

6   Child AM. Microbial taphonomy of archaeological bone. *Studies in Conservation* 1995; **40**: 19–30.

7   Nielsen-Marsh C, Gernaey AM, Turner-Walker G, Hedges REM, Pike AWG, Collins MJ. The chemical degradation of bone (Chapter 26 – this volume).

8   Atkinson RA, Evans JS, Hauschka PV, Levine BA, Meats R, Triffitt JT, Virdi AS, Williams RJP. Conformational studies of osteocalcin in solution. *European Journal of Biochemistry* 1995; **232**: 515.

9   Hauschka PV, Carr SA. Calcium-dependent α-helical structure in osteocalcin. In: Weis A (ed.), *The Chemistry and Biology of Mineralized Connective Tissue*. Amsterdam: Elsevier, 1982: pp. 337–341.

10 Brown K. Ancient DNA applications in human osteoarchaeology: achievements, problems and potential (Chapter 27 – this volume).

11 Fuchs TM. Molecular mechanisms of bacterial pathogenicity *Naturwissenschaften* 1998; **85**: 99–108AB.

12   Hagelberg E, Sykes B, Hedges REM. Ancient bone DNA amplified. *Nature* 1989; **342**: 485.

13   Paabo S. Molecular cloning of ancient Egyptian mummy. *Nature* 1985; **314**: 644–645.

14   Nerlich AG, Haas CJ, Zink A, Szeimies U, Hagedorn HG. Molecular evidence for tuberculosis in an ancient Egyptian mummy. *Lancet* 1997; **350**: 1404.

15   Taylor GM, Rutland P, Molleson T. A sensitive polymerase chain reaction method for the detection of *Plasmodium* species DNA in ancient human remains. *Ancient Biomolecules* 1997; **1**: 193–203.

16   Lassen C, Hummel S, Herrmann B. Comparison of DNA extraction and amplification from ancient human bone and mummified soft tissue. *International Journal of Legal Medicine* 1994; **107**: 152–155.

17   Waite ER, Child AM, Craig OE, Collins MJ, Gelsthorp K, Brown TA. A preliminary investigation of DNA stability in bone during artificial diagenesis. *Bulletin de la Societe Géologique de France* 1997; **168**: 547–554.

18   Stratz M, Mau M, Timmis KN. System to study horizontal gene exchange among microorganisms without cultivation of recipients. *Molecular Microbiology* 1996; **22**: 207–215.

19   Wang GCY, Wang Y. Frequency of formation of chimeric molecules is a consequence of PCR co-amplification of 16S rRNA genes from mixed bacterial genomes. *Applied and Environmental Microbiology* 1997; **63**: 4645–4650.

20   Wintzingerode F, Göbel UB, Stackebrandt E. Determination of microbial diversity in environmental samples: pitfalls of PCR-based rRNA analysis. *FEMS Microbiology Reviews* 1997; **21**: 213–239.

21   Delvig AA, Robinson JH. Two T cell epitopes from the M5 protein of viable *Streptococcus pyogenes* engage different pathways of bacterial antigen processing in mouse macrophages. *Journal of Immunology* 1998; **160**: 5267–5272.

22   Zavyalov VP, Abramov VM, Cherepanov PG, Spirina GV, Chernovskaya TV, Vasiliev AM, Zavyalova GA. pH6 antigen (rPsaA protein) of *Yersinia pestis*, a novel bacterial FC-receptor. *FEMS Immunology and Medical Microbiology* 1996; **14**: 53–57.

23   Collins MJ, Child AM, van Duin ACT, Vermeer C. Ancient osteocalcin: the most stable bone protein? *Ancient Biomolecules* 1998; **2**: 223–233.

24   Collins MJ, Walton D, King A. The geochemical fate of proteins. In: Stankiewicz BA, van Bergen PF (eds), Nitrogen-containing macromolecules in the biosphere and geosphere. *ACS Symposium Series* 1998; **707**: 74–86.

25   Krokoszynska I, Otlewski J. Thermodynamic stability effects of single peptide-bond hydrolysis in protein inhibitors of serine proteinases. *Journal of Molecular Biology* 1996; **256**: 793–802.

26   Quiquampoix H, Abadie J, Baron MH, Leprince F, MatumotoPintro PT, Ratcliffe RG, Staunton S. Mechanisms and consequences of protein adsorption on soil mineral surfaces. *ACS Symposium Series* 1995; **602**: 321–333.

27   Tissot BP, Welte DH. *Petroleum Formation and Occurrence* (2nd edn). Berlin: Springer, 1984.

28   Steinberg SM, Venkatesan MI, Kaplan IR. Organic geochemistry of sediments from the continental margin off southern New England. *Marine Chemistry* 1987; **21**: 249–265.

29   Cowie GL, Hedges JL. Carbohydrate sources in a coastal marine environment. *Geochimica et Cosmochimica Acta* 1984; **48**: 2075–2087.

30   Collins MJ, Westbroek P, Muyzer G, DeLeeuw JW. Experimental evidence for condensation reactions between sugars and proteins in carbonate skeletons. *Geochimica et Cosmochimica Acta* 1992; **56**: 1539–1544.

31   Moers MEC. *Occurrence and fate of carbohydrates in recent and ancient sediments from different environments of deposition*. Doctoral dissertation, University of Delft, 1980.

32   Evans K, Heron C. Glue, disinfectant and chewing gum – natural products chemistry in archaeology. *Chemistry and Industry* 1993; **12**: 446–449.

33   Stankiewicz BA, Hutchins JC, Thomson R, Briggs DEG, Evershed RP. Assessment of bog-body tissue preservation by pyrolysis gas chromatography mass spectrometry. *Rapid Communications in Mass Spectrometry* 1997; **11**: 1884–1890.

34   Stott AW, Evershed RP. δC13 analysis of cholesterol preserved in archaeological bones and teeth. *Analytical Chemistry* 1996; **68**: 4402–4408.

35   Basile F, Beverly MB, Voorhees KJ, Hadfield TL. Pathogenic bacteria: their detection and differentiation by rapid lipid profiling with pyrolysis mass spectrometry. *Trends in Analytical Chemistry* 1998; **17**: 95–109.

36   Glickman SE, Kilburn JO, Butler WR, Ramos LS. Rapid identification of mycolic acid patterns of mycobacteria by high performance liquid chromatography using pattern recognition software and a mycobacterial library. *Journal of Clinical Microbiology* 1994; **32**: 740–745.

37   Donoghue HD, Spigelman M, Zias1 J, Gernaey-Child AM, Minnikin DE. Demonstration of *Mycobacterium tuberculosis* complex DNA in calcified pleura from remains 1400 years old. *Letters in Applied Microbiology* 1998; **27**: 265–269.

38   Gernaey AM, Minnikin DE, Copley MS, Power JJ, Ahmed, AM, Dixon RA, Roberts, CA, Robertson DJ, Nolan J, Chamberlain A. Detecting ancient tuberculosis. *Internet Archaeology* 5: http://intarch.ac.uk/journal/issue5/gernaey_index.html

39   Tohme JF, Seibel MJ, Silverberg SJ, Robins SP, Bilezikian JP. Biochemical markers of bone metabolism. *Zeitschrift fur Rheumatologie* 1991; **50**: 133–141.

40   Salen G, Shefer S, Berginer VM. Familial disease and storage of sterols other than cholesterol; cerebroteninous xanthomatosis and sitosterolemia with xanthomatosis. In: Stanbury JB, Wyngaarden JB, Fredrickson DS, Goldstein JL, Brown MS (eds), *Metabolic Basis of Inherited Disease* (5th edn). New York: McGraw-Hill, 1983: pp. 713–730.

41   Jones AKG, Hutchinson AR, Nicholson C. The worms of Roman horses and other finds of intestinal parasite eggs from unpromising deposits. *Antiquity* 1988; **62**: 275–276.

42   Warnock PJ, Reinhard KJ. Methods for extracting pollen and parasite eggs from latrine soils. *Journal of Archaeological Science* 1992; **19**: 261–264.

43   Beveridge WIB. The chronicle of influenza epidemics. *History and Philosophy of the Life Sciences* 1991; **13**: 223–235.

44   Tomkins SM. The failure of expertise – public health policy in Britain during the 1918–19 influenza epidemic. *Social History of Medicine* 1992; **5**: 435–454.

45   Taubenberger JK, Reid AH, Krafft AE, Bijwaard KE, Fanning TG. Initial genetic characterization of the 1918 'Spanish' influenza virus. *Science* 1997; **275**: 1793–1796.

46   Dobson G, Minnikin DE, Minnikin SM, Parlett JH, Goodfellow M, Ridell M, Magnusson M. Systematic analysis of complex mycobacterial lipids. In: Goodfellow M, Minnikin DE (eds), *Chemical Methods in Bacterial Systematics*. London: Academic Press, 1985: pp. 237–265.

47   Goodfellow M, O'Donnell AG. *Handbook of New Bacterial Systematics*. London: Academic Press, 1993.

48   Minnikin DE. Lipids: complex lipids, their chemistry, biosynthesis and roles. In: Ratledge C, Stanford J (eds), *The Biology of the Mycobacteria*. London: Academic Press, 1982: pp. 95–185.

49   Brennan PJ, Nikaido H. The envelope of mycobacteria. *Annual Review of Biochemistry* 1995; **64**: 29–63.

50   Domingue GJ, Woody HB. Bacterial persistence and expression of disease. *Clinical Microbiology Reviews* 1997; **10**: 320–347.

51   Wayne LG, Hayes LG. An *in-vitro* model for sequential study of shiftdown of *Mycobacterium tuberculosis* through two stages of non-replicating persistence. *Infection and Immunity* 1996; **64**: 2062–2069.

52   Rasoamanana B, Leroy F, Boisier P, Rasolomaharo M, Buchy P, Carniel, Chanteau S. Field evaluation of an immunoglobulin G anti-F1 enzyme-linked immunosorbent assay for serodiagnosis of human plague in Madagascar. *Clinical and Diagnostic Laboratory Immunology* 1997; **4**: 587–591.

53   Tsukano H, Itoh K, Suzuki S, Watanabe H. Detection and identification of *Yersinia pestis* by polymerase chain reaction (PCR) using multiplex primers. *Microbiology and Immunology* 1996; **40**: 773–775.

54   Heath DG, Anderson GW, Mauro JM, Welkos SL, Andrews GP, Adamovicz J, Friedlander AM. Protection against experimental bubonic and pneumonic plague by a recombinant capsular F1-V antigen fusion protein vaccine. *Vaccine* 1998; **16**: 1131–1137.

55   Anderson GW, Leary SEC, Williamson ED, Titball RW, Welkos SL, Worsham PL, Freidlander AM. Recombinant V antigen protects mice against pneumonic and bubonic plague caused by F1-capsule-positive and F1-capsule-negative strains of *Yersinia pestis*. *Infection and Immunity* 1996; **64**: 4580–4585.

56   Roggenkamp A, Geiger AM, Leitritz L, Kessler A, Heesemann J. Passive immunity to infection with *Yersinia* spp mediated by anti-recombinant V antigen is dependent on polymorphism of V antigen. *Infection and Immunity* 1997; **65**: 446–451.

57   Leary SEC, Griffin KF, Garmory HS, Williamson ED, Titball RW. Expression of an F1/V fusion protein in attenuated *Salmonella typhimurium* and protection of mice against plague. *Microbial Pathogenesis* 1997; **23**: 167–179.

58   Drygin YF, Sakhuriya IB, Vorobev II, Dikhanov GG, Podladchikova ON. Detection of *Yersinia pestis* and *Y. pseudotuberculosis* by PCR amplification of 16S rRNA and its genes. *Molecular Biology* 1995; **29**: 791–797.

59   Cruickshank R. *Medical Microbiology*. Edinburgh:Livingston, 1965.

60   Blanco DR, Miller JN, Lovett MA. Surface antigens of the syphilis spirochete and their potential as virulence determinants. *Emerging Infectious Diseases* 1997; **3**: 11–20.

61   Shevchenko DV, Akins DR, Robinson EJ, Li MY, Shevchenko OV, Radolf JD. Identification of homologs for thioredoxin, peptidyl prolyl cis-trans isomerase, and glycerophosphodiester phosphodiesterase in outer membrane fractions from *Treponema pallidum*, the syphilis spirochete. *Infection and Immunity* 1997; **65**: 4179–4189.

62   MullerAlouf H, Geoffroy C, Geslin P, Bouvet A, Felten A, Gunther E, Ozegowski JH, Alouf JE. Streptococcal pyrogenic exotoxin A, streptolysin O, exoenzymes, serotype and biotype profiles of *Streptococcus pyogenes* isolates from patients with toxic shock syndrome and other severe infections. *Zentralblatt für Bakterologie* 1997; **286**: 421–433.

63   Phillips GN, Flicker PF, Cohen C, Manjula BN, Fishetti VA. Streptococcal M protein; alpha-helical coiled coil structure and arrangement on the cell surface. *Proceedings of the National Academy of Sciences, USA* 1981; **78**: 4689–4693.

64   Fishetti VA, Parry DAD, Trus BL, Hollingshead SK, Scott JR, Manjula BN. Conformational characteristics of the complete sequence of group A streptococcal M6 protein. *Proteins: Structure, Function and Genetics* 1988; **3**: 60–69.

65   Norgren M, Eriksson A. Streptococcal superantigens and their role in the pathogenesis of severe infections. *Journal of Toxicology – Toxin Reviews* 1997; **16**: 1–32.

66   Debriel D, Couderc F, Riegel P, Jehl F, Minck R. High performance liquid chromatography of corynemycolic acids as a tool in the identification of *Corynebacterium* species and related organisms. *Journal of Clinical Microbiology* 1992; **30**: 1407–1417.

67   Cervino ACL, Curnow RN. Testing candidate genes that may affect susceptibility to leprosy. *International Journal of Leprosy and other Mycobacterial Diseases* 1997; **65**: 456–460.

68   Abrahams EW. Original mycobacterial sin. *Tubercle* 1970; **51**: 316–321.

69   Grange JM. *Mycobacteria and Human Disease* (2nd edn). London: Edward Arnold, 1996.

70   Richards P. Leprosy: myth, melodrama and mediaevalism. *Journal of the Royal College of Physicians of London* 1990; **24**: 55–62.

71   Manchester K, Roberts CA. The palaeopathology of leprosy in Britain: a review. *World Archaeology* 1989; **21**: 265–272.

72   Ell SR. Leprosy and social class in the middle ages. *International Journal of Leprosy* 1986; **54**: 300–305.

73   Minnikin DE (1987) Chemical targets in cell envelopes of the leprosy bacillus and related bacteria. In: Hooper M (ed.), *Chemotherapy of Tropical Diseases*. Critical Reports on Applied Chemistry, Vol. 21. New York: Wiley, 1987: pp. 19–23.

74   Ridley, DS. *Pathogenesis of Leprosy and related diseases*. London: Wright, 1988.

75   Manchester K. Tuberculosis and leprosy: evidence for the interaction of disease. In: Ortner D and Aufderheide A (eds), *Human Paleopathology. Current Syntheses and Future Options*. Washington, DC: Smithsonian Institution Press, 1991: pp. 23–25.

76   Fine PEM, Smith PG. Vaccination against leprosy – the view from 1996 *Leprosy Review* 1996; **67**: 249–252.

77   Wilson GS, Miles AA. Tuberculosis. In: Wilson GS (ed.), *Topley and Wilson's Principles of Bacteriology and Immunity* (3rd edn). London: Edward Arnold, 1946; pp. 1289–1357.

78   Gernaey-Child AM, Minnikin DE, Copley MS, Dixon RA, Middleton, J, Roberts CA. Detection of mycolic acids confirms DNA evidence for tuberculosis in medieval human skeletal remains. *Proceedings of the National Academy of Sciences, USA* (in preparation).

79   Gernaey AM, Minnikin DE, Copley MS, Robertson DJ, Nolan J, Power JJ, Chamberlain A. Mycolic acids are biomarkers for ancient tuberculosis *Ancient Biomolecules* (in preparation).

80   Krishnamurthy T, Ross PL, Rajamani U. Detection of pathogenic and non-pathogenic bacteria by matrix-assisted laser desorption/ionization time-of-flight mass spectrometry. *Rapid Communications in Mass Spectrometry* 1996; **10**: 883–888.

16

AN INTRODUCTION TO PALAEOHISTOPATHOLOGY

Lynne Bell and Kim Piper

INTRODUCTION

This chapter deals with histopathology of archaeological skeletal remains and excludes remnant soft tissue histopathology. The main purpose here is briefly to introduce, and demonstrate the usefulness of, skeletal palaeohistopathology to palaeopathology, both at the level of diagnosis and as a bridge to modern clinical interpretations of disease states. To this end, the general aims and objectives of modern medicine and palaeopathology are initially contextualized and discussed, with the latter part of the chapter focusing on histopathological examples. The examples given are intended to be illustrative of the pathology itself and of post-mortem agencies, which can complicate, but not exclude, histopathological analysis. The maxillo-facial region is given some weight here since pathologies in this area can be both informative of a specific localized pathology, or of a larger condition affecting the individual. This latter consideration is often overlooked. It also serves as a vehicle to explore future avenues of research.

The chapter is not intended to be a methodological chapter or a review of past work, but references are given throughout that provide for more technical and detailed reading. The scope is then an 'introduction', which assumes a basic understanding of skeletal microstructural biology and pathology.

Histopathology

In the context of modern medicine, histopathology plays a vital role, particularly where diseases present similar clinical and radiographical features, and where a definitive diagnosis often depends on the histological examination of a biopsy specimen. However, it is acknowledged that in a modern clinical setting histopathology provides information at a cellular and structural level only and usually forms part of a larger clinical picture including patient history, radiology and blood chemistry. In the context of archaeological material where, as is usually the case, the body has completely skeletonized, then only the cellular product, namely the mineralized tissues and any residual or complexed organics, will remain as evidence of any pathology that once affected the individual during life. If the skeleton itself was unaffected by the pathology, then obviously there will be no record at the microstructural level.

Disease classification: the surgical sieve

Disease is broadly defined as either developmental or acquired, and is further subdivided into traumatic, degenerative, infective, idiopathic, metabolic and neoplastic. This system of disease classification is known in the medical literature as the surgical sieve. At the level of radiological presentation, pathological lesions present as radiopacities and radiolucencies or combinations of both. Many pathologies may be initially radiolucent but mature to become radiopaque. This is clearly a cellular process, and consideration of what has been identified on a radiograph, a biopsy in a modern context, or aligned section for archaeological material, would enable greater elucidation of any abnormal cellular activity and/or mineralization defects at the level of microstructure at that anatomical site.

Brief examples of some common diseases in relation to the surgical sieve are given in Table 1. This is not intended to be exhaustive and serves only as an illustration. We also include dental pathologies, and a separate discussion of such pathology follows below.

Hardware

Histopathology is simply a way of looking at pathological material using microscopy. Three technological advancements in microscopy have been particularly significant over the past 150 years. The first is the development of the earliest microscope, the normal and polarizing light microscope. It allows examination of thin section material, illuminated by a single or dual light source of mixed or single wavelengths, and is still the general workhorse microscope of hospital laboratories. Other light microscopes of similar design are configured for use with fluorescent stains.

The development of the electron microscope enabled much greater magnification than was previously possible using traditional light microscopy, and has several modes of operation. The scanning electron microscope (SEM) has facilitated a better understanding of three-

Table 1 – Surgical sieve: examples.

Congenital	Odontogenic cysts
	Cherubism
Traumatic	Fractures
	Aneurysmal bone cyst
	Solitary bone cysts
Infective	Syphilis
	Tuberculosis
	Chronic and acute osteomyelitis
Idiopathic	Fibrosseous and cementosseous lesions
	Giant cell lesions
Metabolic	Hyperparathyroidism rickets/osteomalacia
	Osteoporosis
	Scurvy
Neoplastic	Primary bone and cartilage tumours
	Odontogenic tumours

dimensional morphology, e.g. trabecular microstructure and orientation with regard to say osteoporosis.[1,2] The SEM operated in backscattered electron mode can provide information on both the elemental constituents of the substance being imaged, and also on the relationship between skeletal microstructure and density.[3] Transmission electron microscopy provides a way of imaging at greater magnification still, e.g. internal cell structures and proteins at the nanometer level.[4]

The most recent development in microscope technology has been the development of confocal reflecting scanning laser light microscope. This microscope gives information at the micron and submicron levels, where light returns only from one point in space. This method of imaging allows high precision micron stepped focusing into, for example, bone, living tissues or cells, where the image can be captured and stored digitally, then re-stacked to recreate a three-dimensional image.[5] This microscope is still very much a research tool of biomedical science.

Finally, as a caveat, and although not discussed here, it is important to note that other imaging methods exist as powerful diagnostic tools in modern medicine and include computed tomography, ultrasound and magnetic resonance imaging. Each has a particular use with regard to the imaging of a disease process, and is usually used in association with other tests.[6]

Stain technology

The purpose of a stain is to identify either a mineral or organic component in a living preparation or section. There are many stains but the main histological stain used in current histopathological diagnosis remains the haematoxolin and eosin (H&E) stain. Modern histopathological diagnosis also uses a variety of special stains, many based on the antigen–antibody reaction, where polyclonal and monoclonal antibodies elucidate the origin of seemingly undifferentiated tissue in tiny biopsy fragments. Polyclonal antibodies are less specific than monoclonals, and can be used to determine cell lineage (e.g. epithelial from mesenchymal). However, in an archaeological context polyclonals should be used with some caution, as diagenetic alterations and/or inclusions may invalidate results (see correspondence between Rothschild and Nieberger concerning the identification of syphilis in a Pleistocene bear[7-9]). The use of modern staining regimes has thus far been little attempted using archaeological skeletal tissue, and we currently have little information on how the preservation process will alter any tissue remnants that may be examined with these monoclonal stains.[7-11] It is conceivable that some soft tissue remnants at the remnant cell level may be preserved within the skeleton. In the future, it might be possible to determine whether, for example, a radiolucency is due to an epithelial-lined cyst, rather than a metastatic haematological malignancy, both of which may look similar radiographically.

What are we doing and why?

Studies of disease in archaeology have different objectives to those of modern medicine. The main objective of modern medicine is to make a diagnosis so that a course of treatment can be decided upon. An archaeologist, however, wants to understand as much as possible about past peoples, and skeletal remains form an important part of this overall picture. Such remains constitute primarily a biological resource of information, and secondarily a socio-cultural one.

This type of information can be usefully described as a biocultural matrix. Disease forms one part of this matrix both at the level of the individual or populations, with co-implications at the level of subgroups, be they climatic, spatial, familial, sex or age related.

Interpreting disease states in the past is closely akin to epidemiology, although the epidemiologist is attempting to 'deconstruct' known data sets from individuals and/or populations to gain an understanding of a particular disease, based on reliable diagnostic criteria. In contrast, the palaeopathologist is attempting to 'reconstruct' similar understanding from partial or incomplete data sets or populations,[12] and so archaeological material will always fall short of the level of sampling required for modern epidemiological investigation. This lack of information in terms of skeletal recovery and poorly defined archaeological populations is part of the challenge of palaeopathological enquiry. By adopting and adapting other methods that are routinely employed in modern medicine, such as, in this instance, histopathology, the resulting information can usefully increase our understanding of disease states in the past.

A useful model of diagnostic criteria for clinical and palaeopathological assessment is given by Rogers and Waldron[13] (Figure 1a and b). These Venn diagrams demonstrate that the only line of evidence that currently ties archaeological material to modern material, and therefore modern interpretative criteria, is radiographic evidence. This represents the current theoretical upper limit for palaeopathological diagnosis. However, if histopathology were to be incorporated into Figure 1b, this upper limit would be significantly extended to include histopathology within the palaeopathological diagnostic model. Figure 1c illustrates this alteration of the model, whereby pathology becomes connected to the radiological evidence.

Given the clear increase in diagnostic power, it is curious that histopathology is rarely undertaken on archaeological material. The reasons for this probably fall broadly into two main areas. One is the understandable resistance by curators and osteologists to the sectioning of bone and teeth; the other is a general lack of understanding and training in histopathology itself. Invasive analysis is often considered and described as destructive, and falls within museum sampling protocols for such analyses.[14] A truly destructive analysis usually involves the total combustion of a sample for dating or isotopic studies.[15] While histopathology is undoubtedly invasive, it is not destructive in this way, since a section may be preserved and archived indefinitely. This is an extremely important distinction, not just in terms of the management of skeletal collections, but also as a recoverable resource or archive of palaeopathological information. In a modern context, diseases are often reclassified and retrievable palaeohistopathological sections would allow for similar re-adjustments, even at the level of informing present-day reclassification. Perhaps the biggest obstacle, however, is the lack of training for palaeohistopathological study, and this alone probably accounts for its perceived lack of utility among palaeopathologists. For the present, the study of disease states remains at the level of Figure 1b.

Application of microscopy to archaeological and fossil material

For the purposes of discussion, a distinction is made between the microscopic study of non-pathological skeletal material, here referred to as 'palaeohistology', as distinct to the

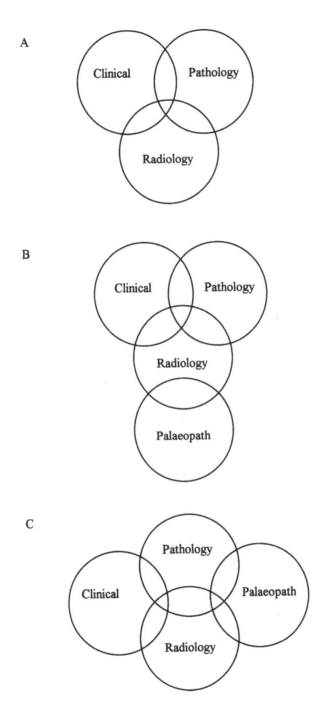

Figure 1 – (a) Venn diagram after Rogers and Waldron[13] illustrating the interconnected relationship of diagnostic criteria used in modern medicine. (b) Current relationship between palaeopathology and clinical diagnosis via the use of radiology.[13] (c) Our suggestion for greater unity of diagnostic criteria for palaeopathology by connecting pathology via the use of palaeohistopathology.

microscopic study of pathological material, here referred to as 'palaeohistopathology'. This distinction is present in the published literature, but can be confusing when used together or interchangeably.

Palaeohistological analysis of skeletal remains is not uncommon from the late 1850s.[16,17] Much early work documented the microstructural organization of fossil material, and latterly workers have extended these studies to teeth and more taphonomic considerations.[16–21] What is clear from these studies is that microstructural information from bone and teeth can survive many millions of years from differing environmental contexts.

Considerable work has also accumulated on the microstructural changes which occur postmortem either during soft tissue decomposition or within sediments.[22,23] Such changes are usually referred to as diagenetic but may equally be included within taphonomy. Diagenetic changes will often obscure the anatomical microstructural arrangement of the skeletal tissues, and such changes can effect other methods at the mineral and organic level, including DNA,[24] trace element[25] and isotopic analyses.[15]

As stated, there has been little palaeohistopathology published, relative to the vast number of macroscopic studies in palaeopathology. A recent chapter on palaeohistology by Martin[26] outlined the wider uses of microscopy in skeletal material, beyond that which is purely pathological. She points out that all processes involved during growth and bone turnover reflect the general health of the individual and of the population. She complains, however, of the lack of utilization of histology for the examination of disease in archaeological material. Authors such as Jarcho,[27] Blumberg and Kerley,[28] Stout and Simmons,[29] Race et al.[30] and Garland[11] have made the case, as have others, for the application of histopathology more generally in the study of archaeological skeletal remains. Others have successfully identified such conditions as Pagetic bone in archaeological material[31,32] and some of this work is presented below as a palaeohistopathological case study. De la Rua et al.[33] and Grupe[34] examined the histology of metastatic carcinoma in Neolithic and Medieval material in association with radiography. Schultz, who has published more than anyone in this area,[35–40] recently assessed the frequency of bony tumours in an archaeological population using macroscopic, radiologic, endoscopic and microscopic examination.[36] Of the student textbooks that exist on the subject of palaeopathology, only Aufderheide and Rodriguez-Martin[41] include the histological appearance of some pathologies, and these are text descriptions with no images. Rothschild and Martin[42] give histopathology a brief mention at the level of histotechnology, and Roberts and Manchester[43] place palaeohistopathology into the next 10 years of new developments in the study of skeletal palaeopathology.

HISTOPATHOLOGICAL EXAMPLES: ARCHAEOLOGICAL AND MODERN

An archaeological illustration: pathology, preservation and diagenesis

The study that follows is intended to illustrate the best and worst scenarios potentially faced by the palaeohistopathologist, and discusses diagenetic alteration in association with pathological change. A histological study of two putative cases of Paget's disease was undertaken using backscattered electron imaging in a scanning electron microscope (BSE-SEM).[31] This method of analysis was chosen as BSE-SEM imaging has proved a superior tool to detail skeletal microstructure and related density changes, be they ante- or post-mortem.[22,44]

In brief, Paget's disease was originally described as 'osteitis deformans' by Sir James Paget in 1877.[45] It is a disease of considerable antiquity, usually affecting those over 40 years and has an unknown aetiology. Recent immunohistochemical studies have demonstrated viral inclusions within osteoclasts[46] and these inclusions have been connected to the paramyxovirus group. It affects most bones of the body and radiologically the bones appear expanded with an irregular sclerotic and porous appearance. The advancing edge of a lesion has been described as 'flame-like'.[47] The histological appearance at a purely microstructural level is characterized by excessive and rapid resorption and formation of bone, combined with abnormal mineralization and poor collagen organization. Consequently there is a higher frequency of immature forms of bone, greater number of reversal lines, larger poorly defined osteocyte lacunae, Haversian canals of varying size, which combined provide the mosaic appearance characteristic of Pagetic bone. However, in the early stage of the disease, bone may not have this mosaic appearance.[48]

Two specimens were provided for this study and on a macroscopic level one section was taken from a complete well-preserved skeleton, while the other section was provided by a chalky friable bone which exfoliated on handling and came from an incomplete skeleton. The complete skeleton came from St Margaret *in combusto* (SM),[49] Norwich, the second came from Sandwell Priory (SP), both of which are English medieval cemetery sites. Sections were embedded in a plastic, polished, carbon-coated and examined using BSE-SEM imaging.[22] Radiological evidence and the distribution of lesions for SM was post-cranial[49], while the SP distribution, such as it was, was cranial.

The results demonstrated what had been seen previously, in that macroscopic preservation bears little relationship to microstructural preservation.[22] In brief, the SM specimens, which were macroscopically the best preserved, had extensive bacterial-type post-mortem remodelling[19,50,51] with little original bone remaining. While the SP specimen, a poor specimen macroscopically, had near perfect microstructural preservation.

Sandwell Priory histology

The specimen had the appearance of a high bone turnover condition not dissimilar to the early stages of Paget's disease.[48] There is evidence of increased vascularity (Figure 2a), with irregularly defined vascular canals (Figure 2b) and enlarged osteocyte lacunae within poorly organized collagen lamellae with an overall increase in cement lines (Figure 2d–f). Small diagenetic lesions were evident on the endocranial aspect only, located on likely sites of osteocyte lacunae (Figure 3a).

St Margaret in combusto histology

The SM specimen (radius) had been extensively affected by a common diagenetic process associated with bacterial ingress and consequent alteration,[19,22,50,51] and had little original bone

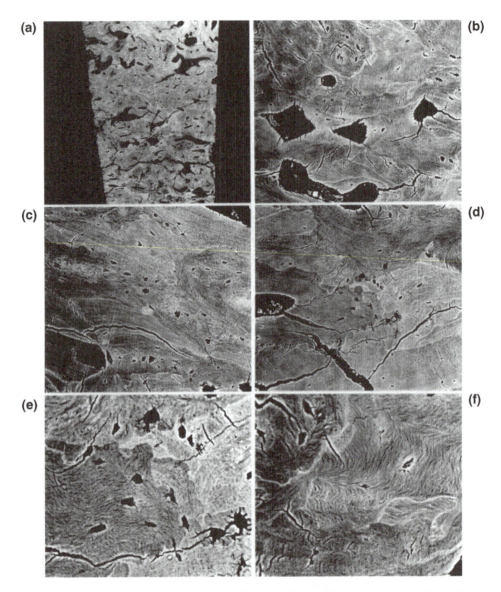

Figure 2 – (a) Sandwell Priory specimen (SP). Sagittal section of occipital bone. Increased vascularity with irregularly defined vascular canals evident among poorly organized and mineralized bone (less well-mineralized bone is darker in tone than relatively more highly mineralized bone). Field width (FW) 2600 μm. (b) SP specimen showing irregularly defined vascular canals, among many reversal lines that are hypermineralized (whiter) compared with the surrounding bone. FW 440 μm. (c) SP specimen. Centre field shows irregular and enlarged osteocyte lacunae within poorly mineralized collagen. FW 440 μm. (d) SP specimen. Two osteonal systems are seen bordering each other and at an earlier maturation state than the interstitial bone. Centre field the osteonal lamellae are poorly organized with irregularly shaped, large osteocyte lacunae. FW 440 μm. (e) SP specimen. Higher power of previous field. A hypermineralized reversal line can be seen clearly with the characteristic scalloped outline of osteoclastic resorption lacunae. The irregular osteocytes are more clearly evident, as is the arrangement of collagen, particularly in the less mature bone centre field. FW 185 μm. (f) SP specimen. An area of bone showing rapid remodelling as evidenced by several hypermineralized reversal lines close together, and the generally lower state of mineralization of bone packets. FW 185 μm.

tissue remaining. However, the specimen had the classic mosaic pattern of Pagetic bone, which had been coarsely replicated by the diagenetic process itself (Figure 3b). Similarly the left humerus exhibited large irregular vascular canals within a field of diagenetic bone (Figure 3c). The periosteal circumferential lamellae of both specimens often survived intact (Figure 3d). Internally, many osteoclastic resorption lacunae could be identified (Figure 3e). Although the density of these specimens had been profoundly altered, the diagenetic alteration had a strong orientation with the long axis of gross collagen direction (Figure 3d and f).

The two examples given above illustrate the limits of what can be gained from archaeological material at its best and worst. At its best, even bone that is incomplete and poorly preserved at a macroscopic level can provide an enormous amount of information on the underlying pathology. The SP histology suggests the early stages of developing Paget's disease within the skeleton. While the SM skeleton by comparison had good macroscopic presentation of Paget's disease with X-rays which fitted the Pagetic picture, the histopathology was severely obscured by diagenetic alteration, but Haversian organization and osteoclastic activity could still be identified, which indicated increased vascularity and bone turnover. Not only that, the microstructural changes in density do not appear to invalidate gross X-rays, since the bacterial alteration tracked and replicated the gross collagen orientation (and therefore mineral) along its long axis. Hence, the palaeohistopathological analysis in these two examples of Paget's disease has greatly aided differential diagnosis, even where the macroscopic and microstructural preservation was poor.

Modern illustrations: common pathologies affecting the maxillo-facial region

This section will cover, albeit briefly, some of the more common maxillo-facial pathologies, some of which are not exclusive to this part of the skeleton. The salient features of the pathologies discussed below include brief detail, where relevant, on age, sex and ethnic distributions, together with their radiological and histopatholgical appearance. The histopathology is drawn from modern biopsy material because there is limited comparative palaeohistopathological material currently available.

Many pathologies that present within the maxilla and mandible present as radiolucencies or radiopacities or an initial radiolucency that matures to become a radiopacity. Within modern populations, a considerable amount of pathology is picked up as an incidental finding during routine dental panoramic radiograph examination. Thus, it is possible that unless radiographic survey was being undertaken routinely, pathology would be missed. Many radiolucencies may be macroscopically visible in an archaeological specimen as periapical cavities in the alveolar bone. These cavities, whether large or small, single or multiple, are normally described within archaeological literature as abscess cavities. This is probably an oversimplification of the array of pathologies that can present in this way.[52] Thus, in an archaeological context a tentative diagnosis is often reached on the basis of the macroscopic and radiographic appearance alone, whereas in a modern clinical setting, this level of information would only provide a similar broad differential diagnosis. A subsequent 'definitive' diagnosis would normally follow further histological examination of a biopsy specimen, a process not normally undertaken on archaeological material.

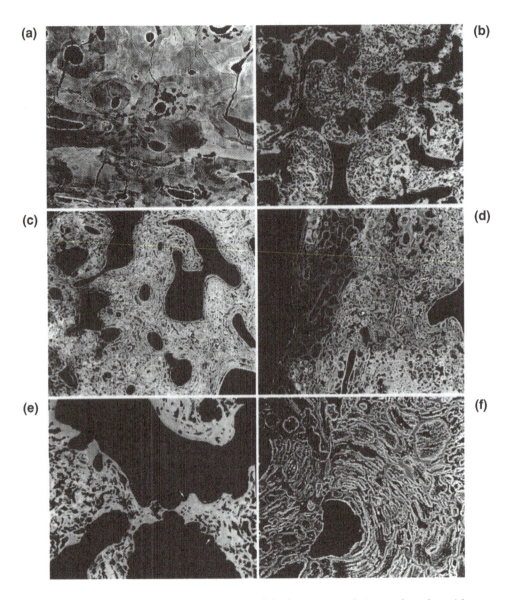

Figure 3 – (a) Sandwell Priory (SP) specimen with small focal post-mortem lesions on the endocranial aspect of the section. The diagenetic foci all had this type of morphology, located mostly within osteonal systems. FW 875 μm. (b) St Margaret *in combusto* (SM) left radius midshaft transverse section (TS). The classic 'mosaic' pattern of Paget's disease replicated by the diagenetic process. Very little of the original bone remains. FW 1900 μm. (c) SM left humerus midshaft TS. Enlarged vascular canal characteristic of increased bone turnover found in a small area of the humeral cortex. Again diagenetic ingress is almost total. FW 1660 μm. (d) SM left humerus midshaft TS. The subperiosteal circumferential lamellae in both specimens often remained intact. However, regions just below the lamellae were entirely reorganized both at a level of microstructure and density. FW 800 μm. (e) SM left radius midshaft TS. Osteoclastic resorption lacunae clearly evident as scalloped edging at the periphery of enlarged vascular spaces, even though diagenesis is prevalent. (f) SM left humerus midshaft TS. The process of diagenetic ingress is seen to orientate itself strongly with general collagen direction. Also a reversal line (top left centre field) is highlighted by two different orientations of diagenetic ingress. FW 400 μm.

Radiolucencies

Radiolucencies that occur at the apex of a tooth root are most often described as abscess cavities in the archaeological literature.[52] These may in fact be periapical granulomas or odontogenic cysts.[53] Periapical granulomas are inflammatory in origin and related to a decayed or dead tooth and are composed of reactionary mesenchymal tissue and inflammatory cells. In some instances epithelial remnants from tooth root development proliferate within the reactionary mesenchymal tissue and form a cyst, which is lined by epithelium; these are known as radicular cysts. Larger radiolucencies mimicking a radicular cyst, even if they appear to be related to a tooth root, may be due to proliferating embryonic remnants of the dental lamina, known as odontogenic keratocysts. Such cysts may be missed during macroscopic survey alone as they tend to manifest late clinically, spreading preferentially through the cancellous bone before causing appreciable bony expansion. Definitive diagnosis in a modern context is made on the basis of the histopathological examination of a biopsy specimen. A keratocyst has a thin fibrous wall which is often firmly adhered to the bony cavity and an epithelial lining about two-to-five cells thick (Figure 4). It is possible that parts of this lining may be retained within an archaeological specimen and would provide a definitive diagnosis if examined histologically. Keratocysts are linked to the syndrome Gorlin–Goltz or basal cell naevus syndrome[54] in which patients may develop multiple keratocysts of the jaws together with basal cell carcinomas of the skin and other skeletal stigmata such as bifid ribs. This syndrome has allegedly been observed in an Egyptian archaeological specimen.[55]

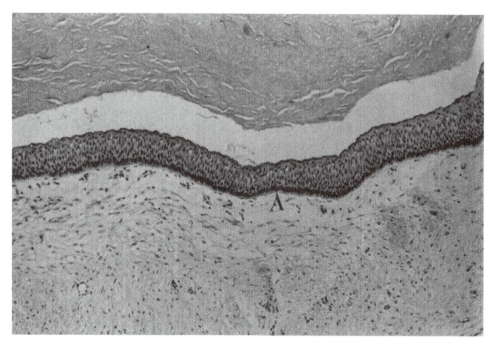

Figure 4 – Odontogenic keratocyst. The cyst comprises a fibrous wall and a parakeratinized epithelial lining (two-to-five cells thick) with columnar and hyperchromatic basal cells (arrow). Magnification ×25.

Many radiolucencies, however, may not be true cysts because they are not lined by epithelium but instead represent a vast array of different pathological processes. Such pathological processes may be divided using a surgical sieve as indicated in Table 1. Examples that may present under the relevant subdivisions as radiolucencies are: traumatic (e.g. aneurysmal bone cysts), idiopathic (e.g. central giant cell granulomas), metabolic (e.g. hyperparathyroidism) or neoplastic (e.g. multiple myeloma). Many may not be picked up on gross macroscopic examination alone and only become apparent during detailed radiological investigation with further definitive diagnosis dependant on both the experience of examiner and histopathological analysis. The salient features of their radiographic and histological features are described briefly to provide the non-specialist pathologist or archaeologist with an outline of how they may appear, should radiographic survey be undertaken and if a biopsy sample of the pathology were obtained.

The *aneurysmal bone cyst* appears radiographically as a uni- or multilocular radiolucency and occurs more commonly in the mandible during the first three decades of life. In life it is a cystic space filled with blood and lined by fibroblastic tissue. No epithelium is seen. The fibroblastic tissue of this cyst may potentially be preserved within the archaeological record and visible during a histopathological examination.[56]

Central giant cell granulomas are uncommon intra-osseous lesions that occur mainly in adolescents and young adults with a 68% female preponderance. They occur principally in the tooth-bearing areas anterior to first permanent molars, more commonly in the mandible, and are not seen in the axial skeleton. In the later stages the jaw may be obviously enlarged with exfoliation and loosening of teeth, and during initial examination of the skeleton a neoplastic or odontogenic cause may be suggested. However, radiographically a well-defined, often multilocular, radiolucent area is seen; a feature not normally associated with a neoplastic cause but which may be seen in cases of odontogenic keratocysts. Histologically, however, an absence of an epithelial lining would exclude an odontogenic keratocyst and the features visible would be delicate trabeculae of osteoid and bone together with numerous multinucleate cells embedded within a vascular fibrous stroma (Figure 5). Some of these features may be retained within the archaeological record and available for careful examination.[57]

Hyperparathyroidism is a relatively common metabolic disease today in which there is excessive parathyroid hormone secretion. It is likely that it was also present in the past.[58] It affects the middle years of life, with a female preponderance. A quote often used to describe the signs and symptoms of the disease is 'bones, stones and abdominal groans'. A generalized osteoporosis may be seen together with focal areas of resorption within the jaws and elsewhere within the axial skeleton (so called brown tumours). Kidney stones are also often present[59] and these may be retained in the archaeological record. Histopathological examination, if carried out on the bony cavity contents, should reveal an absence of an epithelial lining and together with other skeletal features, may allow a diagnosis of hyperparathyroidism to be made.

Neoplasms that affect the skeleton may be primary or secondary. On the whole, primary bony or cartilaginous neoplasms tend to present as mixed radiolucencies and radiopacities, some of which are discussed below. However, a neoplasm that shows multiple or diffuse bony

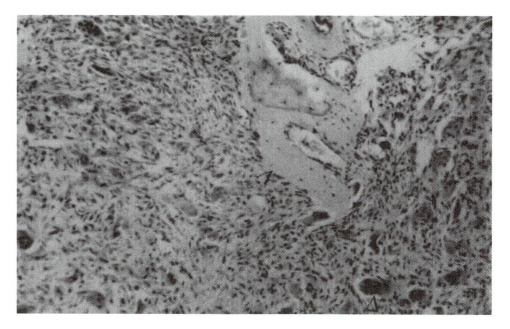

Figure 5 – Central giant cell granuloma. Islands of woven bone (arrow) together with numerous multinucleate giant cells (triangle) embedded in a fibrous stroma. Magnification ×25.

involvement is a known as a *myeloma,* which is a malignant tumour composed of mature plasma cells that occurs in older age groups (50–70 years) and is four-to-five times more common in males. The skull is involved in 70% of cases and the jaws in 30%. Radiographically 'punched-out' defects are seen which would, in life, have contained masses of plasma cells, some of which could be retained in the smaller lytic areas and therefore potentially be detectable using a polyclonal or monoclonal antibodies. A speculative suggestion would be to apply the V538 antibody (a common antigen to mature plasma cells).

Thus, not all radiolucencies are abscesses; many may be true cysts with the prominence of those in a radicular relationship being periapical granulomas or radicular cysts. However, some radiolucencies may be due to other pathologies as indicated above.

Radiopacities

Radiopacities are also relatively common within the facial skeleton and are often identified in modern populations during routine radiographic examination. They fall largely into a group of fibro- and cemento-osseous lesions that comprise both true neoplasms and dysplasias. These lesions present initially as radiolucencies, which may mature to become radiopacities. Primary bone or cartilaginous neoplasms also present as mixed radiolucent and radiopaque lesions. Examples of some of the pathologies that present as radiopacities follow.

The *cementoblastoma* is a benign odontogenic neoplasm that presents in a young age group and is more common in males. It appears as a mass of calcified material 'cementum' attached to a tooth root and is often described as Pagetoid in appearance (Figure 6). Unlike the hypercementoses seen in Paget's disease, this condition only affects a single tooth.

Another benign neoplasm is the *cemento-ossifying fibroma*. This tends to affect adults in the 20–40-year age group and is more common in females. The lesion appears similar to cases of fibrous dysplasia although it occurs in an older population. The lesion presents as a slow-growing swelling surrounded by a fibrous capsule, unlike fibrous dysplasia where the lesional tissue merges with the surrounding normal bone. Radiographically, it presents as a well defined radiolucent area containing varying amounts of calcification, which comprises metaplastic bone and cemental-like tissue (Figure 7), which may remain identifiable in the archaeological record.[60]

Other radiopaque lesions are classified as dysplasias.[61] These tend to present in older age groups and are usually multifocal. Even in modern populations they are often mistaken for multiple periapical granulomas or radicular cysts; the definitive diagnosis being made after vitality testing of the teeth, something clearly not possible in an archaeological setting or after biopsy.

Periapical cemental (fibrous) dysplasia affects females more commonly than males in the > 50-year age bracket. It affects one or more of the mandibular incisor teeth, which in life usually remain vital and without symptom. The initial radiographic changes are visible as small radiolucent areas, and as the lesion matures over time, it becomes a dense radiopaque mass.

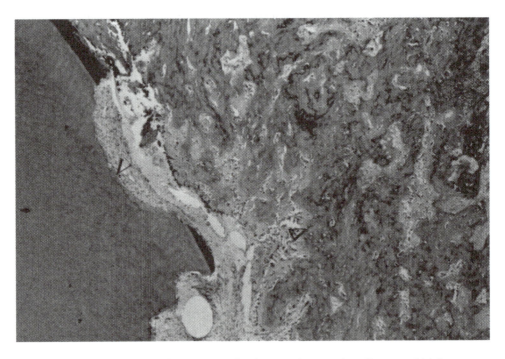

Figure 6 – Cementoblastoma. Tooth root (arrow) showing extensive resorption adjacent to which large islands of Pagetoid cemental-like tissue (triangle) are seen. Magnification ×25.

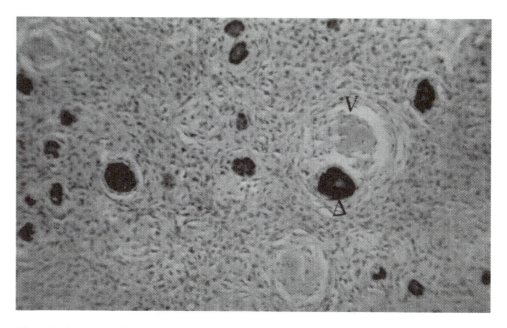

Figure 7 – Cemento-ossifying fibroma. Scattered islands of metaplastic woven bone (arrow) and smaller islands of more darkly staining cemental-like tissue (triangle) embedded in a fibrous stroma. Magnification ×40.

Histologically, replacement of normal bone with cellular fibrous tissue and progressive deposition of metaplastic bone and basophilic cemental-like tissue (Figure 8) is seen, which ultimately becomes a dense mineralized mass.

Florid cemento-osseous dysplasia (gigantiform cementoma) presents more commonly in middle aged female negroids. It occurs equally within the mandible and maxilla and is usually present in more than one quadrant, especially in the molar region. The lesions present as poorly demarcated painless swellings, which appear as dense radiopacities on radiographs. Histologically, bone is replaced by cellular fibrous tissue, which is gradually replaced by dense sheets of basophilic cemental-like tissue with little stroma (Figure 9). Both these lesions may be histologically distinguishable in skeletal remains.

The most common malignant tumour of bone is *osteosarcoma*, which has peak incidence in the 10–30-year age group in the long bones. While it is rarer within the jaws, it usually occurs much later in the > 30-year age group. It is found equally in both sexes and tends to be more common in the maxilla. It is seen within an older population as a complication of Paget's disease. A large swelling is seen with obvious signs of tooth resorption. The classical radiographic appearance is described as sunray, but this appearance varies depending upon the amount of neoplastic bone formed. Histologically, poor tumour bone is formed by malignant and pleomorphic osteoblasts[62] (Figure 10), and this microstructural arrangement would be retained within skeletal remains.

The previous examples have illustrated how radiolucent and radiopaque lesions that present within the maxillo-facial region may not be visible on macroscopic examination

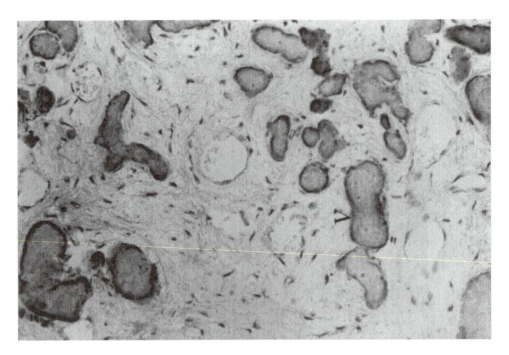

Figure 8 – Periapical cemental (fibrous) dysplasia. Rounded islands of cemental-like tissue (arrow) in a fibrous stroma. Magnification ×40.

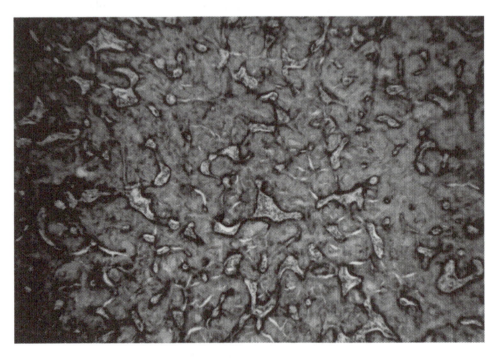

Figure 9 – Florid cemento-osseous dysplasia (gigantiform cementoma). Fused islands of cemental-like tissue. Magnification ×25.

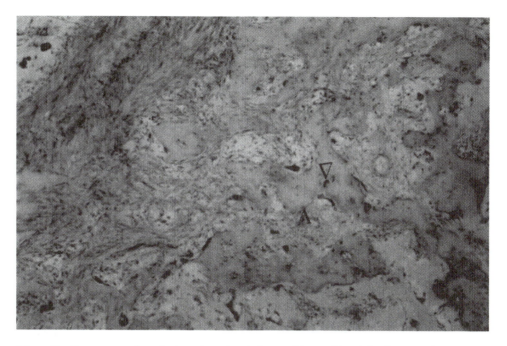

Figure 10 – Osteosarcoma. Irregular bone (arrow) and pleomorphic osteoblasts (triangle). Magnification ×25.

alone, and how their radiographic appearance, in some instances, may be inconclusive. Hence, histological examination of biopsy specimens is essential to provide a definitive diagnosis, be it in a modern clinical or an archaeological setting.

CONCLUSIONS

We have attempted to introduce palaeohistopathology, demonstrating its usefulness to the entire skeleton through case studies. Even where diagenetic change has obscured much of the internal arrangement of the original bone, such change often replicates the gross collagenous arrangement of the tissue and leaves the Haversian canals and resorption lacunae intact. Where microstructure is unaffected, the gains are large and a full assessment could be made to add significantly to the diagnostic picture. This underscores what has been demonstrated repeatedly by previous authors. It seems to us everything is to be gained from using and experimenting with this technology, where diagnostic criteria can be significantly extended, and that palaeopathology itself can, through its use, modernize at both a practical and theoretical level.

REFERENCES

1   Boyde A, Maconnachie E, Reid SA, Delling G, Mundy GR. Scanning electron microscopy in bone pathology: review of methods, potential and applications. *Scanning Electron Microscopy* 1986; **4**: 1537–1554.

2   Wakely J, Manchester K, Roberts C. Scanning electron microscopic study of normal vertebrae and ribs from early medieval human skeletons. *Journal of Archaeological Science* 1989; **16**: 627–642.

3   Jones SJ, Glorieux R, Traver R, Boyde A. The microscopic structure of bone in normal children and patients with osteogenesis imperfecta: a survey using backscattered electron imaging. *Calcified Tissue International* 1999; **64**: 8–17.

4   Warley A. *X-Ray Microanalysis for Biologists*. Practical methods in Electron Microscopy, 16. London: Portland, 1997.

5   Vesely P, Boyde A. Video rate confocal laser scanning reflection microscopy in the investigation of normal and neoplastic living cell dynamics. *Scanning Microscopy. Supplement* 1996; **10**: 201–211.

6   Stoker DJ. Imaging procedures in orthopaedic pathology. In: Salisbury JR, Woods CG, Byers PD (eds), *Diseases of Bones and Joints: Cell Biology, Mechanisms, Pathology*. London: Chapman & Hall Medical, 1994: pp. 40–59.

7   Rothschild BM. Treponemal infection in a Pleistocene bear. *Nature* 1987; **329**: 61–62.

8   Neiburger EJ. Syphilis in a Pleistocene bear. *Nature* 1988; **333**: 603.

9   Rothschild BM. Existence of syphilis in a Pleistocene bear. *Nature* 1988; **335**: 595.

10   Cook M, Molto E, Anderson C. Fluorochrome labelling in Roman period skeletons from Dakhleh Oasis, Egypt. *American Journal of Physical Anthropology* 1989; **80**: 137–143.

11   Garland AN. Microscopical analysis of fossil bone. *Applied Geochemistry* 1989; **4**: 215–229.

12   Waldron T. *Counting the Dead: The Epidemiology of Skeletal Populations*. New York: Wiley, 1994.

13   Rogers J, Waldron T. *A Field Guide to Joint Disease in Archaeology*. Chichester: Wiley, 1995.

14   Historic Scotland. *The Treatment of Human Remains in Archaeology*. Operational Policy Paper 5. Edinburgh: Historic Scotland, 1997.

15   Bell LS, Lee-Thorp JA. Advances and constraints in the study of human skeletal remains: a joint perspective. In: Cox. M (ed.), *Grave Concerns: Death and Burial in England 1700–1850*. London: Council for British Archaeology, 1998: pp. 238–246.

16   Schaffer J. Über den feineren bau fossiler knocken. *Sitzungberichte (Kais. Akademie der Wissenschaften in Wien) Mathematik, Naturwissenschaften III* 1890; **99**: 149–152.

17   Enlow DH, Brown SO. A comparative histological study of fossil and recent bone tissues, Part 1. *Texas Journal of Science* 1956; **8**: 405–443.

18   Wedl C. Über einen im zahnbein und knochen keimenden pilz. *Akademie der Wissenschaften in Wien. Sitzungungsberichte Naturwissenchafiliche Klasse ABI, Mineralogie, Biologie Erdkunde* 1864; **50**: 171–193.

19   Bell LS, Boyde A, Jones SJ. Diagenetic alteration to teeth in-situ illustrated by backscattered electron imaging. *Scanning* 1991, **13**: 173–183.

20   Falin LI. Histological and histochemical studies of human teeth of the Bronze and Stone ages. *Archives of Oral Biology* 1961; **5**: 5–13.

21   Piepenbrink H. Two examples of biogenous dead bone decomposition and their consequences for taphonomic interpretation. *Journal of Archaeological Science* 1986; **13**: 417–430.

22   Bell LS. Palaeopathology and diagenesis: an SEM evaluation of structural changes using backscattered electron imaging. *Journal of Archaeological Science* 1990; **17**: 85–102.

23   Hackett CJ. Microscopical focal destruction (tunnels) in excavated human bones. *Medicine Science and the Law* 1981; **21**: 243–265.

24   Hagelberg E, Bell LS, Allen T, Boyde A, Jones SJ, Clegg JB. Analysis of ancient bone DNA: techniques and applications. *Philosophical Transactions of the Royal Society of London Series B, Biological Sciences* 1991; **333**: 399–407.

25   Sillen A, Sealy JC, van der Merwe. Chemistry and paleodietary research: no more easy answers. *American Antiquity* 1989; **54**: 504–512.

26   Martin DL. Bone histology and paleopathology: methodological considerations. In: Ortner DJ, Aufderheide AC (eds), *Human Paleopathology: Current Syntheses and Future Options*. Washington, DC: Smithsonian Institution Press, 1991: pp. 55–59.

27   Jarcho S. The development and present condition of human paleopathology in the United States. In: Jarcho S (ed.), *Human Paleopathology*. New Haven: Yale University Press, 1966: pp. 3–42.

28   Blumberg JM, Kerley ER. A critical consideration of roentgenology and microscopy in palaeopathology. In: Jarcho S (ed.), *Human Paleopathology*. New Haven: Yale University Press, 1966: pp. 150–170.

29   Stout S, Simmons DJ. Use of histology in ancient bone research. *Yearbook of Physical Anthropology* 1979; **22**: 229–249.

30   Race GJ, Wendorf F, Humphreys SB, Fry EI. Paleopathology of ancient Nubian human bone studied by chemical and electron microscopic methods. *Journal of Human Evolution* 1972; **1**: 263–279.

31   Bell LS, Jones SJ. Macroscopic and microscopic evaluation of archaeological pathological bone: backscattered electron imaging of putative Pagetic bone. *International Journal of Osteoarchaeology* 1991; **1**: 179–184.

32   Aaron JE, Rogers J, Kanis JA. Paleohistology of Paget's disease in two medieval skeletons. *American Journal of Physical Anthropology* 1992; **89**: 325–331.

33   De la Rua C, Baraybar JP, Etxeberria F. Neolithic case of metastasizing carcinoma: multiple approaches to differential diagnosis. *International Journal of Osteoarchaeology* 1995; **5**: 254–264.

34   Grupe G. Metastasizing carcinoma in a medieval skeleton: differential diagnosis and etiology. *American Journal of Physical Anthropology* 1988; **75**: 369–374

35   Schultz M. Nature and frequency of bony tumors in prehistoric and historic populations. *In Vivo* 1990; **6**: 439–441.

36   Schultz M. Results of osteologic studies of medieval pediatric skeletons with special reference to the population of Anatolia. *Anthropologischer Anzeiger* 1989; **47**: 39–50.

37   Schultz M. Acute and chronic middle ear pathology in mediaeval man. *HNO; Zeitschrift für Hals-, Nasen-, und Ohrenheilkunde.* 1979; **27**: 77–85.

38   Schultz M. Malformations of odontogenic tissue in prehistoric human bone material. A contribution to the differential diagnosis of odontomas. *Deutsche Zahnarztliche Zeitschrift* 1978; **33**: 715–724.

39   Schultz M. Dysplastic changes in the skull of a pre-Columbian Mimbres-Indian from New Mexico. *Zeitschrift für Morphologie und Anthropologie* 1978; **69**: 43–56.

40   Schultz M. New studies and considerations on the pathology of the primate skull. A contribution to the 'Gundu' problem. *Folia Primatologica* 1977; **28**: 81–108.

41   Aufderheide AC, Rodriguez-Martin C. *The Cambridge Encyclopedia of Paleopathology*. Cambridge: Cambridge University Press, 1998.

42   Rothschild M, Martin LD. *Paleopathology: Disease in the Fossil Record*. Boca Raton: CRC Press, 1993.

43   Roberts C, Manchester K. *The Archaeology of Disease*. New York: Cornell University Press, 1997.

44   Boyde A, Jones SJ. Back-scattered electron imaging of skeletal tissues. *Metabolic Bone Disease and Related Research* 1983; **5**: 145–150.

45   Paget J. On a form of chronic inflammation of bones (osteitis deformans). *Transactions of the Medico-Chirurgical Society.* 1877; **60**: 37–64.

46   Cartwright EJ, Gordon MT, Freemont AJ *et al.* Paramyxovirus and Paget's disease. *Journal of Medical Virology* 1993; **40**: 133–141.

47   Woods CG. Metabolic bone diseases. In: Salisbury JR, Woods CG, Byers PD (eds), *Diseases of Bones and Joints: Cell Biology, Mechanisms, Pathology*. London: Chapman & Hall Medical, 1994: pp. 236–285.

48   Tillman HH. Paget's disease of bone. *Oral Surgery, Oral Medicine, Oral Pathology* 1962; **15**: 1225–1234.

49   Stirland A. Paget's disease (osteitis deformans): a classic case? *International Journal of Osteoarchaeology* 1991; **1**: 173–177.

50   Bell LS, Skinner MF, Jones SJ. The speed of post mortem change to the human skeleton and its taphonomic significance. *Forensic Science International* 1996; **82**: 129–140.

51   Yoshinio M, Kimijima T, Miyasaka S, Sato H, Sueshige S. Microscopical study on estimation of time since death in skeletal remains. *Forensic Science International* 1991; **49**: 143–158.

52   Dias G, Tayles N, 'Abscess cavity' – a misnomer. *International Journal of Osteoarchaeology* 1997; **7**: 548–554.

53   Shear M. *Cysts of the Oral Regions* (3rd edn). Bristol: Wright, 1992.

54   Gorlin RJ. Naevoid basal cell carcinoma syndrome. *Medicine* 1987; **66**: 98–113.

55   Satinoff MI, Wells C. Multiple basal cell naevus syndrome in ancient Egypt. *Medical History* 1969; **13**: 294–297.

56   Vergel Am, Bond JR, Shives TC, McLeod RA, Unni KK. Aneurysmal bone cyst: a clinicopathologic study of 228 cases. *Cancer* 1992; **69**: 2921–2931.

57   Whittaker SB, Waldron CA. Central giant cell lesions of the jaws. A clinical, radiologic and histopathological study. *Oral Surgery, Oral Medicine, Oral Pathology* 1993; **75**: 199–208.

58   Cook M, Molto E, Anderson C. Possible case of hyperparathroidism in a Roman period skeleton form the Dakhleh Oasis, Egypt, diagnoses using bone histomorphometry. *American Journal of Physical Anthropology* 1988; **75**: 23–30.

59   Silverberg SJ, Shane E, Jacobs TP, Siris ES, Gartenberg F, Seldin D, Clemens TL, Bilezikian JP. Nephrolithiasis and bone involvement in primary hyperparathyroidism. *American Journal of Medicine* 1990; **89**: 327–334 .

60   Eversole LR, Leider As, Nelson K Ossifying fibromas: a clinical pathologic study of sixty-four cases. *Oral Surgery, Oral Medicine, Oral Pathology* 1985; **60**: 505–511.

61   Waldron CA Fibro-osseous lesions of the jaws. *Journal of Oral and Maxillofacial Surgery* 1993; **51**: 828–835.

62   Clark JL, Unni KK, Dahlin DS, Devine KD. Osteosarcoma of the jaws. *Cancer* 1983; **51**: 2311–2316.

Section IV

Human variation

This section focuses on the metric and non-metric study of normal skeletal variation. Simon Mays discusses reasons for the decline of interest among British workers over the past few decades in craniometry for the study of ancient migrations. He makes the case for a renewal of interest in craniometry, citing the fact that the potential of craniometric analyses to examine migrations of peoples and other aspects of population history fits neatly with the recent prominence enjoyed by issues such as early migrations and ethnicity in archaeological theory. Such work may act as a spur to enhance the integration of osteological evidence with material culture. Andrew Tyrell provides a much-needed review of the role of non-metric traits in the assessment of inter- and intra-population diversity. This area of research likewise has enormous potential to contribute to current archaeological debates about ancient population dynamics. He warns against an over-simplistic use of non-metric traits to determine relatedness within cemetery assemblages, while displaying optimism that further research may elucidate their significance and causation.

Moving away from such studies, James Steele provides an interesting overview of human handedness, firmly placing it in its evolutionary and cultural context. He discusses skeletal indicators of handedness, focusing on asymmetries in paired elements in the upper limb and shoulder girdle. The study of skeletal asymmetry clearly has great value for investigating handedness patterns in past populations and for helping individualise remains in forensic cases.

The final chapter by Richard Neave discusses the reconstruction of facial appearance from skull morphology. He considers methodological issues, both relating to traditional modelling techniques and to more recently developed computer-based methods. He also reminds us that what is produced using techniques of facial reconstruction is in fact an approximation of the facial appearance of the living subject rather than an exact portrait. Facial reconstruction is clearly of great utility in assisting personal identification of unknown remains in forensic cases, but its use on archaeological skeletal material is also of value, particularly when presenting archaeological work to the public, as it may help to individualize a past that may otherwise seem rather remote and impersonal.

17

BIODISTANCE STUDIES USING CRANIOMETRIC VARIATION IN BRITISH ARCHAEOLOGICAL SKELETAL MATERIAL

Simon Mays

INTRODUCTION

A survey of recent osteoarchaeological publications[1] indicates that the study of normal skeletal variation has been rather neglected by British workers compared with those in some other countries. In particular, very few biodistance studies using cranial variation have recently been conducted. There are a number of possible reasons for this dearth of craniometric biodistance work. In part it may simply reflect the observation that most British osteologists are rather more interested in the study of pathological lesions than in normal skeletal variation.[1] However, it can also be viewed, in the broader context, as being linked with the general decline in interest in population history witnessed in the last few decades in British archaeology. The ultimate causes of this decline in the archaeological study of population history in the UK are complex and are likely embedded in the cultural and political milieu in which we work,[2,3] however, an important proximate factor is the theoretical shift which has taken place within archaeology as a whole during recent decades. Until the 1960s, major changes in material culture and other aspects of the archaeological record in the UK were generally explained in terms of invading or immigrant peoples. Within this framework craniometry played a central role, as skulls were measured in an effort to find evidence for ancient migrations. In the 1960s, radiocarbon dating forced a re-think of this traditional framework, as many cultural developments in the UK and other parts of western Europe were found to predate their supposed antecedents in south-east Europe and the Near East.[4] At this time there was also a general theoretical re-orientation, as it became widely acknowledged that explanations for culture change in the past were likely much more complex than simple migrations and replacements of peoples. There was a general movement away from particularistic approaches to the past, in which changes visible archaeologically were ascribed to specific historical events (such as migrations), towards an emphasis on the study of process, influenced by the rise of the so-called 'New Archaeology' in North America. The result was a reaction against 'migrationism' and a growing tendency to favour explanations involving continuity of populations and indigenous cultural development over those invoking migrations or invasions. In Britain this reaction in favour of stressing continuity was particularly strong among prehistorians, so that in recent decades little work has been done on the study of prehistoric migrations.

However, there have recently been signs of a revival of interest among British prehistorians in ancient migrations. At a theoretical level, the recent rise of post-processual archaeology may have created an academic environment more favourable to the study of early migrations; post-processual approaches place an emphasis on constructing a historically specific account of past societies in which events as well as processes assume importance.[5] It has also been emphasized[6,7] that the analysis of migrations can be accommodated within a processual framework, by treating them as patterned, dynamic human behaviour, explicable through general principles, rather than unique, one-off events. In addition, there is currently an increasing interest in the archaeological study of ethnicity,[8,9] of which biological relationships are an important component. The recent recognition among archaeologists of the potential of linguistics and modern population genetics to inform us about population history[10–12] has acted as a further spur to renewed study of ancient migrations.

This recent rise in interest in early migrations among British archaeologists has not led to an increase in craniometric work. It might be suggested that this is a reflection of the lack of integration between human osteoarchaeology and the rest of archaeology, which has been evident since the 1960s. Since then much osteological work has been of a palaeopathological nature driven by medico-historical rather than archaeological questions. However, the increasing adoption by British osteologists in recent years of a 'biocultural' approach, which emphasizes the integration of biological and cultural evidence, has led to an osteoarchaeology better equipped to address questions of mainstream archaeological importance, rather than of mainly specialist interest, but this has not led to a revival of craniometry. There has been little stimulus from mainstream archaeology for craniometric biodistance studies. This reflects the rather jaundiced view of craniometry held by many archaeologists whose training is not in osteology. The value of craniometric work for investigating ancient migrations is denigrated, and it appears to be seen as a rather old-fashioned and politically questionable pursuit. Indeed one prominent British archaeologist has asserted that craniometry has recently 'enjoyed about as much prestige in scientific circles as phrenology' (p. 4).[13] Given this erroneous but (in the UK) distressingly widespread view of craniometry, it is perhaps worth at this point summarizing briefly its value for biodistance studies.

VALUE OF CRANIOMETRY IN BIODISTANCE STUDIES

Both genetic and non-genetic factors influence skull form.[14] Among the non-genetic factors which exert an influence are diet, nutrition and climate. In some instances patterning in craniometric data in skeletal series has been understood in these terms.[14] However, despite the undoubted influence of extraneous factors, it is clear that there is a strong genetic component in cranial variability. The evidence for this comes from animal breeding studies, and also from work on man, in the form of family studies using cephalometry or anthropometry. Reviewing this literature, Kohn[15] indicates that a high degree of inheritance of cranial dimensions has been a consistent finding. Large-scale studies using human populations whose biological relationships are known or can reasonably be inferred, have provided confirmation that the degree of genetic causation in cranial variation is sufficient to render craniometry useful for investigating biological relationships among human populations. Studies have shown that there is a strong correlation between biological relationships among human groups revealed by biochemical genetic markers and those inferred from anthropometric measurements.[16,17] Anthropometric traits have enabled successful discrimination between groups living in different villages within restricted geographical areas.[18] They have also enabled historical population relationships to be reconstructed between groups living over broader geographical zones.[19–21]

In archaeology, the value of craniometric analyses has been amply demonstrated, as they have made major contributions to some important questions and debates. Studies of cranial variation in various skeletal series around the world have helped shed light on modern human origins and affinities between different populations.[22–24] Craniometric work has also aided the study of patterns of dispersal of human groups into new lands – for example the first human settlement of South America.[25,26] Regional studies have helped shed light on questions as diverse as the origins of intensive rice agriculture in Japan,[14] the rise of the Oxus civilization in south-west Asia,[27] and in North America, prehistoric migrations of Amerindian groups[28] and ingress of European traders during the historic era.[29]

METHODOLOGICAL ISSUES

Linear measurements between landmarks have long been the mainstay of craniometry. During the early 19th century measurements, and the measuring instruments to take them, began to be devised in order that differences in cranial morphology might be quantified. During the late 19th and early 20th century, attempts at standardization of cranial landmarks, measurement techniques and nomenclature were made, and these culminated in the production of osteometric textbooks[30] which are still in use today, or at least form the basis for more recent works.

There are clearly limitations in using simple linear measurements and angles to describe the morphology of a complex three-dimensional object such as a skull. In recent years, computer-linked methods for capture and analysis of three-dimensional coordinate[31] or surface[32] data have been devised. Although these have made an impact in some areas of human osteoarchaeology (e.g. in studies of artificial cranial deformation[33]), their impact on craniometric biodistance studies has been negligible. The continued primacy of linear measurement data in this field may be associated with a number of factors. Callipers are relatively inexpensive and readily portable so that a researcher can easily travel around museums collecting data. Linear measurement data tend to be normally distributed. This renders them tractable to analysis using standard multivariate techniques, and amenable to parametric significance testing. Statistical treatment of three-dimensional morphometric data may be rather more problematic.[31] Three-dimensional morphometric data presumably provide more encompassing measures of morphology than do simple combinations of linear measurements. Although it seems intuitively likely that these more sensitive measures of cranial form would yield improved inferences when applied to population historical studies, this has yet to be demonstrated. One suspects that only when it can be shown that three-dimensional morphometric techniques offer decisive advantages by revealing insights into population history which would remain hidden to conventional multivariate analysis of linear dimensions, will they make a significant impact on craniometric biodistance studies.

CONTRIBUTION OF CRANIOMETRIC ANALYSES TO THE STUDY OF BRITISH POPULATION HISTORY

The role of migration of farming peoples in the spread of agriculture throughout most of Europe in the Neolithic, has long been debated.[34] In recent years, studies of genetic and linguistic aspects of modern European populations have made an important contribution to this debate. For example, Renfrew and co-workers have used modern gene frequencies[11] and language distributions[10] to argue for the expansion of Neolithic farming peoples northwards and westwards from a centre in the Near East into regions previously occupied by hunter-gatherers. However, analysis of mitochondrial DNA in modern Europeans[12] seems to suggest that the great majority of maternal lineages stretch back to the Palaeolithic and do not derive from some advancing wave of Neolithic farmers. The apparent conflict between these results has yet to be resolved.

Craniometric analysis of excavated skeletal material clearly has the potential to make a contribution to this debate, and indeed some work has been done in this direction although progress has been hampered by shortage of suitable skeletal material, especially from Mesolithic contexts. A general metric study of European Neolithic crania[35] revealed no evidence for a south-east to north-west clinal pattern in morphology that might be indicative of demic diffusion of Neolithic colonists from a centre in the Near East. However, different models of Neolithization may apply in different areas of Europe. Osteological evidence supporting the idea of Neolithic migrants has emerged for some regions in which both Mesolithic and Neolithic material are available for comparison. Fox[36] found evidence for cranial morphological change between Mesolithic and Neolithic groups in Iberia. He argues that the nature of the changes observed is not consistent with that which might be expected simply as a result of a change from hunter-gatherer to agricultural diets, but rather indicates population replacement (but see Jackes *et al.*[37] for an alternative viewpoint). Analysis of material from the Iron Gates region of Serbia,[38] suggested the influx of a new population there in the Neolithic. In Britain, the dearth of Mesolithic human remains means that it is difficult to use skeletal evidence to analyse the role, if any, played by colonization in the introduction of agriculture at the start of the Neolithic period. However, the skeletal evidence does make an important contribution to the study of culture change at the end of the British Neolithic.

At the Neolithic–Bronze Age transition in the UK, a change in burial practices occurred, with the appearance of single inhumations, covered by a round barrow and accompanied by distinctive grave goods, particularly finely decorated pottery beakers (Figure 1). This period also saw the introduction of metalwork.[40,41] Within the traditional explanatory framework, which held sway in British archaeology until the 1960s, the changes observed at the

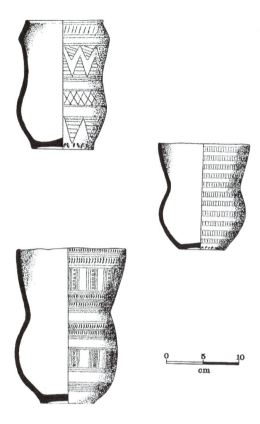

Figure 1 – Beaker pottery from various British sites. After Critall.[39]

Neolithic–Bronze Age transition were ascribed to invaders or immigrant peoples – the so-called 'Beaker Folk'. This idea seemed to be supported by the observation of a marked difference in cranial form between Neolithic and Bronze Age specimens, those from the Neolithic having a lower cranial index than the more rounded Bronze Age skulls (Figure 2). From the 1960s, when migration hypotheses started to fall from favour, they were replaced as explanations for the Beaker phenomenon with various hypotheses involving the movement of goods rather than people. Workers who suggested these 'non-migrationist' explanations built their hypotheses mainly or entirely around the cultural evidence; the osteological data was generally accorded only cursory discussion if it was considered at all.

The visual difference in cranial form between British Neolithic and Beaker period material, which has been noted since the 19th century, has been confirmed metrically. Brothwell and Krzanowski[42] conducted a multivariate analysis of cranial vault measurements in British material, and found a good separation between Neolithic and Bronze Age skulls. Twenty years later, Brodie[43] conducted another multivariate study. Unlike Brothwell and Krzanowski, he had access to crania with facial bones intact for measurement, and he demonstrated that differences between Beaker and Neolithic crania were essentially restricted to differences in vault length and breadth.

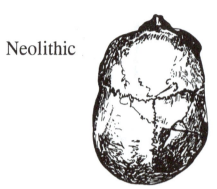

Neolithic

Beaker

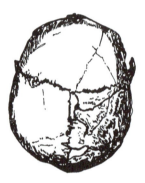

Figure 2 – Superior view of typical long-headed Neolithic and round-headed Beaker skulls from Britain. After Harrison.[41]

Many writers[44] who have argued against migration playing a major role in the Beaker phenomenon in the UK, have emphasized that most British Neolithic bones come from early or middle Neolithic contexts. Several centuries separate them from the Beaker period, plenty of time, they claim, for morphological changes to occur in the absence of population movements. Brodie[43] did have access to a small number of late Neolithic crania, which had not been available to earlier workers. The late Neolithic material grouped with the early and middle Neolithic crania, suggesting that the change in cranial form can indeed be dated to the transition to the Bronze Age, although this inference must remain tentative due to the small number of late Neolithic skulls upon which it is based.

It might be argued that some non-genetic factor such as climate or diet might be behind the change in cranial form; however, there is no independent evidence for major changes in these parameters at the Neolithic–Bronze Age transition in the UK. In addition, the nature of the cranial changes observed is inconsistent with those expected if these non-genetic factors were playing an important role. For example, although there is some evidence for an association between cranial index and climate, other areas of the skull which are known to be climate-sensitive (e.g. the nasal aperture) show no change at the Neolithic–Bronze Age transition.[43] There is also no sign of any change in the morphology of the jaws and other areas directly associated with the chewing apparatus[43,45] as might be expected if dietary change were an important cause of the alterations in cranial morphology in this instance.

Although it can hardly be said that the craniometric data provide an unequivocal answer to the problem of the Beaker Folk, the balance of the evidence would at present seem to favour a migration hypothesis. Although one could argue that some, as yet unidentified, non-genetic factors might be responsible for the change in cranial form, arrival of migrants does seem to be the most parsimonious explanation for the discontinuities observed in the oste-ological and the cultural evidence during the Neolithic–Bronze Age transition. The picture would perhaps be clarified further if British crania could be compared with series from Continental Europe, particularly the Lower Rhine area, from whence any Beaker migrants into Britain are traditionally thought to have come. Analyses of dental metrics, and dental and osteological non-metric data would also be helpful, both to determine whether discon-tinuities exist in these aspects at the Neolithic–Bronze Age transition in the UK, and to form additional comparisons with any suitable Continental material.

One of the few 'migration explanations' for culture change that survived the upheavals of the 1960s in British prehistoric archaeology relates to the Iron Age Arras culture. The Arras culture is known mainly from burials, and is confined to a small area of eastern Yorkshire.[46] Arras culture burials date from the 4th to 1st century BC, and are inhumations, generally crouched, placed beneath square barrows. The burials are often accompanied by grave goods; sometimes these may be quite elaborate, as in the cart or chariot burials (Figure 3) which are occasionally found.[47,48] Arras culture burials often occur in large cemeteries, containing several hundred graves, and as such are the earliest large inhumation cemeteries in England.

The Arras culture shows strong continental parallels in both burial practices and material culture.[49] In addition, there is also some documentary evidence that may support a conti-nental origin. Ptolemy, in the 2nd century AD, described a tribe he called the Parisi occu-pying the area of east Yorkshire now associated with archaeological finds of the Arras culture. Given the continuity of the Yorkshire Arras culture until the Roman conquest, the tribal name Parisi may date back to the dawn of the Arras culture here.[49] A tribe of the same name were settled in northern France, at least by Caesar's time, and in preceding centuries vehicle burials are known from this area.[50] This may support the idea that a group origi-nating from northern France gave rise to the Arras culture in east Yorkshire, indeed the historical and archaeological evidence as a whole is such that it has long been believed that the insular Arras culture was the product of colonisation from this area of Continental Europe.[51] Although some writers[52] have interpreted it as a local development, the prevailing view[49] still seems to favour some sort of intrusion by migrants from mainland Europe. Whether this took the form of a small-scale initial colonization, which then resulted in the transmission of an alien culture to the indigenous inhabitants, or was a larger scale migra-tion is at present unclear.

As with the Beaker example, the debate over the role of colonization in the rise of the Yorkshire Arras culture has centred on the cultural evidence, not the osteological remains of the people themselves. One problem with the osteological evidence is the dearth of

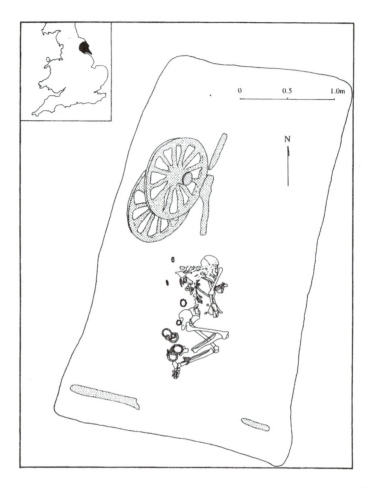

Figure 3 – An Arras Culture burial accompanied by a cart and other grave goods. After Stead.[48] The inset shows the location of Arras Culture burials in England.

contemporary Iron Age skeletal material from England with which to compare the remains from Arras culture sites. However, Arras culture material has been included in two fairly recent craniometric studies. Leese[53] found that crania from a number of Arras culture sites formed a fairly homogenous group. Dawes[54] included Arras culture material from Wetwang Slack and from Danes' Graves, Driffield, in a multivariate cranial study. She found that the Danes' Graves and Wetwang Slack material clustered together, and was distinct from Roman and Anglian crania from York, and from material from the Yorkshire Bronze Age. This might be interpreted as supporting the idea of the Arras people as migrants, but such a conclusion would be premature at this stage; further osteological work is needed before firm inferences can be made.

The reaction against explanations for culture change involving migrations was not nearly as strong among those studying the archaeology of the historic eras as it was among prehistorians. One reason for this is that the influence of changes in archaeological theory, particularly the advent of the American New Archaeology, was much less than it was on prehistorians, perhaps because of the close ties that archaeological period specialists dealing with the historic eras have with the historical disciplines. Another was that the sheer weight of non-archaeological evidence meant that the occurrence of migrations could hardly be denied, and they could not be ignored if an adequate understanding of these periods was to be obtained. For example, it is clear from written sources, and from linguistic and place name evidence that, following the end of Roman occupation in the 5th century AD, there was settlement in the UK by migrants from northern Germany and southern Scandinavia; the archaeological evidence also supports this.[55,56] However, the scale of this migration, and its patterning in time and space are unclear. Despite the existence of more than 5000 5th–7th-century AD skeletons excavated from sites in England,[57] few investigations of early Saxon migration into Britain using osteological evidence have been done. Richards *et al.*[58] attempted, without much success, to address the issue using ancient DNA. Härke[59,60] investigated cultural and osteological (but not craniometric) aspects of early Saxon male burials accompanied by weapons, and suggested that 5th–6th-century AD weapon burials may have been of individuals of Germanic origin. Lloyd-Jones[61] investigated non-metric variation in some Romano-British and early Saxon period skeletons from south-east England, and found that results generally supported biological continuity with no evidence for large numbers of incomers in early Saxon times. No recent large-scale craniometric studies investigating population history in the 5th–7th centuries AD in the UK appear to have been published.

CONCLUSIONS

For a long period the study of ancient migrations has been deeply unfashionable in British archaeology. In the minds of many, the analysis of migrations in archaeology was tainted by its past association with simplistic ideas of culture change. However, this attitude is fading, and changes in theory and practice in British archaeology in recent years have created a climate much more conducive to studying population history in general, and ancient migrations in particular. No one would advocate a return to the days when a simple sequence of migrations and invasions was held to account for the changes visible in the archaeological record. However, the study of ancient migrations and population history in general is an important area of academic enquiry in other disciplines,[7] and ought not to be neglected in archaeology. Population movement can be incorporated as a variable in general models which attempt to account for change and to describe periods of transition in the past. In this way a more complete picture of change in past cultures can be obtained. Adequate analysis of ancient migrations will involve both cultural and osteological evidence. Osteological analyses can aid the recognition of population movements in the archaeological record, and when evidence is found for them may aid the elucidation of the nature of these events or processes and their temporal and geographical extent. One would hope, therefore, that the scientific analysis of human remains will once more play a significant role in the study of ancient migrations in the UK, and indeed no adequate analysis of the phenomenon, particularly in the prehistoric past, can be conducted without analysing the remains of the people themselves. Although a variety of biochemical and morphological analyses are likely to be useful in this respect, the fact that genetic factors make a major contribution to cranial form ought to ensure that craniometry plays a major role.

REFERENCES

1   Mays S. A perspective on human osteoarchaeology in Britain. *International Journal of Osteoarchaeology* 1997; **7**: 600–604.

2   Clark G. The invasion hypothesis in British archaeology. *Antiquity* 1966; **40**: 172–189.

3   Härke H. Archaeologists and migrations, a problem of attitude. *Current Anthropology* 1998; **39**: 19–24.

4   Renfrew C. *Before Civilisation*. Harmondsworth: Pengiun, 1973.

5   Champion T. Migration revived. *Journal of Danish Archaeology* 1992; **9**: 214–218.

6   Anthony DW. Migration in archaeology: the baby and the bathwater. *American Anthropologist* 1990; **92**: 895–914.

7   Anthony D. Prehistoric migration as social process. In: Chapman, J, Hamerow, H (eds), *Migrations and Invasions in Archaeological Explanation*. British Archaeological Reports, International Series, No. 664. Oxford: Archaeopress, 1997; 21–32.

8   Shennan S (ed.), *Archaeological Approaches to Cultural Identity*. London: Routledge, 1989.

9   Jones S. *The Archaeology of Ethnicity*. London: Routledge, 1997.

10 Renfrew C. Archaeology, genetics and linguistic diversity. *Man* 1992; **27**: 445–478.

11 Barbujani G, Pilastro A, DeDominico S, Renfrew C. Genetic variation in North Africa and Eurasia: Neolithic demic diffusion vs. Palaeolithic colonisation. *American Journal of Physical Anthropology* 1994; **95**: 137–154.

12 Richards M, Corte-Real H, Forster P, Macauley V, Wilkinson-Herbots H, Demaine A *et al*. Palaeolithic and Neolithic lineages in the European mitochondrial gene pool. *American Journal of Human Genetics*, 1996; **59**: 185–203.

13 Renfrew C. *Archaeology and Language: The Puzzle of Indo-European Origins*. London: Cape, 1987.

14 Mays S. *The Archaeology of Human Bones*. London: Routledge/English Heritage, 1998.

15 Kohn LAP. The role of genetics in craniofacial morphology and growth. *Annual Review of Anthropology* 1991; **20**: 261–278.

16 Salzano FM, Callegari J, Franco MHLP, Hutz MH, Weimer RSS, da Rocha FJ. The Caingang revisited: blood genetics and anthropometry. *American Journal of Physical Anthropology* 1980; **53**: 513–524.

17 Vecci F, Coppa A, Priori R. Morphological distance between four ethnic groups in southern Mexico. *Rivista di Antropologia (Roma)* 1987; **65**: 223–234.

18 Spielman RS, Smouse PE. Multivariate classification of human populations I. Allocation of Yanomama Indians to villages. *American Journal of Human Genetics* 1976; **28**: 317–331.

19 Heathcote GM. Population history reconstruction, based on craniometry I. The backtracking approach and initial results. *Human Evolution* 1994; **9**: 97–119.

20 Rightmire GP. Metric versus discrete traits in African skulls. In: Giles E, Friedlaender JS (eds), *The Measures of Man: Methodologies in Biological Anthropology*. New York: Peabody, 1976; pp. 383–407.

21 Zegura S. Taxonomic congruence in Eskimoid populations. *American Journal of Physical Anthropology* 1975; **43**: 271–284.

22 Howells WW. *Skull Shapes and the Map*. Papers of the Peabody Museum of Archaeology and Ethnology, Harvard University, vol. 79. Harvard: Harvard University Press, 1989.

23 Hanihara T. Comparison of craniofacial features of major human groups. *American Journal of Physical Anthropology* 1996; **99**: 389–412.

24 Relethford JH, Harpending HC. Craniometric variation, genetic theory, and modern human origins. *American Journal of Physical Anthropology*, 1994; **95**: 249–270.

25 Neves WA, Pucciarelli HM. Morphological affinities of the first Americans: an exploratory analysis based on early South American human remains. *Journal of Human Evolution* 1991; **21**: 261–273.

26 Munford D, Zanni AD, Neves WA. Human cranial variation in South America: implications for the settlement of the New World. *Brazilian Journal of Genetics* 1995; **18**: 673–688.

27   Hemphill, BE. Biological affinities and adaptations of Bronze Age Bactrians: IV. A craniometric investigation of Bactrian origins. *American Journal of Physical Anthropology* 1999; **108**: 173–192.

28   Steadman DW. The population shuffle in the central Illinois Valley: a diachronic model of Mississippian biocultural interactions. *World Archaeology* 1998; **30**: 306–326.

29   Janz RL, Owsley DW. White traders in the upper Missouri: evidence from the Swan Creek site. In: Owsley DW, Janz RL (eds), *Skeletal Biology of the Great Plains: Migration, Warfare, Health and Subsistence*. Washington, DC: Smithsonian Institution Press, 1994: pp. 189–201.

30   Martin R. *Lehrbuch der Anthropologie in Systematische Darstellung*. Jena: Fischer, 1928.

31   Richtsmeier JT, Cheverud JM, Lele S. Advances in anthropological morphometrics. *Annual Review of Anthropology* 1992; **21**: 283–305.

32   Dean D. The analysis and collection of coordinate data in physical anthropology. In: Boaz NT, Wolfe LD (eds), *Biological Anthropology: The State of the Science*. Corvallis: IIHER, 1995; pp. 169–181.

33   Kohn LAP, Leight SR, Cheverud JM. Asymmetric vault modification in Hopi crania. *American Journal of Physical Anthropology* 1995; **98**: 173–195.

34   Childe VG. *The Prehistory of European Society*. London: Penguin, 1958.

35   Harding RM, Rösing FW, Sokal RR. Cranial measurements do not support neolithisation of Europe by demic expansion. *Homo* 1989; **40**: 45–58.

36   Fox CL. Physical anthropological aspects of the Mesolithic–Neolithic transition in the Iberian Peninsula. *Current Anthropology* 1996; **37**: 689–695.

37   Jackes M, Lubell D, Meikeljohn C. On Physical anthropological aspects of the Mesolithic–Neolithic transition in the Iberian Peninsula. *Current Anthropology* 1997; **38**: 839–846.

38   Menk R, Nemeskéri J. The transition from Mesolithic to Early Neolithic in Southeastern and Eastern Europe: An Anthropological Outline. In: Hershkovitz I (ed.), *People and Culture in Change*. British Archaeological Reports, International Series No. 508. Oxford: Tempus Reparatum, 1989; pp. 531–539.

39   Critall E. *A History of Wiltshire*, vol. 1, part 2. London: Victoria County History, University of London Institute for Historical Research, 1973.

40   Parker-Pearson M. *Bronze Age Britain*. London: Batsford/English Heritage, 1993.

41   Harrison RJ. *The Beaker Folk*. London: Thames & Hudson, 1980.

42   Brothwell DR, Krzanowski W. Evidence of biological differences between early British populations from Neolithic to mediaeval times as revealed by eleven commonly available cranial vault measurements. *Journal of Archaeological Science* 1974; **1**: 249–260.

43   Brodie N. *The Neolithic–Bronze Age Transition in Britain*. British Archaeological Reports, British Series, No. 238. Oxford: Tempus Reparatum, 1994.

44   Burgess C, Shennan S. The Beaker phenomenon: some suggestions. In: Burgess C, Miket R (eds), *Settlement and Economy in the 3rd and 2nd Millenia BC*. British Archaeological Reports, British Series, No. 33. Oxford: Tempus Reparatum, 1976; pp. 309–331.

45   Moore WJ, Lavelle CLB, Spence TF. Changes in the size and shape of the human mandible in Britain. *British Dental Journal* 1968; **125**: 163–169.

46   Dent JS. Cemeteries and settlement patterns of the Iron Age on the Yorkshire Wolds. *Proceedings of the Prehistoric Society* 1982; **48**: 437–457.

47   Dent JS. Three cart burials from Wetwang, Yorkshire. *Antiquity* 1985; **59**: 85–92.

48   Stead, IM. *Iron Age Cemeteries in East Yorkshire*. Archaeological Report No. 22. London: English Heritage, 1991.

49   Cunliffe B. *Iron Age Communities in Britain* (3rd edn). London: Routledge, 1991.

50   Stead IM. *The Arras Culture*. York: Yorkshire Philosophical Society, 1979.

51   Whimster R. *Burial Practices in Iron Age Britain*. British Archaeological Reports, British Series No. 90. BAR: Oxford, 1981: p193.

52   Higham N. Brigantia revisited. *Northern History* 1987; **23**: 1–19.

53   Leese M. A preliminary statistical survey. In: Stead IM (ed.), *Iron Age Cemeteries in East Yorkshire*. Archaeological Report No. 22. London: English Heritage, 1991; pp. 171–178.

54   Dawes JD The human bones. In: Dawes JD, Magilton JR. *The Cemetery of St Helen-on-the-Walls, Aldwark*. The Archaeology of York 12/1. York: Council for British Archaeology, 1980; pp. 19–120.

55   Hamerow H. Migration theory and the Anglo-Saxon 'identity crisis'. In: Chapman, J, Hamerow, H (eds), *Migrations and Invasions in Archaeological Explanation*. British Archaeological Reports, International Series, No. 664. Oxford: Archaeopress, 1997; pp. 33–44.

56   Scull C. Archaeology, early Anglo-Saxon society and the origins of Anglo-Saxon kingdoms. *Anglo-Saxon Studies in Archaeology and History* 1993; **6**: 65–82.

57   Mays S. A computer database of sites yielding human bone in England. London: English Heritage (unpublished).

58   Richards M, Smalley K, Sykes B, Hedges R. Archaeology and genetics: analysing DNA from skeletal remains. *World Archaeology* 1993; **25**: 18–28.

59   Härke H. 'Warrior Graves'? The background of an Anglo-Saxon burial rite. *Past and Present* 1990; **126**: 22–43.

60   Härke H. Changing symbols in a changing society: the Anglo-Saxon weapon burial rite in the seventh century. In: Carver MOH (ed.), *The Age of Sutton Hoo*. Woodbridge: Boydell, 1992; pp. 149–165.

61   Lloyd-Jones J. Calculating biodistance using dental morphology. In: Anderson S, Boyle K (eds), *Computing and Statistics in Osteoarchaeology*. Proceedings of the 2nd Meeting of the Osteoarchaeological Research Group, 1995. Oxford: Oxbow, 1997; pp. 23–30.

18

SKELETAL NON-METRIC TRAITS AND THE ASSESSMENT OF INTER- AND INTRA-POPULATION DIVERSITY: PAST PROBLEMS AND FUTURE POTENTIAL

Andrew Tyrrell

INTRODUCTION

Biological anthropology is largely the analysis of human diversity and variation. Skeletal non-metric traits are one type of human variation which can provide useful data for insight into processes of assortative mating, levels of interbreeding, gene flow, drift and population dissimilarity. Further, with other phenotypic markers, they inform on the nature of the interaction between human genotype and environment. Much confusion currently exists in the archaeological community as to what exactly non-metric traits mean, or can be used for. They are often used to denote 'family groups' within cemeteries,[1] cited as 'ethnic' indicators,[2] or simply used to indicate some type of vaguely defined 'relationship'.[3] This has been due to the misconception derived from some studies that traits are equivalent to genes, in both the type, and level, of information that they can convey.

There are several important topics which, for completeness, should be discussed in relation to the use of non-metric traits to determine ancient population dynamics. Three especially relevant areas of study are those of quantitative anthropological genetics, phylogenetics and population genetic theory. The limited space available means that it has not been possible to discuss these issues in any detail. The reader who wishes to contextualize the use of morphology to elucidate population relations should consult these suggested texts.[4-7] This chapter takes the form of a review of the current state of thinking concerning the use of non-metric traits in archaeology with some suggestions for further work. It will review the models suggested for trait manifestation, trait development and heritability, and discuss pragmatic issues that affect recording and analytical procedures. It will also briefly touch upon the mean measure of divergence, a statistical method used for the analysis of data after collection, but to gain further insights into this and other statistical approaches to non-metric traits and biodistance the reader is referred to other works.[8,9]

NON-METRIC TRAITS IN CONTEXT

Early developments

Non-metric traits are minor variants of phenotypic expression. They can be present in all human tissues, but those which are expressed in the skeleton are most suitable for archaeological studies, because of the greater preservation potential of bones and teeth. Non-metric traits have had a long history of classification; the Dutch anatomist Kerkring first described anatomical variants in the human skeleton in 1670[10] in his studies of human skull morphology (cited in Hauser and de Stefano[11]).

However, a reasonable understanding of the developmental and genetic basis for non-metric traits had to wait until the 1950s with the work of Grüneberg,[12] the first person to postulate the quasi-continuous nature of these traits. What Grüneberg noted in his extensive testing of the effect of cross breeds on the skeletal phenotype of mice, was that the genetic basis for non-metric traits did not follow the usual Mendelian pattern of inheritance. He could find no regular correlation between the distribution of traits within parent and offspring. Grüneberg took this to mean that those individuals with, and individuals without, a trait in an inbred strain could be genetically similar. He postulated that the part of the genome responsible for non-metric traits was likely to be polymorphic (consisting of loci acting additively).

The non-occurrence of third molars in mice (a non-metric trait which Grüneberg became particularly interested in) can, like other non-metric traits, be ultimately reduced in its expression to either a present or absent condition, unlike stature for example, which has a continuous phenotypic expression between a theoretical maximum and minimum value. Thus, if a third molar tooth germ does not reach a critical size in development, it is rendered ontogenetically unviable (at about 5 days after birth in the mouse[13]) and the hard tissues of the tooth will not form. Grüneberg called this type of developmental pattern 'quasi-continuous'; there is a continuous genetic basis to the trait, but its expression is discontinuous, i.e. the tooth is either present or absent. Although the processes of development for osseous and dental traits are dissimilar, the principal of quasi-continuity remains the same for both.

Grüneberg's work had hinted at the presence of developmental thresholds within the genome, such that the manifestation of certain phenotypic variants was determined by sufficient weighting within the genome to cross the relevant threshold for a particular trait. The concept of a developmental threshold was to be confirmed by Falconer,[14] who proposed that the distribution of qualitative morphological traits within a population was a consequence of the constituent individuals' inherited genetic propensity to develop a trait, plus the series of consequences that occur throughout the ontogeny of those individuals that make them more or less likely to do so, i.e. all other environmental factors. This series of factors (both genetic and otherwise) was said by Falconer to be normally distributed for any given trait within a population (Figure 1). The point along that distribution, after which all individuals in the population manifest the trait, Falconer named the 'population threshold'. The relative position on the distribution of a single individual in relation to the threshold was termed their 'liability', defined by Falconer as a graded 'attribute immediately related to the causation'. For Falconer's model to work successfully all the genes that act

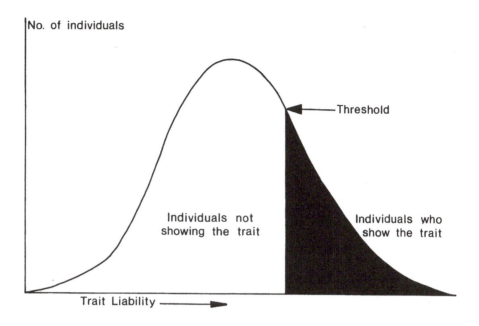

Figure 1 – Falconer's[14] threshold model adapted for a hypothetical non-metric trait. The distribution represents all factors that could potentially affect trait manifestation for each individual within a single population. After the marked threshold, the combined genetic and environmental loading is such that all individuals who fall in this part of the distribution must express the trait. The threshold is not fixed and will vary according to different populations, different traits and different environmental factors.

together towards the trait's manifestation are said to be equal and additive in their contribution, i.e. they are equivalent in (generally small) size of effect regardless of whether the effect is positive or negative. Nevertheless, it is worth bearing in mind that polymorphic genes are in reality often linked, or pleiotropic, and alleles may be shared, epistatic or complementary.

In addition to genetic loading, the variation in the reaction between the genome and different types, and levels, of environmental stimuli means that an individual who does not reach the threshold of expression in one particular environmental situation, might well do so in another, as environmental effects push them into the 'affected' region of the distribution. These problems with the threshold model and the gauging of the relative influence of environmental factors on the development of traits have in part led to the controversial nature of non-metric variation as a means of studying population relations. It is these factors which are the likely cause of fluctuations in the heritability of the same trait between different individuals (and thus by extension over populations too).

The renaissance of non-metric studies

During the late 1960s there was a considerable renewal of interest in the use of non-metric traits for archaeological study, motivated, in part, by Berry and Berry's paper 'Epigenetic variation in the human cranium'.[15] At the time that this was published, it was thought that the frequency of skeletal non-metric traits might provide important information about the relative relationship between contemporaneous and temporally disjunct human populations in the archaeological past. Since biomolecular studies were very much in their infancy at the time, this possible avenue of investigation seemed highly attractive to many scholars. Berry and Berry described epigenetic variants (or non-metric traits) as 'an expression of the genes affecting development'.[15] Their use of the term 'epigenetic' was meant in part to emphasize the likelihood of modification during development and the non-Mendelian nature of trait inheritance, i.e. that there is no specific single gene to single character relationship. Thus, the Berrys' hypothesis was that any change in the frequency of non-metric characters within a population was unlikely to be due to changes within any single gene, but to reflect larger scale processes. Also included in this seminal paper was a statistical technique, which Berry and Smith had been working on previously,[16] called the mean measure of divergence, which allowed the measurement of a non-Euclidean dissimilarity measure (see below) from non-metric trait frequencies.

The low cost, the ease of recording for relatively unskilled practitioners, the added advantage that non-metric traits can be used effectively on fragmentary remains (to which they are still eminently suited) and the development of a distance measure which could be tested for statistical significance, meant that the use of non-metric traits for past human population studies was to become academically fashionable for a brief period. The dominant theoretical environment of the late 1960s and 1970s, with its emerging emphasis on the logico-positivist 'New Archaeology', was highly conducive to the development of esoteric analytical techniques. Studies of biological distance and intra-group variation based on non-metric traits were taken up with gusto. The plethora of case studies which emerged[17–22] (but cf. Allen and Richardson[23]) seemed to indicate that certainly by the late 1990s the study of biological distance would be well established in American and British biological anthropology.

So what has happened to the study of non-metric traits in the UK? Although the Berrys'[15] paper is often seen as providing a turning point for the re-popularization of non-metric studies, which led to an adoption of these techniques, principally by scholars in the USA, it can also be seen as partly responsible for the tone and content of much of the ensuing debate and controversy which has ultimately been responsible for the decline in the use of non-metric traits in current archaeological work.[24] The Berrys' claim that metric traits were less suitable as population measures than non-metric traits has not only proved as fruitless as the single versus polygenic debate which raged in biomolecular genetics,[25] but also it has led to the concentration in the majority of papers and studies that followed on methodological issues. Important though these are, there have been few successful, rigorous studies of biological distance on archaeological populations from Britain.

Invariably non-metric traits can be found recorded in recent skeletal reports from the UK, with varying quality in recording and trait selection. The trait lists often include mechanically modified morphologies, such as the third trochanter, and occasional pathological lesions (the author has even seen cribra orbitalia included in a non-metric trait list!). Furthermore there is a distinct tendency to record only those traits present, and to ignore absent traits. One wonders why non-metric trait data are included in what are already overcrowded documents, since this information is now so rarely used or properly under-stood, and is almost never standardized in terms of trait description and recording. Preservation by record has been the norm for the majority of British archaeology, but unfortunately for non-metric traits the quality of the record is normally poor. The re-burial issue, which is likely to catalyse the development of biological anthropology in the UK, will mean that standards of recording will have to be enforced. Although one is currently likely to go straight to the original material when conducting a study of non-metric traits, usually ignoring published data totally, this may not be an option in the near future for any newly excavated material, and possibly for some existing collections.

ISSUES FOR CONSIDERATION

The main areas of controversy relating to the use of non-metric traits have, almost without exception, still to be resolved. Insufficient work on the nature of individual trait develop-ment and the undetermined level of trait heritabilities are still the main issues which cause investigators concern over the use of traits for population analyses. However, age depend-ency, sex correlation, asymmetry, inter-trait correlation, recording accuracy and trait selec-tion are other issues which ultimately have their roots in the uncertain nature of development and heritability, but which are more immediate issues for investigators working at the 'front line' of practical human osteology. The next section will review each issue and will discuss current options for trying to overcome their associated problems.

Embryology and development

For a few traits there exists an extensive and well-developed listing of their development (e.g. the hypoglossal canal[26] and atlas bridging[27]) but unfortunately for most traits their embryology remains poorly understood. At its most basic level, the general progression of bone growth in the human organism suggests that the fundamental factor in osseous (cranial and infra-cranial) trait expression lies in the soft tissues and organs which surround the osteogenic tissues.[28] Embryologically, the differentiation and primary development of functioning soft tissue structures tends to precede the development of connected skeletal structures. An individual's locally acting genes determine the potential of skeletogenic cells through the control of cell structure, by specifying the proteins and polysaccharides involved in skeletogenesis, and selecting enzymatic control of the metabolism of relevant cells. Other external factors that act on this development are classified as epigenetic. The word 'epigenetic' has now come to mean something slightly different from the Berrys' use in 1967.[15] Waddington[29] proposed the term 'epigenotype' to refer to the total developmental system of the organism, along with the developmental pathways through which the adult form is reached (Figure 2). Following from this, Hall[30] suggests that the epigenotype is a stable, heritable characteristic whose mode of expression is not directly dependent on the base sequence of DNA. Conventionally,[31] epigenetic factors are seen to originate from embryonic inductions involving cells or tissues from other developing organs or anatomical systems (neural, muscular, vascular, etc.). Other effects that potentially bear on the pheno-typic development of individuals include maternal performance, litter size, uterine envi-ronment, maternal metabolism, blood supply, placental efficiency, postnatal maternal

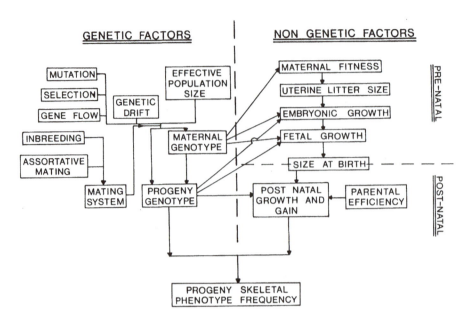

Figure 2 – Flow-chart illustrating the groups of factors, and the pathways linking them, that affect the skeletal form of an individual. The diagram is divided into genetic and non-genetic factors and pre- and post-natal environments. After Atchley *et al.*[31]

performance, etc. These are modulated by the maternal and foetal genomes and environments during the course of the development of an individual. The skeleton continually adjusts its form in relation to the surrounding soft tissues throughout development.[32]

The implication of this style of development for the majority of osseous non-metric traits (associated with other soft tissue structures and influenced by epigenetic and non-heritable environmental factors) is that to get the most information regarding genotype, the investigator must choose those traits which are associated with highly canalized soft tissue structures. This includes those structures that develop in relation to vascular, and to a lesser extent neurological structures (Table 1). The cranial complex is highly canalized during the early part of an individual's development, and for this reason cranial traits are preferable to include in studies over infra-cranial traits. However, as a caveat, once dental eruption and more especially occlusion are achieved, the jaws and facial skeleton are subject to powerful stresses. For functionally modified traits in particular (e.g. zygomatic tubercle) this new regime is likely to influence expression. Infra-cranial traits may well be potentially good reflections of the genome, but their increased susceptibility to remodelling and functional modification, along with a relatively low canalization trajectory means that they are far less suitable for use in biodistance studies, and are likely to remain so until their developmental basis is better understood.

Dental traits may be considered highly advantageous in this respect since the mammalian gnathic complex is well buffered against influence from maternal effects *in utero*.[31] The majority of development of the human permanent dentition takes place post-partum,[33,34]

Table 1 – Selection of osseous cranial traits and the types of anatomical structures with which they are associated. Traits with checks in the functional column are those that are either the site of tendinous insertions or are affected by increased biomechanical loading on the relevant skeletal element.

Trait	Arterial	Venous	Neural	Sutural or Ontogenetic	Functional
Auditory exostoses					×
Clinoid bridging	×				
Condylar canals		×			
Coronal ossicles				×	
Divided parietal				×	
Divided temporal squama				×	
Epipteric bone				×	
Ethmoidal foramina			×		
Foramen ovale incomplete	×	×	×		
Foramen spinosum incomplete	×		×		
Fronto-temporal articulation				×	
Highest nuchal line					×
Divided hypoglossal canal	×	×	×		
Infra orbital foramina		×			
Jugular foramen bridge		×	×		
Lambdoid ossicles				×	
Mandibular and maxillary tori					×
Mastoid foramina	×	×			
Median basilar canal		×			
Metopic suture				×	
Meningeal artery emissaries	×				
Mental foramen			×		
Nasal foramina			×		
Occipital foramina		×			
Os inca, asterion and japonicum				×	
Ossicle at lambda and bregma				×	
Palatine bridge			×		
Palatine foramina			×		
Palatine torus					×
Paracondylar process					×
Parietal foramina	×	×			
Parietal notch bone				×	
Petrosquamous emissaries		×			
Pterygo-basal bridge			×		
Pterygo-spinous bridge	×		×		
Retromastoid process					×
Sagittal ossicles				×	
Supra-meatal spine					×
Supra-orbital structures			×		
Trochlear spine					×
Tympanic dehiscence			×	×	
Zygomatico-facial foramen			×		
Zygomaxillary tubercle					×

which in effect means that the impact of environmental effects on the development of dental traits is limited to those that occur after an individual is born. Dental traits have other properties that make them valuable for use in biodistance studies: they evolve slowly, are probably selectively neutral, are likely to be linked tightly to a small and stable portion of the genome, show little sexual dimorphism, and have a low level of intercorrelation.[35,36] They are not, however, totally without drawback. Tooth wear is often a limiting factor in recording accuracy, as indeed is the preservation of sufficient teeth.

The genetics and heritability of traits

Concrete statements about the genetic basis of skeletal non-metric traits are fraught with difficulties. There are three main areas of investigation, but all are based on indirect evidence:

- Distance matrix concordance.
- Experimental animal data.
- Twin, familial and pedigree studies.

Common to all these studies is the hypothesis that non-metric traits are inherited, either because they share a similar pattern of distribution to known heritable material, or because they can be shown to have a probable genetic basis in humans, by measuring the level of additive genetic variance in other mammal species. Heritability is defined as the proportion of the total genotypic variance to the total phenotypic variance (broad sense heritability). However, for quantitative studies it is more usual to use the proportion of the additive portion of the genotypic variance to the phenotypic variance.[37] The reason for this is to minimize the effect of epistasis, dominance and other 'internal' effects that affect the variance of an individual's genotype.[38,39]

All traits can potentially be understood in terms of the threshold model developed by Falconer.[14] If genealogies are present for a sample, it is possible to determine approximate heritabilities for traits using the threshold model, assuming that the liabilities for trait manifestation within a population are normally distributed.[38–40] But there are problems with heritability studies, not least being that work on human populations is very limited (although see Nichol[41]). Second, the underlying assumption that the liability is normally distributed could be highly erroneous if there are single genes acting with large effect, as there are for instance in relation to the dentition of the mouse.[42] Third, heritability studies often have large standard errors that tend to diminish the reliability of a study's results.[38,39] Finally, and most importantly, heritabilities are always unique to populations. If we assume that the liability/threshold model is correct, small changes in environment and loading can alter the heritability of a trait *without affecting its mean frequency within a population*. This has dramatic implications for the basic model as popularized by Berry and Berry,[15] and reiterated by Irish,[43] which is that trait distances have a proportional relationship with gene frequency change, such that phenetic expression is an approximation of genetic variation.

Distance matrix concordance

Berry[44] indicated that using 30 uncorrelated traits would involve the screening of about 300 loci. Saunders[13] suggested that if this model is accurate then traits could be used to infer gene flow, admixture, evolutionary trees, etc. However, as she also points out, success with the model has been very variable, which is surprising when one considers that most allozymic comparisons are made with far fewer loci but meet with much higher success rates. One test of the 'gene frequency/trait equivalence' model has been to use comparisons between frequency data for traits, both non-metric and genetic, for parent and hybrid populations. Ideally the parent populations should show a linear distance and the hybrid should lie somewhere along this vector. Where studies have been done[45] the results are slightly inconclusive, partly because the distance measure used (mean measure of divergence) was non-linear, but in general the pattern of distances falls into that expected (cf. Corrucini *et al.*[46]).

Distance matrices drawn up between populations based on allelomorphic data often share a great deal of similarity with those based on morphometric[47] or non-metric data.[48] Comparisons between matrices of metric and non-metric data also, relatively unsurprisingly, show high levels of concordance.[49,50] The correlation between morphometrics and non-metric traits is almost certainly caused in part by the strong relationship first noted by Grüneberg[12] between size of skeletal, or dental, element and the development of a particular trait, especially the association between hyperostotic traits and increased size of element, and hypostotic traits with decreased size of element.[44] It may well be that the debate about relative merits of using metrical and non-metric methods to determine biological relationships between population groups has always been sterile, since the development of non-metric traits is highly dependent on size and form (the fundamental measurement objectives of nearly all metric studies).

Experimental animal data

These studies have in general concentrated on either mouse or primate skeletons, partly because human skeletal samples of sufficient size, with genealogies to establish pedigrees, are not widely available. Self and Leamy's[51] study of randombred house mice showed heritabilities to be low for a series of 11 traits. Cheverud and Buikstra's[38,39] work on the Cayo Santiago Macaques showed that heritabilities ranged from $h^2 = -0.22$–1.12, although they calculated that at least half of the heritabilities for all traits were > 0.5. They claimed that this showed a high level of 'genetic variation'. It may not be possible, however, to partition out variance with any reliability, unless one can test the consistency of heritability across different types of relatives, which has been a general failing of most studies.[13] Cheverud's[52] work on a selection of 20 primate samples showed that for these groups morphological skeletal traits have an average heritability (i.e. h^2) $= 0.35$. Atchley *et al.*[31] have shown that in mice at least, progeny genotypes have a strong bearing on their skeletal development. Their experiments showed that there is likely to be a significant level of non-additive genetic effect in an individual's skeletal development. Given then, that the progeny genotype is effective in the expression of phenotype, this means that there will nearly always be some reflection of genotype in phenotype. However, even if this is the case, all other empirical studies indicate that the actual proportion of genetic variance reflected in the phenotype is low; on average between 0.35 and 0.5.

Twin, familial and other pedigree studies

Twin studies have offered some of the most potentially revealing information about the heritability of phenotypic traits, particularly through comparisons of the variation in expression between monozygotic and dizygotic twins. Unsurprisingly monozygotic twins have a higher concordance than dizygotic twins in the frequencies of dental traits which they exhibit.[53] Jordan *et al.*[54] have shown crown morphology similarities in triplets whereby the monozygotic partners show greater similarities with each other than with their dizygotic partner. Almost all twin studies have shown that traits are inherited polygenically and that there is at least in part a significant genetic component in the expression of some traits – notably shovelling and upper molar and lower premolar cusp number.[55]

METHODOLOGICAL PROBLEMS

The fundamental methodological problems associated with the use of non-metric traits are those relating to biases produced by the possible correlations of trait frequency with age and sex, with other traits, and with side for bilateral traits. These biases along with the respective inconsistencies of recording associated with bilateral traits, recording accuracy of trait state, and trait selection are the areas into which most of the research into non-metric traits has been undertaken over the past 20 years. The reason for this is that so much of the nature of trait heritability, development, etc. is uncertain. Maximizing the usefulness of the data by trying to eliminate all known bias is thus a crucial part of any study based on non-metric trait data.

Age dependency and sex correlations

If the threshold model is correct, then one should assume that size differences caused by sexual dimorphism should alter the frequency of trait occurrence between the biological sexes. Traits that are sex correlated have been infrequently noted in non-metric studies (although the foramen of Hüschke does merit mention as a trait correlated with sex in a small number of studies).[56] The low number of non-metric traits that appear to be correlated with sex has occasionally been cited as one reason to utilize them over metric traits, which require correction for sexual dimorphism. Those studies that have shown evidence for sexual dimorphism in non-metric traits have tended to be very inconsistent, and, as Berry says, this 'confirm(s) the idea that they are the outward manifestation of the activity of genetic, epigenetic and even overtly environmental forces, thus being a long way from the primary site of gene action'.[57] Hauser and De Stefano suggest that if any variation between the sexes in trait frequency is biologically meaningful, then 'one would expect each to show parallel trends in the two sexes unless there is good reason'.[11] If this is not the case, as it appears not to be (except for a very few traits with any consistency across large numbers of populations), then either the trait is differently influenced in the two sexes, or there is an inadequacy in the sample size or statistical analysis. As far as testing for sex correlation is concerned, all traits should be tested by sex using the chi-square test. There are three methods of dealing with sex linked traits if they occur. These are:

- Remove them from the study after testing shows their presence.
- Perform all distance studies by sex.
- Keep the sex ratio in the sample at an artificially uniform level.

The selection of any of these solutions is really dependent on the context of study. Removal of traits is a certain loss of information. For example, in those studies that attempted to determine intra-site variation in trait frequency between the sexes,[58] one stage in the analysis was to remove sex linked traits, to avoid artificially skewing the frequency differences. By removing the very information the investigator was looking for, that is those traits that are the expression of intra-site variation between the sexes, the study became a self-defeating exercise. This author's preference is to try and keep the level of the sexes relatively balanced within the sample, purely because it is less of a dilution of intra-population heterogeneity than the alternatives (first and second options).

Age variation in trait appearance has been much more commonly noted than sex correlations in human populations, although analyses investigating this type of data bias are made more difficult by the lack of precision in skeletal ageing criteria. Korey[59] examined 124 Haida crania from several sites in British Columbia for the occurrence of the supra orbital foramen. He noted that the prevalence of its bilateral form increased with developmental age, in turn postulating that its unilateral manifestation was of 'no genetic significance'. This has led some authors to suggest that the inclusion of non-adults into any analyses of population affinity may well be methodologically unsound, although Kitagawa et al.[60] have performed such studies, apparently successfully, on the deciduous dentition of individuals from the Pacific region. If traits are age progressive, it implies that they continue to develop their expressions through development and possibly into adulthood. Buikstra[61] has suggested that all hyperostotic traits may be age regressive, and as such all pre-pubertal material should be discarded from study (apart perhaps from those permanent dental crowns that have reached a sufficient state of development). It seems as if the overall trend for osseous traits is for hyperostotic traits to be age dependent and for hypostotic traits to be age regressive. The use of dental traits on the permanent dentition bypasses this problem (assuming that tooth wear is sufficiently light to allow traits to be recorded from more mature specimens).

Symmetry

As with all other paired characteristics in bilaterally symmetrical organisms there is a tendency for the occurrence of bilateral traits to be strongly correlated. The presence of a trait on one side is not always a guarantee of its appearance on another (i.e. it is not a perfect correlation); however, it is nearly always the case with non-metric traits that bilateral occurrences or absences of paired traits are more common than would be expected by chance, or if the two sides were expressed independently of each other. There are several potential methods of dealing with this, first calculating trait incidence by individual (number of individuals expressing the trait regardless of side or symmetry divided by the total number of individuals), and second, recording traits by side (number of traits on either left or right side divided by the total number of left or right sides). The 'individual' technique tends to underestimate the true population frequency in badly preserved material and the side technique assumes side independence (which is strongly refuted by researchers[59,62]).

The actual meaning of asymmetry in bilateral traits is uncertain, but seems to be related either to age[59] or to fluctuating asymmetry produced by random non-genetic disruptions in development, proportional to ontogenetic homeostasis.[62] Should the fluctuating asymmetry hypothesis prove to be correct, then bilateral traits should be expressed randomly on either side, and measuring by side is unlikely to overestimate frequency. One partial solution to this problem is to use the randomization procedure suggested first by Konigsberg.[58] Where both sides of a skeletal element that could potentially express a particular trait are present, then the trait is scored as present when both of the sides express that trait. The trait is scored as absent when neither side expresses the trait. If one side expresses the trait and the other does not, then the score is randomized to determine whether a present or absent score is given. Single sides are recorded according to the usual manner (present for present, and absent for absent).

Recording and trait selection

These two issues have a heavy impact on the quality of any study that uses non-metric traits for population analysis. The recording of non-metric traits requires a broad level of standardization between investigators to enable a greater level of precision for large-scale studies. This is one reason why over-arching studies from published material are generally impossible.

Traits are normally recorded using a presence/absence system. There has however, been a recent trend to divide up the expression of traits into multiple states of expression (see Turner et al.,[35] for example). The use of multiple state trait expressions is potentially very useful, because it may provide an increased amount of information about levels of genome/environment interaction. At the very least it should enable much of the statistical 'noise' from non-metric trait based studies to be cut out. On the other hand, using multiple expressions increases error in recording greatly. This is particularly true for the partial expressions of traits (e.g. with bridging and sutural traits), where degrees of bridge completion, etc. must be determined. The use of casts has certainly improved the situation for dental traits, but at present no casts are forthcoming for osseous traits. To improve accuracy further between observers a far more rigorous approach needs to be taken with intra- and inter-observer error protocols, which are currently almost never implemented in British recording procedures (or at least the results are never included when trait frequencies and results are presented). The Phi coefficient is very easy to use and can prevent large inconsistencies from occurring in the data set.[63]

Trait selection for specific studies can cause problems, especially when the majority of investigators copy previous trait lists from other authors, with little regard for the applicability of the traits selected to the study they are undertaking. A standardized trait list for recording from skeletons found in the British Isles would be very useful in terms of allowing direct comparison of trait frequencies from a wide number of sites, but distance studies should still be performed on the basis of the most appropriate traits from such a hypothetical list. To maximize the efficiency of the statistical techniques, traits which show a low difference in variability between the populations under study should be excluded, since they are likely to contribute more 'noise' than signal to the distance measure.[64]

BIODISTANCE ANALYSIS

Non-metric traits have been used mainly for the determination of biodistance, which is a measure of the relative similarity between skeletal population samples. Their polymorphic nature, and the uncertain environmental contribution to their expression, makes non-metric traits unsuitable as measures of relatedness between individuals. Ideally each sample being tested would consist of a large number of individuals, in order to minimize biases induced from small sample sizes, but also to get a representative sample of the phenome for that population. To improve further the quality of the analysis, it is useful to compare populations on a broad spectrum of traits. However, it should be noted that statistically significant distances have been obtained from relatively few individuals and traits. How valid these studies are when extrapolated to a population level is open to question.

The mean measure of divergence

Although there have been other methods developed to determine population distances, the one traditionally associated with non-metric traits is the mean measure of divergence. The mean measure of divergence is based around the measure of a distance based on the divergence between the average frequency of a series of traits recorded for each population. There are other more traditional multivariate methods for measuring the difference between two sample frequencies, but the quasi-continuous nature of non-metric traits makes these unsuitable. This is because the distribution of presence/absence data is binomial. To bypass this problem, trait frequencies are normally standardized using a transformation. That illustrated here is the Anscombe transformation:[65]

$$p = \frac{x + 3/8}{n + 3/4} \tag{1}$$

where p is relative frequency of a trait in the sample, x is absolute frequency of that trait (i.e. the number of incidences recorded) and n is sample size (all individuals, or sides, see above).

This transformation is performed to make the variance of p proportional to $1/n$ instead of being proportional to p. It also has the advantage of standardizing the variances between the traits which are at a maximum when P is at 0.5 decreasing towards 0 when P approaches either 0 or 1, where P is the real proportion of the traits in the 'true' population, not that given by p which is the frequency observed from the sample.

The mathematical working in the following section is taken largely from Sjøvold.[9] For two hypothetical populations 1 and 2 with p for each trait given as p_1 and p_2 the mean measure of divergence (MMD) is measured using the following equation:

$$MMD = 1/r \sum_{i=1}^{r} \left[(\theta_{1i} - \theta_{2i})^2 - V_{12i} \right] \tag{2}$$

where

$$\theta_{1i} = \arcsin(1 - 2p_{1i}) \tag{3}$$

Equation 3 is known as the angular transformation. The frequency of the ith trait in population 1 is denoted by p_{1i}, where i is the trait in question and r is total number of traits studied. The consequence of the angular transformation is to project the trait frequencies onto a theoretical sphere of many dimensions: a hypersphere (Figure 3), along the surface of which the distance between the frequencies is measured. V_{12i} is a measure of the variance for the means based on n and is used to ensure that the MMD is independent of sample size. V_{12i} is given as:

$$V_{12i} = (1/n_{1i} + 0.5) + (1/n_{2i} + 0.5) \tag{4}$$

MMD is regarded as significant if it is equal to more than twice its standard deviation, which is given as:

$$\text{standard deviation of the } MMD = \sqrt{2/r^2} \sum_{i=1}^{r} V_{12i}{}^2 \tag{5}$$

MMD is a measure of dissimilarity, so that values close to 0 show high similarity and values close to 1 show a low similarity. When the distance between two populations is not very large, the surface of the sphere onto which they are projected (Figure 3) by the angular transform, is almost planar and in such cases Euclidean geometry holds to all intents. When the divergence increases then Euclidean space is obviously not applicable, but in some cases the triangular inequality holds, although this implies that the points all lie in a straight line along the sphere. Sjøvold,[21] demonstrated that the difference between two populations may be regarded in terms of an intermediate third population, i.e. from populations 1 to 2 can be expressed in terms of 1–3 + 2–3 if 3 is considered as an intermediate between 1 and 2. This is realised in terms of MMD as:

$$MMD_{12} \equiv MMD_{13} + MMD_{23} - 2(\theta_1 - \theta_3)(\theta_2 - \theta_3) + 2/n_3 \tag{6}$$

The triangular inequality is not fulfilled when the q differences are positive and $< 1/n_3$. If, however, the product is negative (population 3 is between populations 1 and 2; i.e. population 3 lies on a line between populations 1 and 2) then the inequality is satisfied. To help minimize this the MMD can be squared.

CONCLUSIONS

The re-popularization of non-metric traits by the Berrys[15] led to many new studies being undertaken, but the Berrys' original hypothesis that trait manifestation was a long way away from the site of actual gene action has largely been ignored in subsequent studies. Many studies have treated trait frequencies as if they were an archaeological typology, using a mix and match approach to determine if skeletons in a cemetery belonged to related individuals, or to determine the 'ethnic' group to which an individual skeleton belonged. This is unacceptable since not only does it lead to misleading conclusions, but also it promises access to information which morphological studies cannot at present ascertain. However, despite these controversies (e.g. 'Kennewick man', see Goodman[66] for a good critique), the amount of research into fundamental aspects of non-metric traits remains very limited. Basic

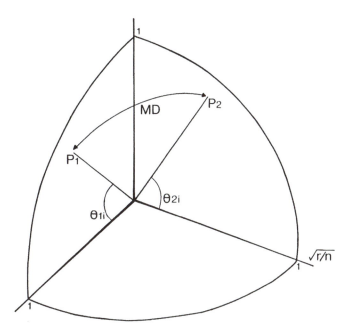

Figure 3 – Biological distance between two populations as based on the frequency of a single trait within those populations. Where q_{1i} and q_{2i} are trait frequencies which have been submitted to the angular transformation. P_1 and P_2 are the transformed frequencies projected onto the surface of a hypersphere. An average distance based on the chord subtended between P_1 and P_2, for a number of traits, is used to produce the mean measure of divergence (see Equation 2). The axes are the square root of trait frequency.

questions about the viability of the threshold model and the level of heritability of traits remain to be addressed.

It may well be that much of the hesitancy in the application of morphological approaches to broader archaeological questions and issues arises from the confusion between ethnicity and biological affiliation. Scholars are occasionally, and understandably, reticent to confront these issues, especially in the current theoretical climate which is, quite rightly, highly antagonistic to biological determinism in any of its forms. However, this is no reason to ignore a critical part of the development and variation of human group constitution as a valid area for study. It does mean, however, that when investigating the assignation of group affiliation, ethical issues should be paramount in the minds of researchers. So, while this chapter is in large part a technical review of current thinking and opinions on the practical use of non-metric traits (just one of the methodological avenues for the investigation of archaeological population relationships), it should be born in mind that investigations of this type are not (or should not) be conducted in isolation. Hopefully, with the use of more nuanced study and increased communication between social theorists, biological anthropologists, archaeologists and population biologists we can begin to approach a situation where biological anthropologists can define themselves, in the words of Jonathan Marks, as 'first rate anthropologists, and not as second rate biologists'.[67]

ACKNOWLEDGEMENTS

This chapter was written during my doctoral research, which was partly funded by a NERC studentship and carried out at the Department of Archaeology and Prehistory, University of Sheffield. I thank Dr Andrew Chamberlain for his work as my supervisor. I also thank Bill Frazer, Jeremy Ottevanger and two anonymous peer reviewers for their incisive criticism and constructive advice on the initial versions of this chapter. Finally I am very grateful to Drs Margaret Cox and Simon Mays for inviting me to contribute to this volume.

REFERENCES

1   Alt, KW, Pichler S, Vach W, Klíma B, Vlcek E, Sedlmeier J. Twenty-five thousand-year-old triple burial from Dolni Vestonice: an ice age family? *American Journal of Physical Anthropology* 1997; **102**: 123–131.

2   Härke H. 'Warrior graves?' The background of the Anglo-Saxon weapon burial rite. *Past and Present* 1990; **126**: 22–43.

3   Chapman A. Blackmills Northampton, an early Iron Age torc. *Current Archaeology* 1998; **159 XIV**(3): 92–95.

4   Cavalli-Sforza LL, Menozzi P, Piazza A. *The history and geography of human genes*. Princeton: Princeton University Press, 1994.

5   Chakraborty R. Quantitative traits in relation to population structure: why and how are they used and what do they imply? *Human Biology* 1990; **62**: 147–62.

6   Sokal RR, Rohlf FJ. *Biometry* (3rd edn). New York: WH Freeman, 1995.

7   Falconer DS. *Introduction to Quantitative Genetics* (2nd edn). London: Longman, 1981.

8   Tyrrell AJ, Chamberlain AT. Non-metric trait evidence for modern human affinities and the distinctivness of the Neanderthals. *Journal of Human Evolution* 1998; **34(5)**: 549–554.

9   Sjøvold T. Non metrical divergence between skeletal populations. *Ossa* 1977; **4** (suppl. 1): 1–117.

10 Kerkring, T. *Spicilegium anatomicum*. Amsterdam: Andreas Frisius, 1670.

11 Hauser G, De Stefano GF. *Epigenetic Variants of the Human Skull*. Stuttgart: Schweizerbartsche, 1989.

12 Grüneberg, H. Genetical studies on the skeleton of the mouse IV. Quasi-continuous variation. *Journal of Genetics* 1952; **51**: 95–114.

13 Saunders S. Nonmetric skeletal variation. In: Isçan MY, Kennedy KAR (eds), *Reconstruction of Life from the Skeleton*. New York: Wiley-Liss, 1989: pp. 95–108.

14 Falconer DS. The inheritance of liability to certain disease, estimated from the incidence among relatives. *Annals of Human Genetics* 1965; **29**: 51–76.

15 Berry AC, Berry RJ. Epigenetic variation in the human cranium. *Journal of Anatomy* 1967; **101**(2): 361–379.

16 Berry RJ, Smith CAB. The genetical characterisation of rat populations from skeletal data. Unpublished MS, 1967.

17 Kaul SS, Anand V, Corruccini RS. Non-metric variation of the skull in samples of four Indian populations. *Journal of Human Evolution* 1979; **8**: 693–697.

18 Lane RA, Sublett AJ. The osteology of social organization: residence pattern. *American Antiquity* 1972; **37(2)**: 186–209.

19 Ossenberg NS. Within and between race distances in population studies based on discrete traits of the human skull. *American Journal of Physical Anthropology* 1976; **45**: 701–709.

20 Ossenberg NS. Congruence of distance matrices based on cranial discrete traits, cranial measuremants, and linguistic–geographic criteria in five Alaskan populations. *American Journal of Physical Anthropology* 1977; **47**: 93–98.

21 Sjøvold T. The occurrence of minor non-metric variants in the skeleton and their quantitative treatment for population comparisons. *Homo* 1973; **24**: 204–233.

22   Sjøvold T. A method for familial studies based on minor skeletal variants. *Ossa* 1976; **314**: 97–107.

23   Allen W, Richardson J. The reconstruction of kinship from archaeological data: the concepts, the methods and the feasibility. *American Antiquity* 1971; **36**: 41–45.

24   Buikstra JE, Frankenberg SR, Konigsberg LW. Skeletal biological distance studies in American physical anthropology: recent trends. *American Journal of Physical Anthropology* 1990; **82**: 1–7.

25   Rogers AR, Harpending HC. Population structure and quantitative characters. *Genetics* 1983; **105**: 985–1002.

26   Dodo Y. Appearance of bony bridging of the hypoglossal canal during the fetal period. *Journal of the Anthropological Society of Nippon* 1980; **88**: 229–238.

27   Saunders S, Popovich F. A family study of two skeletal variants: atlas bridging and clinoid bridging. *American Journal of Physical Anthropology* 1978; **49**: 193–204.

28   Richtsmeier JT, Cheverud JM, Buikstra JE. The relationship between cranial metric and non-metric traits in the rhesus macaques from Cayo Santiago. *American Journal of Physical Anthropology* 1984; **64**: 213–222.

29   Waddington C. Epigenetics and evolution. *Symposia of the Society of Experimental Biology* 1956; **7**: 186–199.

30   Hall BK. Genetic and epigenetic control of connective tissues in the cranio-facial structure. *March of Dimes, Original Articles Series* 1984; **20**: 3–17.

31   Atchley WR, Logsdon T, Cowley DE, Eisen EJ. Uterine effects, epigenetics, and postnatal skeletal development in the mouse. *Evolution* 1991; **45(4)**: 891–909.

32   Moss ML, Moss-Salentijn L. The muscle bone interface: An analysis of a morphological boundary. In: Carlson DS, McNamara J (eds), *Muscle Adaption in the Craniofacial Region*. Ann Arbor: Centre for Human growth and development 1979; pp. 39–71.

33   Schour I, Massler M. The development of the human dentition. *Journal of the American Dental Association* 1941; **28**: 1153–1160.

34   Hillson, S. *Dental Anthropology*. Cambridge: Cambridge University Press, 1996.

35   Turner CG II, Nichol CR, Scott GR. Scoring procedures for key morphological traits of the permanent dentition: The Arizona State University Dental Anthropology System. In: Kelley MA, Larsen CS (eds), *Advances in Dental Anthropology*. New York: Wiley-Liss, 1991: pp. 13–31.

36   Irish J, Turner CG II. West African dental affinity of late Pleistocene Nubians: peopling of the Eurafrican–South Asian Triangle II. *Homo* 1990; **41**: 42–53.

37   Keiser J.A. *Human Adult Odontometrics*. Cambridge Studies in Biological Anthropology 4. Cambridge: Cambridge University Press, 1990

38   Cheverud JM, Buikstra JE. Quantitative genetics of skeletal non-metric traits in the rhesus macaques on Cayo Santiago. I. Single trait heritabilities. *American Journal of Physical Anthropology* 1981; **54**: 43–49.

39   Cheverud JM, Buikstra JE. Quantitative genetics of skeletal non-metric traits in the rhesus macaques on Cayo Santiago. II. Phenotypic, genetic and environmental correlations between traits. *American Journal of Physical Anthropology* 1981; **54**: 51–58.

40   Sjøvold T. A report on the heritability of some cranial measurements and non-metric traits. In: Van Vark GN, Howells WW (eds), *Multivariate Statistical Methods in Physical Anthropology: A Review of Recent Advances and Current Developments*. Boston: D Reidel, 1984: pp. 223–248.

41   Nichol CR. Complex segregation analysis of dental morphological variants. *American Journal of Physical Anthropology* 1989; **78**: 37–59.

42   Thesleff I. Two genes for missing teeth. *Nature Genetics* 1996; **13**: 379–380.

43   Irish J. Ancestral dental traits in recent Sub-Saharan Africans and the origins of modern humans. *Journal of Human Evolution* 1998; **34**: 81–98.

44   Berry RJ. Genes and skeletons, ancient and modern. *Journal of Human Evolution* 1979; **8**: 669–677.

45   Wijsman EM, Neves WA. The use of non-metric variation in estimating human population admixture: a test case with Brazilian blacks, whites and mulattoes. *American Journal of Physical Anthropology* 1986; **70**: 395–405.

46   Corrucini RS, Handler JS, Mutaw RJ, Lange FW. Osteology of a slave population from Barbados, West Indies. *American Journal of Physical Anthropology* 1982; **59**: 443–460.

47   Derish PA, Sokal RR. A classification of European populations based on gene frequencies and cranial measurements: a map quadrat approach. *Human Biology* 1988; **60(5)**: 801–824.

48   Szathmary EJE, Ossenberg NS. Are the biological differences between North American Indians and Eskimos truely profound? *Current Anthropology* 1978; **19**: 673–701.

49   Ossenburg NS. Congruence of distance matrices based on cranial discrete traits, cranial measurements, and linguistic–geographic criteria in five Alaskan populations. *American Journal of Physical Anthropology* 1977; **47**: 93–98.

50   Ossenberg NS. Origins of the native peoples of Northwestern North America: the evidence of cranial non-metric traits. In: Bonnichsen R, Steele DG (eds), *Method and Theory for Investigating the Peopling of the Americas*. Oregon: Center for the Study of the First Americans, Oregon State University, 1994: pp. 79–115.

51   Self SG, Leamy L. Heritability of quasi-continuous skeletal traits in a randombred population of house mouse. *Genetics* 1978; **88**: 109–120.

52   Cheverud JM. A comparison of genetic and phenotypic correlations. *Evolution* 1988; **42(5)**: 958–968.

53   Berry AC. Anthropological and family studies on minor variants of the dental crown. In: Butler PM, Joysey KA (eds), *Development Function and Evolution of Teeth*. London: Academic Press, 1978: pp. 81–98.

54   Jordan RE, Abrams L, Kraus BS. *Kraus' Dental Anatomy and Occlusion* (2nd edn). St Louis: Mosby Yearbook, 1992.

55   Sharma JC, Dental morphology and odontometry of twins and the heritability of dental variation. In: Lukacs JR (ed.), *Culture, Ecology and Dental Anthropology*. Journal of Human Ecology 1992; Special Issue **2**: pp. 49–60.

56   Corruccini RS. An examination of the meaning of cranial discrete traits for human skeletal biological studies. *American Journal of Physical Anthropology* 1974; **40**: 425–446.

57   Berry AC. Factors affecting the incidence of non-metric skeletal variants. *Journal of Anatomy* 1975; **120**: 519–535.

58   Konigsberg LW. Population genetic models for interpreting prehistoric intra-cemetery biological variation. Unpublished PhD dissertation, Northwestern University, Illinois, 1987.

59   Korey KA. The incidence of bilateral non-metric skeletal traits: a re-analysis of sampling procedures. *American Journal of Physical Anthropology* 1980; **53**: 19–23.

60   Kitagawa Y, Manabe Y, Oyamada J, Rokutanda A. Deciduous dental morphology of the prehistoric Jomon people of Japan: comparison of non-metric characters. *American Journal of Physical Anthropology* 1995; **97**: 101–111.

61   Buikstra, J.E. Techniques for coping with the age regressive nature of non-metric traits. *American Journal of Physical Anthropology* 1972; **37**: 431–432 (abstract).

62   McGrath JW, Cheverud JM, Buikstra JE. Genetic correlations between sides and heritability of asymmetry for non-metric traits in rhesus macaques on Cayo Santiago. *American Journal of Physical Anthropology* 1984; **54**: 471–479.

63   Molto JE. Intra-observer scoring precision of cranial discrete traits. *American Journal of Physical Anthropology* 1979; **51**: 333–343.

64   Buikstra JE. Non-metric traits: the control of environmental noise. *American Journal of Physical Anthropology* 1974; **41**: 471 (abstract).

65   Anscombe FJ. The transformation of Poisson, binomial and negative binomial data. *Biometrika* 1948; **35**: 246–254.

66   Goodman, A. Racializing Kennewick Man. *American Anthropological Association Anthropology Newsletter* 1997; **38(6)**: 3.

67   Marks, J. Replaying the race card. *American Anthropological Association Anthropology Newsletter* 1998; **39(5)**: 1–5.

19

SKELETAL INDICATORS OF HANDEDNESS

James Steele

INTRODUCTION: HANDEDNESS IN CONTEMPORARY HUMAN POPULATIONS

For the purposes here, we shall define human handedness as the tendency to prefer consistently to use one hand in skilled tasks. Handedness is of interest to anthropologists for several reasons. First, in an evolutionary context it is related to a more general pattern of lateralization of brain function that also involves language capacities. Some important hypotheses about human brain evolution place great emphasis on the existence of heritable variability in the direction and degree of human cerebral lateralization (both of hand motor skill and of language processing).[1,2] Quantifying frequencies of left- and right-handedness in past populations is useful for testing such models. Second, in a biomechanical context human handedness provides us with a behavioural origin for asymmetries in bone growth in paired bones of the forelimb and shoulder girdle. This means that we can evaluate theories of the effects of mechanical loading on skeletal growth using these paired elements as our experimental model.[3] Finally, as an individuating characteristic with known skeletal markers, variability in human hand preferences enables us to provide useful data contributing to the identification of the deceased in forensic contexts.[4]

In living individuals, handedness can be measured in two ways: as an asymmetry between the right and left hands in skill or performance, and as an asymmetry between the right and left hands in preference. There is debate among psychologists as to which of these is primary.[5] Annett[6] has found that in human populations, pooled data on the degree of individuals' asymmetry of skill between the two hands in precise, rapid aimed movement tasks has a unimodal normal distribution, with a mean biased towards the right hand (although other studies have found some signs of bimodality in the distribution of relative hand skill[7]). Most people are more skilled with the right hand, but of these many have only a slight right-handed skill advantage. Similarly, about 16% of people are more skilled with the left hand; but of these, too, many have only a slight left-handed skill advantage. Preference, measured by Annett using a questionnaire, which asks which hand is preferred in a range of everyday tasks, shows a J-shaped distribution. Most people have a clear preference for using one or other hand fairly consistently across tasks. Annett argues that the asymmetries in performance are primary, and that the development of preferences comes under the joint influence of innate performance biases and of cultural factors. Hand preferences seem to develop quite early in childhood. For individuals with only a slight innate performance advantage in the left hand, only slight cultural biases favouring right hand use are needed to channel the development of a pattern of right-hand preference for a majority of tasks.

This interaction of innate and cultural factors in the development of hand preferences can be seen in secular trends of increased frequency of preferentially left-handed individuals in modern post-industrial societies. For instance, whereas in 1928 a survey of American college students found 4% preferential left-handers, a survey of the same college in 1983 found 13% preferential left-handers.[8] In Australia and New Zealand, a survey of individuals matched for socio-economic status found an increase from about 2% in 1880 to about 13% in 1967.[9] In Norway, this same trend was found in the decreasing prevalence of preferential left-handedness among older age groups surveyed recently, with frequencies of preferential left-handedness ranging from 1% in the oldest adult age group to 10% in the youngest adult age group.[10] In a study of 800 patients at a dental clinic in Guy's Hospital, London, in the mid–1970s, 2.9% of adults in the 55–64-year age range were left-handed writers, while it was 10.8% for adolescents and adults in the 15–24-year age range.[11] Relaxation of cultural pressures to learn to write with the right hand may account for much of this secular variability.

Evidence for an underlying 'natural frequency' of biases towards right- or left-handedness is seen in a meta-analysis of 88 published studies, which found a mean of 8% left-handers and a range of 2–23%, with no geographical pattern to this variability.[7,12] A secular trend was evident; in studies of people born before about 1910, the overall prevalences of left-handed males and females were respectively 4.6 and 3.4%, while for people born since 1960 the overall prevalences were 11.2% left-handed males and 9.1% left-handed females.[12] Across this large sample of survey datasets, males were consistently and significantly more likely to be left-handed than females (the overall ratio of male to female left-handers being 1.27:1). It seems likely that this reflects genetic rather than cultural factors, since there is also correlated variability between the sexes in the prevalence of gross morphological asymmetries of the brain which are determined early in foetal development.[13] Possible explanations of this underlying 'natural frequency' of handedness phenotypes include the action of genes for handedness,[14] the action of genes for cerebral lateralization,[1,2] and the effects of random local disturbances during morphogenesis (or developmental instability).[15] Certainly cross-cultural evidence suggests strongly that human handedness is maintained as a balanced polymorphism with right-handedness always the most frequently observed variant.[16] Cultural pressures for conformity to a right-handed norm can mask these underlying frequencies of innate hand skill asymmetry.[17,18] The causes of the underlying pattern remain, however, incompletely understood.

EFFECTS OF HANDEDNESS ON ASYMMETRIES OF BONE MORPHOLOGY AND OF BONE MINERAL DISTRIBUTION IN PAIRED SKELETAL ELEMENTS FROM THE UPPER LIMB AND SHOULDER GIRDLE

Bone morphology and bone mineral distribution

Annett has found that in rapid, precise aimed movement tasks, one hand (by implication, usually the dominant or preferred hand) is capable of performing more skilfully (with an average speed advantage over the other hand of 4.2% in females and 3.4% in males).[19] It has also repeatedly been observed that in right-handed adults of both sexes, normal grip strength in the dominant hand tends to be about 10% greater than the grip strength of the non-dominant hand.[20–23] A similar pattern of relative pinch strength between the dominant and non-dominant hand has also been reported (with the dominant hand about 10% stronger than the non-dominant hand).[23,24] Further contrasts relating to hand preference have been described for wrist extension, with the dominant side having on average about 10% greater wrist extension strength.[25] Perplexingly, however, left-handed subjects are equally likely to have a stronger grip in either hand[21,22] (perhaps this reflects the need for left-handers to adapt their hand use pattern to the constraints of a right-handed world). An effect of work pattern has been reported;[26] heavy manual workers have the strongest grip and the least strength difference between the two hands, while office workers have the weakest grip and the greatest strength difference between the two hands. Light manual workers were intermediate between these two groups.

These strength differences reflect the greater use of the dominant or preferred hand in the active or 'leading' aspects of tool-using behaviour. Evidence suggests that in any particular case, the osteogenic effect of muscle strength on bone density is localized to the specific site of muscle–bone interaction.[27,28] Aspects of skeletal growth which may reflect the greater muscle mass and mechanical loading of the dominant limb include changes in external geometry (dimensions of bones), the differential development of areas of surface attachment of muscles and ligaments, and increased diaphyseal bone mineral formation. Bone mineral may also be differentially distributed within an element as a reaction to mechanical loading patterns. Such changes can be observed in within-pair comparisons of bones of the right and left sides of a single individual.

Bones of the shoulder girdle: scapula and clavicle

The bones of the shoulder girdle (the scapula and clavicle) have been less studied than the long bones of the forelimb, but they often show clear asymmetries related to handedness. In the scapulae, Schulter-Ellis[4] found a correlation between hand preference and the presence of an extensor facet on the dorsal margin of the glenoid fossa on the dominant side. This is presumably due to the head of the humerus on the dominant side riding up onto that margin during extension, causing it to have a bevelled appearance. It is usual to find a greater range of motion in the gleno-humeral joint on the side of the preferred hand,[29] and both men and women tend also to have a larger angle of retroversion of the humeral head on the dominant side, consistent with an increased range of external rotation.[30] Professional handball players have been shown to develop a significantly greater retrotorsional angle on the dominant (throwing) side;[31] but the osteological correlates of these more specific variations in the mobility of the shoulder joint are unknown. Stewart,[32] however, has noted that the plane of the glenoid cavity of the right scapula tends to be more dorsally inclined than that of the left bone, and that this is associated with increased torsion of the proximal end of the right humerus.

In the clavicles, the right bone tends to be both shorter and more robust than the left. Mays *et al.*,[33] in a study of the clavicles from the predominantly medieval population of Wharram Percy, have found this same pattern. They have also found a tendency for the areas of attachment of the costoclavicular ligament (the site of a feature known as the rhomboid fossa) and of the trapezoid ligament to be more developed on the right side. Mays *et al.* give evidence in support of the hypothesis that loading of the dominant limb exerts greater axially compressive forces on the ipsilateral clavicle, leading both to shape changes (greater robusticity) and to greater development of the attachment sites of those ligaments that stabilize the clavicle within the shoulder girdle during axial compression. Inter-population contrasts have been reported in the prevalence of the rhomboid fossa. In a recent English urban sample Parsons[34] found the fossa to be present in only 10% of instances, while in Indian populations characterized by heavier manual labour the observed prevalence has been as high as 95%.[35,36] In the latter cases, as at Wharram Percy, North Yorkshire, the fossa tends to be more developed on the right clavicle (suggesting a link to handedness).

Risk for asymmetrical development of degenerative shoulder joint diseases appears to vary with working pattern. 'Coalmen', and other workers such as millers whose occupations involved carrying sacks on the left shoulder, used to have very strong left arms even though they were right-handed.[37] A recent study of construction workers (brick layers, rock blasters and foremen) found an elevated risk for osteoarthrosis in the acromioclavicular joint in the heavy manual labourers, with an unusually high incidence of bilateral involvement (since the pattern of work loads both sides equally). However, there was a further independent effect of high level of participation in sports activities that produced a marked increase in risk of arthrosis on the right side.[38,39]

Long bones of the forelimb: humerus, radius and ulna

In right-handed adolescents and adults, muscle mass tends to be greater in the arm on the dominant side.[40–43] It is also well established that the right humerus and radius tend to be slightly longer and heavier than their counterparts on the left.[44,45] Ingelmark, in a pioneering radiographic study,[46] found that greater forelimb length (as measured by the sum of the lengths of the humerus and radius) was correlated with the side of the preferred hand in children. In this study he classified as left-handers all children who reported the use of their left hands in at least two of seven everyday tasks. Consistent with modern behavioural data on handedness, females are also more likely than males to have longer long bones in the right forelimb. Faulkner *et al.*[47] also found, in children in the age range 8–16 years, that the dominant arm tends to have greater bone mineral content and density, and also greater bone-free lean tissue. Reichel *et al.*,[48] in a radiographic study of normal adults, also found a correlation between handedness and the side of greater bone mineral density and bone width in the radius in its midshaft and distal segments

There have been recent radiographic studies of professional racket sports players and other athletes (who may begin their training early in childhood, and whose dominant arms tend to experience unusually large mechanical loads during the playing years).[49–53] These studies have concentrated on differences between the long bones of the two forelimbs in bone mineral content, bone mineral density and cross-sectional cortical area, with repeated observations of greater bone mineral density and content in the long bones (humerus, radius, ulna) on the dominant side (a pattern also found, but less markedly, in normal control samples). Two recent studies of tennis players and normal controls also go some way to replicating, among adults, Ingelmark's finding in children of an effect of handedness on long bone length.[54,55] These modern radiographic studies converge on the finding that activity stresses produce adaptive responses in the bones of the dominant forelimb, which ought to be discernible as measurable asymmetries in paired skeletal elements in individuals from archaeological populations. Evidence from the adult skeletons of an American Indian ossuary in Kleinburg, Ohio (n = about 400 adults) suggests that these stresses continue to produce responses in the bones of the forelimb through adulthood.[56] In a comparison of the bones of the younger and older adults in this sample (where young adults were classified by the presence of a visible proximal humeral epiphyseal line), the older adults had significantly greater dimensions of the right humerus (but not the left) at a number of locations where continuing subperiosteal appositional growth would have occurred in response to loading. These included the humeral diaphysis at the midshaft, the humeral head, and the humeral epicondyles.

In addition to length, diaphyseal cross-sectional shape and area, and the dimensions of the articular surfaces, there exist some aspects of long bone morphology which probably reflect activity and handedness. The intertubercular sulcus of the humerus, situated between the greater and lesser tubercles, functions as the canal for the tendon of the long head of the biceps brachii muscle (which maintains the alignment of the humeral head with the glenoid cavity of the scapula during movements of the upper extremity). This sulcus was more often wider in the right humerus, and with a more acute angle between its medial wall and the plane of its floor,[57] presumably due to the greater pressure of the taut biceps head on the humerus on the dominant side. It has also been reported that the diaphyseal nutrient foramen of the right humerus tends to be larger than that of the left, perhaps reflecting vascular responses to loading of the dominant arm.[58] In the radius, it has been proposed that several dimensions that are characteristically greater on the right side are therefore indicative of handedness.[59] These include the side with greater distance between the dorsal tubercle and the styloid process, and the side with greater dorso-palmar diameter of the carpal articular surface opposite the dorsal tubercle.

The ulna appears to be the bone with least bilateral asymmetry of the three long bones in the arm. In professional racket sports players, the effect of prolonged unilateral loading on increase in bone mineral content and bone mineral density in these bones is slightest at sites in the ulnar shaft and the distal ulna.[28,51] Presumably this reflects its lesser role in distributing mechanical load in these tasks. However, Kennedy has observed preferential development of the ulnar supinator crest in the right arms of males in certain populations, apparently reflecting the stresses involved in overarm throwing (as, for example, of a hunting spear).[60] Additionally, where osteoarthritis occurs asymmetrically in the elbow joint it tends to occur on the right side,[32] with ulnar involvement very common.[61]

Certain fractures of the distal left forearm (in particular, in the ulna) in archaeological populations have been interpreted as 'parry fractures' relating to defence against a right-handed face-to-face attacker wielding a weapon.[62] Although this pattern of behaviour may well have occurred in the past, it is relevant that, in modern clinical populations, fractures and dislocations of the long bones of the arm also occur most frequently on the left side (for a variety of other reasons).[63–65] Where these fractures are due to falls, the left arm bias seems to reflect a preference to use the left hand to parry the fall.

Mechanical loading has been shown (in clinical radiographic studies) to affect the degree of lateral asymmetries of bone shape, size and mineral content. Archaeological evidence for inter-population contrasts in activity patterns has also been reported. This evidence should constitute a caveat against using a single set of absolute reference standards for inferring handedness without first considering past variation in activity type and level. Ruff[3] has compared the differences between the bending and torsional strengths of the dominant and non-dominant humeri in tennis players with that seen in the paired humeri from two archaeological populations with differing activity regimes, in order to emphasize that activity regime affects the degree of development of such asymmetries. A hunting–gathering–fishing sample from prehistoric California had higher levels of humeral asymmetry in the males than in the females, while in an historic Georgia coast sample, this sexual dimorphism was virtually absent and male humeral asymmetry was reduced to a level similar to that seen in the California females. This observed pattern of reduced sexual dimorphism in this character is consistent with the hypothesis that male and female subsistence tasks became very similar in the historic Georgia coast population due to the effects of contact at the time of Spanish colonization, and of missionary influence.

Several other archaeological studies have reported diachronic and inter-regional contrasts in the prevalence of arm bone asymmetries which may be due to activity pattern.[66–69] Wada[68] found a significantly greater asymmetry in the cross-sectional dimensions of the radius in male adults from rural agricultural/pastoral sites in protohistoric and early Islamic Iraq, compared with that found in male adult skeletons in two Japanese anatomy collections derived from modern urban populations. This contrast was less apparent in the adult females. He too interpreted this in terms of contrasting activity patterns. Huggare and Houghton[69] found a significant tendency for the right arm bones (especially the humerus) to be longer in a sample of adult Polynesian Maoris (both sexes combined), while no such significant asymmetries existed in the lengths of the clavicles, humeri, radii and ulnae from a sample of adults from prehistoric central Thailand (again, both sexes combined). They interpret this in terms of lower levels of heavy physical activity in the sedentary Thai population as opposed to the Maori coastal fishing population.

Some other interesting activity-related contrasts have been reported by Stirland,[70] who has compared the degree of humeral asymmetry in two male adult samples from medieval England. She found greater development of the humeral head and of the greater tubercle in the left bones of individuals from King Henry VIII's flagship, the *Mary Rose*, than in the left bones of individuals from the parish churchyard of St Margaret *in combusto*, Norwich. This pattern she interprets as due to the practice by the *Mary Rose* complement of archery with the weighty medieval longbow, which heavily loads the bow or non-drawing shoulder and arm, usually on the left side.

Work on morphological changes at the site of attachment of muscles and ligaments is entering a new phase of development, with several recent studies of lateral asymmetries in the arm and shoulder girdle complex.[33,71–74] This research promises to add a new dimension to the study of activity-related change, which will complement the more conventional focus on overall adaptive changes of bone shape and size.

Bones of the hand

Another repeated clinical observation is that the bones of the right hand tend to be larger than those of the left hand, as does the volume of the hand itself.[75] This has been seen in radiographs,[76] although in the earliest studies of side differences in the second metacarpals by Garn et al.[77] and by Plato et al.[78] no correlation was found with handedness (as measured either by hand preference or by grip strength). A correlation of relative hand size with handedness has been reported for right-handers, although not for left-handers.[75] Most recently, Roy et al.[79] have reported a finding of bilateral asymmetry of bone area in the second metacarpal correlated with hand dominance, in which handedness was assessed by the subject's own personal impressions of which handedness group they belonged to.

Singh[80] has recorded significant left-right differences in the direction of rotation of the head of the first metacarpal, as well as in the torsion of the metacarpal bones of the second to fifth digital rays. This pattern is interpreted as representing a 'lateral shift' in the degree of torsion of the metacarpals on the right side, facilitating efficient grips by preventing crowding of the fingers during flexion. Given both the importance of the thumb and index finger in many grip types, and the magnitude of normal asymmetries of pinch strength favouring the dominant hand (about 10%), we would expect to find some morphological correlates of handedness in the bones of the thumb as well as in those of the index finger. Bimson et al.[81] found that thumb flexion strength at the interphalangeal joint can be predicted with reasonable accuracy ($r = 0.73$) from the interaction of two measurements of the pollical distal phalanx, maximum length and joint depth. Osteological study of right-left differences in these measures might therefore provide information about relative thumb flexion strength in the two hands at this joint. Marsk[82] reports that the thumb of the dominant hand has a reduced range of extension at the metacarpophalangeal joint, which he interpreted as a sequel to adaptations to increased flexion in the same joint in most grip types. Of 66 subjects tested from each of two handedness categories, he found a relative reduction of extension in the dominant hand in 40 cases (right-handers), with only three having less extension in the non-dominant thumb. In the left-handers, the proportions were more equal (less extension in the left thumb in 23 cases, and in the right thumb in 21 cases). However, no examination has yet been made of side differences in the articular surfaces of the first metacarpophalangeal joint to test whether these contrasts in range of motion have any osteological signature.

Other studies have also focused on arthritic changes to the hand skeleton and their possible relationship with handedness. The severity of erosive lesions in rheumatoid arthritis appears to be influenced by hand dominance, with the dominant hand tending to show significantly greater radiographic changes.[83,84] With regard to osteoarthritis, Buckland-Wright et al.[85] found in a clinical study that in osteoarthritic hands, osteophyte formation was greatest at those sites corresponding with those for the largest forces exerted in the hand: the dominant side, and the finger tripod used in the precision grip, power grip, and pulp–pinch respectively. Waldron[86] studied the distribution of osteoarthritis of the hands in a series of 168 skeletons (77 males, 87 females, four of unknown sex) from 12 medieval and post-medieval archaeological sites in England. He reported that the only significant differences between the hands were seen in the second and third metacarpophalangeal joints, which were more often affected on the right side. Osteoarthritic changes at these sites are not seen so commonly in modern populations, and Waldron interprets the contrast as most likely being due to the higher levels of manual activity undertaken in the past. This interpretation is confirmed by modern clinical data showing an elevated incidence of metacarpophalangeal joint OA in men who undertook heavy manual labour for more than 10 years, among whom the typical site was in the second and third fingers, most often in the dominant hand.[87]

Hand injuries appear to be influenced by hand preference. In an audit of 4873 hand and wrist injuries seen in six accident and emergency clinics in Northern Ireland over 4 months, and in the about 50% of cases where the patient's handedness was recorded, right handers were injured in the right hand and wrist 55% of the time and in the left hand or wrist 45% of the time.[88] For left-handers, in contrast, the ratio was 58% left side injuries to 42% right side injuries.

ADDITIONAL PROCESSES WHICH MIGHT PRODUCE SKELETAL ASYMMETRIES INDEPENDENT OF HANDEDNESS

Some other processes may affect the development of asymmetry in paired skeletal elements in the forelimb and shoulder girdle, and these should be taken into account in any analysis of the markers of handedness. These other processes include both fluctuating asymmetry, and directional asymmetries favouring growth in one member of a pair of bones when these are due to innate developmental biases and not to mechanical loading history. Pathological development of elements of one side of the body is a third potentially complicating variable.

Fluctuating asymmetry

Fluctuating asymmetry occurs in paired bones and teeth due to random, local genetic or external environmental disturbances during morphogenesis.[89] Because the development on each side of a bilateral character is the product of a common gene complex, and because these disturbances are random, at the population level we expect a normal distribution of signed asymmetry scores about a mean of zero (or symmetry). The extent of such fluctuating asymmetry in a character, and the incidence of similar fluctuating asymmetries in other characters in any one individual, give a measure of developmental instability. Developmental instabilities may be expressed in an individual as deviations from symmetry in any paired skeletal element (for instance, in the length of the long bones). In principal, this may occur independently of the factors affecting the development of hand preferences. We should therefore expect to see some contribution from such developmental disturbances to the development of asymmetry in paired bones (e.g. in the length of the humeri), and this may be in the opposite direction to that predicted from hand preference.

Directional asymmetry in developmental gradients

Another possible source of developmental asymmetries is some innate biasing factor, such as a right-left gradient in oxygen tension in the blood supply to paired skeletal elements.[90] Evidence for such mechanisms is inconclusive, but it has been argued that foetal asymmetries in the long bones of the forelimb may reflect such a process. Bareggi *et al.*[91] found that in 58 aborted embryos and foetuses with developmental ages between 8 and 14 weeks, the right humerus was longer in 39 cases (and the left in four); the right radius was longer in 23 cases (and the left in three); and the right ulna was longer in 30 cases (and the left in seven). Schultz[92] found by dissection of 100 foetuses that by the beginning of the fourth month, foetal humeri showed asymmetric growth with the right humerus the longer of the pair in 52% of cases, the left longer in 21% of cases, and the remainder equal in length to within measurement precision. He argued that this refuted the suggestion that adult humeral length asymmetries were due to loading history and to handedness (although recent ultrasound findings[93] indicate that 85% of foetuses at 10 weeks of gestational age move their right arm more than their left arm, which might represent an osteogenic stimulus favouring the dominant arm). Pande and Singh[94] also found that in nine out of ten foetuses with crown rump lengths in the range 195–290 mm, muscle and bone weight in the upper limb was greater on the right side.

However, other findings have been contradictory. Bagnall *et al.*[95] found, in a study of a large sample of foetuses ($n = 728$) with gestational ages in the range 8–26 weeks, that on average the left humerus was significantly longer then the right, while no significant length asymmetry existed in the foetal radius and ulna. Ingelmark[46] found a tendency for the humerus to be longer on the left side and the ulna on the right in full-term foetuses, although he subsequently cast doubt upon the significance of this finding when account was taken of measurement error. Steele and Mays,[96] who measured the humeri of 14 neonatal infants from the deserted medieval village of Wharram Percy, found that in 12 cases the left humerus was longer. A more recent anthropometric study by Dangerfield[97] of 211 live, full-term neonates found the same result; namely, that the left upper arm (and the dorsum of the hand) tends to be slightly longer at this early stage of development, although in the forearm the right side tends to be longer.

It is probably wise to conclude that the issue is unresolved. However, osteological findings from full-term foetuses and anthropometric findings from live full-term neonates are more likely to be representative of the normal pattern of development than are studies of aborted embryos and foetuses with younger gestational ages. Findings from the former class of study suggest that if anything, the left humerus tends to be longer in full-term neonates. Pre-existing developmental biases of this kind are therefore unlikely to account for the greater development of the arm and hand bones on the right side in the majority of juvenile and adult human skeletons.

Pathological asymmetry

Pathological processes, leading either to hemihypertrophy or hemiatrophy, can also affect growth of the upper limb bones. Syndromes of hemihypertrophy include the Proteus syndrome and Russel–Silver dwarfism, while hemihypertrophy is also often associated with a predisposition to malignant disease.[97] Asymmetry can also be caused by angiodysplasias and by the congenital absence of the pectoralis major muscle on one side of the body (Poland's syndrome).[97] Congenital unilateral limb reduction deficits can also occur in apparent association with early unilateral brain lesions.[98–100] Finally, asymmetrical bone remodelling can occur as a result of unilateral disuse atrophy. Abnormally large asymmetries of the forelimb long bones (the left arm bones being smaller), have been identified in an adult male from the Upper Palaeolithic in Liguria, Italy.[101] These have been interpreted as a consequence of entrapment neuropathy, of direct trauma to one or more of the muscles of the shoulder, or of glenohumeral joint instability on the left side.

INCIDENCE OF SKELETAL ASYMMETRIES RELATED TO HANDEDNESS IN PAST POPULATIONS

Some hypotheses concerning the selective advantages of human handedness are predicated on estimates of the prevalence of handedness phenotypes in human populations.[1,2,14] Several studies of handedness in archaeological populations have used artefact variability as the index. Other studies have inferred cognitive laterality from morphological brain asymmetries in skulls and endocasts, and have discussed inter-population contrasts. These studies are reviewed elsewhere.[102–104] In this context, we shall focus only on handedness as it has been inferred from skeletal indicators of asymmetrical mechanical loading of the forelimb and shoulder girdle.

Fossil hominid remains have been studied from this perspective. The skeleton of the Nariokotome boy, WT–15000 (*Homo ergaster*), has greater development of the clavicular area of attachment of the right deltoid muscle and greater length of the right ulna, consistent with right handedness.[105] Humeral diaphyseal asymmetry consistent with right arm dominance is also prevalent in Neanderthal skeletons; of six skeletons in which the relevant measurements could be taken bilaterally, all were more robust in the right arm.[106]

In early Holocene (Mesolithic) skeletal samples of modern *Homo sapiens sapiens*, mostly from northern Europe, most individuals have longer right forelimbs, a pattern seen slightly more strongly in females.[107] Twenty-four adult males had longer right arms (summed lengths of the humerus and radius), and nine had longer left arms. For the females, the ratio was 19 with longer right arms to 5 with longer left arms. A study of asymmetries in bone mineral content and mid-shaft bone width in the radii in a Neolithic sample of 27 individuals from three sites in the Middle Elbe-Saale region found a right-dominant pattern in 70% of individuals, with 15% left-handed and 15% 'ambidextrous'.[48] However, the discriminant function used to predict handedness in this study is likely to have somewhat inflated the estimated frequencies of non-right handedness. Thould and Thould[108] examined 416 adult skeletons from Romano-British Poundbury and found in a pilot study that the arm bones were longer on the right side in 210 individuals and on the left in 65 (the rest were not measurably asymmetrical). They give no further details of their results.

Steele and Mays' study of asymmetry in the summed lengths of the humerus and radius in the medieval Wharram Percy cemetery population[96] found a pattern in adults very similar to that reported by Annett for the distribution of manual performance asymmetries in the modern British population. Their results were 81% showing the right-handed pattern, 3% showing no significant asymmetry, and 16% showing the left-handed pattern. These frequencies of arm length asymmetry were almost identical to those recorded by Schultz[109] in anatomy collections in the USA, where the percentages of instances falling into each of the same categories were 80:4:16 in a pooled sample of 232 Americans of European ancestry. Schultz recorded data on long bone length asymmetries for the humerus, radius, and for both combined, partitioned by sex and also by population (his sample also included 233 Americans of African origin, 122 Alaskan Eskimo-Inuit, 118 North American Indians, and smaller samples of Chinese and of Aboriginal Australians). The overall prevalence for the complete pooled sample is 79% longer right arms, 3% equal to measurement precision, and 18% longer left arms. For all the populations for which the information was tabulated, the females were always less likely to have longer left arms and more likely to have longer right arms (which is consistent with sexual dimorphism in the prevalences of right and left hand preference[12]).

In a more recent skeletal study,[110] side dominance in musculo-stress markers in 25 adults of a Hudson Bay Eskimo-Inuit population showed 20 with right side dominance, two with left side dominance, and three with no discernible asymmetry. Allowing for chance effects of such a small sample size, this is quite comparable with Schultz's findings of a ratio of arm length asymmetry in his larger Eskimo-Inuit sample ($n = 122$) of 82.5% right arm longer, 3% symmetrical to measurement precision and 14.5% left arm longer. Although in individual cases these measures may be unreliable as an indicator of handedness, it seems plausible that these prevalences give reasonable broad indications of underlying prevalences of right and left handedness in the populations sampled. However, account should be taken of the complicating effects of developmental fluctuating asymmetry in long bone length which, because it is equally likely to result in greater dimensions on the left or on the right sides, will tend to inflate the apparent prevalence of left-handedness.

We should also note that all these studies focus on only a small set of measures or a single skeletal element. The search for correlations among measurements of asymmetry at different sites in the forelimb and shoulder girdle complex may not yield simple and consistent results.[71] A recent study by Sakaue[111] of asymmetry in the humerus in 63 modern Japanese and 40 Jomon-period individuals found no correlation between asymmetry of humeral length and asymmetry of transverse diaphyseal cross-sectional area. Sakaue interprets this as reflecting the different effects of mechanical loading bias before epiphyseal fusion, and more immediately before death. However, this really needs to be tested on a skeletal sample with many individuals who died in childhood and adolescence, since it predicts that in these age groups the longitudinal and diaphyseal asymmetries will be more convergent.

FUTURE RESEARCH

Implications for forensic work

For forensic contexts, where accurate diagnosis of the hand preferences are required to aid in identification, the potential clearly exists for such diagnoses, and these are likely to be more reliable when a number of different measures converge on the same right- or left-handed pattern. However, there are important caveats. We should recall that until recently there has been some cultural pressure for natural left-handers to switch to right hand use in tasks such as handwriting, and we do not know how that contradictory pattern might look in terms of skeletal asymmetries. The handedness of a deceased individual as reported by his/her familiars may not correspond exactly to that individual's own perception of his/her hand preferences, since these patterns can be complex. Additionally, we do not always know how far the relatively low levels of manual activity of many modern individuals will affect the expression of gross morphological asymmetries of the forelimb elements. (Although the studies cited do suggest that measures such as humeral diaphyseal asymmetry and asymmetry in the size of the second metacarpal appear to be fairly reliable diagnostic indicators.) There is, finally, the additional problem that left-handers are often less consistent in their patterns of lateralization (for instance of grip strength and hand volume, as noted earlier). While these complications add spice to the challenge of recognizing the effects of handedness in human skeletal material, they also mean that simple forensic diagnosis of the hand preference of a deceased individual will not always be possible.

Research potential of large cemetery collections

This review has concentrated on right-left asymmetries in bones of the shoulder, arm and hand that may reflect preferential mechanical loading of the dominant side. In some cases, their associations with behavioural handedness have been tested explicitly. In many other cases, the inferred association of a particular skeletal asymmetry with behavioural handedness has still to be tested by studies of the pattern in individuals of known handedness. In the meantime, the inference of handedness from such features must remain provisional, and dependent on the lack of any other clearly identified causal mechanism that might produce asymmetrical development of such a skeletal character on the right side in most individuals. Further correlational studies of skeletal asymmetries and handedness in living subjects are therefore needed.

Future work should also focus on indirect confirmation of these associations, by testing for correlations among measures of handedness at different sites in the forelimb and shoulder girdle complex, and among different types of measure (external morphology, morphology of muscle and ligament attachment sites, and radiographic measures of bone mineral density and distribution). Such work will enable us to discern the effects of handedness, and mechanical loading bias, from those of fluctuating asymmetry in the development of particular paired skeletal elements. This work will be best carried out on large, well-preserved cemetery populations with good representations of individuals from all age and sex classes (since it may take large sample sizes to satisfy the requirements of valid statistical inference).

Future work might also focus on contrasts between populations in the degree of development of asymmetric characters, as a measure of activity regime. Such work, if it provides a good cross-cultural coverage of different populations with different economies, may ultimately provide a test of the hypotheses of a constant underlying proportion of right and left handers, and of an innate tendency for males to be more often left-handed than females, in all human groups.

ACKNOWLEDGEMENTS

I am grateful to Margaret Cox and Simon Mays for providing the opportunity for me to compile this review. I am also particularly grateful to Marian Annett, Tim Crow, Chris McManus and Marjorie LeMay, who have each been sources of regular encouragement for my and my collaborators' studies of these unwritten records of past human variability.

REFERENCES

1   Annett M. The right shift theory of a genetic balanced polymorphism for cerebral dominance and cognitive processing. *Current Psychology of Cognition* 1995; **14**: 427–480.

2   Crow TJ. Relative hand skill predicts academic ability: global deficits at the point of hemispheric indecision. *Neuropsychologia* 1998; **36**: 1275–1282.

3   Ruff C. Biomechanical analyses of archaeological human skeletal samples. In: Saunders SR, Katzenberg A (eds), *Skeletal Biology of Past Peoples: Research Methods*. New York: Wiley-Liss, 1992: pp. 37–58.

4   Schulter-Ellis FP. Evidence of handedness on documented skeletons. *Journal of Forensic Sciences* 1980; **25**: 624–630.

5   McManus IC. Handedness. In: Beaumont JG, Kenealy PM, Rogers MJC (eds), *The Blackwell Dictionary of Neuropsychology*. Oxford: Blackwell, 1996: pp. 367–376.

6   Annett M. The distribution of manual asymmetry. *British Journal of Psychology* 1972; **63**: 343–358.

7   McManus IC. The inheritance of left-handedness. In: *Biological Asymmetry and Handedness*. Ciba Foundation Symposium 162. Chichester: Wiley, 1991: pp. 251–281.

8   Spiegler BJ, Yenikomshian GH. Incidence of left-handed writing in a college population with reference to family patterns of hand preference. *Neuropsychologia* 1983; **21**: 651–659.

9   Brackenridge CJ. Secular variation in handedness over ninety years. *Neuropsychologia* 1981; **19**: 459–462.

10 Tambs K, Magnus P, Berg K. Left-handedness in twin families – support of an environmental hypothesis. *Perceptual and Motor Skills* 1987; **64**: 155–170.

11 Fleminger JJ, Dalton R, Standage KF. Age as a factor in the handedness of adults. *Neuropsychologia* 1977; **15**: 471–473.

12 Seddon BM, McManus IC. The incidence of left-handedness: a meta-analysis. MS (n.d.).

13 de Lacoste M-C, Horvath DS, Woodward DJ. Possible sex differences in the developing human fetal brain. *Journal of Clinical and Experimental Neuropsychology* 1991; **13**: 831–846.

14 Raymond M, Pontier D, Dufour A-B, Moller AP. Frequency-dependent maintenance of left-handedness in humans. *Proceedings of the Royal Society of London, Series B* 1996; **263**: 1627–1633.

15 Yeo RA, Gangestad SW, Daniel WF. Hand preference and developmental instability. *Psychobiology* 1993; **21**: 161–168.

16 Connolly KJ, Bishop DVM. The measurement of handedess – a cross-cultural comparison of samples from England and Papua New Guinea. *Neuropsychologia* 1992; **30**: 13–26.

17 Dawson JLMB. An anthropological perspective on the evolution and lateralization of the brain. *Annals of the New York Academy of Science* 1977; **299**: 424–447.

18 Bryden MP, Ardila A, Ardila O. Handedness in native Amazonians. *Neuropsychologia* 1993; **31**: 301–308.

19 Annett M. The stability of handedness. In: Connolly KJ (ed.), *The Psychobiology of the Hand*. Clinics in Developmental Medicine 147. Cambridge: Cambridge University Press, 1998: pp. 63–76.

20 Thorngren K-G, Werner CO. Normal grip strength. *Acta Orthopaedica Scandinavica* 1979; **50**: 255–259.

21 Petersen P, Petrick M, Connor H, Conklin D. Grip strength and hand dominance: challenging the 10% rule. *American Journal of Occupational Therapy* 1989; **43**: 444–447.

22 Crosby CA, Wehbe MA, Mawr B. Hand strength: normative values. *Journal of Hand Surgery – American Volume* 1994; **19**: 665–670.

23   Chau N, Remy E, Petry D, Huguenin P, Bourgkard E, Andre JM. Asymmetry correction equations for hand volume, grip and pinch strengths in healthy working people. *European Journal of Epidemiology* 1998; **14**: 71–77.

24   Brorson H, Werner CO, Thorngren KG. Normal pinch strength. *Acta Orthopaedica Scandinaviva* 1989; **60**: 66–68.

25   Richards RR, Gordon R, Beaton D. Measurement of wrist, metacarpophalangeal joint, and thumb extension strength in a normal population. *Journal of Hand Surgery – American Volume* 1993; **18A**: 253–261.

26   Josty IC, Tyler MP, Shewell PC, Roberts AH. Grip and pinch strength variations in different types of workers. *Journal of Hand Surgery – British Volume* 1997; **22**: 266–269.

27   Madsen OR, Schaadt O, Bliddal H, Egsmose C, Sylvest J. Relationship between quadriceps strength and bone mineral density of the proximal tibia and distal forearm in women. *Journal of Bone Mineral Research* 1993; **8**: 1439–1444.

28   Kannus P, Haapasalo H, Sievanen H, Oja P, Vuori I. The site-specific effects of long-term unilateral activity on bone mineral density and content. *Bone* 1994; **15**: 279–284.

29   Bonci CM, Hensal FJ, Torg JS. A preliminary study on the measurement of static and dynamic motion at the glenohumeral joint. *American Journal of Sports Medicine* 1986; **14**: 12–17.

30   Kronberg M, Brostrom LA, Soderlund V. Retroversion of the humeral head in the normal shoulder and its relationship to the normal range of motion. *Clinical Orthopaedics* 1990; **253**: 113–117.

31   Pieper, HG. Humeral torsion in the throwing arm of handball players. *American Journal of Sports Medicine* 1998; **26**: 247–253.

32   Stewart, TD. *Essentials of Forensic Anthropology*. Springfield: Charles C Thomas, 1979.

33   Mays S, Steele J, Ford M. Directional asymmetry in the human clavicle. *International Journal of Osteoarchaeology* 1999; **9**: 18–28.

34   Parsons FG. On the proportions and characteristics of the modern English clavicle. *Journal of Anatomy* 1916; **51**: 71–93.

35   Longia GS, Agarwal AK, Thomas RJ, Jain PN, Saxena SK. Metrical study of rhomboid fossa of clavicle. *Anthropologische Anzeiger* 1982; **40**: 111–115.

36   Jit I, Kaur H. Rhomboid fossa in the clavicles of North Indians. *American Journal of Physical Anthropology* 1986; **70**: 97–103.

37   Spenneman D, personal communication, 1998.

38   Stenlund B, Goldie I, Hagberg M, Hogstedt C, Marions O. Radiographic osteoarthrosis in the acromioclavicular joint resulting from manual work or exposure to vibration. *British Journal of Industrial Medicine* 1992; **49**: 588–593.

39   Stenlund B. Shoulder tendinitis and osteoarthrosis of the acromioclavicular joint and their relation to sports. *British Journal of Sports Medicine* 1993; **27**: 125–130.

40   Chhibber SR, Singh I. Asymmetry in muscle weight in the human upper limbs. *Acta Anatomica* 1972; **81**: 462–465.

41   Schell LM, Johnston FE, Smith DR, Paolone AM. Directional asymmetry of body dimensions among white adolescents. *American Journal of Physical Anthropology* 1985; **67**: 317–322.

42   Neumann S. Händigkeit im Vergleich zur Asymmetrie der oberen Extremität. *Zeitschrift für Morphologie und Anthropologie* 1992; **79**: 183–195.

43   Taaffe DR, Lewis B, Marcus R. Quantifying the effect of hand preference on upper limb bone mineral and soft tissue composition in young and elderly women by dual-energy X-ray absorptiometry. *Clinical Physiology* 1994; **14**: 393–404.

44   Latimer HB, Lowrance EW. Bilateral asymmetry in weight and in length of human bones. *The Anatomical Record* 1965; **152**: 217–224.

45   Ruff CB, Jones HH. Bilateral asymmetry in cortical bone of the humerus and tibia – sex and age factors. *Human Biology* 1981; **53**: 69–86.

46   Ingelmark BE. Über die Längenasymmetrien der Extremitäten und ihren Zusammenhang mit der Rechts-Linkshändigkeit. *Upsala Läkareförenings Förhandlingar N.F.* 1946; **52**: 17–82.

47   Faulkner RA, Houston CS, Bailey DA, Drinkwater DT, McKay HA, Wilkinson AA. Comparison of bone-mineral content and bone-mineral density between dominant and nondominant limbs in children 8–16 years of age. *American Journal of Human Biology* 1993; **5**: 491–499.

48   Reichel H, Runge H, Bruchaus H. Die seitendifferenz des mineralgehaltes und der breite am radius und ihre bedeutung für die händigkeitsbestimmung an skelettmaterial. *Zeitschrift für Morphologie und Anthropologie* 1990; **78**: 217–227.

49   Buskirk ER, Andersen KL, Brozek J. Unilateral activity and bone and muscle development in the forearm. *Research Quarterly* 1956; **27**: 127–131.

50   Jones HH, Priest JD, Hayes WC, Tichenor CC, Nagel DA. Humeral hypertrophy in response to exercise. *Journal of Bone and Joint Surgery* 1977; **59A**: 204–208.

51   Haapasalo H, Kannus P, Sievanen H, Heinonen A, Oja P, Vuori I. Long-term unilateral loading and bone mineral density and content in female squash players. *Calcified Tissue International* 1994; **54**: 249–255.

52   Kannus P, Haapasalo H, Sankelo M, Sievanen H, Pasanen M, Heinonen A, Oja P, Vuori I. Effect of starting age of physical activity on bone mass in the dominant arm of tennis and squash players. *Annals of Internal Medicine* 1995; **123**: 27–31.

53   Tsuji S, Tsunoda N, Yata H, Katsukawa F, Onishi S, Yamazaki H. Relation between grip strength and radial bone mineral density in young athletes. *Archives of Physical Medicine and Rehabilitation* 1995; **76**: 234–238.

54   Krahl H, Michaelis U, Pieper HG, Quack G, Montag M. Stimulation of bone growth through sports. A radiologic investigation of the upper extremities in professional tennis players. *American Journal of Sports Medicine* 1994; **22**: 751–757.

55   Haapasalo H, Sievanen H, Kannus P, Heinonen A, Oja P, Vuori I. Dimensions and estimated mechanical characteristics of the humerus after long-term tennis loading. *Journal of Bone and Mineral Research* 1996; **11**: 864–872.

56   Pfeiffer S. Age changes in the external dimensions of adult bone. *American Journal of Physical Anthropology* 1980; **52**: 529–532.

57   Vettivel S, Indrasingh I, Chandi G, Chandi SM. Variations in the intertubercular sulcus of the humerus related to handedness. *Journal of Anatomy* 1992; **180**: 321–326.

58   Carroll SE. A study of the nutrient foramina of the humeral diaphysis. *Journal of Bone and Joint Surgery* 1963; **45B**: 176–181.

59   Holla SJ, Vettivel S, Chandi G. Bony markers at the distal end of the radius for estimating handedness and radial length. *Anatomische Anzeiger* 1996; **178**: 191–195.

60   Kennedy KAR. Morphological variation in ulnar supinator crests and fossae as identification markers of occupational stress. *Journal of Forensic Science* 1983; **28**: 871–876.

61   Wells C. The human burials. In: McWhirr A, Viner L, Wells C (eds), *Romano-British Cemeteries at Cirencester*. Cirencester: Cirencester Excavation Committee, 1982: pp. 134–202.

62   Webb S. *Palaeopathology of Aboriginal Australians*. Cambridge: Cambridge University Press, 1995.

63   Meals RA. The laterality of fractures and dislocations with respect to handedness. *Clinical Orthopaedics* 1979; **143**: 158–161.

64   Mortensson W, Thonell S. Left-side dominance of upper extremity fracture in children. *Acta Orthopaedica Scandinavica* 1991; **62**: 154–155.

65   Borton D, Masterson E, O'Brien T. Distal forearm fractures in children: the role of hand dominance. *Journal of Pediatric Orthopaedics* 1994; **14**: 496–497.

66   Fresia AE, Ruff CB, Larsen CS. Temporal decline in bilateral asymmetry of the upper limb on the Georgia coast. In: Larsen CS (ed.), *The Archaeology of the Mission Santa Catalina De Guale*, 2: *Biocultural Interpretations of a Population in Transition*. Anthropological Paper 68. New York: American Museum of Natural History, 1990: 121–132.

67   Hiramoto Y. Right-left differences in the lengths of human arm and leg bones. *Kaibogaku Zasshi* 1993; **68**: 536–543.

68   Wada Y. Morphological assessment of ethnic, sex and side differences in the human radius based on intra-regional and side ratios. *Anthropological Science* 1998; **105**: 193–210.

69   Huggare I, Houghton P. Asymmetry in the human skeleton: a study on prehistoric Polynesians and Thais. *European Journal of Morphology* 1995; **33**: 3–14.

70   Stirland AJ. Asymmetry and activity-related change in the male humerus. *International Journal of Osteoarchaeology* 1993; **3**: 105–113.

71   Wilczak CA. Consideration of sexual dimorphism, age, and asymmetry in quantitative measurements of muscle insertion sites. *International Journal of Osteoarchaeology* 1998; **8**: 311–325.

72   Steen SL, Lane RW. Evaluation of habitual activities among two Alaskan Eskimo populations based on musculoskeletal stress markers. *International Journal of Osteoarchaeology* 1998; **8**: 341–353.

73   Stirland AJ. Musculoskeletal evidence for activity: problems of evaluation. *International Journal of Osteoarchaeology* 1998; **8**: 354–362.

74   Peterson J. The Natufian hunting conundrum: spears, atlatls, or bows? Musculoskeletal and armature evidence. *International Journal of Osteoarchaeology* 1998; **8**: 378–389.

75   Purves D, White LE, Andrews TJ. Manual asymmetry and handedness. *Proceedings of the National Academy of Sciences, USA* 1994; **91**: 5030–5032.

76   McLeod DR, Coupland SG. Asymmetry quantification utilizing hand radiographs. *American Journal of Medical Genetics* 1992; **44**: 321–325.

77   Garn SM, Mayor GH, Shaw HA. Paradoxical bilateral asymmetry in bone size and bone mass in the hand. *American Journal of Physical Anthropology* 1976; **45**: 209–210.

78   Plato CC, Wood JL, Norris AH. Bilateral asymmetry in bone measurements of the hand and lateral dominance. *American Journal of Physical Anthropology* 1980; **52**: 27–31.

79   Roy TA, Ruff CB, Plato CC. Hand dominance and bilateral asymmetry in the structure of the second metacarpal. *American Journal of Physical Anthropology* 1994; **94**: 203–211.

80   Singh I. Torsion in metacarpal bones and bilateral asymmetry. *Journal of Anatomy* 1979; **129**: 343–349.

81   Bimson B, Ottevanger J, Roberts N, Macho G, Percy D, Whitehouse GH. Hominid thumb strength predicted by high-resolution magnetic resonance imaging and force measurements in living subjects. *Magnetic Resonance Imaging* 1997; **15**: 899–908.

82   Marsk A. Studies on weight-distribution upon the lower extremities in individuals working in a standing position. *Acta Orthopaedica Scandinavica* 1958; **27** (suppl. 31).

83   Mody GM, Meyers OL, Reinach SG. Handedness and deformities, radiographic changes, and function of the hand in rheumatoid arthritis. *Annals of the Rheumatic Diseases* 1989; **48**: 104–107.

84   Boonsaner K, Louthrenoo W, Meyer S, Schumacher HR. Effect of dominancy on severity in rheumatoid arthritis. *British Journal of Rheumatology* 1992; **31**: 77–80.

85   Buckland-Wright JC, Macfarlane DG, Lynch JA. Osteophytes in the osteoarthritic hand – their incidence, size, distribution, and progression. *Annals of the Rheumatic Diseases* 1991; **50**: 627–630.

86   Waldron HA. Osteoarthritis of the hands in early populations. *British Journal of Rheumatology* 1996; **35**: 1292–1298.

87   Ulreich A, Klein E. Frequency of arthritis of metacarpophalangeal joints – a degenerative disease linked to manual heavy work. *Zeitschrift für Rheumatologie* 1991; **50**: 6–9.

88   Hill C, Riaz M, Mozzam A, Brennen MD. A regional audit of hand and wrist injuries. *Journal of Hand Surgery – British Volume* 1998; **23B**: 196–200.

89   Moller AP, Swaddle JP. *Asymmetry, Developmental Stability, and Evolution.* Oxford: Oxford University Press, 1997.

90   Brown NA, Hoyle CI, McCarthy A, Wolpert L. The development of asymmetry: the sidedness of drug-induced limb abnormalities is reversed in situs inversus mice. *Development* 1989; **107**: 637–642.

91   Bareggi R, Grill V, Zweyer M, Sandrucci MA, Narducci P, Forabasco A. The growth of long bones in human embryological and fetal upper limbs and its relationship to other developmental patterns. *Anatomy and Embryology* 1994; **189**: 19–24.

92   Schultz AH. Fetal growth of man and other primates. *Quarterly Review of Biology* 1926; **1**: 465–521.

93   Hepper PG, McCartney GR, Shannon EA. Lateralised behaviour in first trimester human foetuses. *Neuropsychologia* 1998; **36**: 531–534.

94 Pande BS, Singh I. One-sided dominance in the upper limbs of human fetuses as evidenced by asymmetry in muscle and bone weight. *Journal of Anatomy* 1971; **109**: 457–459.

95 Bagnall KM, Harris PF, Jones PRM. A radiographic study of the longitudinal growth of primary ossification centers in limb long bones of the human fetus. *The Anatomical Record* 1982; **203**: 293–299.

96 Steele J, Mays S. Handedness and directional asymmetry in the long bones of the human upper limb. *International Journal of Osteoarchaeology* 1995; **5**: 39–49.

97 Dangerfield PH. Asymmetry and growth. In: Ulijaszek SJ, Mascie-Taylor CGN (eds), *Anthropometry: The Individual and the Population*. Cambridge: Cambridge University Press, 1994: pp. 7–29.

98 Aram DM, Ekelman BL, Satz P. Trophic changes following early unilateral injury to the brain. *Developmental Medicine and Child Neurology* 1986; **28**: 165–170.

99 Iloeje SO. Trophic limb changes among children with developmental apraxia. *Developmental Medicine and Child Neurology* 1988; **30**: 791–796.

100 Dlugosz LJ, Byers T, Msall ME, Marshall J, Lesswing A, Cooke RE. Relationships between laterality of congenital upper limb reduction deficits and school performance. *Clinical Pediatrics* 1988; **27**: 319–324.

101 Churchill SE, Formicola V. A case of marked bilateral asymmetry in the upper limbs of an upper palaeolithic male from Barma Grande (Liguria), Italy. *International Journal of Osteoarchaeology* 1997; **7**: 18–38.

102 Spennemann DHR. On the origins and development of handedness in humans – some remarks on past and current theories. *Homo* 1985; **36**: 121–141.

103 LeMay M. Left-right dissymmetry, handedness. *American Journal of Neuroradiology* 1992; **13**: 493–504.

104 Steele J. Evolution of laterality in hominids, including humans: archaeological perspectives. *Laterality* (in press).

105 Walker A, Leakey R. The postcranial bones. In: Walker A, Leakey R (eds), *The Nariokotome Homo erectus Skeleton*. Berlin: Springer, 1993: pp. 95–160.

106 Trinkaus E, Churchill SE, Ruff CB. Postcranial robusticity in Homo. II: Humeral bilateral asymmetry and bone plasticity. *American Journal of Physical Anthropology* 1994; **93**: 1–34.

107 Constandse-Westermann TS, Newell RR. Limb lateralization and social stratification in western European Mesolithic societies. In: Hershkovitz I (ed.), *People and Culture in Change, Part ii*. British Archaeological Reports. International Series 508(i). Oxford: British Archaeological Reports, 1989: pp. 405–433.

108 Thould AK, Thould BT. Arthritis in Roman Britain. *British Medical Journal* 1983; **287**: 1909–1911.

109 Schultz AH. Proportions, variability, and asymmetries of the long bones of the limbs and the clavicles in man and apes. *Human Biology* 1937; **9**: 281–328.

110 Hawkey DE, Merbs CF. Activity-induced musculoskeletal stress markers (MSM) and subsistence strategy changes among ancient Hudson Bay Eskimos. *International Journal of Osteoarchaeology* 1995; **5**: 324–338.

111 Sakaue K. Bilateral asymmetry of the humerus in Jomon people and modern Japanese. *Anthropological Science* 1998; **105**: 231–246.

20

FORENSIC AND ARCHAEOLOGICAL RECONSTRUCTION OF THE HUMAN FACE UPON THE SKULL

Richard Neave

INTRODUCTION

The existence of a predictable relationship between the skull and its overlying soft tissue structures is a fact well recognized by artists and scientists alike. Emphasizing how central such understanding is to the reconstruction of a face are the words of the celebrated Roman doctor, Galen, who in AD 130 wrote, 'As poles to tents and walls to houses so are bones to all living creatures, for other features naturally take form from them and change with them' (p. 2)[1]. While this is not strictly true for 'all living creatures', certainly as far as the majority of vertebrate animals is concerned it must be so.

The skeleton is therefore the armature for the body, and fundamental to the success of any figurative sculpture (success, that is, in terms of the degree of likeness between the subject and the image) are the proportions. Should the armature be of the wrong proportions then the model will be incorrect and the desired effect will never be achieved regardless of how much attention may be paid to the fine detail. Given that such facts have been well recognized by the majority of artists and scientists for centuries, it is hardly surprising that attempts are constantly being made to use the skeletons of prehistoric animals and hominids to penetrate time. In so far as it is possible, replacing the soft tissue that once clothed the now bare bones gives a good indication as to their probable appearance when alive. All those who are involved in such attempts inevitably run up against the same set of problems with regard to the treatment of particular areas where the skeleton appears not to hold the answer. In the case of our early ancestors, questions such as skin colour, hair colour, shape of the lips, absence or presence of facial hair remain uncertain.

When we turn our attention to more modern people such questions present fewer problems, but the precise shape and form of much finer details may still elude us. None the less, just as the post-cranial bones form the armature for the rest of the body, so the skull forms the armature for the head and face. What more perfect an armature could there be upon which to build someone's face than his/her skull?

The rebuilding of a face over the skull provides us not only with an opportunity to gain an insight into the appearance of our early ancestors, but also of more recent individuals whose remains fall within the preserve of the archaeologist. Valuable as such studies are to our understanding of the past, it is the immediate past, that which falls into the forensic arena, which is where facial reconstruction as an investigative tool is of everyday practical value.

APPROACHES TO THE PROBLEM

Rebuilding a face over a skull may be approached in several different ways, but despite the myths and misunderstandings that surround the subject it must always be understood that an exact portrait can never be achieved. Realistically, an appearance similar to the type of face that the subject had when alive is the best that can be expected in the majority of cases. The most well understood and logical approach is to make a three-dimensional reconstruction using a plastic material such as clay, wax or plasterline. Indeed, this had been the preferred approach until quite recently when the perceived usefulness of rebuilding faces over skulls became a popular avenue of exploration.

Reliance is frequently placed exclusively upon soft tissue measurements to provide the necessary information with which to develop the features of the face. Less frequently, basic anatomy developed over a skull in combination with statistical data is employed as a means of developing a face. The latter option may appear the most logical and represents all that must be understood by any reconstruction practitioner, regardless of which method is adopted. However, there is considerable debate over the need to carry out such detailed preliminary work, as it is unlikely ever to be seen.

The majority of early studies were undertaken by modelling in clay upon a cast of the skull. Measurements of soft tissue thickness were generally used to indicate how much 'tissue' should be laid over the skull while the position, size and approximate shape of the morphological features were determined from the bony landmarks. Among the most notable of these projects was the reconstruction of the face of Johann Sebastian Bach by the German anatomist Wilhelm His. The presumed remains of Bach were exhumed in 1894. In 1896,[2] utilizing a set of soft tissue measurements gathered from fresh corpses, His rebuilt a face over Bach's skull resulting in a face that bore a close resemblance to known portraits of the composer.

Others followed in the footsteps of His. Kollman and Buchley are the best known and often quoted. Kollman, the scientist, and Buchley, the sculptor, collaborated together and produced a reconstruction of the head of a Neolithic female from Auvernier in Switzerland.[3] In 1913, the anatomist Professor von Eggelling, a man who had undertaken numerous studies in the subject, was convinced that racial type could be determined by reconstruction. To test his theory he designed an experiment whereby two sculptors were to work independently upon separate casts of the same skull. The results were then to be compared with a death mask made of the deceased before defleshing. In the event, the reconstructions neither looked alike nor did they resemble the deceased.[4] This result, coupled with the advent of two World Wars, seems to have brought further work to a halt in

Europe. Not until 1946, when the American anatomist Krogman wrote an article promoting the technique and describing a method of facial reconstruction that could be usefully undertaken, was any serious attention again paid to the subject. It is interesting to note that Krogman, like others before him, employed a sculptor to undertake the practical work of making the face.[5] The method required a series of measured markers indicating the thickness of the soft tissue to be attached to the skull. Strips of plasticine were then laid in a latticework over the skull joining all the measured points. In this way a basic face was formed.

The anatomical approach, promoted by the anthropologist Gerasimov in Russia between 1930 and 1970, relied upon the logical building of the musculature upon the skull to form the shape of the face. This method also relied upon the bony landmarks to determine the shape of many of the features. Gerasimov undertook all the modelling himself, developing the necessary skills to allow him to carry out his own ideas without having to rely on a third party. Not surprisingly, the anatomical approach is referred to as the Russian method.[6] Both these methods required a degree of technical skill that frequently fell outside the range of would-be practitioners. One compromise is to use a commercially produced 'plasterline/plasticine' material, which, unlike clay, has the advantage of remaining soft.[7] By combining the use of such material with modelling directly upon the original skull, the complex tasks of making a mould and casting the skull are avoided. There are both advantages and disadvantages in working with plasticine. There are, however, very few advantages and many serious disadvantages when working directly on to the original specimen; these are discussed below.

Two-dimensional reconstruction has been used in forensic investigations with some success in the USA. In this approach, soft tissue thickness markers are glued to the skull and photographs from the lateral and antero-posterior projections are made with the skull mounted in the Frankfurt plane. Prints of the skull are then covered with a sheet of tracing paper and the artist draws/reconstructs the face accordingly.[5]

The approach that is currently being pursued with great intensity by workers in the field is computer/digitally generated facial reconstruction. In common with all of the methods referred to thus far, digital reconstruction relies upon basic tissue thickness data. However, while it will undoubtedly become the preferred method in the future, there remain many areas and features for which no data exist. In the absence of such information a digital reconstruction is unlikely to be any more precise in its depiction of a face than any of the other methods already discussed. The advantages will be considerable when accurate digital reconstruction becomes a reality, for a whole range of possible appearances in terms of weight, build and age, together with different hairstyles, etc. can be catered for relatively swiftly by 'morphing'. The relative speed with which such work can be carried out, together with the lack of any specialist manual skills, makes it a very attractive option.

Currently the most credible computer-generated reconstructions rely upon laser scanning the skull to create a digital image in the computer.[8] A suitable digital face compiled from a data bank of living faces, obtained in the same manner as the skull, is morphed over the digitized skull. Controlled by the soft tissue thickness measurements and the underlying skull, the digitized face is modified to conform to this new data. It can be argued that this and other similar approaches consist of forcing an 'average' face over a skull instead of allowing the features to develop from the bone. Although this is true, it is the proportions that are among the vital elements in recognition and therefore such an approach represents a valid starting point.[9] The finer elements of the face that give specific individuality may be missing but as a tool to spark 'recognition', computer-generated reconstructions potentially represent an interesting alternative to the more conventional three-dimensional methods.

Seductive and compelling though it is, a computer is no more accurate or certain in its results than many of the other techniques. It is for this reason that the author has continued to explore three-dimensional reconstruction instead of following the digital approach, in the firm belief that one approach is complimentary to the other and that ultimately it will be a fusion of the two that will provide the complete answer.

BASIC PRINCIPLES

Regardless of the methods or techniques that are being explored, developed or considered, there remain some basic elements central to the whole process that must be recognized and understood.

The availability of a skull is naturally the first element; however, direct access to the original specimen may not always be an option. Circumstances may arise, particularly in the archaeological field when dealing with artificially preserved remains (mummies), where it would be inappropriate to expose the skull. The same will apply in naturally preserved remains, be they wet (bog bodies), or dry (naturally preserved or frozen). In such situations, indirect access may be available by working from either a comprehensive set of radiographs or using techniques such as CT scanning. Digital data gathered from CT scans form an image of the skull within the computer ideal for those considering computer-generated reconstructions. A solid three-dimensional model employing one of several differing technical processes controlled by the same digital information is also an option. It would be inappropriate to provide anything more than a brief overview of some of these processes in this chapter. None the less, a superficial understanding of what each entails can be enormously helpful when planning different procedures and assessing the feasibility of a project.

The most difficult method is working from radiographs alone. The preparation of a 'model' skull requires a considerable grasp on how to interpret the data[10] and build a model in three dimensions based upon those data.[11] With the advent of modern scanning techniques, such exercises are likely to be required only in situations where it is not possible to bring the specimen to an appropriate scanning facility. Currently the types of equipment likely to be employed for the preparation of models using digital data fall in to three main categories. The most frequently used is a computer controlled milling system, which carves the desired shape from styrene foam. The results are a strong, light and dimensionally accurate copy of the skull. A more complex system uses two laser beams projected into a container of liquid plastic that polymerize at the point where the beams cross (stereo-lithography), producing a model in which all the inter-osseous spaces are present. The surface detail produced by some of the more advanced systems is limited only by the resolution of the scan data. Geometrically such models are accurate, although for the very subtle details one may have to refer to pictures of the specimen. All three-dimensional models are sufficiently robust for the reconstruction to be built directly upon them.

In forensic reconstructions the evidence is routinely available for examination, but although a skull may be sufficiently robust it is inadvisable to work directly onto an original specimen for several reasons. Investing a forensic specimen in a layer of material such as clay or plasterline is likely to cause considerable inconvenience to those undertaking further studies of the specimen at a later date. Not only does the specimen become inaccessible, the potential for damage to occur to original evidence is very real and should not be ignored, particularly if the bone has become brittle. The handling of any archaeological material in such a way would, of course, be totally unacceptable, as in many cases the bones are very fragile and porous. Although the preparation of a mould and the making of a cast may be the first step in the exercise of facial reconstruction, the reassembly of fragmented skulls and the preparation of fragile specimens frequently precedes the task.

The conservation of archaeological material is the preserve of the conservator, and in many instances the repair and reassembly of damaged specimens will not necessarily be the responsibility of the individual who will be undertaking the facial reconstruction. In some situations specialist staff may also undertake the preparation of moulds and the making of casts, although this is not generally the case. When dealing with forensic material, on the other hand, the repair and reassembly of the specimen is normally the responsibility of the reconstructor, as is the making of casts.

REPAIR, REASSEMBLY AND CASTING

A forensic specimen will be used in many ways and serves different purposes but it is seldom required to be a permanent object for display or research. For this reason a different approach to repair and reassembly can be adopted from that of an archaeological specimen. The use of wax has proven to be extremely effective for cementing bone fragments together. It allows for their almost unlimited readjustment and repositioning, particularly of large sections, by softening the wax where required. It also enables one to rebuild those areas where bone may be missing. Should it be necessary for the entire skull to be disassembled, this can be achieved with very little difficulty using either hot air or, in some cases, hot water.

The making of a cast of a skull is a complex and delicate task, which should be approached with care and attention to detail. The correct preparation of a skull whether complete, reassembled from fragments or still in pieces, is critical, for if it is not handled correctly there is a danger of damaging the original specimen or, at the very least, making an imperfect cast. The skull, in common with many bones in the human body, does not lend itself to being cast easily. The many undercuts, foramina, arches, delicate areas, and fine surface detail, create hazards for the caster, such as air traps. An engineer designing a mould for casting takes great care to avoid such potential hazards.

Preparation of the specimen requires that all foramina are blocked, and areas that will form an undercut must also be packed. In the majority of circumstances a single cast is all that is required, in which case a 'waste mould' can be made from alginate. More permanent moulds of skulls can be prepared using such materials as silicone rubbers for the moulds and methylmethacrylate for the casts.[12] Permanent moulds allow for multiple copies of the specimen to be made.

Areas such as the orbits are partially filled so that they become less deep. First tissue or cotton wool is placed into the orbit and then a layer of Plasterline, supported on the inner soft packing, is pressed into the orbit and teased against the bony rim. It should not be over-looked that enough space and depth should remain to accommodate an eyeball at a later stage. The piriform opening (nasal aperture) can be treated in a similar manner to the orbits. Foramina, from the foramen magnum downwards in size, can be filled by merely placing an appropriately sized ball or pellet of material over the space and pressing it until it holds. It is not advisable to smooth everything down as it makes removal later more difficult and it also makes it less easy to ascertain the filled areas on the cast. The zygomatic arch must be filled so that the space between the arch and the temporal and sphenoid bones is eliminated.

For archaeological specimens such direct handling may be inappropriate, particularly in the case of very delicate or porous specimens. There are conflicting views as to just how certain archaeological specimens should be handled, but if the expense of scanning and milling are too great or impractical the only alternative is to make a cast. The following is a brief outline of a method, both safe and effective, for producing casts of skulls or parts of the cranium upon which reconstructions can be made.

Specimens that are particularly likely to suffer damage from being crushed can be filled firmly with polyester waste. This soft light material remains springy when packed into a small space giving light pressure in the inside of the cranium to counter any external pressures during casting. To safeguard further the specimen fine aluminium foil (7 [mu]m thick) can be burnished over the surface of the bone. Strips (about 40 × 80 mm) are tacked very lightly with a sliver of tape and burnished down with a soft cloth revealing most of the surface detail. This effectively puts a waterproof barrier between the specimen and the moulding medium. The specimen remains protected when in the mould and can be taken from the mould very easily when the moulding medium has cured, sometimes leaving the aluminium sheet in the mould. This is peeled off before taking a cast.

A mould made from alginate is the simplest and quickest way to obtain an accurate cast, using the traditional two-part 'split mould'. The mould is designed to be divided along a line chosen to offer the least resistance when it comes to removal of the specimen. Each half of the mould is made by applying a reasonably firm mixture of alginate over the surface of the specimen to a thickness of about 10–15 mm, allowing it to flow over any broken edges so that their surfaces are also recorded. The alginate will be too flexible to maintain its shape accurately away from the skull; therefore, a supporting jacket of plaster 10–15 mm thick should be layered over the alginate immediately after setting. The two layers are best separated by a thin membrane of plastic or foil to prevent hydrostatic changes in the moisture levels of the two materials which could in turn compromise the dimensional accuracy of the final cast.

When cured, the plaster jacket is removed and the alginate mould lifted off the specimen then returned to the supporting jacket. The halves of the mould, looking like the halves of a walnut, may be first filled with a small quantity of plaster of Paris, which can be run around the inside until set. This helps to stabilize the soft mould against the outer supporting case of plaster. One-half is then filled with fresh plaster; the halves are reunited and strapped quickly together and then the mould is rotated continuously until the plaster of Paris ceases to flow. The rotation ensures an even coating over the inside of the mould producing a hollow cast. When the mould has been stripped away the dimensional accuracy should be checked against the original specimen.

SOFT TISSUE REPLICATION

The completed cast should be mounted securely on a suitable stand in the Frankfurt plane. Routinely the mandible will be cast separately and is important when attaching it to the cranium to place the mandible in cuspal occlusion with the maxilla. This will automatically indicate the space in the temporomandibular joint. By filling this space with some soft material and then rotating the mandible in the joint, until a 3–4 mm freeway space between the occlusal molar surfaces is achieved, the lower jaw is correctly aligned.

It is essential before any further work is undertaken that the age, sex, ethnic group, and build of the subject are established. The appropriate tables of soft tissue measurements can then be selected.[13–16] A series of small holes are drilled at specific anatomical sites where they relate to the measurements. The holes should be at right angles to the bony surface. Small pegs of the correct length are then inserted indicating the thickness of soft tissue at the chosen sites.

Eyeballs (between 25 and 27 mm in diameter) may be fixed in to the eye sockets. Their position can be determined by locating the medial and lateral canthae. The medial canthus is in line with the upper part of the lacrimal crest, and the lateral canthus in line with a small tubercle on the zygomatic bone, just within the orbital margins. A horizontal line drawn through these two points will indicate the angle of the eye slit. Placing the pupil of the eye at the mid-point of this line will put the eyeball in the correct position. The degree of projection of the eyeball is subject to considerable variation depending upon the shape of the skull. A useful guide is a vertical line drawn through the pupil from the inferior orbital margin to the superior orbital margin, which should just touch the cornea of the eye.

The following is an outline of the reconstruction techniques as practised by the author. All other techniques will inevitably utilize the same or similar information to a greater or lesser degree, although they will not necessarily apply it in the same way.

In the case of skulls where bone may be missing, due either to congenital abnormality, disease, or as a result of trauma, soft tissue measurements become meaningless. Under such circumstances one has to understand how the anatomy may have altered to accommodate such abnormalities or changes, reconstructing accordingly. Clearly this presents major problems when utilizing methods that rely solely upon statistical data to guide a reconstruction. Work currently in progress indicates that facial abnormalities can be recreated on a skull with surprising accuracy if a logical development of the anatomical soft tissue structures is undertaken in an objective manner. By noting the origins and insertions of the basic muscle groups that form the face it is possible to build them quite quickly so that the face is seen to grow from the surface of the skull outwards. The choice of materials is up to the individual, although modelling clay is regarded by the author as being superior to other materials for the reconstruction of the soft tissue.

It is advisable to start by blocking in the neck, noting the level at which the hyoid bone would lie and the size and direction of the sternocleidomastoid muscle. The temporalis and masseter muscles can then be developed followed by buccinator, orbicularis oris, mentalis, depressor anguli oris and depressor labii inferioris. Lines drawn from the lateral borders of the canine teeth can determine the width of the mouth. The mouth slit will lie about one-third of the way up the enamel of the upper incisors. The width of the philtrum will be about equivalent to the distance between the centres of the upper incisors.

At this point the nose may be blocked in, ideally following the anatomical pattern of the nasal cartilage. Routinely the width of the piriform opening will be three-fifths of the overall distance between the outer borders of the nasal alae. A line tangent to the last one-third of the nasal bone, projected down to bisect a second line which follows the general direction of the anterior spine, will indicate the distance that the nose projects from the surface of the skull.[6] The muscles that are modelled to form the upper half of the face include the levator anguli oris, levator labii superioris, zygomaticus major and minor, the obicularis oculi, the depressor supercilii and the occipito frontalis. Others, such as procerus and the lavator labii superioris alaeque nasi, can be used to allow the tissue to grow in a more explicable way, but are not likely to have any significant effect on the final reconstruction.

In life, all the spaces surrounding the muscles are filled with connective tissue, fat, nerves, blood vessels, glands etc. In the course of reconstruction, therefore, it is useful to fill these areas to ensure that the structures already built do not collapse when the final superficial layer is applied. If everything has been done accurately and the fatty areas developed to give an overall evenness to the anatomical face there will be little of the measuring pegs left showing, particularly in the upper half of the face. Finally, the ears may be attached. There are few clues as to ear shape. A mastoid process that projects forward is likely to be associated with a non-adherent lobe. Apart from its position, indicated by the external auditory meatus, and the fact that elderly individuals tend to have rather longer ears, there is little guidance from the skull.

By taking strips of soft clay (about 30 mm wide and 5 mm thick) and laying them over the anatomical face the final surface of the reconstruction can be formed. The clay strips should be allowed to follow the contours of that which lies below but not come above the level of the tissue measurement pegs. This final stage is where so many problems lie, and not just with this technique. Up to this point there has been a logical development, but to make the reconstruction look like a real person all the superficial details have to be added. In some forensic cases there may exist details of hair and scars or details of the lips, eyes or the tip of the nose. The manner in which these features are depicted will depend upon the skill of individual workers, their knowledge of how features are formed, and their experience in observing faces.

It is impossible to produce an exact likeness, as there are too many variables, but routinely the method outlined produces a face that will be broadly similar to the type of face the subject had when alive.

CONCLUSION

The techniques of facial reconstruction when applied to archaeological studies may highlight anatomical abnormalities, racial differences and the appearance of wounds. They are a potent communication tool.

In forensic work, facial reconstruction provides a valuable investigative technique that can be used in situations where the identity of a body is unknown and where no other avenue of investigation exists. Making unrecognizable remains recognizable may elicit recognition from a member of the public, which in turn may lead to a positive identification of the deceased by the use of conventional forensic techniques.

REFERENCES

1   Galen. *De Anatomicis Administrationibus*, i2.218, translated by Singer C: *Galen on Anatomical Procedure*. London: Oxford University Press, 1956.

2   His W. Anatomische forschungen über Johan Sebastian Bach gebeine und antlitz nebst bemerkung uber dessen bilder. *Abhandlungen der mathematisch-physischen Classe der Königlich Sächsischen Gesellschaft der Wissenschaften* 1895; **22**: 381–420.

3   Kollman J. and Buchley W. Die persistenz der rassen und die rekonstruktion der physiognomie prähistorischer schädel. *Archiv für Anthropologie* 1898; **25**: 329–359.

4   Von Eggeling H. Die leistungsfahigkeit physiognomischer rekonstruktionsversuche auf grundlage des schädels. *Archiv für Anthpopologie* 1913; **12**: 44–47.

5   Krogman WM, Iscan MY. *The Human Skeleton in Forensic Medicine* (2nd edn). Springfield: Charles C Thomas, 1986: pp. 413–457.

6   Gerasimov MM. *The Face Finder*. London: Hutchinson, 1971: pp. 52–61.

7   Gatliff BP, Snow CC. From skull to visage. *Journal of Biocommunication*. 1979; **6**: 27–30.

8   Linney A, Coombs AM. Computer modelling of facial form. In: Clement JG, Ranson DL (eds), *Craniofacial Identification in Forensic Medicine*. London: Arnold, 1998: pp. 187–198.

9   Vanezis P, Blowes RW, Linney A, Tan AC, Richards R, Neave R. Application of 3D computer graphics for facial reconstruction and comparison with sculpting techniques. *Forensic Science International* 1989; **42**: 69–84.

10 Neave RAH. The reconstruction of skulls for facial reconstruction using radiographic techniques. In: David AR (ed.), *Science in Egyptology*. Manchester: Manchester University Press, 1986: pp. 129–133.

11 Neave RAH. Reconstruction of the skull and soft tissues of the head and face of Lindow Man. *Canadian Society of Forensic Science Journal* 1989; **22(1)**: 43–53.

12 Taylor RG, Angel C. Facial reconstruction and approximation. In: Clement JG, Ranson DL (ed.), *Craniofacial Identification in Forensic Medicine*. London: Arnold, 1998: pp. 177–185.

13 Suzuki T. On the thickness of the soft parts of the Japanese face. *Journal of the Anthropological Society of Nippon* 1948; **60**: 7–11.

14 Rhine JS, Moore CE. *Reproduction Tables of Facial Tissue Thicknesses of American Caucasoids*. Forensic Anthropology, Maxwell Museum Series. 1. Albuquerque: Maxwell Museum of Anthropology, 1984.

15 Rhine JS, Campbell HR. Thickness of facial tissue in American blacks. *Journal of Forensic Sciences* 1980; **29**: 847–858.

16 Helmer R. *Schaedelidentifizierung durch Electronische Bildmischung*. Heidelberg: Kriminalistik , 1984.

Section V

Assaults on the skeleton

This section considers aspects of physical change to bone that may occur, either before or after death, as a result of a variety of external agents. These agents include patterns of mechanical loading, accidental or deliberate injury, surgical intervention, post-mortem ritual or other mutilations, and the act of cremating bone as a funerary rite.

Charlotte Roberts' chapter focuses primarily on fractures in archaeological bone. She covers diagnostic criteria, methodological approaches to the recording of fractures and the cultural significance of patterning in such injuries in earlier populations. The treatment of fractures in the past is also discussed, as are trepanation and amputation. Anthea Boylston provides a thorough review of evidence for weapon-related trauma in Britain. She discusses the significance of trauma patterning, and a range of weapon injuries is described. Emphasis is placed on the value of a multidisciplinary approach to understanding trauma in ancient bones.

Chris Knüsel tackles the topic of bone adaptation to physical activity. He discusses the various ways in which bone responds to mechanical loading and considers studies of cortical bone remodelling, enthesial changes, joint surface morphological adaptations, and osteoarthritic lesions in a biomechanical perspective.

Jacqueline McKinley discusses the analysis of cremated bone. She gives an account of the cremation process, both in relation to pyre cremation and burning in a modern crematorium. The form and nature of cremated bone is described and the academic objectives of scientific analysis of such material are considered.

21

TRAUMA IN BIOCULTURAL PERSPECTIVE: PAST, PRESENT AND FUTURE WORK IN BRITAIN

Charlotte Roberts

INTRODUCTION

'Investigation of injury morbidity and mortality facilitates the assessment of environmental, cultural and social influences on behavior' (p. 9).[1] The aims of this chapter are to review the types of information that are potentially retrievable from a study of trauma in antiquity, and summarize the range of published research already extant on trauma. Further, it seeks to document the range and quality of work already completed on British material, and to recommend the way forward and best practice. It will not be possible to include all aspects of trauma but the more common approaches will be considered. Emphasis is placed on the study of both biological (skeletal) evidence for trauma, and the cultural context from which it is derived (i.e. the biocultural approach).

A holistic approach to studying any health problem is recommended, i.e. consideration of multiple forms of evidence to reconstruct health and disease patterning. While much of the emphasis in the study of trauma in British contexts has been on individual case studies, in North America the 'population-based biocultural approach' has been developed. If palaeopathological study in Britain is to advance, this latter approach is recommended.

BACKGROUND

Trauma can be defined as any bodily injury or wound, and it may affect bone, soft tissue, or both.[2] Fractures are the result of any traumatic event that leads to a complete or partial break in the continuity of bone. Trauma covers many different areas and, as such, is commonly seen in archaeologically derived human skeletal material along with joint and dental disease. Of course, trauma may also affect only the soft tissues and will not, therefore, necessarily be observed in the skeleton. In addition, traumatic lesions may be so long-standing that the evidence could have been remodelled away before the person died, e.g. a fracture in child-hood may be invisible by adulthood.

Trauma is regularly reported in skeletal material and can potentially provide data on a variety of aspects of past population behaviour. Some areas to be considered include domestic accidents (which may reflect physical environment and, for example, the climate), interpersonal violence (which may reflect sedentism, competition for resources, social inequalities and complexity, and increased trade and contact), and occupationally related trauma (e.g. environments and their effects on lifestyle). In addition, subsistence strategy (hunter-gathering versus agriculture), male and female differences, availability of treatment and nutritional status at the time of the fracture and throughout the healing phase (indicated by the end result of the healing process), are also areas of potential study with respect to occurrence and patterning of trauma. While, in general, the vast majority of work in palaeopathology has concentrated on injuries resulting from interpersonal violence, there is also research published on less dramatic lesions.

Trauma can be classified into four categories:[3] a partial or complete break in a bone (fracture), abnormal displacement or dislocation of a bone, disruption of nerve or blood supply (which may be a complication of a fracture), and artificially induced abnormal shape or contour (e.g. artificial deformation of the head). For the purposes of this chapter fractures and dislocations to the post-cranial skeleton will be considered, as the majority of injuries to the head and neck region are due to intra- and intergroup violence rather than accidental injury, and are covered elsewhere (see Boylston, chapter 22, in this volume). In addition, the evidence for trauma in the form of amputation and trepanation will be considered, as well as the treatment of post-cranial fractures; decapitation, scalping, weapon and soft tissue injuries, cannibalism and dental trauma are beyond the scope here.

PREVIOUS WORK

Many excellent books, chapters, and major review articles have been written on trauma in antiquity,[1-8] their content ranging from very clinically based diagnostic approaches, to bioculturally interpretative considerations. Perhaps most work published in trauma has tended to consist of the 'case study',[9,10] or focus on trauma to particular parts of the body.[11] While interesting in themselves, they do not necessarily contribute to reconstructions of trauma patterning through time, although collectively considered they are helpful. Rarely have researchers dealt with issues of gender, status or economic, geographic or chronological differences in trauma patterns on a large scale (although see Cohen and Armelagos[12] on hunter-gatherer/agricultural differences, see Grimm[13] on gender differences, and see Angel[14] on chronological change in Greece). Other papers have contributed studies on developing a methodology for recording fractures in archaeological material,[2,15-18] while some have concentrated on treatment of trauma.[17,19-22] There is a lack of population studies of trauma patterning and prevalence, although over the past few years more have been published,[1,15,16,23-25] which describe very useful bioculturally relevant population studies. While trauma is common and easily recognizable in the archaeological record, and can potentially inform us of many aspects of past human behaviour, this potential has sadly not been exploited fully in published literature worldwide. As has been stated, 'The sparseness of a population perspective in this literature, however, precludes the realisation of the enormous potential that these kinds of data have for drawing inferences about human behaviour and conflict in earlier societies'[1] (p. 109).

FRACTURES: A GUIDE

There is a considerable literature reviewing this subject.[26–29] Acute injury, repeated stress or an underlying weakness (e.g. osteoporosis in the spine) may induce fractures, but it is acute injury that constitutes the major cause. In addition, fractures may be closed (simple) or open (compound). Compound fractures mean that the fractured bone is exposed to microorganisms infiltrating the fracture site and causing infection, an obvious danger in antiquity without the availability of antibiotics for treatment. In addition, there are many types of fractures that are caused by varying forces. Some are named after the person who originally described them, some are named after occupations that commonly cause them, some names reflect the anatomical part affected, and some indicate the causative force.[6] For example, oblique and spiral fractures are caused by indirect/torsional forces, and transverse fractures by direct force. Comminuted (in many pieces) fractures tend to be associated today with high-impact road traffic accidents, greenstick fractures are seen in young individuals where the bones are malleable and do not break completely, and an impacted fracture results when the two fractured ends are driven into each other. Traction/avulsion fractures are when a fragment of bone is detached due to a sudden contraction of a muscle associated with a bone, and a compression fracture (usually in a vertebra) is the result of compression forces running through the bone(s). These fracture types have been illustrated previously,[7] but a particular problem to note with compression fractures in the spine is their differential diagnoses (Figures 1–3). Specific causes of fractures in archaeological contexts may be hard to identify. However, it is known that particular fractures occur more commonly in some circumstances, for example falls on an outstretched hand often lead to Colles' fractures of the wrist, i.e. an acute injury.

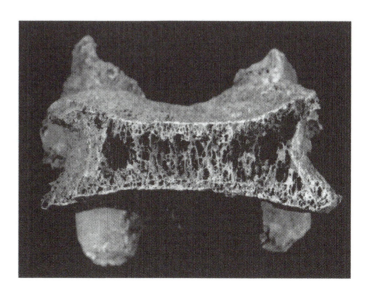

Figure 1 – Osteoporosis underlying a vertebral compression fracture (Romano-British).

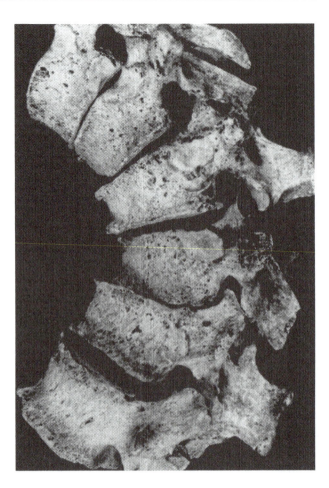

Figure 2 – Compression fractures in vertebral bodies as a result of trauma – no underlying pathology (Romano-British).

In archaeological contexts fractures observed are usually healed, indicating that the bone has undergone the first two stages of the healing process (circulatory/cellular and metabolic) and is into the final (and longest) mechanical phase. In this phase the bone (or bone cells, osteoblasts and osteoclasts) is gradually remodelled back to its normal anatomical shape. There are, naturally, many factors that affect the rate and efficiency of healing, and these include the fracture type and the bone affected. For example, arm fractures heal faster than leg fractures in clinical contexts but it should be remembered that availability of treatment will have an effect on this, for example forearm fractures often need internal fixation, something not readily available in the past. Other factors that may affect the healing process are the age of the person (the young heal faster than the old), whether the fracture has been treated, the presence of infection or other disease, the blood supply to the affected part and the person's diet. Some of these factors may be identifiable in skeletal material or known about the sample under study, but some will not, yet all must be considered with respect to fractures in past human groups. Of course, complications of fractures are many and some have been recorded in archaeological contexts (e.g. non-union[30]). In clinical contexts, infection, shortening and/or angulation of a limb due to a poorly reduced fracture (with or

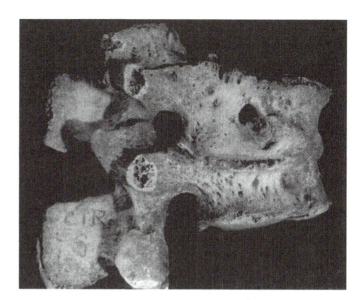

Figure 3 – Compression fractures of lumbar vertebrae due to underlying infection (Romano-British).

without associated osteoarthritis of adjacent joints), death of bone due to severing of blood supply, blood vessel or nerve damage, pseudoarthrosis, and myositis ossificans (ossification of damaged muscle tissue) are the most common. In archaeological contexts there has only rarely been systematic documentation of fracture complications.

In clinical contexts trauma is well documented, and it is from there that information on types of fractures, their causes, complications and healing rates is usually accessed by people working on the palaeopathology of trauma.[26–29,31–33] It is generally easy to apply the principles for studying fractures in modern populations to the dead, although the factors inherent in the aetiology of fractures have changed through time so care must be taken in using some of these data. For example, comparative data from traditional agricultural communities with no access to modern technology do exist and have been used, and these are more appropriate for archaeologically based studies.[34] Furthermore, there is an equal or greater number of papers covering a range of areas in modern fracture studies that can be used as comparative data,[35] although with modern studies the whole patient is being observed and not just fragments (as in an archaeological context).

STUDIES OF TRAUMA IN ARCHAEOLOGICALLY DERIVED SKELETAL MATERIAL

Archaeological studies of trauma range from the case study to the biocultural approach to fracture patterning. For example, individual case studies have been used to investigate prevalence rates of fractures from the 7th millennium BC to the 2nd century AD in Greece.[14] However, population based studies of chronological trends in fractures are rare. A different approach, looking in detail at fractures in a particular sample, was undertaken on skeletal material from Ohio, North America[36] and, although focusing on one medieval population in England, a comparative study of fracture patterns with five other sites of the same period has also been made.[15] A recent issue of a journal in the field, although dealing with issues of trauma in archaeologically derived human remains, was somewhat disappointing in that most papers failed to deliver a truly biocultural approach to trauma patterning, with real fracture prevalence rates.[37]

A survey of trauma reported in published and unpublished skeletal reports from Britain also displays a disappointing amount of useful data; many reports do not describe trauma by actual prevalence rate. It indicates that there are three classes of trauma data in skeletal reports. Some describe fractures by individuals affected with no bone counts available to determine *actual* prevalence rate[38-44] (this assumes all bones for all people were available for examination). Others describe fractures by individuals *and* by bones affected, with[45,46] or without[47] bone counts. Finally, some provide data on individuals affected and bones affected but do not discuss *actual* prevalence rates for each bone, although bone counts are available (i.e. the reader can calculate this using the data provided).[48-52] There clearly needs to be greater consistency in reporting.

Special fractures include the clay shoveller's fracture of the seventh cervical and first thoracic vertebrae, and spondylolysis (detachment of the neural arch at the pars interarticularis), usually of the fifth lumbar vertebra.[53] The latter is more commonly reported than the former, although both are seen in British material.[54,55] Both conditions may be directly related to activity (stress and strain) and need more study. In addition, attention has recently been drawn to the skeletal evidence for child abuse in the form of both fractures at specific sites in the body and periosteal new bone formation on certain bones of the skeleton.[56] Child abuse, and also torture (described in the forensic literature as consisting of mainly soft tissue injuries and possible amputation of parts such as fingers[57]) are frequently described in the media today but are rarely considered in the past. Having so much modern data on these two aspects of human behaviour means that a study in the past potentially has some comparative base, and this is another area that could be considered with respect to British archaeologically derived skeletal material.

Some other traumatically induced conditions reported very occasionally in British material include slipped femoral epiphysis,[58] and dislocation.[59] Similar conditions are also reported from outside Britain.[60-62] The loss of contact between two bones at a joint (dislocation), usually of the hip or the shoulder (which may be either congenitally, traumatically or disease induced) is recognizable only if the bones stay out of alignment for long enough for another joint surface to be created, or if characteristic fractures in peri-articular bone are present,[29] or other related lesions.[63] It is possible, as today, that some dislocations may have eventually naturally reduced themselves.[7]

TREATMENT OF TRAUMA

Arising from a study of trauma is the question of whether, and how, people in the past cared for those who suffered trauma. Trauma, like any other health problem (as today), may have prevented a person from functioning 'normally' within their community. Therefore, care and treatment are likely to have been sought, and communities would have gradually developed care systems. The abundant evidence for beliefs and concepts of disease, diagnosis of disease, anatomical knowledge and its relevance to treatment, and treatment in a general sense in past and contemporary traditional societies, is beyond the scope of this paper; however, there is some evidence of direct treatment of traumatic lesions.

Fractures

Historical, iconographic and ethnographic sources suggest that there was knowledge of how to treat fractures in the past,[64–67] and traditional living populations today also have systems and knowledge for dealing with trauma.[68] Occasionally there is also direct evidence,[69] but there has been little attention paid to determining whether documented knowledge can be displayed in the skeletal evidence for trauma. Correlating evidence and efficiency in healing of long bone fractures with contemporary historical data is possible in some British material but, with some exceptions[2,15–17,21], little attempt has been made to do this worldwide. Although some researchers make comments on how well fractures have healed and whether there may have been therapeutic intervention, few take the data any further, something which should be of interest to biological anthropologists. Figures 4 and 5 illustrate two tibial fractures from different Anglo-Saxon sites which reveal very different healing; does this reflect the availability or not of treatment in different populations?

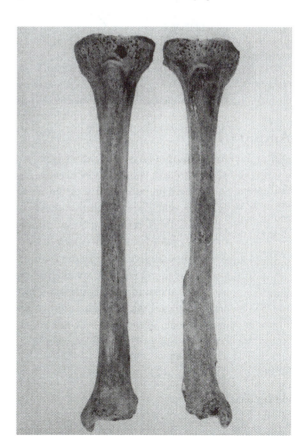

Figure 4 – Fractured right tibia (Anglo-Saxon) with normal left tibia for comparison. Healing is good with no angulation, overlap or lack of apposition; this suggests possible treatment.

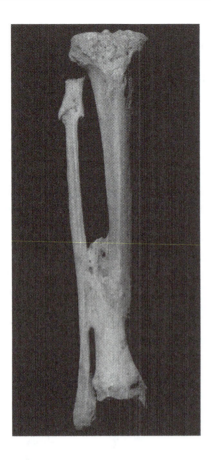

Figure 5 – Fractures to tibia and fibula (Anglo-Saxon).
There is overlap and lack of apposition of the broken ends;
this suggests lack of treatment.

Amputation

Amputations (surgical/accidental) of limbs may be classified as fractures and may have been
performed as a result of complications of a severe fracture. They have also been described
in historical literature and depicted artistically; rarely, however, are they described in skeletal
evidence, and examples almost always have evidence of healing.[19,70-73] This arises from the
problem of differentiating between unhealed peri-mortem (sustained shortly before or at
the time of death) and post-mortem fractures. It is highly probable that many people under-
going amputation in the past died at the time of the operation, probably from blood loss and
shock, and therefore there would be no evidence of healing on the amputated bone. Clearly,
as seen in illustrations, people did undergo amputations and were provided with crutches
and prostheses with which to move around post-operatively.[74] When recording possible
amputations, examination of the edges of the cut is essential to prevent over-diagnosis,
although the problem of 'weathering' of peri-mortem cut edges post-mortem must be
considered.

Trepanation

Trepanations (which cover all surgically induced holes in the skull) or trephinations (which
describe only holes made by a trephine or drill) are the surgical removal of a piece of bone

from the skull and are also a form of treatment. They can also be classified as fractures and their history goes back into the prehistoric period where successful examples are apparent (i.e. the person survived the operation). Many reviews have been published of this remarkable operation.[1,3,4,6–8,75–77] While some cases are associated with head injuries,[20,78] others do not have any indication of why the trepanation was done, although headaches, migraine and epilepsy are claimed to have been treated using trepanation in the past. Trepanations have been documented around the world from all periods[79,80] and have been described and documented historically.[4,67] In British contexts, a prime researcher in the art of, and evidence for, trepanation was Parry[81] but later researchers have also contributed to the collective evidence for trepanation in Britain.[22,82,83] While there are many different types of trepanation (scrape, saw, bore and saw, gouge and drill), it was the more controllable scraping method that seems to have been used the most in British contexts, and it was also the one that appeared to heal, i.e. the person survived the operation. However, in the past, the risk of infection being introduced into the brain tissue via the operation must have been high, and it is likely that cerebral infection post-operatively would have led to the death of the unfortunate individual. When recording trepanations, in addition to the site of operation, type of trepanation, and characteristics of the edges of the opening, it is advisable to note any evidence of infection around the site. Of course the possibility that holes in the skull may be postmortem must be ruled out by considering the characteristics of the edges of the hole. In addition, the consideration of the many differential diagnoses for holes in the skull should be considered, e.g. enlarged parietal foramina and neoplastic disease.[8]

LIMITATIONS OF THE DATA

The limitations of studying fractures in the past need some discussion. As for any other pathological condition, it is preferable to have the whole skeleton for study so that fracture patterning can be observed. For example, if one of the forearm or lower leg bones is fractured, observation of the other bone (and the opposite side to gain an impression of the level of deformity on healing) helps with interpretation. It is particularly important to look at fracture patterning, as in certain circumstances one may expect to see fractures occurring in specific parts of the body as a result of a particular traumatic incident. For example, interpersonal violence may result in head (especially the face), neck and forearm injuries.[84] However, forearm (parry) fractures alone do not necessarily mean interpersonal violence as they can be caused by falls.

Many people publish data on fractures with reference to age at death but it is virtually impossible to ascertain when a person sustained a fracture in life once the fracture is healed; was it 1, 5 or 10 years before death? It is only if the fracture is in the early stages of healing that age at death is directly relevant (of course, the older you are the more fractures you are likely to have sustained, as for any pathological condition). Very few fractures are observed in non-adults recovered from archaeological contexts, even though it is likely that in the past, as today, childhood fractures were a common occurrence. This absence of fractures seen in the young is probably because the skeleton is rapidly growing and if a bone is fractured then the fracture will heal quickly and even become invisible when viewed radiographically. However, the observation of bowing of bones both in adult and non-adult skeletons,[85] or shortened but normal-looking bones, may indicate old fractures. It is, however, interesting to note reports of accidents in children documented in historical data,[86] and it is probably here that more data on trauma (and other health problems) in children may be gleaned. Looking at typical childhood fractures in adult skeletal material may also provide clues to data for the younger part of the population. For example, fractures in the elbow region are common in children but rare in adults,[26] but fractures of the scaphoid and femur neck are uncommon in children. In addition, fractures to the distal radius (Colles' fractures) are the commonest fracture today in people > 40 years, especially females.[26] Observation of the bone elements affected in relation to age may aid us in identifying fracture occurrence in the growing years, even if the hard evidence is unavailable.

As all bones are not radiographed in palaeopathological work, very well healed fractures will not be detected. Recently sustained (peri-mortem) fractures are difficult to identify archaeologically because no healing has taken place. Even taking into account the particular fracture patterning determined by the characteristics of 'fresh' as opposed to archaeological bone[4] can be potentially misleading, as post-mortem breaks occurring while the bone still retains its highly collagenous 'fresh' composition would display similar fracture patterning and colouration to peri-mortem fractures. Also, a problem in identification may arise if the edges of a peri-mortem fracture have been weathered due to burial in the ground. Finally, stress induced fractures may also be hard to identify because they are often manifest as hairline fractures and, even if radiographed, they may not be obvious; tibiae, fibulae and metatarsals are the commonest bones affected.[26] Despite these limitations, there is a wealth of evidence available from a study of trauma.

RECOMMENDATIONS FOR RECORDING FRACTURES

Recommendations for recording fractures should follow published guidelines[17,18] with additional data,[87] according to the question being asked of the material. The initial, general and detailed description of the injury is the pre-requisite for more detailed work (Table 1). There are certain features that should always be recorded. These include fracture position using anatomical terms and type of fracture (e.g. is there any underlying pathology). In addition, the state of healing and any associated deformity, such as apposition, overlap, linear or rotational deformity (describe the distal fragment in relation to the proximal), and infection or joint degeneration (assuming these occur after the fracture and not before, and thus are complications) should be noted. Looking at the types of fracture and bone fractured, and comparing that information with clinical data may give an insight into treatment in the past. For example, forearm fractures and femoral shaft fractures often lead to considerable deformity and need either internal fixation and/or considerable traction to treat them. In archaeological contexts poorly aligned forearm and femoral fractures are recognized, perhaps indicating problems with treatment (Figure 6), but occasionally good results are seen which may reflect either careful and effective therapy or just good luck (Figure 7). Detailed descriptions of the state of healing of the fracture observed may reveal definite healing, non-union or non-union due to the person dying before union could take place. Figures 8 and 9 show examples of what the author believes to be clear non-union, and non-union due to healing being halted by death.

Table 1 – Fracture recording (macroscopic): features to note.

 1 Age and sex of individual
 2 Bone affected
 3 Side affected
 4 Fracture position (proximal, mid, distal for a long bone, for example; use anatomical terms)
 5 Fracture type[7]
 6 State of healing (healed, unhealed, healing, woven/lamellar/mixed bone)
 7 Evidence of infection (pitting, new bone formation, osteomyelitis)
 8 Evidence of underlying pathology
 9 Evidence of joint degeneration in adjacent joints
10 Evidence of linear/rotational deformity in degrees (measure on radiograph[15])
11 Amount of overlap/apposition in millimetres (measure on radiograph[15])
12 Alignment of bone (consider features 10 and 11)

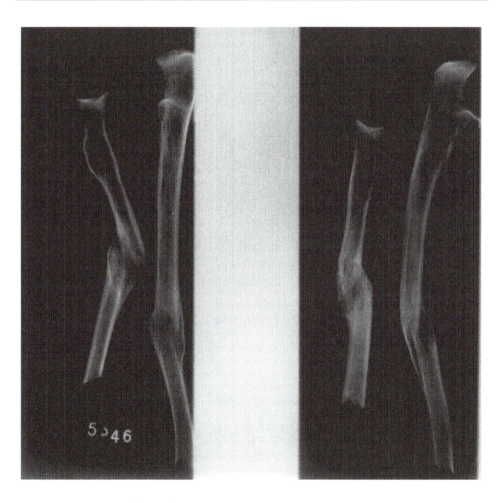

Figure 6 – Poorly aligned forearm fractures (later medieval).

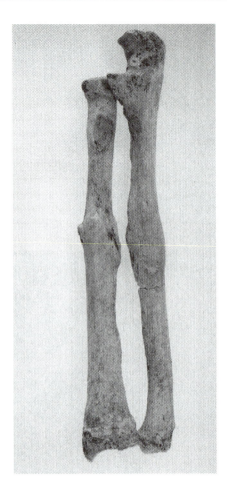

Figure 7 – Well-aligned forearm fractures (post-medieval).

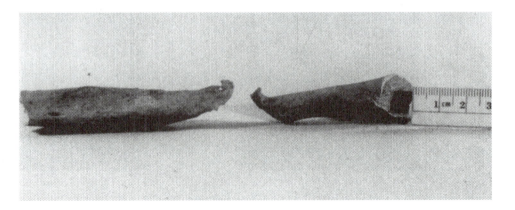

Figure 8 – Non-union of ulna fracture (California, USA).

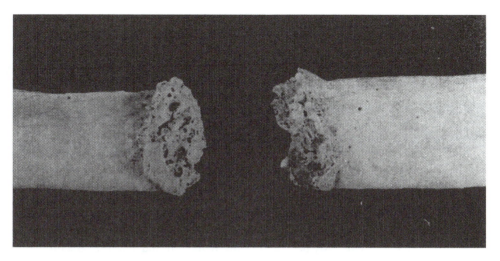

Figure 9 – Non-union of rib fracture, probably due to premature death of the individual – note bone formation at ends (Romano-British).

In addition to macroscopic recording, a radiograph of the fracture should be taken (minimum of two views, antero-posterior and medio-lateral). This aids in collecting the previously described data (particularly state of healing and deformity). For example, the actual type of fracture may not be obvious macroscopically, and the state of healing becomes more visible with a radiograph (e.g. is the fracture line visible?). In addition, measurements of overlap, apposition and linear deformity are most accurately measured on a radiograph,[15] and pseudopathological features visualized and noted. The radiography of trauma, of course, is documented in many excellent texts,[32] which aid in interpretation of archaeological material. Features of the radiographic picture should also be recorded (Table 2).

Table 2 – Fracture recording (radiographic): additional features to note.

1 X-ray view taken: antero-posterior, medio-lateral, etc.
2 Fracture type;[7] may be different from that observed macroscopically
3 Visibility of fracture line (clearly visible, partially obliterated, totally obliterated)
4 Is there cortical and cancellous continuity? (links to features 3 and 5)
5 State of healing; is the bone formed opaque (more recent) or translucent (older and remodelled)? – links to features 3 and 4
6 Evidence of shortening of affected limb (if long bone): measure on radiograph and compare with opposite side
7 Evidence of infection (new bone formation, osteomyelitis)
8 Evidence of underlying pathology (e.g. osteoporosis, neoplastic disease)
9 Evidence of joint degeneration in adjacent joints (e.g. subchondral cysts)
10 Evidence of linear/rotational deformity (measure linear on radiograph)
11 Amount of overlap/apposition of bone fragments (measure on radiograph)
12 Alignment of bone

The most important point to note is that, as for any other pathological lesions in skeletal remains, the total number of bones present for observation for the population sample under consideration should be known so that *actual* prevalence rates can be calculated. Both individuals affected, and bones affected as a percentage of bones should be recorded.[15] Additionally, the portion of the bone present needs to be noted. For example, if Colles' fractures are being recorded, the number of distal radii present is needed to determine prevalence rates. This means that if the original basic data exists for a population then comparisons can be made between groups.[15] Finally, of course, the patterning of trauma should be considered by age, sex and status, and in socio-cultural environmental context which will aid considerably in interpretation; in British contexts there is also an abundance of contemporary historical data for later periods with which to interpret patterns of trauma. The value of the recording system described has been illustrated already and shows the detailed information retrievable from the data recorded about fracture patterning in populations.[15-18]

While the emphasis here is on how to record and interpret fracture data, in the UK (and elsewhere) emphasis must be placed on better cooperation between biological anthropologists and archaeologists, both on and off site. Careful excavation and recovery of all bones,[88] and meticulous informed processing of material, with detailed recording on site, can contribute significantly to the final interpretation of a sample population's trauma patterns. For example, good clear photographs of skeletons *in situ* may give an indication of trauma complications that will probably not be evident once the skeleton has been removed from the ground. Figure 10 shows an individual who had sustained a femoral neck fracture and clearly had a shortened leg. In addition, purely by accurate recording of the skeleton in the ground, fracture complications such as nerve or blood vessel disruption may be revealed. In the case of a supracondylar fracture to the humerus, for example, injury to the brachial artery can occur with Volkmann's ischaemic contracture. Here there can be replacement of affected muscles by fibrous tissue and contracture of the wrists and fingers into flexion; sensory and motor paralysis of the hand can also occur.[26] Flexion contracture may only be recognized in the burial context, although lesions to the phalanges of the hand may be apparent (also seen in leprosy[89]). Loss of function as a result of trauma may also be revealed in the presence of osteoporosis or atrophy of the affected limb.

Most people working on trauma will only have access to macroscopic and radiographic techniques for recording, but there has been some work using more sophisticated methods of analysis. For example, there are problems of diagnosing osteoporosis in archaeological material because of post-mortem changes in bone leading to loss of bone mass. In such cases, the study of microfractures using scanning electron microscopy (SEM) may potentially provide information about osteoporotic fractures in the spine, wrist and hip, as microfractures can occur in osteoporotic bones.[90] It should not be forgotten that microfractures can also occur in bones subject to stress in young adults. Furthermore, computed tomography (CT), i.e. taking cross-sectional images at 1.5–10 mm intervals of a subject, be it of a bone or a body, has been little used in the investigation of trauma (but see Notman[91] for use of this method on identification of rib fractures in a mummy). The identification of non-adult, well healed fractures and stress fractures using CT, and the microscopic evaluation of the surfaces of possible peri-mortem fractures using SEM, may help to solve some of the limitations of trauma study outlined above.

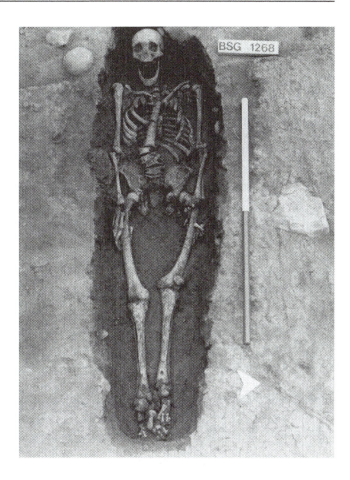

Figure 10 – Skeleton from St Giles by Brompton Bridge, North Yorkshire.

CONCLUSIONS

Clearly there is much to be gained from a study of trauma. However, and not only in British contexts, there needs to be more concentration on the population and not the 'individual' in the future rather than a further proliferation of interesting cases of trauma. In this way more meaningful information about patterns of trauma (and its treatment) may be gained. In Britain, as there has been so little work done at a population level, gaps in knowledge are large and therefore we are only just beginning. Some points need emphasizing for future work in this field:

- Population studies are of prime importance, with a stated hypothesis to test.
- Prevalence rates as a percentage of bones available for study, plus people (individuals) affected, must be stated in any report, or at least data provided to do these calculations.
- Detailed descriptions of traumatic lesions are essential. For fractures interpretations should work from a clinical base, and anatomical position, state of healing, and complications evident, with radiographic supporting evidence, are needed.
- Prevalence rates by age, sex, and status are required, where possible.
- Trauma needs to be considered chronologically and geographically.

- Data should to be interpreted with reference to both the cultural and funerary context. For example, are there differences in trauma between urban and rural, and monastic and lay populations, and are the fractures better healed in a hospital as opposed to non-hospital context?
- Sample representivity must be considered (i.e. is it biased?). For example, if a battlefield cemetery were being considered then many fractures (probably many unhealed) would be expected compared with a general cemetery, and a preponderance of males is also likely.
- Is there any evidence for treatment? For example, are the bones well aligned and healed? Is there contemporary evidence for the period for treatment of fractures?
- Case studies need collating for British contexts.
- Data need comparing to other samples worldwide.
- A consideration of levels of disability associated with traumatic lesions, and how disability was viewed and treated in the past, would be of value in determining attitudes to disability.

Much remains to be done. However, there is a lot of data already extant in published and unpublished skeletal reports, case and the occasional sample study. However, if work on British material could start from a sound base with established and accepted standardized recording methods many of the recommendations above would be achievable. Population prevalence rates of trauma for age, sex, and status, in geographical, funerary, chronological and cultural context are the key areas for consideration with a clinically based macroscopic and radiographic recording system for trauma, and should be a focus of attention for biological anthropologists working in Britain.

ACKNOWLEDGEMENTS

Jean Brown of the Department of Archaeological Sciences, University of Bradford produced the photographs, Figure 7 was provided by Dr Keith Manchester (University of Bradford), Figure 8 by Robert Jurmain of San Jose State University, California, and Figure 10 by Peter Cardwell of Northern Archaeological Associates. The author is extremely grateful to all these people. Finally, acknowledgement goes to the two referees whose comments were extremely useful, and enhanced the final version of this chapter.

REFERENCES

1 Larsen CS. *Bioarchaeology. Interpreting Behaviour from the Human Skeleton*. Cambridge: Cambridge University Press, 1998.

2 Roberts CA. Trauma and treatment in the British Isles in the historical period: a design for multidisciplinary approach. In: Ortner DJ, Aufderheide AC (eds), *Human Paleopathology. Current Syntheses and Future Options*. Washington, DC: Smithsonian Institution, 1991: pp. 225–240.

3 Ortner DJ, Putschar WG. *Identification of Pathological Conditions in Human Skeletal Remains*. Washington, DC: Smithsonian Institution Press, 1981.

4 Aufderheide AC, Rodriguez-Martin C. *The Cambridge Encyclopedia of Human Paleopathology*. Cambridge: Cambridge University Press, 1998.

5   Lovell NC. Trauma analysis in paleopathology. *Yearbook of Physical Anthropology* 1997; **40**: 139–170.

6   Merbs CF. Trauma. In: Işcan MY, Kennedy KAR (eds), *Reconstruction of Life from the Skeleton*. New York: Alan R. Liss, 1989: pp. 161–189.

7   Roberts CA, Manchester K. *The Archaeology of Disease* (2nd edn). Stroud: Sutton, 1995.

8   Steinbock RT. *Paleopathological Diagnosis and Interpretation*. Springfield: Charles C Thomas, 1976.

9   Anderson T, Carter AR. An archaeological example of medieval trauma. *Journal of Paleopathology* 1994; **6(3)**: 145–150.

10 Wells C. Fractures of the heel bones in prehistoric times. *The Practitioner* 1976; **217**: 294–298.

11 Alexandersen V. Evidence for injuries to the jaws. In: Brothwell DR, Sandison AT (eds), *Diseases in Antiquity. A Survey of the Diseases, Injuries and Surgery of Early Populations*. Springfield: Charles C Thomas, 1967: pp. 623–629.

12 Cohen MN, Armelagos GJ. *Paleopathology at the Origins of Agriculture*. London: Academic Press, 1984.

13 Grimm H. Sex differences in the frequency of bone fracture in prehistoric and historic times. In: Schwidetzky I, Chiarelli B, Necrasov O (eds), *Physical Anthropology of European Populations*. The Hague: Mouton, 1980: pp. 347–349.

14 Angel JL. Patterns of fractures from Neolithic to modern times. *Anthropologiai Közlemények* 1974; **18**: 9–18.

15 Grauer AL, Roberts CA. Paleoepidemiology, healing and possible treatment of trauma in the medieval cemetery population of St Helen-on-the-Walls, York, England. *American Journal of Physical Anthropology* 1976; **100**(4): 531–544.

16 Judd M, Roberts CA. Fracture patterns at the medieval leper hospital in Chichester. *American Journal of Physical Anthropology* 1998; **105**(1): 43–55.

17 Roberts CA. Trauma and its treatment in British antiquity. Unpublished PhD thesis, University of Bradford, 1988.

18 Roberts CA. Trauma and treatment in antiquity: a radiographic study. In: Slater E, Tate J (eds), *Science and Archaeology, Glasgow*. British Series 196(ii). Oxford: British Archaeological Reports, 1988: pp. 339–359.

19 Lazenby R, Pfeiffer S. Effects of a 19th century below-knee amputation and prosthesis on femoral morphology. *International Journal of Osteoarchaeology* 1993; **3**: 19–28.

20 McKinley J. A skull wound and possible trepanation from a Roman cemetery at Baldock, Hertfordshire. *International Journal of Osteoarchaeology* 1992; **2**: 337–340.

21 Wells C. Results of bone setting in Anglo-Saxon times. *Medical and Biological Illustration* 1974; **24**: 215–220.

22 Wells C. Probable trephination of five early Saxon skulls. *Antiquity* 1974; **48**: 298–302.

23 Burrell LL, Mass MC, Van Gerven DP. Patterns of long bone fractures in two Nubian populations. *Human Evolution* 1986; **1**: 495–506.

24 Jurmain RD. Paleoepidemiology of trauma in a prehistoric central California population. In: Ortner DJ, Aufderheide AC (eds), *Human Paleopathology. Current Syntheses and Future Options*. Washington, DC: Smithsonian Institution Press, 1991: pp. 241–248.

25 Kilgore L, Jurmain R, Van Gerven D. Palaeoepidemiological patterns of trauma in a medieval Nubian skeletal population. *International Journal of Osteoarchaeology* 1997; **7(2)**: 103–114.

26 Crawford Adams J. *Outline of Fractures*. London: Churchill Livingstone, 1983.

27 Paton D. *Notes on Fractures*. Edinburgh: Churchill Livingstone, 1984.

28 Watson-Jones R. *Fractures and Joint Injuries*. Edinburgh: Churchill Livingstone, 1982.

29 Resnick D, Niwayama G. *Diagnosis of Bone and Joint Disorders* (2nd edn). London: WB Saunders, 1988.

30 Stewart TD. Non-union of fractures in antiquity, with descriptions of five cases involving the forearm. *Bulletin of the New York Academy of Medicine* 1974; **50(8)**: 875–891.

31 Heppenstall RB *Fracture Treatment and Healing*. Philadelphia: WB Saunders, 1980.

32 Rogers LF. *Radiology of Skeletal Trauma*. Edinburgh: Churchill Livingstone, 1992.

33 Sevitt S. *Bone Repair and Fracture Healing in Man*. Edinburgh: Churchill Livingstone, 1981.

34 Judd M. Fracture patterns in two populations from medieval Britain. Unpublished PhD thesis, University of Bradford, 1994.

35 Donaldson LJ, Cook A, Thomson RG. Incidence of fractures in a geographically defined population. *Journal of Epidemiology and Community Health* 1990; **44**: 241–245.

36 Lovejoy CO, Heiple KG. The analysis of fracture patterns in skeletal populations with an example from the Libben site, Ottawa County, Ohio. *American Journal of Physical Anthropology* 1981; **55**: 529–541.

37 Papers in: *International Journal of Osteoarchaeology* 1996; **6**(Issue 1).

38 Lilley JM, Stroud G, Brothwell DR, Williamson MH. *The Jewish Burial Ground at Jewbury*. The Archaeology of York. The Medieval Cemeteries 12/3. York: Council for British Archaeology for York Archaeological Trust, 1994.

39 Miles AEW. *An Early Christian Burial Ground on The Isle of Ensay, Outer Hebrides, Scotland*. British Series 212. Oxford: British Archaeological Reports, 1989.

40 Pinter-Bellows S. The human skeletons. In: Crummy N, Crummy P, Crossan C (eds), *Excavations of Roman and Later Cemeteries, Churches and Monastic Sites in Colchester, 1971–88*. Archaeological Report No. 9. Colchester: Colchester Archaeological Trust, 1993: pp. 62–92.

41 Stroud G, Kemp RL. *Cemeteries of St Andrew, Fishergate*. The Archaeology of York. The Medieval Cemeteries 12/2. York: Council for British Archaeology, 1993.

42 Wells C. The human bones. In: Wade-Martin P (ed.), *Excavations at North Elmham Park 1967–1972*. Report No. 9. Norfolk: East Anglian Archaeology, 1980: pp. 247–372.

43 Wells C. The human burials. In: McWhirr A, Viner L, Wells C. *Romano-British Cemeteries at Cirencester*. Cirencester: Cirencester Excavations Committee, 1982: pp. 135–202.

44 White W. *The Cemetery of St Nicholas Shambles*. London: London and Middlesex Archaeological Society, 1988.

45 Boghi F, Boylston A. The medieval cemetery of Pennell Street, Lincoln, Lincolnshire. Unpublished skeletal report, Bradford, 1997.

46 Mays S. *The Medieval Burials from the Blackfriars Friary, School Street, Ipswich, Suffolk*. English Heritage Ancient Monuments Laboratory Report 16/91, 1991.

47 Waldron T. The health of the adults. In: Molleson T, Cox M. *The Spitalfields Project. The Anthropology. The Middling Sort*. Research Report 86. York: Council for British Archaeology, 1993: 67–89.

48 Boocock P, Manchester K, Roberts C. The human remains from Eccles, Kent. Unpublished skeletal report, Bradford, 1995.

49 Dawes JD, Magilton JR. *The Cemetery of St Helen-on-the-Walls, Aldwark*. The Archaeology of York. The Medieval Cemeteries 12/1. London: Council for British Archaeology, 1980.

50 Molleson TI. The human remains. In: Farwell DE, Molleson TI. *Poundbury*, vol. **2**: *The Cemeteries*. Monograph Series No. 11. Dorchester: Dorset Natural History and Archaeological Society, 1993: pp. 142–214.

51 Wiggins R, Boylston A, Roberts C. Castledyke, Barton-on-Humber. Human Skeletal Report. Unpublished skeletal report, Bradford, 1992.

52 Wiggins R, Boylston A, Roberts C. Report on the human remains from Blackfriars, Gloucester (19/91). Unpublished skeletal report, Bradford, 1993.

53 Merbs CF. Spondylolysis and spondylolisthesis: a cost of being an erect biped or a clever adaptation? *Yearbook of Physical Anthropology* 1996; **39**: 201–228.

54 Knusel CJ, Roberts CA, Boylston A. Brief communication: When Adam delved...An activity-related lesion in three human skeletal populations. *American Journal of Physical Anthropology* 1996; **100**: 427–434.

55 Waldron T. Variation in the rates of spondylolysis in early populations. *International Journal of Osteoarchaeology* 1991; **1(1)**: 63–5.

56 Walker PL, Cook DC, Lambert PM. Skeletal evidence for child abuse: physical anthropological perspective. *Journal of Forensic Science* 1997; **42(2)**: 196–207.

57 Petersen HD, Wandall JH. Evidence of physical torture in a series of children. *Forensic Science International* 1995; **75**: 45–55.

58   Knusel CJ, Chundun Z, Cardwell P. Slipped femoral epiphysis in a priest from the medieval period. *International Journal of Osteoarchaeology* 1992; **2**: 109–119.

59   Wakely J. Bilateral congenital dislocation of the hip, spina bifida occulta and spondylolysis in a female skeleton from the medieval cemetery at Abingdon, England. *International Journal of Osteoarchaeology* 1993; **5(1)**: 37–45.

60   Blondiaux J, Millot F. Dislocation of the hip. Discussion of eleven cases from medieval France. *International Journal of Osteoarchaeology* 1991; 1(3–4): 203–208.

61   Drier FG. The palaeopathology of a finger dislocation. *International Journal of Osteoarchaeology* 1992; **2(1)**: 31–36.

62   Holck P. The occurrence of hip joint dislocation in early Lappic populations of Norway. *International Journal of Osteoarchaeology* 1991; **1**: 199–202.

63   Crawford Adams J. *Outline of Orthopaedics*. London: Churchill Livingstone, 1981.

64   Ackerknecht EH. Primitive surgery. In: Brothwell DR, Sandison AT (eds), *Diseases in Antiquity. A Survey of Diseases, Injuries and Surgery of Earlier Populations*. Springfield: Charles C Thomas, 1967: pp. 635–650.

65   Anderson RT. On doctors and bone setters in the 16th and 17th centuries. *Chiropractic History* 1983; **3(1)**: 11–15.

66   Brennan WA. *Guy De Chauliac on Wounds and Fractures*. Chicago: Translator, 1923.

67   Withington ET (ed.), *Hippocrates*. 3 vols. London: William Heinemann, 1927.

68   Oyebola D. Yoruba traditional bone setters: the practise of orthopaedics in a primitive setting in Nigeria. *Journal of Trauma* 1980; **20(4)**: 312–322.

69   Elliott Smith G. The most ancient splints. *British Medical Journal* 1908; **1**: 732–733.

70   Bloom AI, Bloom RA, Kahila G, Eisenberg E, Smith P. Amputation of the hand in the 3600 year old skeletal remains of an adult male. The first case reported from Israel. *International Journal of Osteoarchaeology* 1995; **5**: 188–191.

71   Brothwell D, Moller Christensen V. Medico-historical aspects of a very early case of mutilation. *Danish Medical Bulletin* 1963; **10(1)**: 21–25.

72   Brothwell D, Moller Christensen V. A possible case of amputation. *Man* 1963; **63**: 192–194

73   Mays S. Healed limb amputations in human osteoarchaeology and their causes: a case study from Ipswich, UK. *International Journal of Osteoarchaeology* 1996; **6**: 101–113.

74   Epstein S. Art, history and the crutch. *Annals of Medical History* N.S. 1937; **9**: 304–313.

75   Backay L. *Early History of Craniotomy from Antiquity to the Napoleonic Era*. Springfield: Charles C Thomas, 1985.

76   Lisowski FP. Prehistoric and early historic trepanations. In: Brothwell DR, Sandison AT (eds), *Diseases in Antiquity. A Survey of Diseases, Injuries and Surgery of Earlier Populations*. Springfield: Charles C Thomas, 1967: pp. 651–672.

77   Margetts EL. Trepanation of the skull by the medicine-men of primitive cultures, with particular reference to present-day native East African practice. In: Brothwell DR, Sandison AT (eds), *Diseases in Antiquity. A Survey of Diseases, Injuries and Surgery of Earlier Populations*. Springfield: Charles C Thomas, 1967: pp. 673–701.

78   Zimmerman MR, Trinkaus E, Lemay M, Aufderheide AC, Reyman TA, Marrocco GR. Trauma and trephination in a Peruvian mummy. *American Journal of Physical Anthropology* 1984; **55**: 497–501.

79   Bennike P. *Palaeopathology of Danish skeletons. A Comparative Study of Demography, Disease and Injury*. Copenhagen: Akademisk, 1985.

80   Stone JL, Miles ML. Skull trepanation among the early Indians of Canada and the United States. *Neurosurgery* 1990; **26(6)**: 1015–1020.

81   Parry TW. Cranial trephination in prehistoric Great Britain. *Medical Press* 1923; November 16th and 23rd: 403–407 and 423–425.

82   Buckley L, O'Donnabhain B. Trephination: early cranial surgery in Ireland. *Archaeology Ireland* 1992; **6(4)**: 10–12.

83   Parker S, Manchester K, Roberts C. A review of British trepanations with reports on two new cases. *Ossa* 1986; **12**: 141–157.

84   Jurmain R. *Stories from the Skeleton. Behavioral Reconstruction in Human Osteology*. New York: Gordon & Breach, 1999 (in press)

85   Stuart-Macadam, P. Glencross B, Kricun M. Traumatic bowing deformities of tubular bones. *International Journal of Osteoarchaeology* 1998; **8(4)**: 252–262.

86   Gordon E. Accidents among medieval children as seen from the miracles of six English saints and martyrs. *Medical History* 1991; **35**: 145–163.

87   Buikstra JE, Ubelaker D (eds), *Standards for Data Collection from Human Skeletal Remains*. Research Series 44. Arkansas: Arkansas Archeological Survey, 1994.

88   McKinley J, Roberts C. *Excavation and Post-Excavation Treatment of Cremated and Inhumed Human Remains*. Technical Paper 13. Birmingham: Institute for Field Archaeologists, 1993

89   Anderson J, Manchester K. Grooving of the proximal phalanx in leprosy: a palaeopathological and radiological study. *Journal of Archaeological Science* 1987; **14**: 77–82

90   Roberts C, Wakely J. Microscopical findings associated with the diagnosis of osteoporosis in palaeopathology. *International Journal of Osteoarchaeology* 1992; **2**: 23–20.

91   Notman DNH Ancient scannings: computed tomography of Egyptian mummies. In: David AR (ed.), *Science in Egyptology*. Manchester: Manchester University Press, 1986: pp. 251–320.

22

EVIDENCE FOR WEAPON-RELATED TRAUMA IN BRITISH ARCHAEOLOGICAL SAMPLES

Anthea Boylston

INTRODUCTION

This chapter discusses the criteria for the recognition of different types of weapon-related trauma and their limitations. Evidence for such injuries in the British archaeological record is reviewed and suggestions are made regarding directions for future research. Consideration is given to healed and unhealed wounds inflicted by bladed weapons, blunt or projectile (including gunshot) injuries to the cranium, in addition to post-cranial injuries inflicted by projectiles and other means. Archaeologists and biological anthropologists are often unfamiliar with the appearance of trauma which occurred at the time of death (peri-mortally), since most of the fractures encountered during research on human remains are well-healed. At most, a cemetery excavation may yield one or two individuals with cut marks or healed depressions in the cranial vault. It is therefore essential that research which was initiated to assist in the conviction of the perpetrators of violent assault in a modern context becomes more widely known to those who are engaged in studying historical populations.[1] In addition, an accumulating body of data in the clinical and forensic anthropological literature relating to the effects of trauma, particularly on the cranium, is assisting us in our ability to recognize and describe it effectively in skeletons from archaeological sites.

Analysis of weapon-related trauma on the human skeleton can provide valuable information on interpersonal relations in the past. Patterns of violence and warfare vary according to social context, and the quality and precision in manufacture of the weapons themselves naturally depend upon the material used in their fabrication and the available technology. For example, Brothwell[2] distinguished an Anglo-Saxon from a Neolithic burial at Maiden Castle, since cut marks on the cranium must have been delivered by an edged weapon rather than a flint implement, indicating that the skeleton came from the more recent of the two periods.

Weapons can be classified into those which are effective at long or short range.[3] Different weapons are required for fighting on horseback from those which are appropriate to the foot soldier, since a horseman would be quickly unseated if his weapon was either too large or too heavy. The repertoire of a medieval knight and his retinue, as documented from historical sources, was quite extensive (Figure 1) and included fearsome objects such as the morning star, whereas Anglo-Saxon weaponry was more restricted. Weapons found in Anglo-Saxon graves include spears and occasionally a sword, axe, seax or battle knife,[4] and we also have evidence from arrowheads found embedded in the vertebral column.[5] During the Neolithic and earlier periods the club, stone-tipped spear and flint arrowhead were employed, in addition to the use of household implements as weapons.[6]

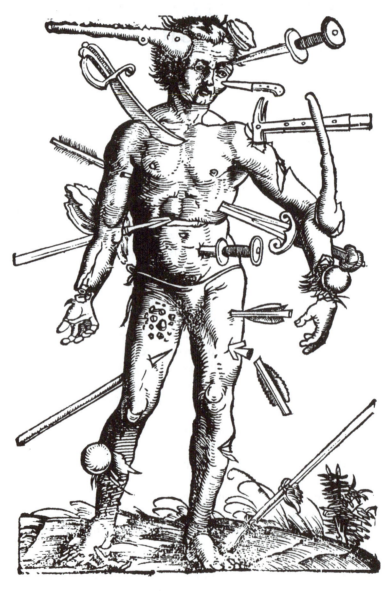

Figure 1 – 'The wound man', from Gerssdorff's Feldbuch der Wundartzney (1517), showing injuries from different weapons Source: Dr Jeremy Burgess/Science Photo Laboratory.

Many weapons can produce more than one type of injury; for example the cut and thrust of a sword or dagger, or the battle-axe, which has both pointed and blunt ends with varying signatures. It is seldom possible, therefore, to match an injury with a particular weapon. The amount of damage that may be caused to bone depends on the force with which the blow is delivered[7] or the velocity of a projectile. It also depends upon whether the victim is protected by armour or other means, such as a brigandine jacket in the case of the medieval soldier. The distribution of injuries on the skeleton may also give indications as to which areas of the body were shielded adequately.[8]

Major advances in weapon manufacture occurred in the late medieval period with the introduction of firearms, which totally changed the way in which battles were fought and caused armour to become obsolete.[9] Firearms were already being developed from the beginning of the 14th century AD.[10]

CLASSIFICATION OF TRAUMA PATTERNS

One of the most confusing aspects of the subject is the many different types of classification system used in the literature to describe weapon trauma. Initially, injuries can be subdivided into three main categories. These are sharp force, blunt force[11] and projectile trauma.[12] Brothwell[13] developed a four-point classification system; two of these categories referred to blunt trauma caused by large or small maces or clubs. Trauma caused by edged weapons might represent a slice with a sword or a broader wound caused by an axe, and pointed weapons might perforate bone. He also described the radiating fractures that might result from blunt trauma. Ortner and Putschar[14] listed the different types of force applied to bone which may result in fracture, namely compression, tension, torsion, bending and shearing. Merbs[15] elaborated on these categories and discussed many types of trauma, including weapon wounds and dental trauma.

Much of the evidence for weapon injury on the skeleton comes from a study of cranial trauma,[16–18] where the patterns are most distinctive. However, recent advances in recognition of the response of bone to insult, developed in order to identify the marks of cannibalism on the human skeleton[19] have facilitated the description and classification of post-cranial injuries which have occurred around the time of death (i.e. those that are peri-mortem).

Pseudopathology

Calvin Wells[20] reminded us that it is always necessary to exclude the artefactual when making palaeopathological diagnoses and of no subject is this truer than the identification of weapon injury on the skeleton. He highlighted particularly the cranial deformation caused by the burial environment. This makes the establishment of diagnostic criteria an essential part of trauma analysis. Buikstra and Ubelaker[21] illustrated the difference between peri-mortem and post-mortem cranial fractures and drew attention to the squareness of the breakage pattern that affects dry bone, once the collagen element has decreased leaving a brittle mineralized framework. Wounds that occur around the time of death are more likely to produce an oblique fracture pattern (Figure 2a and 2b). Sauer[22] describes in detail the differences in the effects on bone of ante-, peri- and post-mortem injury, and elaborates on the different rates of loss of collagen, according to whether the individual is buried in wet, dry or permanently frozen conditions. Loss of water and collagen in the burial environment alters the characteristics of bone, making it harder and stiffer.[23] However, fractures indicating some elasticity may occur up to weeks after death.

The amount of force needed to fracture living bone with the soft tissues intact is between 435 and 900 lb per square inch (psi)[24] which is more than ten times that required to break dry bone (40 psi). Cranial bone averages 0.272 inches in thickness, but is much thicker in some parts than in others. The cranial vault bones are buttressed by thicker osseous tissue

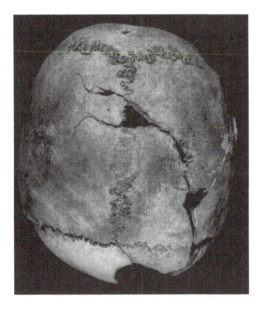

Figure 2a – Blunt force injury to the back of the cranium of a burial from a mass grave at Towton (burial 21) showing the typical oblique radiating fractures which characterize this type of injury. One of these blends with a sharp force injury to the left parietal and frontal bone.[12]

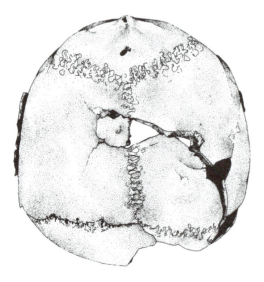

Figure 2b – Drawing of the same injury. Illustrator: Caroline Needham.

in certain areas, for example, a triangular area in the centre of the frontal and occipital bones.[7] Therefore, an explanation is needed when a discrete hole is found in the robust bones of the cranial vault. This may well be provided by studying the endocranial surface, where a bevelled edge with no evidence of healing would suggest an event that occurred around the time of death.[13]

Cut marks produced by edged weapons (sharp force injury)

This type of trauma is the most easily identified on the skeleton. The diagnostic criteria are:[25]

- Linearity.
- A well-defined clean edge.
- A flat, smooth, polished cut surface.
- The presence of parallel scratch marks on the bone surface when viewed by light or scanning electron microscopy.

In addition, it may be possible to recognize the direction from which the cut has been delivered by studying the angle at which it passed through the bone. The opposite side of the cut from the polished surface will show flaking and roughening, except in cases where the weapon has cut cleanly through the skull. Many studies have found that the majority of cranial injuries occur on the left side of the head[26] as a result of face-to-face combat between right-handed combatants. However, in a battle situation the close-packed nature of the conflict may result in injuries to any part of the cranium;[27] this is well illustrated in the skeletal remains from the Battle of Wisby, Sweden, where many of the injuries were to the occipital bone.

Blunt trauma to the cranium

The biomechanics of cranial injury have recently been summarized by Berryman and Haun,[28] who draw attention to the effects of trauma on the skull. In the immediate aftermath of a traumatic event, the outer table of the cranium comes under compression and the inner table under tension (except in the case of a projectile exit wound when the situation would be reversed). If the force of the blow exceeds the elastic limit of the bone, it is the inner table that breaks first in the immediate area of the blow. The outer table is more likely to fracture in a concentric fashion around the affected area.[29] Berryman and Symes[7] emphasize that it is actually the trabecular bone of the diploe which fractures before the breaking of the inner and outer tables.

Blunt trauma can normally be identified by the presence of such concentric or radiating fractures, depending upon the force with which the blow is delivered.[24] A relatively light blow may result in a simple linear fracture. However, one delivered with greater force may produce a comminuted fracture (see below) with radiating fractures in the immediate area around the wound, or a contrecoup fracture in another area of the cranium when the inertial stresses propagate towards the opposite end of the head from the area of impact.[3] For example, a penetrating injury to the parietal bone (Figure 3a) can cause a contrecoup fracture to the base of the skull (Figure 3b).[12] Blunt trauma may dent, crack or splinter bone, in contrast to the incised nature of sharp force injury.[6]

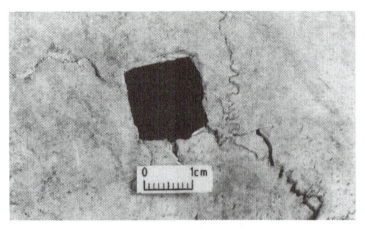

Figure 3a – Square hole in left parietal bone delivered by a blunt weapon such as a poleaxe (Towton 96: inhumation 9).

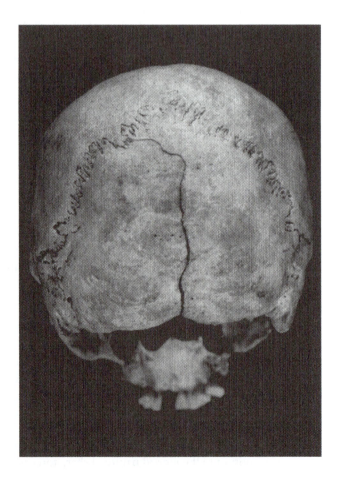

Figure 3b – Contrecoup fracture to posterior cranium resulting from force of blow illustrated in Figure 2a.[12]

King[30] produced a classification system for blunt trauma based on the descriptions in Gurdjian,[3] Burkhardt,[31] Bergeron and Rumbaugh,[32] Polsen *et al.*[33] and Ortner and Putschar[14] which includes expressed and depressed, diastatic and gutter fractures (Figure 4). An expressed fracture occurs when the broken fragments project outside the perimeter of the skull. Diastasis involves a parting of the cranial sutures, which is often seen in children subjected to blunt force injury, and a gutter fracture results from the blade or point of the weapon grazing bone. Depressed fractures (where the incident pushes the bone fragments below the endocranial surface) are subdivided according to whether they are comminuted

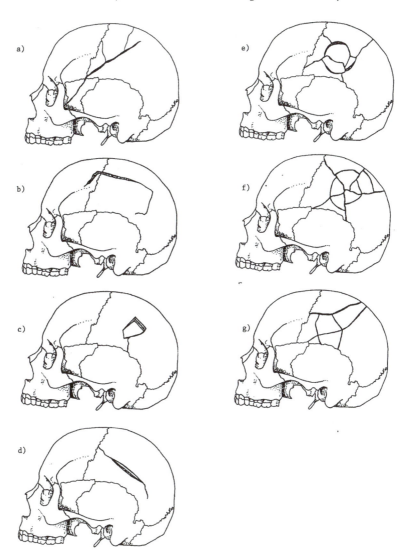

Figure 4 – Different types of blunt force trauma: (a) linear fracture with radiating fissure fractures, (b) depressed fracture, (c) depressed fracture á la signature, (d) depressed fracture produced by a sharp-edged weapon, (e) depressed pond fracture (also comminuted), (f) depressed stellate fracture, (g) comminuted fracture (reproduced by permission of Sarah King[30]).

(the bone is broken into many fragments), or whether a pond or stellate effect is produced by the fracture lines. The bevel of the concentric fracture lines should also be studied as this may vary according to the position of the injury on the cranium.

The effects of injury on the soft tissues should not be forgotten, although in archaeological contexts evidence is usually absent. Quite a small injury can produce a considerable amount of bleeding. The brain may be injured by acceleration or deceleration forces depending upon whether the head is hit by a moving object or a moving head is stopped by a stationary object;[24] therefore, accidental injury may be difficult to distinguish from deliberately inflicted weapon damage. Blood clotting in the subdural, extradural or subarachnoid space may damage the brain and may cause death within hours or days. Blood accumulating in the cranial cavity can lead to alteration of intracranial pressure and meningitis can follow penetrating weapon injuries or compound fractures.

Projectile trauma

The effects on the cranium produced by a missile can be quite devastating. This type of trauma includes not only injuries produced by bullets, but also those produced by arrows and javelin-type weapons. The results of gunshot wounds on the soft tissues and bone are described in detail by Dimaio.[34] An example of early gunshot injury was recently illustrated by Kaufman et al.[35] on the cranium of a soldier from the Battle of Waterloo, whose skull had been destroyed by a musket ball and subsequent osteomyelitis.

Healed lesions of the cranium

Sledzik and Barbian[36] related the sequence of events characterizing the early healing process in documented cranial injuries. This commences with a quiescent period of about 1 week, followed by an osteoclastic (bone-resorbing) phase which then leads to an osteoblastic (bone-depositional) phase where new bone is formed beneath the periosteum around the fracture. The earliest visible change is rounding of the cut edges of bone at the site of the wound. Campillo[37] described cicatrization, which is an early stage in the process of healing in certain types of wound. Walker[38] recently made an extensive study of healed trauma worldwide based on skeletal samples from many different periods and commented on the frequency of healed trauma to the nasal bones.

Healed depressed fractures are quite often described in the archaeological record. They are often quite small and commonly occur on the frontal bone[39–42]. Stirland[43] documented a particular dramatic example of a healed cranial wound from medieval St Margaret *in combusto* in Norwich. It was still possible to see the fracture lines of this blunt force injury, although considerable evidence of healing was present in the joining of adjacent wound edges by remodelled osseous tissue. An unusual healed cranial fracture has been reported from a multiperiod excavation at York Minster.[44] The only Romano-British burial from the site demonstrated a hemispherical healed depression fracture, which covered a large area of the frontal bone. It had caused the inner table of the skull to project inwards, with possible consequences for cerebral function such as unconsciousness or personality change. Manchester[27] described a healed injury from Pontefract Castle, Yorkshire that was so severe that the brain would have been exposed, yet the individual survived. A very characteristic depression, which may have been produced by a slingshot, was found at Romano-British Cirencester, Gloucestershire.[45]

Postcranial injuries

Occasionally a weapon, such as a spearhead or arrow, is found still in place in the abdominal cavity.[27] Postcranial sharp force injuries which took place around the time of death may be recognized by identification of cut marks on bone, but can be difficult to distinguish from pseudopathology if the characteristic polishing is not present.[46] Perimortal blunt force trauma to the long bones may produce the classic 'butterfly' fracture, but this has also been described in a case of post-mortem breakage.[47] White[19] illustrated the peeling, flaking and spiral fractures that distinguish post-mortem trauma.

Gunshot wounds

Crypt excavations in recent years have led to the discovery of weapon injuries inflicted by firearms. Nevertheless, only a few instances of gunshot trauma have been recorded in the British literature on the subject. Bowman *et al.*[48] described the case of a suicide from St Bride's crypt, London. The burial was that of a young man of 25 who had recently married. He was recorded in the burial register as 'suddenly found dead'. Upon examination of his skull, it was found that this individual had shot himself in the mouth at close range and there was an exit wound in the region of the lambdoid suture. The death had been reported in *The Morning Chronicle* of the day, thereby confirming the authenticity of the osteological findings.

Another suicide victim was found among the burials at Christchurch, Spitalfields.[49] The named individual had died in AD 1837. An entrance wound for the bullet was found in the right sphenoid and the much larger exit wound was situated just above lambda on the parietal bones. The bullet had evidently ricocheted off the sella turcica and turned through 100° inside the cranium. Documentary evidence was found for the cause of this individual's suicide in the newspapers of the day. There was also an old wound in the frontal bone where a bullet had grazed the surface during a previous attempt.

King[50] reported a similar tragic event among a group of 82 burials, which were excavated from Glasgow Cathedral cemetery in 1993/94. A young adult male was found, upon excavation, with three lead balls inside his skull. He had a 15 mm gunshot entrance wound in his left frontal bone and an exit wound measuring 24 mm in the posterior right parietal bone. Both wounds displayed radiating fracture lines. The lead balls appeared to have come from a blunderbuss, which became popular during the 18th century for household defence as well as military purposes.[10]

EVIDENCE FOR INJURY IN BRITISH POPULATIONS

Before the 1960s there is little evidence in the literature for weapon injury in British populations. Brothwell[51] reviewed the cases published up to that time and came to the conclusion that injuries to the cranial vault were much more common than instances of trauma to the face. He listed 37 injuries to the frontal and parietal bones, by contrast there were only ten wounds to the facial bones. However, these are commonly shattered by pressure of the soil or collapse during excavation and, unless each skull is completely reconstructed during analysis, it is probable that many craniofacial fractures are missed. Wells[52] discussed the subject of deliberate injury to the skeleton, but did not cite a single example from the British archaeological record. He described the 'nest' of 38 crania exhibiting blunt trauma from Ofnet in Bavaria dating to the Mesolithic period, and the evidence for medieval weapon injury from the Battle of Wisby which took place in AD 1361 on the Swedish island of Gotland. Since that time there has been an increasing number of reports in the British literature on weapon-related trauma to the skeleton. A literature search produced the following examples, which are discussed in chronological order.

Early prehistoric period

The lack of evidence for burial in the Palaeolithic and Mesolithic periods is reflected in a corresponding scarcity of weapon injuries. A Beaker-Age burial with three flint arrowheads embedded in the ribs and breastbone was found at Stonehenge.[53] The presence of cut marks on other ribs enabled the trajectory of each arrow to be reconstructed and the cause of death ascertained. An adult male with a cranial fracture resulting in localized swelling was described by Brothwell[54] in a study of the Bronze Age people of the Yorkshire Wolds. Undoubtedly burial practices in the Bronze Age contributed to the paucity of evidence of trauma from these periods. The cremation rite in the Middle Bronze Age, and random scattering of human remains on settlement sites during the Late Bronze Age, drastically reduces the human remains available for study. However, the hoards of weapons found in rivers and bogs suggest that warfare may have been common in this period.

Iron Age

The Iron Age and Romano-British periods are a time when ritual and violence are evident in the burial record, sometimes involving mutilation and dismemberment. Weapons are occasionally found in Iron Age graves with those who have suffered wounds to the skull and other parts of the body, for example at Burton Fleming on the Yorkshire Wolds (Table 1), suggesting an association with conflict.[55] This is in contrast to the Anglo-Saxon period when many weapons accompanying the dead appear to have been put there for funerary and other purposes.[4]

An interesting series of cranial injuries was found at Danebury[60] including a skull with four perimortal injuries, two of which were depressed fractures with adherent flakes indicating blunt perimortal trauma, and two were holes in the cranial vault. A frontal bone from the disarticulated material showed a clear weapon impression and two perimortal blunt force injuries.

Romano-British period

Typical injuries by bladed weapons to the cranium are described by Wells[45] at Cirencester, one of the largest Roman towns in the UK, where fighting was purported to be

Table 1 – Iron Age burials showing evidence of weapon injury.[55]

Site	Burial No.	Sex	Age (years)	Position	Type of lesion	References
Danes Graves, East Yorkshire	104	–	35–40	Left parietal	1–2 inch cut	Stead[56]
Danes Graves, East Yorkshire	45	?F	about 45	Frontal	2 inch scar or old cut	Stead[56]
Burton Fleming, East Yorkshire	–	–	–	Chest cavity	Spearhead	Stead[56]
Burton Fleming, East Yorkshire	–	–	–	Pelvis	Embedded weapon	Stead[56]
Burton Fleming, East Yorkshire	–	–	–	Vertebrae	Embedded weapon	Stead[56]
Garton Slack, East Yorkshire	11	–	> 60	Skull	6 mm healed puncture	Brewster[57]
Gussage all Saints, Dorset	285	M	YA	Skull and left forearm	Sharp instrument	Whimster[58]
Berwick St John, Wiltshire	512	M	OA	Back of skull	Healed wound	Whimster[58]
Eggington, Bedfordshire	–	M	YA	Right tibia	Partially healed but infected sword cut	Whimster[58]
St Merryn, Cornwall	58	–	–	Head and face	Unhealed sword cuts	Whimster[58]
Wetwang Slack, East Yorkshire	114	M	17–20	Right occipital	Slice by sword	Dent[59]
Wetwang Slack, East Yorkshire	119	M	20–24	Right frontal	Partially healed depression fracture	Dent[59]
Wetwang Slack, East Yorkshire	211	F	25–35	'Stomach region'	Iron spearhead	Dent[59]
Danebury, Hampshire	11	–	Ad	Frontal	Three unhealed, blunt force	Hooper[60]
Danebury, Hampshire	30	–	–	Right orbital rim	Healed blunt force	Hooper[60]
Danebury, Hampshire	47	–	Ad	Left ilium	Unhealed sword cuts	Hooper[60]
Danebury, Hampshire	48	M	30+	Frontal, right and parietal	Unhealed blunt force including two depression fractures	Hooper[60]

Key for Tables 1–4: Age YA – young adult, MA – middle adult, YMA – Young-middle adult, OA – Old Adult, Ad – Adult

commonplace.[45] These included an extensive healed injury, which had partially detached a large triangular area of the right parietal bone. Although this had healed, the depressed fragment would probably have caused neurological complications. The wound appeared to have been augmented by a deliberate trepanation whose rounded edges suggested long-term survival after the event (Table 2).

The problems of differential diagnosis are well illustrated by the cranial injuries at the cemetery of Trentholme Drive in York, which was excavated during the 1950s.[66] On one of the skulls, two oval holes joined by a radiating fracture and the bevelling on the inner table can be clearly seen.[66] A pickaxe driven through the skull after burial would have shattered the cranium, therefore these are most likely to have been peri-mortem injuries. McKinley[67] discusses the problems of differentiating between weapon injuries and trepanation in a case from Baldock and emphasizes the importance of considering both the internal and external bevelling in detail.

Decapitation

The widespread ritual of decapitation before burial represents an entirely different form of trauma, which was practised both during the Romano-British and Anglo-Saxon periods. In 1981 Harman *et al.*[68] assembled all the information on decapitated and prone burials published up to that date and looked in detail at five sites dating to the late Romano-British period. They note that both practices took place in the Romano-British and Anglo-Saxon periods but decapitation was more frequent in the former and prone burial in the latter.

Table 2 – Romano-British burials with evidence of weapon injury

Site	Burial No.	Sex	Age (years)	Position	Type of lesion	References
Snell's Corner, Horndean, Hampshire	RB5	M	OA	Left parietal	Healed depression fracture or trepanation	Cave[61]
Dunstable, Bedfordshire	RP	–	–	Zygoma, maxilla	Unhealed sword cut	Matthews[62]
Cirencester, Gloucestershire	24	M	–	Left frontal	Healed sword cut	Wells[45]
Cirencester, Gloucestershire	58	F	–	Left parietal	Healed ?knife wound	Wells[45]
Cirencester, Gloucestershire	81	–	–	Frontal	Healed graze from arrow or lance	Wells[45]
Cirencester, Gloucestershire	S	M	–	Frontal	Healed dagger thrust	Wells[45]
Cirencester, Gloucestershire	101	M	–	Parietals	Healed sword cuts	Wells[45]
Cirencester, Gloucestershire	305	M	–	Right parietal	Healed sharp and blunt injuries + trepanation	Wells[45]
Cirencester, Gloucestershire	14	M	–	Right humerus	Unhealed sword cut	Wells[45]
Cirencester, Gloucestershire	21	M	–	Right humerus	Two unhealed sword cuts	Wells[45]
Cirencester, Gloucestershire	163	M	–	Left femur	Unhealed sword cut	Wells[45]
Ancaster, Lincolnshire	–	–	Ad	Left frontal	Unhealed sword scoop	Cox[63]
Baldock, Hertfordshire	5779	M	OA	Parietals	Healed ?trepanation	McKinley[64]
Poundbury, Dorset	938	F	Ad	Parietals and occipital	Two unhealed sword scoops	Farwell and Molleson[65]

Decapitation was quite common in rural cemeteries but was only seen in a few urban sites such as at Poundbury in Dorset,[65] Lankhills in Winchester[69] and Cirencester, Gloucestershire.[45] They also determined that the 'normal' means of decapitation was from the front of the neck in most of these burials. Philpott[70] studied the demographic pattern of such unusual burials and came to the conclusion that individuals of both sexes and all age groups were equally affected, although the ritual was less common in children. The wide age distribution militates against the practice having been exclusively reserved for society's outcasts. Occasionally, mutilation also seems to be a factor, as at Dunstable where one burial had the lower legs cut off and placed beside the head.[62] Only a few decapitated infants have been found, including two at Springhead, who appear to have been foundation sacrifices,[71] and one from Bishop Grosseteste College in Lincoln, a neonatal infant burial which was also found beneath the floor of a building.[72]

McKinley[64] describes decapitation at Baldock, Hertfordshire. The burial was that of an adolescent who was probably female. Her axis vertebra demonstrated six cuts on its anterior aspect including two on the odontoid process, and this vertebra had eventually been severed through the body. A very similar decapitation is one of 12 from the late Romano-British cemetery of Kempston in Bedford. There are also six cut marks on the anterior aspect of the axis with eventual transection of the vertebra. This was also the burial of a female.[73]

A rather different form of ritual is described by Mays and Steele[74] in the context of a skull found in a pit at Folly Lane, St Albans, dating to the second century AD. There was a 1 cm hole in the left part of the lambdoid suture with bevelled internal edges. A further three holes in the left side of the skull also appeared to be perimortal in nature. In addition, there were knife marks, clustered in groups, on the parietal bones. The authors discuss the possibility of the cut marks having been caused by scalping or mutilation wrought by a desire for retribution, perhaps an echo of early Iron Age practices.

Anglo-Saxon period

Injuries from bladed weapons are the most common signs of interpersonal violence recorded in the archaeological record during the Anglo-Saxon period (Table 3). Weapon injuries have been reported from a number of sites, but a blunt instrument delivered only one of these.

Weapon injuries from Eccles, Kent

Wenham[25,83] studied six victims of weapon injury from the early Christian site of Eccles using scanning electron microscopy. The burials concerned were part of a group of 176 inhumations dating to the 7th century AD.[84] Four of the six individuals displayed a single injury to the cranial vault; however, the other two had evidence of multiple wounds, both affecting the cranium and other regions of the body. One of these cases has been reported by Manchester and Elmhirst[5] and involved a cut measuring 96 mm to the posterior part of the occipital bone (Figure 5). The polished edges with no evidence of healing showed that it had been administered at the time of death, and indeed the severity of the injury was such that it would undoubtedly have proven fatal. The nature of the wound suggested that it had been carried out with a sword, the sharpness of which was attested to by the lack of terminal fractures at the limits of the injury. Manchester ascertained from the direction of the cut that the assailant would probably have been at the same level as the victim, who would have been upright at the time of the attack.

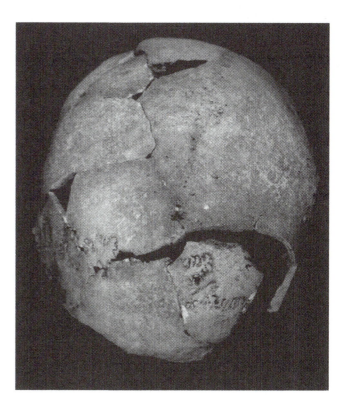

Figure 5 – Blade wound to the posterior cranium of an Anglo-Saxon from Eccles in Kent. Reproduced by permission of Dr Keith Manchester.

Table 3 – Anglo-Saxon burials showing weapon injuries.[75]

Site	No.	Sex	Age (years)	Position	Type of lesion	References
North Elmham Park, Norfolk	171	M	Ad	Right and left temporals	Three unhealed sword cuts	Wells and Cayton[76]
Burgh Castle, Norfolk	43	M	35+		Unhealed sword cut	Anderson & Birkett[77]
Burgh Castle, Norfolk	92	?F	25–35		Unhealed sword cut	Anderson & Birkett[77]
Finglesham, Kent	94	M	Ad		Unhealed sword cut	Hawkes[78]
Eccles, Kent	I	M	25–35	Frontal and left parietal	Unhealed linear wound (?blunt)	Wenham[25]
Eccles, Kent	II	M	20–25	Most cranial bones	Unhealed sword cuts and scoops	Wenham[25]
Eccles, Kent	III	M	35+	Right parietal, lumbar spine	Unhealed sword cut; iron projectile	Wenham[25]
Eccles, Kent	IV	M	25–35	Left frontal, left parietal	Three unhealed sword cuts	Wenham[25]
Eccles, Kent	V	M	25–35	Left parietal	Unhealed sword cut	Wenham[25]
Eccles, Kent	VI	M	20–25	Left frontal and parietal	Unhealed sword cut	Wenham[25]
Staunch Meadow, Brandon, Suffolk	3079	–	Ad	Right frontal	Healed sword cut	Anderson[39]
Staunch Meadow, Brandon, Suffolk	4038	M	YMA	Right humerus, left femur, left parietal and parietals	Unhealed sword cuts	Anderson[39]
Staunch Meadow, Brandon, Suffolk	4055	?M	YA	Right frontal > left parietal, two on right parietal	Unhealed sword cuts and scoop	Anderson[39]
Staunch Meadow, Brandon, Suffolk	8007	F	MA	Left parietal	Unhealed sword cut	Anderson[39]
Caister-on-Sea, Norfolk	108	F	Ad	Occipital and left parietal	Unhealed sword cut	Anderson[40]
Great Chesterford, Essex	75	M	45+		Healing sword cut	Waldron[41]
Great Chesterford, Essex	101	M	45+		Healing blunt weapon	Waldron[41]
Buckland, Kent	303b	M	30–35	Left parietal	Healing axe blow	Anderson[75]
Buckland, Kent	348	M	30–35	Left parietal	Unhealed sword cut	Anderson[75]
Addingham, West Yorkshire	106	?F	Ad	Cranial fragments	Unhealed sword cuts	Boylston[79]
Ailcey Hill, Ripon, North Yorkshire	1043			Right frontal and parietal	Two unhealed sword cuts	Langston[80]
Butler's Field, Lechlade, Gloucs.	65	M	45+	Frontal and facial bones	Multiple healed injuries	Harman[81]
Butler's Field, Lechlade, Gloucs.	87	M	45+	Left frontal	Hollow 25 × 20	Harman[81]
Butler's Field, Lechlade, Gloucs.	178	M	45+	Right temporal	Hollow lesion	Harman[81]
Butler's Field, Lechlade, Gloucs.	55	M	Ad	Left parietal	Unhealed sword cut	Harman[81]
Butler's Field, Lechlade, Gloucs.	21	M	–	Left parietal and frontal	Healed sword scoop, unhealed sword cut	Harman[81]
Barrington, Cambridgeshire	148	M	25–35	Left parietal	Healed sword scoop	Duhig[82]
Barrington, Cambridgeshire	447A	M	25–35	Right parietal	Healed sword scoop	Duhig[82]
Barrington, Cambridgeshire	451A	M	50–59	Left parietal	Shallow indentation ?trepanation	Duhig[82]
Barrington, Cambridgeshire	553	M	45+	Both parietals	Shallow sword scoop	Duhig[82]

Cox Lane killing and Maiden Castle murder

Two case studies, published in the 1960s and 70s, represent a departure from the previous, largely descriptive, approach to the study of palaeopathology. A detailed examination of the entire skeleton was required to determine the cause and manner of death and a reconstruction of a possible course of events was forthcoming, particularly in the Cox Lane case.[85]

Wells describes the case of a victim of extensive peri-mortal trauma from Cox Lane, Ipswich, in the late Saxon/medieval period. The injuries include a sword cut which transected the cranium vertically parallel to the coronal suture, suggesting that the blow was delivered from an individual on horseback or that the victim was on his knees at the time. In addition, there was a sword cut to the left femur, delivered from below, which would have severed the quadriceps muscles. Other perimortal injuries are represented by an amputation of the right wrist and hand and cut marks on the right eighth and ninth ribs.

In 1971 Brothwell[2] reanalysed the human remains excavated by Wheeler from a prehistoric long barrow at Maiden Castle and first described by Morant and Goodman[86] as belonging to the Windmill Hill Culture. Since the inhumation had been placed on the long axis of the burial mound it was thought to have been the primary interment. However, the male individual had suffered eight injuries to the skull including a possible trepanation and a wound from a bladed weapon to the occipital bone. Attempts had also been made to cut off the victim's limbs, and there were cut marks on all the extremities apart from the right arm in the region of the joints. It became obvious from the incisive nature of the cut marks that the attack could only have been carried out with a metal weapon, and therefore the burial was intrusive. An estimate of 635 AD was subsequently forthcoming with radiocarbon dating.

Cemetery of St Andrew, Fishergate

Stroud and Kemp[26] describe a group of burials from Fishergate, which included 29 males with one or more weapon injuries. These include sharp-edged incisions to the cranium, as well as post-cranial injuries, particularly cuts on the ribs and vertebrae. There are also cut marks on the femora and a smaller number on the bones of the upper extremity. The most unusual form of trauma is a projectile injury in the iliac fossa of a left pelvic bone. Composite diagrams of the skull, spine and long bones with superimposition of cut marks from the entire group enabled the pattern of injuries to be studied. Sixteen of the burials have suffered cranial injuries, often multiple, and 19 had cut marks on one or more ribs. Numerous blows to the back of the body suggest less 'formalized fighting' than hand-to-hand combat.

Many of these burials date to the 10th and 11th centuries AD. The battles of Fulford and Stamford Bridge were fought at this period[87] and it is possible that these burials may result from one of these conflicts. The town of York was subjected to periodic violence just before the Norman Conquest as part of William the Conqueror's 'Harrying of the North' in AD 1069 and 1070. The trauma victims have been interred as a distinctive group with some double burials.[26] In addition, they were all male and quite young. A total of 152 injuries are documented from the 10th–11th centuries AD and 58 injuries on those from the 12th–16th centuries.[87] Analysis of the distribution pattern of wounds between the anterior and posterior aspects of the skeleton has demonstrated a pattern, which may be very helpful in reconstructing the type of warfare that led to these horrific injuries.[87]

Late medieval warfare

Many site reports give details of small numbers of individuals who have been the victims of weapon injury, either healed or unhealed. At Jewbury, in York, six examples of deliberate trauma were found, one represented by cut marks to a tibia and the other five consisting of blade injuries to the head and, in one case, to the face and jaw.[88] A variety of injuries are displayed by six trauma victims at the Blackfriars cemetery, School Street, Ipswich,[42] including the tip of an iron projectile embedded in a frontal bone and guttering caused by a surface weapon graze. A slicing injury to the left parietal in a young man from Stratford

Langthorne Abbey, London is accompanied by cut marks on the clavicle and a cervical vertebra, suggesting an attempted decapitation.[89]

There is a much wider variety of weapon injuries from this period, reflecting a greater diversity of weapon types (Table 4). The perimortal nature of the injury to an individual from St Nicholas Shambles, London[94] is well illustrated by the adherent flake and bevelling of the inner table of the cranium. Eleven cranial injuries are mentioned at St Helen-on-the-Walls, York.[90]

An interesting series of injuries dating to the late medieval period came from the Whithorn Church excavations in south-west Scotland.[96] Thirteen crania were affected by depressed fractures, linear wounds, injuries involving removal of a thin slice of bone or possible trepanations. More males than females were involved and the left parietal was the most frequent site of injury.

Table 4 – Injuries dating to the medieval period

Site	No.	Sex	Age (years)	Position	Type of lesion	References
St Helen-on-the-Walls, York, North Yorkshire	5281	M	30+	Right side	Healed contusion	Dawes and Magilton[90]
St Helen-on-the-Walls, York, North Yorkshire	5607	–	30+	Occipital	Healed sword injury	Dawes and Magilton[90]
St Helen-on-the-Walls, York, North Yorkshire	5423	M	40+	Left parietal	Healed blunt injury	Dawes and Magilton[90]
Chester, Cheshire	B42	–	–	Occipital	Large depression fracture	West[91]
Chelmsford, Essex	76	–	–	Occipital	Healed cut	Bayley[92]
Chelmsford, Essex	106/7	–	–	Frontal	Healed cut	Bayley[92]
Hulton Abbey, Staffordshire		M	–	Right scapula, left radius, right femur	Unhealed cut marks	Browne[93]
Stratford Langthorne Abbey, London		M	YA	Left parietal, clavicle, cervical vertebra	Unhealed cut marks	Stuart-Macadam[89]
St Nicholas Shambles, London	5047	M	17–25	Right frontal	Blow from edged weapon	White[94]
St Nicholas Shambles, London	5096	–	–		Puncture wound – adherent flake	White[94]
St Nicholas Shambles, London	5201	–	Ad		Projectile wound	White[94]
Ipswich, Suffolk	992	–	–	Left frontal and parietal	Healed weapon injury	Mays[42]
Ipswich, Suffolk	1749	–	–		Unhealed weapon injury	Mays[42]
Ipswich, Suffolk	1978	–	–	Frontal	Linear gully	Mays[42]
Jewbury, York, North Yorkshire	3050	M	40+		Unhealed cut marks	Lilley *et al.*[88]
Jewbury, York, North Yorkshire	2695	F	50+	Right parietal	Healing blade injury	Lilley *et al.*[88]
Jewbury, York, North Yorkshire	2475	M	40–50		Healed sword scoop	Lilley *et al.*[88]
Jewbury, York, North Yorkshire	1409	F	–	Right orbit	Healed blade injury	Lilley *et al.*[88]
Jewbury, York, North Yorkshire	2590	F	15–20	Left parietal, occipital, left mastoid, maxilla and mandible	Unhealed blade injuries	Lilley *et al.*[88]
St Margaret *in combusto*, Norwich, Norfolk	1	M	Ad	–	Puncture wound	Stirland[43]
St Margaret *in combusto*, Norwich, Norfolk	59	M	Ad	Left frontal and parietal	Healed sword injury	Stirland[43]
St Margaret *in combusto*, Norwich, Norfolk	374	M	YA	Right parietal and frontal	Unhealed blunt force	Stirland[43]
St Margaret *in combusto*, Norwich, Norfolk	392	–	Ad	Left temporal and parietal	Healed blunt injuries	Stirland[43]
Stonar, Kent	19	–	–	Left parietal, two on right parietal	Healed sword cuts	Eley and Bayley[95]

Lincoln Castle

A group of 16 burials, consisting of 14 males and two females, was excavated near the west gate of Lincoln Castle in an area labelled 'the entrenchments of King Stephen' on a 19th-century map.[97] One male from a double burial showed evidence of three cranial injuries. There was a gaping wound on the occipital bone behind the left mastoid process with a terminal fracture demonstrating that a heavy weapon such as an axe had been used in the assault. This injury showed evidence of healing with recent, porous new bone formation, but it had evidently been delivered only a short time before death (Figure 6a). In addition, the point of an armour-piercing bodkin arrow[98] had perforated the outer table of the cranial vertex and the 'coup de grace' was also delivered to the same region (Figure 6b). This was oval in cross-section and had penetrated both bone and soft tissues. Bevelling of the endocranial surface of the skull proved it to have been a perimortal injury.[12] This individual may have been killed in the civil war that took place between King Stephen and Queen Matilda in AD 1140.

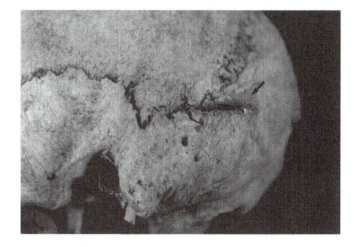

Figure 6a – Wound from a sharp-edged weapon, probably an axe, from a late medieval burial found near the west gate of Lincoln Castle. There is new bone formation, indicative of healing, around the wound (arrow).

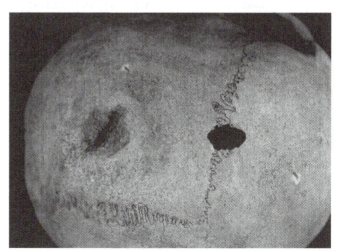

Figure 6b – Wound from a bodkin arrow and an oval entry wound in the cranium of the individual illustrated in Figure 6a.

St Margaret in combusto, Norwich

Stirland[43] describes an unusual group of individuals with cranial trauma from a large parish cemetery. Eleven cases of cranial trauma were detected, eight of which showed evidence of healing – even of quite severe injuries; a further five individuals demonstrated slicing injuries inflicted by sharp-edged weapons. These wounds are contrasted with those exhibited by the occupants of the wreck of the *Mary Rose* (Henry VIII's flagship) who exhibited 11 healed, depressed cranial fractures and one injury from a bodkin arrowhead.

Battle of Towton, AD 1461

It is unusual to find an assemblage of human remains derived from a known battle and therefore securely dated. A total of 37 burials were recently recovered from a mass grave in the village of Towton.[99,100] Twenty-seven of the 29 preserved crania show evidence of weapon injury, sometimes involving as many as 14 separate blows to the head and face.[101] There was evidence of both healed and unhealed injury on these individuals and all three of the main categories of trauma (blunt force, sharp force and projectile) were exhibited.

Trauma due to bladed weapons

Wounds administered to the head took the form of small, superficial incisions or, in one case, a heavy blow from a sword, which had removed the posterior part of the cranium. These may have been delivered by a double-edged sword, such as the Castillon sword, which was commonly used during the 15th century, or by a pommel dagger in the case of some of the stabbing wounds. Sometimes there is a small terminal fracture at the end of the cut, but often it had passed cleanly through the bone and the limits of the injury were obvious. In total, 17 battle casualties had suffered more than 70 blade wounds to the cranium and mandible, four of which show evidence of healing.[101]

Trauma from blunt weapons

The presence of radiating or concentric fractures often indicate a blunt injury which may have been caused by a percussive weapon such as a mace or the handle of a battle-axe. The lesions are either circular in shape or have a branching pattern of radiating fractures from the point of impact (Figure 2a and b). A particularly notable example was a penetrating wound probably caused by one of the spikes of a poleaxe or medieval war hammer (Figure 3a). More than 30 injuries to the skull from blunt weapons were sustained by 19 individuals.[101]

Piercing injuries

Sometimes it is difficult to distinguish between a penetrating injury that has been caused by a projectile and one that has been delivered by the point of a weapon such as a poleaxe or battle-axe. Only one injury can be definitely attributed to piercing by an arrow[101] and there was no evidence of gunshot trauma, although there could have been handguns available for use at Towton. It is thought that the snowstorm at the time of the battle may have inhibited their use by making the ammunition damp.

Healed injuries

The presence of healed wounds to the cranium and mandible suggest that these individuals had been injured in previous battles and survived. The rounded edges of a wound delivered by a sharp-edged weapon are evidence of a healed injury, which may have occurred a long time previously.

The evidence for trauma to the post-cranial skeleton is much more infrequent than it was at the Battle of Wisby in Sweden a century previously.[8] One individual from Towton (Inhumation 30) had severe wounds to both arms, and there were some defence injuries to the hands and minor cut marks on the vertebrae. However, the lower extremities have remained almost entirely unscathed.

FUTURE POTENTIAL

There is much scope for further research in this area, including a review of all the injuries still available for study using modern forensic techniques[87] to make detailed comparisons between different sites and periods. Scanning electron microscopy of blunt force trauma patterns, particularly shear force and crushing injuries would help with the definition of this type of fracture. Experiments are required to test the effects of different types of weapons on the cranium and long bones and also to investigate further the diagenesis of collagen and the time it takes for bone to lose its elasticity under different conditions.

Recently there has been much more collaboration between archaeologists and biological anthropologists in the planning of a cemetery excavation, which is helping to ensure that adequate recording takes place on site. The employment of an osteologist who can train the excavation team in optimum excavation and recovery techniques is important so that any unusual features of the burial can be noted at an early stage. The excavation at Towton in 1996 was unique in that all the participants were trained human osteoarchaeologists and the burials were therefore recovered as individuals from the mass grave.

LIMITATIONS TO THE STUDY

Recognition of trauma patterns depends upon the reconstruction of fragmentary material.[101] Otherwise injuries that have occurred around the time of death may easily be missed. Unfortunately, cranial reconstruction is very time-consuming, particularly the refitting of delicate facial bones, and there is seldom funding available for each skull to be repaired before it is studied. At present, blade injuries are identified much more commonly than blunt or projectile trauma, and it is difficult to ascertain whether this is a true reflection of patterns of injury in the past. Healed weapon injury is also more easily recognizable than an unhealed wound and may be over-represented by comparison.

Detailed recording of weapon injuries is essential and should include diagrams, descriptions and measurements. Reports must indicate the age and sex of the victim, the situation of the wound by skeletal element (not just region of the body) and any indication of the direction of the blow. In the case of injury from a bladed weapon, both acute and obtuse sides of the injury should be described, including patterns of flake removal, bevelling and polishing or chatter marks. Greater attention should be paid to the presence or absence of terminal fractures that may indicate the force of a blow. Where possible, scanning electron microscopy should also be performed. Blunt trauma analysis should include descriptions and measurements of concentric and radiating fractures. Recent studies on two prehistoric mass graves have considerably increased our awareness of this type of trauma.[102,103]

The classification of fracture patterns resulting from both sharp and blunt force trauma should enable biological anthropologists to differentiate between peri-mortem and post-mortem damage in many cases. Excavation damage, often unavoidable with fragile bone, will produce an entirely different fracture pattern from a perimortal weapon injury and the broken edges will be unstained and rectangular. The historical and cultural framework should also be considered[46] and, therefore, interdisciplinary studies are as important as they are in reconstructing activity patterns on the skeleton. Collaboration with specialists in related areas, such as weapons experts and battle re-enactors, is essential if we are to understand not only the injuries themselves, but also the means by which they were inflicted and their consequences for the individual.

ACKNOWLEDGEMENTS

This chapter would not have been possible without the collaborative work of those involved in the Towton project, namely Malin Holst, Tim Sutherland, Jennifer Coughlan, Christopher Knusel and Shannon Novak (who analysed the perimortal trauma on the individuals from the mass grave and taught us how to analyse cranial trauma from the standpoint of the forensic anthropologist), in addition to the valued contributions of the Deputy County Archaeologist of North Yorkshire County Council, Veronica Fiorato, and Andrea Burgess from West Yorkshire Archaeology Service. John Waller, Graham Rimer and Thomas Richardson from the Royal Armouries, Andrew Boardman (a freelance military historian) and Kevin Hicks (a battle re-enactment specialist) are also thanked for their enthusiasm for the project. The author is grateful to Jean Brown and Eric Houlder for their expert photography and to Charlotte Roberts, Christopher Knüsel and Malin Holst for reading and commenting on the manuscript. The comments of both referees were invaluable.

REFERENCES

1   Roberts CA. Forensic anthropology 2: Positive identification of the individual; cause and manner of death. In: Hunter JR, Roberts CA, Martin A (eds), *Studies in Crime: An Introduction to Forensic Archaeology*. London: Batsford, 1996: pp. 122–138.

2   Brothwell D. Forensic aspects of the so-called Neolithic skeleton Q1 from Maiden Castle, Dorset. *World Archaeology* 1971; **3**: 233–241.

3   Gurdjian ES. *Impact Head Injury.* Springfield: Charles C Thomas, 1975.

4   Härke H. Warrior graves? The background of the Anglo-Saxon weapon burial rite. *Past and Present* 1990; **126**: 22–43.

5   Manchester K, Elmhirst OEC. Forensic aspects of an Anglo-Saxon injury. *Ossa* 1980; **7**: 179–188.

6   Knowles AK. Acute traumatic lesions. In: Hart G (ed.), *Disease in Ancient Man*. Toronto: Charles Irwin, 1983: pp. 61–83.

7   Berryman HE, Symes SA. Recognizing gunshot and blunt cranial trauma through fracture interpretation. In: Reichs KJ (ed.), *Forensic Osteology* (2nd edn). Springfield: Charles C Thomas, 1998: pp. 333–352.

8   Ingelmark BG. The skeletons. In: Thordeman B (ed.), *Armour from the Battle of Wisby 1361*. Stockholm: Vitterhets Historie Och Antikvitets Akademien, 1939: pp. 149–210.

9   Keegan J. *The Face of Battle: A Study of Agincourt, Waterloo and the Somme*. London: Pimlico, 1976.

10   Blair C. *Pollard's History of Firearms*. Feltham: Country Life, 1983.

11   Spitz WU, Fisher, RS. *Medicolegal Investigation of Death*. Springfield: Charles C Thomas, 1980.

12   Novak S, personal communication.

13   Brothwell D. *Digging Up Bones*. London: British Museum (Natural History), 1963.

14   Ortner DJ, Putschar WGJ. *Identification of Pathological Conditions in Human Skeletal Remains*. Washington, DC: Smithsonian Institution Press, 1981.

15   Merbs C. Trauma. In: Iscan MY, Kennedy KAR (eds), *Reconstruction of Life from the Skeleton*. Springfield: Charles C Thomas, 1989: pp. 161–189.

16   Courville CB. Cranial injuries in prehistoric man. In: Brothwell D, Sandison AT (eds), *Diseases in Antiquity: A Survey of the Diseases, Injuries and Surgery of Early Populations*. Springfield: Charles C Thomas, 1967: pp. 606–622.

17   Courville CB. Split fractures of the skull produced by edged weapons and their accompanying brain wounds. *Bulletin of the Los Angeles Neurological Society* 1964; **29**: 32–39.

18   Courville CB. War wounds of the cranium in the battle of Wisby. *Bulletin of the Los Angeles Neurological Society* 1965; **30**: 27–44.

19   White, T. *Prehistoric Cannibalism at Mancos 5MTUMR–2346*. Princeton: Princeton University Press, 1992.

20   Wells C. Pseudopathology. In: Brothwell D and Sandison AT (eds), *Diseases in Antiquity: A Survey of the Diseases, Injuries and Surgery of Early Populations*. Springfield: Charles C. Thomas, 1967: pp. 5–19.

21   Buikstra J, Ubelaker DE (eds), *Standards for Data Collection in Human Skeletal Remains*. Arkansas Archaeological Survey Research Series 44. Fayetteville Archaeological Survey, 1994.

22   Sauer NJ. The timing of injuries and manner of death: distinguishing among antemortem, perimortem and postmortem trauma. In: Reichs KJ (ed.), *Forensic Osteology* (2nd edn). Springfield: Charles C Thomas, 1998: pp. 321–332.

23   Maples WR. Trauma analysis by the forensic anthropologist. In: Reichs, KJ (ed.), *Forensic Osteology: Advances in the Identification of Human Remains*. Springfield: Charles C Thomas, 1986: pp. 218–228.

24   Gurdjian ES, Webster JE, Lissner HR. The mechanism of skull fracture. *Journal of Neurosurgery* 1950; **7**: 106–14.

25   Wenham S. Anatomical and microscopic interpretations of ancient weapon injuries. Unpublished BSc dissertation, University of Leicester, 1987.

26   Stroud G, Kemp RL. *Cemeteries of the Church and Priory of St Andrew, Fishergate*. The Archaeology of York, 12: The medieval cemeteries, vol. 2. York: Council for British Archaeology, 1993.

27   Manchester K. *The Archaeology of Disease*. Bradford: University Press, 1983.

28   Berryman HE, Haun SJ. Applying forensic techniques to interpret cranial fracture patterns in an archaeological specimen. *International Journal of Osteoarchaeology* 1996; **6**: 2–9.

29   Knight B. *Forensic Pathology*. New York: Oxford University Press, 1991.

30   King S. Violence and death during the fall of the Roman Empire: interpretations of a late 4th century/early 5th century AD charnel deposit from Arras, France. Unpublished MSc dissertation, University of Bradford, 1992.

31   Burkhardt L. *Pathologische Anatomie des Schadels*. Handbuch der speziellen pathologischen Anatomie und Histologie 9(7). Berlin: Springer, 1970.

32   Bergeron RT, Rumbaugh CL. Skull trauma. In: Newton, TH, Potts, DG (eds), *Radiology of the Skull and Brain: The Skull*, vol. 1. St Louis: Mosby, 1971: pp. 763–818.

33   Polson CJ, Gee DJ, Knight B. *The Essentials of Forensic Medicine*. Oxford: Pergamon, 1985.

34   Dimaio VJM. *Gunshot Wounds: Practical Aspects of Firearms, Ballistics and Forensic Techniques*. Boca Raton: CRC Press, 1983.

35   Kaufman MH, Whitaker D, McTavish J. Differential diagnosis of holes in the calvarium: application of modern clinical data to palaeopathology. *Journal of Archaeological Science* 1997; **24**: 193–218.

36   Sledzik, P., Barbian, L. Healing following cranial trauma. Presentation at the annual meeting of the Paleopathology Association, St Louis, Missouri, 1–2 April 1997 (unpublished).

37 Campillo D. Healing of the skull bone after injury. *Journal of Paleopathology* 1991; **3**: 137–149.

38 Walker PL. Wife beating, boxing and broken noses. In: Martin DL, Frayer DW (eds), *Troubled Times: Violence and Warfare in The Past*. Amsterdam: Gordon & Breach, 1997: pp. 145–179.

39 Anderson S. *The Human Remains from Staunch Meadow, Brandon, Suffolk*. English Heritage Ancient Monuments Laboratory Report 99/90, 1990.

40 Anderson S. *The Human Remains from Caister-On-Sea, Norfolk*. English Heritage Ancient Monuments Laboratory Report 9/91, 1991.

41 Waldron T. *The Human Remains from Great Chesterford, Cambridgeshire*. English Heritage Ancient Monuments Laboratory Report 89/88, 1988.

42 Mays S. *The Medieval Burials from the Blackfriars Friary, School Street, Ipswich, Suffolk (Excavated 1983–85)*. English Heritage Ancient Monuments Laboratory Report 16/91, 1991.

43 Stirland A. Patterns of trauma in a unique medieval parish cemetery. *International Journal of Osteoarchaeology* 1996; **6**: 92–100.

44 Lee F. The pathological report on selected skeletons from the Anglo-Saxon levels at York Minster. Unpublished bone report, University of Bradford, 1988.

45 Wells C. The human burials. In: McWhirr A, Viner L, Wells C (eds), *Romano-British Cemeteries at Cirencester. Vol. 2. Cirencester excavations*. Cirencester: Corinium Museum, 1981: pp. 135–202.

46 Larsen CS. *Bioarchaeology: Interpreting Behaviour from the Human Skeleton*. Cambridge: Cambridge University Press, 1997.

47 Ubelaker DH, Adams BJ. Differentiation of perimortem and postmortem trauma using taphonomic indicators. *Journal of Forensic Sciences* 1995; **40**: 509–512.

48 Bowman JE, MacLaughlin SM, Scheuer JL. Burial of an early 19th century suicide in the crypt of St Bride's Church, Fleet Street. *International Journal of Osteoarchaeology* 1992; **2**: 91–94.

49 Cox M, Molleson T, Waldron T. Preconceptions and perceptions: the lessons of a 19th century suicide. *Journal of Archaeological Science* 1992; **17**: 573–581.

50 King S. The human skeletal remains from Glasgow Cathedral excavations 1992–93. Unpublished bone report, 1994.

51 Brothwell DR. The palaeopathology of early British man. *Journal of the Royal Anthropological Institute of Great Britain and Ireland* 1961; **91**: 318–344.

52 Wells C. *Bones, Bodies and Disease*. London: Thames and Hudson, 1964.

53 Evans JG, Atkinson RJC, O'Connor T, Green HS. Stonehenge – the environment in the late Neolithic and Early Bronze Age and a Beaker-age burial. *Wiltshire Archaeological and Natural History Magazine* 1984; **78**: 7–30.

54 Brothwell DR. The Bronze Age people of Yorkshire: a general survey. *The Advancement of Science* 1960: 311–322.

55 Dent JS. Weapons, wounds and war in the Iron Age. *Archaeological Journal* 1983; **140**: 120–128.

56 Stead IM. *The Arras Culture*. York: Yorkshire Philosophical Society, 1979.

57 Brewster, TCM. *The Excavation of Garton and Wetwang Slacks*. Prehistoric Excavation Reports 2. Wintringham: East Riding Archaeological Research Committee, 1980.

58 Whimster R. *Burial practices in Iron Age Britain: A Discussion and Gazetteer of the Evidence c.700 B.C.–A.D.43*. British Series 90. Oxford: British Archaeological Reports, 1981.

59 Dent JS. Cemeteries and settlement patterns of the Iron Age on the Yorkshire Wolds. *Proceedings of the Prehistoric Society* 1982; **48**: 437–457.

60 Hooper B. Anatomical considerations. In: Cunliffe B (ed.), *Danebury: An Iron Age Hillfort in Hampshire*, vol. **2**: *The Excavations, 1967–1978: The Finds*. Research Report 52. London: Council for British Archaeology, 1984: pp. 463–474.

61 Cave AJE. Report on human remains from Snell's Corner, Horndean, Hants. *Proceedings of the Hampshire Field Club and Archaeology Society* 1955; **178**: 148–170.

62 Matthews CL. A Romano-British inhumation cemetery at Dunstable, Bedfordshire. *The Archaeological Journal* 1981; **15**: 1–73.

63 Cox M. *The Human Bones from Ancaster*. English Heritage Ancient Monuments Laboratory Report 93/89, 1989.

64 McKinley JI. A decapitation from the Romano-British cemetery at Baldock, Hertfordshire. *International Journal of Osteoarchaeology* 1993; **3**: 41–44.

65 Farwell D, Molleson T. *Poundbury*, vol. **2**: *The Cemeteries*. Monograph series 11. Dorchester: Dorset Natural History and Archaeological Society, 1993.

66 Warwick R. The skeletal remains. In: Wenham LP. *The Romano-British Cemetery at Trentholme Drive, York*. London: HMSO, 1968: pp. 113–176.

67 McKinley JI. A skull wound and possible trepanation from a Roman cemetery at Baldock Hertfordshire. *International Journal of Osteoarchaeology* 1992; **2**: 337–340.

68 Harman M, Molleson TI, Price JL. Burials, bodies and beheadings in Romano-British and Anglo-Saxon cemeteries. *Bulletin of the British Museum (Natural History). Geology* 1981; **35**: 145–188.

69 Clarke G. *The Roman Cemetery at Lankhills*. Oxford: Clarendon, 1979.

70 Philpott R. *Burial Practices In Roman Britain: A Survey of Grave Treatment and Furnishing A.D. 43–410*. British Archaeological Reports British Series 219. Oxford: Tempus Reparatum, 1991.

71 Penn WS. Archaeological excavations at Springhead. *Archaeologia Cantiana* 1960; **74**: 113–140.

72 Boylston A. Report on the analysis of two infant burials from Bishop Grosseteste College, Lincoln (BGB95). Unpublished bone report, University of Bradford, 1997.

73 Boylston AE, Roberts CA, Knüsel CJ, Dawson M. Investigation of a Romano-British rural ritual in Bedford, England. *Journal of Archaeological Science* (in press).

74 Mays S, Steele J. A mutilated human skull from Roman St Albans, Herts, England. *Antiquity* 1996; **70**: 155–160.

75 Anderson T. Cranial weapon injuries from Anglo-Saxon Dover. *International Journal of Osteoarchaeology* 1996; **6**: 10–14.

76 Wells C, Cayton H. The human bones. In: Wade-Martins P. *Excavations at North Elmham Park 1967–1992*. East Anglian Archaeology Report 9, 1980: pp. 247–374.

77 Anderson S, Birkett D. *The Human Skeletal Remains from Burgh Castle, Norfolk*. English Heritage Ancient Monuments Laboratory Report 27/89, 1989.

78 Hawkes SC (ed.), *Weapons and Warfare in Anglo-Saxon England*. Monograph 21(7). Oxford: Oxford University Committee for Archaeology, 1989.

79 Boylston A. Human skeletal remains. In: Adams M (ed.), Excavation of a preconquest cemetery at Addingham, West Yorkshire. *Medieval Archaeology* 1996; **44**: 151–191.

80 Langston J. Analysis of human skeletal material. In: Hall RA, Whyman M. Settlement and monasticism at Ripon, North Yorkshire, from the 7th to 11th centuries AD. *Medieval Archaeology* 1996: **44**; 93–99.

81 Harman M. The human remains. In: Boyle A, Jennings, D, Miles D, Palmer S. *The Anglo-Saxon Cemetery at Butler's Field, Lechlade, Gloucestershire*. Thames Valley Landscapes Monograph 10. Oxford: Oxford University Committee for Archaeology, 1998: pp. 43–52.

82 Duhig C. The Anglo-Saxon skeletal remains. In: Malim T, Hines J (eds), *The Anglo-Saxon cemetery at Edix Hill (Barrington A), Cambridgeshire: Excavations 1989–1991*. Research Report 112. London: Council for British Archaeology, 1998; pp. 154–199.

83 Wenham S. Anatomical interpretations of Anglo-Saxon weapon injuries. In: Hawkes S (ed.), *Weapons and Warfare in Anglo-Saxon England*. Oxford: Oxford University Committee for Archaeology Monograph 1989; **21**: 123–139.

84 Detsicas A. Excavations at Eccles, 1972. *Archaeologia Cantiana*, 1973; **88**: 119–134.

85 Wells C. The human skeleton from Cox Lane, Ipswich. *Proceedings of the Suffolk Institute of Archaeology* 1963; **29**: 329–333.

86 Morant GM, Goodman CN. Human bones. In: Wheeler REM (ed.), *Maiden Castle, Dorset*. Reports of the Research Committee of the Society of Antiquaries of London, 17. London: Society of Antiquaries of London, 1943: pp. 337–360.

87   McKinnon G. 'Where Swords Seek to Shatter . . .: a study of deliberate trauma in the medieval cemeteries of St Andrew, Fishergate. Unpublished MSc dissertation, University of Bradford, 1998.

88   Lilley JM, Stroud G, Brothwell DR, Williamson MH. *The Jewish Burial Ground at Jewbury.* The Archaeology of York: the medieval cemeteries. Vol. 12/3. York: Council for British Archaeology, 1994.

89   Stuart-Macadam P. Health and disease in the monks of Stratford Langthorne Abbey. *Essex Journal* 1986; **21**: 67–71.

90   Dawes JD, Magilton JR. *The Cemetery of St Helen-on-the-Walls, Aldwark.* The Archaeology of York: the medieval cemeteries. Vol. 12/1. London: Council for British Archaeology, 1980.

91   West BA. Human bones. In: Ward SW (ed.), *Excavations at Chester: The Lesser Medieval Religious Houses. Sites Investigated 1964–1983.* Grosvenor Museum Archaeological Excavation and Survey Reports 6. Chester: Chester City Council, Department of Leisure Services, 1990: pp. 127–137.

92   Bayley J. *Chelmsford Dominican Priory: Human Bone Report.* English Heritage Ancient Monuments Laboratory Report 1890, 1975.

93   Brown S. Report on the human bone. In: Wise P (ed.), *The Archaeology of Hulton Abbey – A Century of Excavation.* Staffordshire Archaeological Studies, Vol. 2. Stoke-on-Trent: City Museum and Art Gallery, 1985: pp. 7–19.

94   White W. *The Cemetery of St Nicholas Shambles.* London: Museum of London and Middlesex Archaeology Society, 1988.

95   Eley J, Bailey J. *Stonar, Kent: Human Bone Report.* English Heritage Ancient Monuments Laboratory Report No. 1903, 1975.

96   Cardy A. The human bones. In: Hill P (ed.), *Whithorn and St Ninian: The Excavation of a Monastic Town 1984–91.* Stroud: Sutton, 1997: pp. 519–562.

97   Boylston A, Roberts C. *Lincoln Excavations 1972–87: Report on the Human Skeletal Remains.* English Heritage Ancient Monuments Laboratory Report 13/97, 1997.

98   Quinn S, personal communication.

99   Boylston A, Holst M, Coughlan J, Novak S, Sutherland T, Knusel C. Recent excavations of a mass grave from Towton. *Yorkshire Medicine* 1997; **9**: 25–26.

100 Boylston A, Novak S, Sutherland T, Holst M, Coughlan, J. Burials from the battle of Towton. *Royal Armouries Yearbook*, 1997; **2**: 36–39.

101 Novak, S. Battle related trauma. In: *The Battle of Towton: Archaeology of Mediaeval Warfare* (forthcoming).

102 Wahl J, König HG. Anthropologische-traumatologische Untersuchung der menschlichen Skelettreste aus dem bandkeramischen Massengrab bei Talheim, Kreis Heilbronn. *Fundberichte aus Baden-Württemberg* 1987; **12**: 65–193.

103 Frayer, DW. Ofnet: evidence for a Mesolithic massacre. In: Martin DL, Frayer, DW (eds), *Troubled Times: Violence and Warfare in the Past.* Amsterdam: Gordon & Breach, 1997.

23

BONE ADAPTATION AND ITS RELATIONSHIP TO PHYSICAL ACTIVITY IN THE PAST

Christopher Knüsel

INTRODUCTION

The past 30 years have observed a revived interest in the identification of occupational specialists from skeletal remains. The functional understanding of skeletal anatomy required to undertake such studies, however, is not part of most archaeology and anthropology courses. It is a subject left largely uncovered in skeletal biology textbooks. This apparent silence disguises a growing body of research that has the potential to contribute much to our understanding of human lifeways in the distant, and more recent, past. This potential, though, has been tempered by both methodological and theoretical problems. At a conference in 1988, Stirland presented a paper entitled 'Diagnosis of occupationally related paleopathology: can it be done?' and concluded that 'In an archaeological sample, it will never be possible to extrapolate from the general to the particular and assign an individual's occupation from a group study' (p. 46).[1] Stirland's presentation, and the published discussion that followed it, suggested that the determination of occupation from skeletal remains, if it could be accomplished, would require further group comparisons and radiological studies of modern individuals of known occupation. It was also made clear that group comparisons require some contextual evidence to provide clues as to what sorts of occupations might be expected among specific human populations.

A year later, Kennedy published a review article on 'Skeletal markers of occupational stress', an annotated compendium of bony changes linked to posture and activity which continues to hold pride of place among the citations of more recent studies.[2] From early on, this type of research seems to have generated differing opinions as to its relevance from both sides of the Atlantic. One reviewer commented upon the great length of Kennedy's contribution to *Reconstruction of Life from the Skeleton*, noting that the publishers devoted a 16-page table and 32 pages of the book to an 'anecdotal' and minor aspect of skeletal biology.[3] A second reviewer noted the need for more photographs clearly depicting the traits discussed in Kennedy's contribution.[4] These responses highlight areas that continue to plague more recent studies. The first relates to the situation of such studies within anthropology and archaeology, and the second relates to the replicability of such studies, the methods employed in the analysis of the traits, and the format of their dissemination to the wider intellectual community. An *Atlas of Occupational Markers on Human Remains*, recently published by Capasso et al.,[5] provides good photographs and descriptions of some traits, yet as these researchers note the aetiology of them remains poorly understood. They note that 'a specific modification … may not be attributable to a single activity pattern, but rather a wide range of habitual behaviours. Thus, a proper diagnosis may be limited to stating that an individual had engaged in strenuous labour …' (p. 5).[5]

Other researchers are less sanguine. In 1992 Dutour published a problem-oriented critique of such studies, in which he questioned the specificity of individual skeletal markers, noting similarities between those of activity and other conditions.[6] He also highlighted analytical problems, such as those which arise from differences in the manner in which the same activities were performed among people in the past and by modern practitioners, the lack of modern clinical evidence linking a particular activity with a particular skeletal marker, and the sheer lack of analogues caused by a particular activity being present in the past but absent today. More recently, even the possibility that one could determine occupation from skeletal remains has been denied. Waldron writes that he 'could wish that the hope of being able to determine the occupation of a person long dead from his (or her) skeleton will finally be extinguished … it is very easy to show that the probability of being able to do is so remote that the only sensible thing to do is to abandon hope altogether' (p. 22).[7]

Waldron's criticism and cynicism are not without justification. Studies directed at identifying occupational specialists can be criticized for their loosely drawn analogies, their lack of precision in the application of osseous criteria for the identification of specific specialists (the redundancy of osseous response) and their lack of functional morphological understanding. They can also be criticized for their over-reliance on archaeological context in order to support a particular assessment when others are equally possible and, perhaps most importantly, the lack of documented out-groups of sufficient size with which to compare unknown skeletal material. In addition, one might add that both pronouncements for, and against, the utility and possibility of identifying occupations, suffer from an underdeveloped awareness of the place of such studies within interpretations of past peoples and their societies. Whatever the impetus for such studies, in order for them to be placed on a firmer empirical footing they must move away from a typological identification to one based on the mechanical functions of bones.

SKELETAL ADAPTATION IN RESPONSE TO ACTIVITY

The study of activity-related change in human remains cannot be divorced from biometrical considerations, which provide the basis for understanding population variation. It is against the backdrop of variation that one identifies osseous adaptation to activity. Adaptation is defined as any change that allows an organism to cope better with its environment; adaptations can be morphological, genetic, and behavioural. Biometrical studies were developed in an atmosphere of typology in the 19th century, a perspective which seems to have over-ridden observations made toward the end of that century concerning bone morphology and its malleability during growth and development. Subsequently, biometrical data have been used with increasing frequency to characterize not only biological variation, but also functional differences among human populations. Recent studies emphasize not only the innate or genetic component of physical make-up, but also the importance of bone plasticity in understanding morphology.

By the 1930s many of our modern understandings of bone behaviour were already in place, e.g. that bone responds to mechanical stress, and that this response is greatest under cyclic loading (i.e. when bone is rapidly stressed and unstressed, as in movement).[8] Bone deforms, or changes its dimensions, when it is loaded. The amount bone deforms before fracture relates to its strength (the load at failure) and is governed by its stiffness or rigidity (the load required to deform it by a given amount). The extent to which bone recovers its original shape and dimensions after loading is referred to as 'elasticity'. When the load reaches a critical point, the outermost fibres yield and a certain amount of deformation is retained even after the load is removed. This is referred to as 'plastic' change. Plasticity relates to the 'the capability of being moulded',[9] i.e. the malleability of organ systems in response to environmental stimuli, among which one can count climate, topography, diet and physical activity. Therefore, in modern use, plasticity refers to specific adaptations made during growth and development that are irreversible and not inherited;[10] they are thus part of the phenotype, where the phenotype is defined as an expression of the genotype in a particular environment.[11]

The musculature has an essential and fundamental role in the development and alteration of bone in that it contributes to the element's strain (i.e. load), the response within bone to an externally applied stressor that causes force to be transmitted through it. Bone is said to be anisotropic because it responds differently when loaded from different directions; like wood, it has a grain.[12] Bone is thus best understood as a living, dynamic and plastic material that forms (models) during growth and reforms (remodels) during development in response to activity.[13,14] Bone is relatively flexible and tough in that it resists crack propagation, but weak when compared with other materials. Mechanically it is closest to oak wood, which is as flexible but somewhat less strong than bone.[15,16]

Recent research has further substantiated and clarified the relationship between bone morphology and activity. Bone changes in response to the magnitude of the force exerted upon it (i.e. the load) and the frequency and direction of loading. Repetitive, strenuous movements elicit bone formation.[17–19] Increased mechanical loading inhibits remodelling (cellular turnover) while promoting modelling (growth), especially of the periosteal surface. This process produces a net increase in bone dimensions (hypertrophy) which better accommodate greater loads. Thus, larger bones with a greater cross-sectional area, more cortical bone and reduced medullary canal are reflections of increased load bearing. Net bone loss is stimulated by a reduction in loading or a disruption to normal bone metabolism that elicits endosteal and intracortical remodelling but inhibits periosteal modelling (i.e. growth or size increase). The result is a less robust bone with reduced cross-sectional area, less cortical bone and a proportionally enlarged medullary canal. The strain threshold for bone formation may be lower if the manner of loading (i.e. its direction) is different from the pattern experienced more commonly.[20] Abnormal strain distributions, such as those encountered in strenuous exercise, elicit adaptive bone response that has a disproportionate effect on bone morphology. Essentially, these relationships maintain the body's integrity throughout the lifetime of the individual.[21]

Differing responses of adult and juvenile bone demonstrate that the greatest impact on bone morphology is made before physiological maturity when the bones discontinue growth but continue to remodel at a reduced rate.[22–24] This difference appears to be a consequence of the increased plasticity of children's bones as compared with those of adults.[25] The process commences *in utero* from 7 weeks when ligaments, tendons and muscles begin to influence the newly developed bone.[26,27] From work to date, it is clear that the diameters of the long bones are most influenced by activity, and this proclivity is most developed before skeletal maturity. Ruff *et al.* demonstrate that long bone articular surfaces possess a reduced ability to adjust their dimensions to activity after skeletal maturity is attained.[28] Articular dimensions and long bone lengths follow a similar growth pattern that distinguishes them from the more slowly developing cross-sectional diaphyseal dimensions.[29] This means that diaphyseal diameters and cross-sectional areas are susceptible to activity-related growth for a longer period and are thus best for capturing activity-related alterations. Strenuous activities that commence early in the lifetime of the individual will present the greatest osseous response. Asymmetrical changes in articular dimensions in adults are the product of reduced activity before physiological maturity (Figure 1). Thus, limb disability in juveniles will be reflected in both diaphyseal and articular dimensions; whereas, disabilities occurring in adulthood will more greatly affect diaphyseal measurements, sparing the articular processes (i.e. joint surfaces). External bone dimensions, as well as subperiosteal

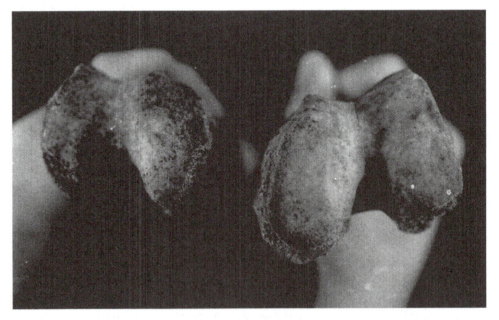

Figure 1 – Femoral condyles of BSG 1423, a medieval priest from the chapel associated with the hospital site at Brough, North Yorkshire, who suffered a slipped proximal femoral epiphysis of his right limb in adolescence.[119] The disparity in size of these paired elements attests to this being an injury sustained before physiological maturity and reduced weight-bearing of the affected, right side.

area, increase with age while cortical area decreases with age,[30,31] especially if exercise is not maintained.[24] Therefore, age-at-death profiles of samples for comparison should be considered when interpreting bone dimensions.

In summary: activity-related changes can be identified through a range of alterations in surface morphology, hypertrophy or atrophy of enthesial development and bone dimensions; asymmetry of homologous structures as reflected in cross-sectional cortical area and medullary canal dimensions; alterations in bone density, mineral content and shape, such that elements are best able to withstand the applied stress of repeated movement.

REMODELLING IN THE POST-CRANIAL SKELETON

Although exercise appears to influence bone density throughout the body in active individuals,[32] elements that are repeatedly used in a strenuous manner demonstrate increased skeletal hypertrophy (size increase). Among the cases of skeletal hypertrophy found in archaeological remains are those found in the upper limbs of a group of individuals thought to have been archers aboard Henry VIII's flagship, the *Mary Rose* (AD 1545). Stirland noted asymmetrical increase in bone dimensions of the left shoulder (greater tubercle of the humerus) when compared with near-contemporaries from the medieval church of St Margaret *in combusto*, Norwich.[33] The *Mary Rose* individuals thus demonstrated a reduced humeral asymmetry due to larger dimensions of the left arm. Stirland attributed the increased hypertrophy of the left arms and reduced asymmetry to a more equal use of the limbs as one might expect to encounter in the performance of archery. Bridges has noted a similar reduction in asymmetry in the arms in a sample of bow-using Mississippian (about 14–15th century AD) males that distinguishes them from the preceding Archaic period males who possess greater asymmetry from atlatl (throwing stick) use.[34]

The complex shape and the number of adhering muscles and ligaments make the pelvic girdle a difficult entity to study from a functional perspective. In one study, however, Roberts noted a hypertrophic alteration, an expansion of cortical bone, between the attachments for the reflected head of *M. rectus femoris* and *M. gluteus minimus*. These were noted in one middle and two older adult female skeletons, dating from the Iron Age/Early Romano-British (1st century BC to 1st century AD) and Anglo-Saxon (6th century AD) periods, respectively.[35] Rader and Peters[36] describe a similar thickening of bone in a robust male, from the King site, north-west Georgia. These researchers noted that this thickening is similar to the large acetabulo-cristal buttress of *os coxae* KMN-ER 3228 and OH24, from east Africa,[37,38] which are from early representatives of the genus *Homo*.[39] Since the muscles in the vicinity of this bony buttress are involved in abduction and medial rotation and flexion of the thigh, as well as in stabilizing the hip joint during the swing phase in walking (i.e. when one foot is unsupported by the ground), exaggerations of these movements may be implied. All of these individuals' femora are platymeric (flattened antero-posteriorly in the subtrochanteric area) which may indicate an alteration or exaggeration of the medio-lateral loading pattern, which is highest in this region.[31] The frequency and causes of this anomaly remain to be clarified.

GEOMETRICAL STUDIES OF LONG BONES

Perhaps the greatest insights into activity variants in the past have come from cross-sectional analysis of long bones. Biomechanical studies of limb bones indicate that many features of the infra-cranium of earlier hominids were influenced by plastic (i.e. non-genetic) changes in response to strenuous physical activity commenced before physiological maturity.[28,40–43] The general decrease in bone robusticity through time is thought to result from a reduction in activity levels, perhaps as a consequence of social and cultural innovations.

Neanderthals have increased humeral cortical area, especially in the medio-lateral plane, when compared with early anatomically modern individuals. Ben-Itzhak *et al.* suggest these individuals were engaging in strenuous medio-lateral arm movements to an extent not seen in more recent groups.[44] More recently, though, Trinkaus *et al.* have associated pronounced bilateral asymmetry present in Neanderthals (24–57%)[41] with activity-related morphological change that is of a magnitude similar to that found in professional tennis players (28–57%).[45] This is more than double the amount found in modern Euroamericans, prehistoric and early historic Amerindians, and prehistoric Japanese. This study revealed a right-sided dominance in the Neanderthal sample, a finding that agrees with studies of a preponderance of right-handed stone tools found in Pleistocene contexts[46] and from studies of scratches on the labial surfaces of anterior teeth of Neanderthals. These scratches have been associated with paramasticatory (e.g. non-dietary) behaviours, the majority involving the right hand.[47,48]

Analyses of the lower limbs are frequently used as a measure of mobility among human populations in the past. Ruff *et al.* have argued that a general reduction in cortical thickness occurs through time among hominid populations as a response to a reduction in strenuous activity and decreased mobility.[43] However, this trend can be reversed to some extent in individual populations. Increased cross-sectional cortical area can also result from increased body mass.[49] It can also occur as a consequence of a transition from a hunting and gathering subsistence base to one based on agricultural production,[50–52] or to one based on mission life.[53] However, in their study of the transition from hunting and gathering to agriculture on the Georgia coast, Ruff *et al.* found that a decrease in geometric femoral dimensions occurred, which suggests that increased cortical dimensions should not be taken as a general rule for all similar transitions.[51] Bridges also noted that males and females were differentially affected in this transition; females among the agricultural sample showed increased strength of their upper limbs bilaterally, while males showed increased lower limb strength.[50] Both of these changes were considered to have resulted from increased activity, those of the females relating to the use of the upper limbs in corn grinding. These results suggest that in some places the transition to agriculture and to mission life was more physically demanding than hunting and gathering and, moreover, that these transitions were not made because these subsistence regimes were easier or more 'civilized'.

Bilateral asymmetry of limb bones can also be used to study the effects of injury on limb bone dimensions and to assess the extent of limb use in such cases. Among these applications is Lazenby and Pfeiffer's study of the executed criminal, Marion ('Madie') 'Peg Leg' Brown, a below-the-knee amputee from the latter half of the 19th century, whose femora show considerable asymmetry due to hypertrophy of the right in compensation for the incapacity of the left.[54] Similar analyses can reveal disability in specimens with less obvious manifestations. Churchill and Formicola assessed the limb function of the Barma Grande 2 fossil remains of an Upper Palaeolithic male from Liguria, Italy.[55] This individual possesses a level of humeral asymmetry that is in excess of that noted for other Middle and Upper Palaeolithic specimens. The percent cortical area asymmetry of the mid-distal (35% of the length measured from the distal end) and mid-proximal humeri (65% from the distal end) is roughly two times (68.4%) and four times (83.5%) greater than those of the next highest means for the late Upper Palaeolithic (29.2%) and Neanderthal (21.3%) samples, respectively. Although there are no visible signs of pathology, this degree of asymmetry would suggest an entrapment neuropathy of the left shoulder nerves or direct trauma that caused paralysis of the shoulder musculature.[55]

ENTHESIAL ACTIVITY-RELATED CHANGE AND NON-METRIC TRAITS

Common activity-related changes are found in modifications to tendonous and ligamentous attachments (entheses) from increased development of muscles (hypertrophy) as they are continuously recruited in the performance of a task.[56,57] Entheses are of two types: those that result in bone deposition and are represented by crests or spicules of bone, and those that are sulcus-like excavations in cortical bone (Figures 2 and 3). Recent studies of enthesopathies, also called musculoskeletal markers of stress, enthesophytes (ossified entheses), and cortical defects, indicate that their appearance and frequency are age-related.[58–60]

Shaibani *et al.*, in their study of the autopsy-derived Todd collection, found that enthesophytes (bone spicules at ligamentous and tendinous attachments) increased with age in

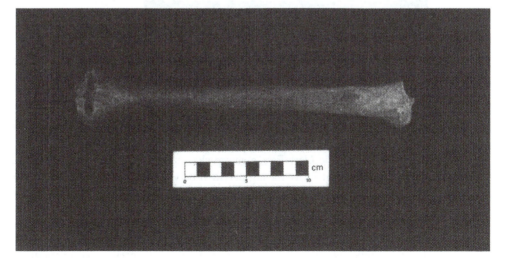

Figure 2 – Cortical defect in the vicinity of the attachment of *M. pectoralis major* of the right humerus of an adolescent (an archaeological specimen).

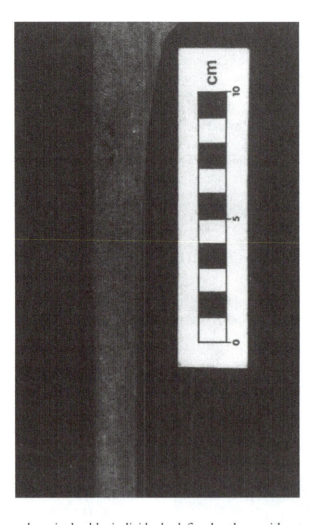

Figure 3 – Close-up of the cortical defect seen in Figure 2 (an archaeological specimen).

otherwise healthy individuals, defined as those without clinical signs of arthritic conditions. Most enthesophytes occurring before the age of 60 were noted in healthy individuals. Of those noted, 18% were at the iliac crests, 13% were of plantar fascia attachment on the anterior and inferior portion of the calcaneal tuberosity, 45% at the calcaneal tuberosity, the site of attachment for the Achilles tendon, and 25% at the attachment of the patellar ligament.[61] Stirland noted a high frequency of vertebral ostephytes (a type of enthesopathy) in the individuals from the *Mary Rose*, a group characterized by their relatively youthful age-at-death profile, the majority having perished between 15 and 25 years, but who performed strenuous activities.[62] Age distributions of the samples, therefore, must be considered for these manifestations as much as in cross-sectional studies of long bone cortical thickness and osteoarthritis (see below).

Further studies of musculo-skeletal stress (entheseal) markers have sought to standardize the scoring and description of such features. For the most part these studies concentrate on the pectoral girdle and upper appendages to provide insights into the sexual division of labour and to monitor activity variation across socio-economic transitions. Hawkey and Merbs present such a study on Thule (Inuits of Hudson Bay) populations, about AD 1000 to present, a period which saw major changes in population density, settlement pattern and subsistence activities.[63] McGhee postulates that these shifts resulted from the ravages of disease rather than environmental change, as previously argued.[64] Munson Chapman recently conducted a similar study of male and female inhabitants of Pecos Pueblo, New Mexico. These populations span the period from AD 1200 to 1838 and include the period of Spanish contact beginning in 1598.[65] Lai and Lovell apply similar muscle markings in other parts of the body, as well as the pectoral girdle and upper limbs in an analysis of a group of fur trader *voyageurs*.[66]

In their study, Hawkey and Merbs note that male activity patterns appear to increase through time, perhaps due to the elevated importance of caribou hunting.[63] This activity relied on the use of kayaks and thrusting spears, which are argued to produce alterations to the attachment site of the costoclavicular ligament on the inferior surface of the sternal end of the clavicle and rugose attachments for *M. pectoralis major* and *M. teres major* at their attachments on the anterior surface of the proximal humerus. Several features allowed the authors to identify the use of *umiaks* (circular rowing boats) among females where none were recorded at contact. A lack of alterations associated with bow use indicates that these were not employed, probably due to the inefficiency of this method for caribou hunting.

Munson Chapman finds significant change in strenuous activities; especially those linked with the processing of maize by both males and females and burden carrying by males among the inhabitants of Pecos Pueblo after contact with the Spanish. Conversely, she notes no statistically significant changes in the flexors and extensors of the wrist and hands to support the suspected increased importance of weaving among males after Spanish contact.[65]

Lai and Lovell offer evidence of strenuous lifestyles among four fur traders, three Métis (people of mixed Native American and European ancestry) and one European. These include Schmorl's nodes (lesions formed during compression of the vertebral column), and hypertrophic enthesial changes associated with the *linea aspera* and similar changes to the gluteal muscles, *M. gastrocnemius*, and *M. soleus* of the lower limbs and to *M. latissimus dorsi, M. deltoideus, M. pectoralis major,* and *M. teres major* of the pectoral girdle and upper limbs as well as similar alterations to the manual flexors in the phalanges and the supinator and pronator crests of the forearm. In addition, they note accessory articular facets on the dorsal surfaces of the metatarsals and pedal phalanges, which may relate to hyperdorsiflexion of the toes during kneeling in a canoe over many hours, as has been historically documented for those involved in the fur trade.[65]

Molleson identifies similar lesions of the first metatarsal in the remains of both younger and older individuals of both sexes from the Epipalaeolithic and Neolithic site of Abu Hureyra in northern Syria. These lesions are accompanied by osteoarthritic changes in the lower segments of the vertebral column and of the knee, well-developed bilateral deltoid tuberosities of the humeri and radial tuberosities of the radii, and a buttress of bone in the popliteal space of the femur. Together they indicate hyperdorsiflexion of the toes, strong flexion of the knees, as well as the heavy use of the upper limbs requiring abduction of the arm and flexion of the forearm. Molleson associates this pattern with the prolonged use of saddle querns for grain preparation. Since some of these remains derive from Epipalaeolithic contexts, this evidence may suggest that grain was being gathered and prepared before its domestic cultivation.[67,68]

Ubelaker identified similar changes in first and second metatarsals from prehistoric coastal Ecuador; among protohistoric Arikara from the Mobridge Site, South Dakota; among recent Alaskan Inuits, and among the ancestors of the Zuni Pueblo from Hawikuh, New Mexico; and in a low frequency in the Terry Collection of recent origin. Ubelaker considered that such changes resulted from habitual kneeling, with the toes hyperdorsiflexed, among these peoples,[69] because of their co-occurrence with one of the traits Trinkaus[70] confirms as likely to be the result of squatting (facets on the postero-superior femoral condyles). No examples were seen of the second trait discussed by Trinkaus, a groove on the femoral intercondylar line that marks the passage of the posterior cruciate ligament when the knee is hyperflexed. It seems very likely, then, that these dorsal facets relate to hyper-dorsiflexion of the toes in a variety of circumstances.

Except in those studies based on the presence or absence of a particular trait, studies of musculo-skeletal stress markers have been directed at assessing intra-population comparisons. Therefore, it is possible that one population's most extreme expression for a particular muscle attachment is only moderate in another. In order for these studies to be applied more generally across populations, a size-related robusticity measurement will be required to provide standards for comparison. Researchers would then be in a position to provide insights into the relative activity levels of populations across geographic space and through time during major social and economic transitions. Such studies would be more comparable to approaches used to assess work performance in modern populations for which height and weight of experimental subjects are measured and controlled.[71]

ACTIVITY-RELATED PATHOLOGY OF THE VERTEBRAL COLUMN

Strenuous loading of the vertebral column produces a condition called intervertebral osteochondrosis (degenerative disc disease) of the lower thoracic and lumbar vertebrae. Lesions of the vertebral plate (the forming epiphysis of the vertebral body) develop in younger individuals in the second or third decade of life, perhaps eventually becoming *spondylosis deformans*, an osteophyte-forming degenerative condition. Kelley distinguishes the crescent-shaped lesions of intervertebral osteochondrosis, placed anteriorly on the body of the vertebrae, from Schmorl's nodes, which are smooth-walled depressions that are centrally placed on the body of the vertebra.[72] (Intervertebral osteochondrosis is not to be confused with Scheuermann's disease, which affects the vertebral plates and is believed to have a different aetiology.) In a comparison of the commingled skeletal remains from the *Mary Rose* with a group of medieval males from St Margaret *in combusto*, Norwich, Stirland and Waldron note an increased prevalence of Schmorl's nodes in the

Norwich males in the thoracic (2.1 times) and lumbar (2.2 times) vertebrae. As the Norwich sample contains older individuals, this suggests that Schmorl's nodes are more commonly associated with older individuals, unlike intervertebral osteochondrosis, which is found in younger individuals.[62]

Spondylolysis, a fracture of the *pars interarticularis* or occasionally of the pedicle of the vertebral neural arch of L4 and or L5, occurs in a high frequency in athletes. For example, it is three times more common in young Japanese athletes (20.67%) than in the general adult population,[73] which Waldron reports as between 3 and 7%. This latter frequency is similar to that found in Romano-British (3.74%), Anglo-Saxon (4.55%) and early modern (1.42%) skeletal populations from Britain.[74] Modern individuals affected include female gymnasts,[75] male cricket bowlers,[76,77] and male American-football players.[78] Many of these individuals experience no pain, and the increased movement allowed by the separation of the arch and the formation of a ligamentous joint has been considered an adaptation to accommodate movement. Merbs documented similar high frequencies in Inuits (51 individuals, 13% from 110 affected sites), males being more affected than females.[79] Bridges reports a similar high frequency in Archaic period Amerindians (18.5%) with females over 40 being slightly more affected than the mostly younger males in her sample.[50] Merbs considered that kayaking was probably responsible for the presence of this defect in Inuits, an activity that requires rotation and lateral flexion of the upper body,[79] while Bridges attributed it to twisting and bending of the lumbar spine; in other words, to a similar aetiology.[50] Studies of more recent individuals do not seem to support a strong sexual dimorphism, probably due to the increasing similarity in male and female participation in sport.

The high frequency of spondylolysis in some skeletal populations, especially among Inuit, meant that some researchers ascribed a genetic origin to it, exacerbated by reputedly small breeding populations.[80] Some individuals may be more predisposed to the condition due to an inherited anatomical architecture in the lower spine. Farfan *et al.* noted that in a group of 35 individuals with lysis of the fifth lumbar vertebra, 34 had long spinous processes on this vertebra. The length of the spinous process is a predisposing factor in shoveller's fractures (see below),[81] sufferers of which have a relatively longer and more slender spinous processes on the seventh cervical vertebra.[82] The aetiology of both is now considered to be largely traumatic and inversely related to age and age-at-death. Further support for this interpretation comes with Merbs' documentation of a number of cases of incomplete spondylolysis and instances of healed defects in archaeological remains.[83] McCarroll *et al.* also noted that in their sample of American-footballers, the defect appeared in the adolescent years with few developing after this period.[78] As in archaeological instances, repetitive twisting or rotation of the torso on the pelvis is considered the predisposing movement associated with a primary stress fracture. A fracture of the right pedicle of right-handed bowlers is a feature of Weatherley *et al.*'s patient, and others in their experience. They consider that a fracture of the right pedicle may be due to a right-sided dominance in turning and throwing in cricket bowling (i.e. their bowlers are right-handed).[76] That fast bowlers are affected, as well as javelin throwers[83] and baseball players,[84] provides an indicator of throwing activities, especially in conjunction with unilateral limb hypertrophy.[85–87]

Shovelling, a form of more generalized labour, can be inferred from the analysis of skeletal changes of the vertebral column. Shovelling is a highly strenuous activity, on par with lifting water and threshing grain.[88] Shovelling heavy clayey soils produces fractures of the seventh cervical vertebra and first thoracic vertebra from traction of the neck and shoulder musculature.[89,90] In Britain, this condition has been found mainly in males from Romano-British, Anglo-Saxon and medieval periods.[91,92] Importantly, it is also reported in modern metal-dippers,[82] which highlights another possible aetiology that may be of use in the context of tracing the development of metalworking in the Old World. Owing to mechanization, shovelling is less common today than it was in the past, although in many places it is still the norm.[93] The shift away from manual shovelling may explain the apparent higher prevalence among past groups than of those today.

CRANIOFACIAL REMODELLING

The cranium is an extremely complex mechanical structure, and studies of cranial function have developed more slowly in comparison to those of the post-cranial skeleton. Despite early work which questioned the effect of mechanical forces on human cranial vault morphology,[16,20] it appears cranial bone and cartilage respond in the same way to mechanical loads as do those of the better-studied long bones of the skeleton.[94] In a test of the relationship between strenuous exercise and cranial bone thickness, Lieberman found increased cranial vault thickness in a group of strenuously exercised juvenile pigs, despite the fact that the cranial vault was not heavily loaded during such activity as measured by inserted strain gauges.[95] He suggests that a general increase in bone thickness may occur throughout the bodies of those engaged in strenuous activities, perhaps through the mediation of growth hormones. Although the mechanisms by which cranial morphology is influenced by mechanical loads have yet to be fully elucidated, there is increasing evidence to suggest that response to mechanical loading occurs in ways that can contribute to considerable morphological change.

Washburn produced morphological change due to reduced masticatory stress of the jaws and cranial vault through excision of the *M. temporalis*,[96] while Hohl has done similarly by transposition of *M. masseter* and *M. temporalis* in experimental animals.[97] Ingervall and Bitsanis demonstrated that increased intensity of chewing produced facial changes in a group of children with long-face morphology and associated weak facial muscles.[98] These long-face children are characterized by large anterior facial heights, small posterior facial heights, steep mandibular planes, and large gonial angles that produce malocclusion problems, including an open bite.

Building on this research, Kiliaridis provides evidence that individuals suffering from myotonic dystrophy, a disorder that affects the speed of muscle contraction, are characterized by a vertical growth pattern of the face, producing a long-face morphology, and a high incidence of malocclusion, as well as reduced bite force and masticatory muscle activity. Individuals with more powerful bite force are characterized by a relatively short face, small gonial angle, and flat mandibular planes (a square-jawed morphology).[99] Carlson and van Gerven reported similar morphological changes in time-successive Nubian populations spanning the transition from hunting and gathering to agricultural production. Agriculturalists also possess a more globular cranial vault, which they interpret as evidence for reduced masticatory demands in this population (Figures 4 and 5).[100] It seems then, that both facial and cranial vault morphology may be affected by a reduction in strenuous muscular activity considered to occur at major subsistence transitions.

OSTEOARTHRITIS AND ACTIVITY

For many years, researchers have postulated that there is a relationship between strenuous activity and an increased prevalence of osteoarthritis in joints. Some other factors are also considered to contribute to the development of osteoarthritis, including heredity, trauma, increased body weight, loss of bone mass, and age-related loss of fine musculo-skeletal control, as well as bony architectural changes to joints as a consequence of injury, inactivity, or old age.[101-104] Indeed, there is no clear-cut relationship between strenuous activity alone, and the onset of osteoarthritic change. Studies of long-term athletes show that some do not

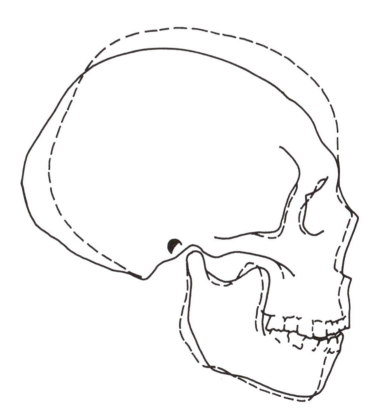

Figure 4 – Schematic representation of the cranial changes in Nubian populations before (solid line) and after (dotted line) the transition to agriculture. Reprinted from Carlson DS and van Gerven DP, Masticatory function and post-Pleistocene evolution in Nubia, *American Journal of Physical Anthropology* 1977; 46: 495–506, figure 4 (p. 502). Wiley-Liss, Inc., a subsidiary of John Wiley and Sons, Inc.

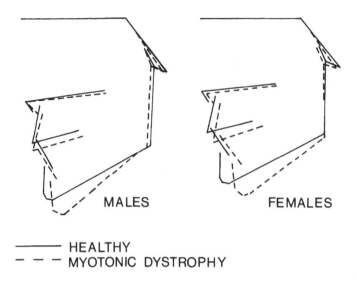

MALES   FEMALES

——— HEALTHY
– – – MYOTONIC DYSTROPHY

Figure 5 – Mean facial diagrams of males and females with myotonic dystrophy (a form of muscular atrophy) compared with healthy normal individuals. The changes noted in the jaws are similar to those noted by Carlson and van Gerven (1977) in Nubian populations making the transition to agriculture and its reduced masticatory demands (Figure 4). Reprinted from Kiliaridis S, Masticatory muscle influence on craniofacial growth, *Acta Odontologica Scandinavica* 1995; **53**: 196–202, figure 2 (p. 199).

develop osteoarthritis, or do so at rates lower than for those who do not engage in such activities.[105–107] There also appears to be a sex bias, whereby women are more often affected than men by a ratio of 2:1.[108]

Biomechanically related skeletal alterations (as measured by limb element robusticity) and osteoarthritic changes appear to respond to different factors.[50,109] Hunter-gatherers in samples from the south-eastern USA have a greater prevalence of osteoarthritis than agriculturalists, though this difference is not statistically significant. Conversely, however, Bridges observes that the agriculturalists demonstrate greater bone robusticity, suggesting that the work associated with agriculture made more demands on the musculo-skeletal system. As increased robusticity is considered to develop as a consequence of strenuous physical activity, this would seem to support the argument that osteoarthritis and strenuous activity are not closely related phenomena. There is the possibility that they are inversely related when age of commencement of activity is considered,[110] greater robusticity being a consequence of strenuous labour commenced at a young age, before physiological maturity, which also confers an adaptive advantage against the development of osteoarthritis. This possibility has yet to be addressed.

From studies of archaeological human remains, there is increasing evidence demonstrating that activity is not reflected in osteoarthritic changes of the vertebral column.[111,112] In fact, in a small sample from the crypt at Christchurch, Spitalfields, London, Waldron and Cox noted a statistically significant association between *non-manual* workers and osteoarthritis of the vertebral column.[113] Rather than reflecting activity differences, the vertebral column appears to reflect the mechanical stresses placed on it as a consequence of bipedal gait and the adoption of certain postures over prolonged periods.[114,115] To demonstrate increased severity of osteoarthritis due to activity, it seems that the forces must be of considerable magnitude and reliant on particular postures over a considerable period, perhaps like those postulated by Lovell to be affecting the cervical vertebrae of ancient Harappans who were using their heads for weight-bearing.[116]

In summary, it seems that physiologically mediated activity may have an important role to play in the development of osteoarthritis. However, multiple etiological factors obscure direct correlation between strenuous activity and the onset of osteoarthritis in both modern and past human groups.

CONCLUSIONS: ACTIVITY AND OCCUPATION

It is clear from the above that research in activity-related change is a developing area in human osteology. In part the subject has been hampered by its historical development, which emphasized the identification of occupations from skeletal remains. Occupational specialization requires that land and labour be treated as commodities, the outcome of a process that develops after a considerable period of social inequality.[117] Such studies, then, can only be meaningful for societies with identifiable social and economic inequality most fully developed in class-based states. Such societies make up only a small percentage of human social groupings until the modern era. To attempt to find occupational specialists in pre-state societies is, at best, an unprofitable venture but, far worse, to assume their existence prevents us from studying the processes by which specialization developed. This view of occupational specialization owes more to modern Western, post-industrial views of labour and working practices than it does to cross-cultural social reality. Interestingly, Hadler echoed similar sentiments in his criticism of studies in occupational medicine that concentrated on types of occupations rather than on individuals and usage. He argued that this practice obscured the relationship between pattern of usage and musculoskeletal disorders, except in cases of overt trauma.[118]

Both occupational medicine and human osteological studies are limited by the amount of documentation that can be brought to bear on individual cases and populations. Modern clinical studies are made from increasingly well-documented groups, matching individuals by age, sex, and experience. Human osteologists have also attempted to control for similar effects in their examination of skeletal populations; age, sex and the social and cultural context of the population are increasingly considered and explicitly stated. These parameters should be considered as a starting point for such studies. Further insights into activity-related change will come from anthropological and human biological studies of modern individuals in a variety of cultural, economic, and social circumstances. As traditional trades and crafts are increasingly mechanized, we face the loss of the very individuals upon whom to base our studies of the origins and developments of various specialisms. This threat is one shared with all ethnographic research and should occasion studies (from youth, if possible) of those specialists that remain in traditional societies, and those of physically active individuals, such as athletes, enthusiastic amateurs, and military personnel, in industrialized societies.

Further study of documented populations, especially those that can be divided on the basis of manual as opposed to non-manual labour are, at the present time, likely to be most fruitful. This is because the biometry of these populations will be the baseline from which more specific studies can be directed in the future. In one of the few published studies of documented individuals, Cunha and Umbelino[60] could not discriminate between different types of manual labour, perhaps because their groupings included manual labourers who may have engaged in similar ranges of movements and activity levels, or because the recorded occupation may not be representative of an individual's lifetime activities. Significant differences may be found when this sample is compared with a more recent sample of clerical workers. These studies should include individuals less than 25 years of age who were excluded from Cunha and Umbellino's study, a group that might be expected to demonstrate the greatest osseous change from activity commenced at a youthful age.

In addition to these recommendations, the following are other pressing concerns in activity-related studies:

- The goal of such studies should be to reconstruct movements and motions, not occupations. These reconstructed movements may reveal sexually dimorphic or population-based activity variants, such as asymmetrical limb use or mobility differences, some of which may be linked to craft or activity specialization, disability, or social standing.
- Increased use of robusticity indices and long bone lengths to control for size-related factors. One would predict that large skeletal elements require larger muscles to move them and this relationship alone may account for a considerable amount of variation and correlation.
- There is a great need for a means by which to accurately gauge body mass from skeletal remains. A large body mass produces abnormally large forces on joints, the muscles which act across them and the tendons and ligaments that support these structures. Therefore, high body mass may mimic strenuous activity. At the present time limb bone lengths are used as controls for size, although these are not necessarily adequate reflections of body mass. Ruff *et al.*[49] suggest that cross-sectional area of the femoral diaphysis is roughly correlated with body mass from their study of 80 individuals. Further research in this area would be much welcomed.

ACKNOWLEDGEMENTS

Carol Palmer has read, commented upon, listened to and edited successive versions of this paper. Her skills in clarity of thought and as an assiduous 'inside-outsider' made this a much more coherent piece. Amanda Forster redrew figures 4 and 5. The substantial comments of two anonymous reviewers, and Anthea Boylston, are also much appreciated; they helped to make this contribution briefer and better organized. These people are, of course, not responsible for any errors or oversights that remain. I bear the burden of those.

REFERENCES

1   Stirland AJ. Diagnosis of occupationally related palaeopathology: can it be done? In: Ortner DJ, Aufderheide AC (eds), *Human Paleopathology: Current Syntheses and Future Options*. Washington, DC: Smithsonian Institution Press, 1991: pp. 40–47.

2   Kennedy KAR. Skeletal markers of occupational stress. In: Isçan MY, Kennedy KAR (eds), *Reconstruction of Life from the Skeleton*. New York: Alan R. Liss, 1989: pp. 129–160.

3   Chamberlain AT. Skeletal studies: an approach to a state-of-the-art assessment. *Current Anthropology* 1991; **32**: 95–96.

4   Hinkes MJ. A review of *Reconstruction of Life from the Skeleton*. *Journal of Forensic Science* 1990; **35**: 1504–1506.

5   Capasso L, Kennedy KAR, Wilczak C. *Atlas of Occupational Markers on Human Remains*. Teramo: Edigrafital SPA, 1998.

6   Dutour O. Activités physiques et squelette humain: le difficile passage de l'actuel au fossile. *Bulletin et Mémoirs de la Société d'Anthropologie de Paris*, n.s. 1992; **4**: 233–241.

7   Waldron T. Population studies. *Paleopathology Society Newsletter* 1997; **100**: 22.

8   Martin RB, Burr DB. *Structure, Function, and Adaptation of Compact Bone*. New York: Raven, 1989.

9   Roberts DF. The pervasiveness of plasticity. In: Mascie-Taylor CGN, Bogin B (eds), *Human Variability and Plasticity*. Cambridge: Cambridge University Press, 1995: pp. 1–17.

10 Schell LM. Human biological adaptability with special emphasis on plasticity: history, development and problems for future research. In: Mascie-Taylor CGN, Bogin B (eds), *Human Variability and Plasticity*. Cambridge: Cambridge University Press, 1995: pp. 212–237.

11 Bock WJ, von Wahlert G. Adaptation and the form–function complex. *Evolution* 1965; **19**: 269–299.

12 Nordin M, Frankel VH. Biomechanics of bone. In: Nordin M, Frankel VH (eds), *Basic Biomechanics of the Skeletal System* (2nd edn). Philadelphia: Lea and Febiger 1989: pp. 3–29.

13 Enlow DH. The remodelling of bone. *Yearbook of Physical Anthropology* 1976; **20**: 19–34.

14 Burr DB, Martin RB. Errors in bone remodelling: toward a unified theory of metabolic bone disease. *American Journal of Anatomy* 1990; **186**: 186–216.

15 Gordon JE. *The New Science of Strong Materials or Why You Don't Fall Through The Floor*. Harmondsworth: Penguin, 1968.

16 Currey JD. *The Mechanical Adaptations of Bone*. Princeton: Princeton University Press, 1984.

17 Lanyon LE, Goodship AE, Pye CJ, MacFie JH. Mechanically adaptive bone remodelling. *Journal of Biomechanics* 1982; **15**: 141–154.

18 Lanyon LE, Rubin CT. Static vs dynamic loads as an influence on bone remodelling. *Journal of Biomechanics* 1984; **17**: 897–905.

19 Lanyon LE. The success and failure of the adaptive response to functional load-bearing in averting bone fracture. *Bone* 1992; **13**: S17–21.

20 Lanyon LE. Functional strain in bone tissue as an objective, and controlling stimulus for adaptive bone remodelling. *Journal of Biomechanics* 1987; **20**: 1083–1093.

21 Rubin CT, McLeod KJ, Bain SD. Functional strains and cortical bone adaptation: epigenetic assurance of skeletal integrity. *Journal of Biomechanics* 1990; **23**: 43–54.

22 Kiiskinen A. Physical training and connective tissues in young mice – physical properties of Achilles tendons and long bones. *Growth* 1977; **41**: 123–137.

23 Woo SL-Y, Kuei SC, Amiel D, Gomez MA, Hayes WC, White FC, Akeson WH. The effect of prolonged training on the properties of long bone: a study of Wolff's Law. *Journal of Bone and Joint Surgery* 1981; **65A**(5): 780–787.

24 Anderson JJB. Development and maintenance of bone mass through the life cycle. In: Anderson JJB, Garner SC (eds), *Calcium and Phosphorus in Health and Disease*. Boca Raton: CRC Press, 1996: pp. 265–288.

25 Currey JD, Butler G. The mechanical properties of bone tissue in children. *Journal of Bone and Joint Surgery* 1975; **57A**: 810–814.

26 Carter DR, Orr TE, Fyrie DP, Schurman DJ. Influences of mechanical stress on prenatal and postnatal skeletal development. *Clinical Orthopaedics and Related Research* 1987; **219**: 237–250.

27 Carter DR, Orr TE. Skeletal development and bone functional adaptation. *Journal of Bone and Mineral Research* 1992; **7**: 389–395.

28 Ruff CB, Walker A, Trinkaus E. Postcranial robusticity in *Homo*. III: Ontogeny. *American Journal of Physical Anthropology* 1994; **93(1)**: 35–54.

29 Humphrey L. Growth patterns in the modern human skeleton. *American Journal of Physical Anthropology* 1998; **105**: 57–72.

30 Pfeiffer S. Age changes in the external dimensions of adult bone. *American Journal of Physical Anthropology* 1980; **52**: 529–532.

31 Ruff CB, Hayes WC. Cross-sectional geometry of Pecos Pueblo femora and tibiae – a biomechanical investigation: II. Sex, age, and side differences. *American Journal of Physical Anthropology* 1983; **60**: 383–400.

32 Schoutens A, Laurent E, Poortmans JR. Effects of inactivity and exercise on bone. *Sports Medicine* 1989; **7**: 71–81.

33 Stirland AJ. Asymmetry and activity-related change in the male humerus. *International Journal of Osteoarchaeology* 1993; **3**: 105–113.

34 Bridges PS. Osteological correlates of weapon use. In: Buikstra JE (ed.), *A Life in Science: Papers in Honor of J. Lawrence Angel*. Scientific Papers no. 6. Center for American Archaeology, 1990: pp. 87–98.

35 Roberts C. Bars of bone on hip bones in antiquity: pathological, occupational or genetic? *Human Evolution* 1987; **2**: 539–545.

36 Rader WT, Peters CR. Hypertrophy of the acetabulo-cristal buttress in *Homo sapiens*. *American Journal of Physical Anthropology* 1993; **92**: 149–153.

37 Rose MD. A hominine hip bone, KNM-ER 3228 from East Lake Turkana, Kenya. *American Journal of Physical Anthropology* 1984; **63**: 371–378.

38 Day MH. Postcranial remains of *Homo erectus* from Bed IV, Olduvai Gorge, Tanzania. *Nature* 1971; **232**: 383–387.

39 Rightmire GP. Variation among early *Homo* crania from Olduvai Gorge and the Koobi Fora region. *American Journal of Physical Anthropology* 1993; **90**: 1–33.

40 Trinkaus E. Neandertal postcrania and the adaptive shift to modern humans. In: Trinkaus E (ed.), *The Mousterian Legacy – Human Biocultural Change in the Upper Pleistocene*. Oxford: British Archaeological Reports S164 (International Series), 1983: pp. 165–200.

41 Trinkaus E, Churchill SE, Ruff CB. Postcranial robusticity in *Homo*. II: Humeral bilateral asymmetry and bone plasticity. *American Journal of Physical Anthropology* 1994; **93**: 1–34.

42 Ruff CB. Biomechanics of the hip and birth in early *Homo*. *American Journal of Physical Anthropology* 1995; **98(4)**: 527–574.

43 Ruff CB, Trinkaus E, Walker A, Larsen CS. Postcranial robusticity in Homo. I: Temporal trends and mechanical interpretation. *American Journal of Physical Anthropology* 1993; **91(1)**: 21–53 .

44 Ben-Itzhak S, Smith P, Bloom RA. Radiographic study of the humerus in Neandertals and *Homo sapiens sapiens*. *American Journal of Physical Anthropology* 1988; **77**: 231–242.

45 Jones H, Priest JD, Hayes WC, Tichenor CC, Nagel DA. Humeral hypertrophy in response to exercise. *Journal of Bone and Joint Surgery* 1977; **59A**(2): 204–208.

46 Toth N. Archaeological evidence for preferential right-handedness in the Lower and Middle Pleistocene, and its possible implications. *Journal of Human Evolution* 1985; **14**: 607–614.

47 Bermúdez de Castro JM, Bromage TG, Jalvo YF. Buccal striations on fossil human anterior teeth: evidence of handedness in the Middle and Early Upper Pleistocene. *Journal of Human Evolution* 1988; **17**: 403–412.

48   Fox CL, Frayer DW. Non-dietary marks in the anterior dentition of the Krapina Neanderthals. *International Journal of Osteoarchaeology* 1997; **7**: 133–149.

49   Ruff CB, Scott WW, Liu AY-C. Articular and diaphyseal remodeling of the proximal femur with changes in body mass in adults. *American Journal of Physical Anthropology* 1991; **86**: 397–414.

50   Bridges PS. Changes in activities with the shift to agriculture in the southeastern United States. *Current Anthropology* 1989; **30**: 385–393.

51   Ruff CB, Larsen CS, Hayes WC. Structural changes in the femur with the transition to agriculture on the Georgia Coast. *American Journal of Physical Anthropology* 1984; **64**: 125–136.

52   Larsen CS. *Bioarchaeology: Interpreting Behavior from the Human Skeleton*. Cambridge: Cambridge University Press, 1997.

53   Larsen CS, Ruff CB. The stresses of conquest in Spanish Florida: structural adaptation and change before and after contact. In: Larsen CS, Milner GR (eds), *In The Wake of Contact: Biological Responses to Conquest*. New York: Wiley-Liss, 1994: pp. 21–34.

54   Lazenby RA, Pfeiffer SK. Effects of a nineteenth century below-knee amputation and prosthesis on femoral morphology. *International Journal of Osteoarchaeology* 1993; **3**: 19–38.

55   Churchill SE, Formicola V. A case of marked bilateral asymmetry in the upper limbs of an Upper Palaeolithic male from Barma Grande (Liguria), Italy. *International Journal of Osteoarchaeology* 1996; **7**: 18–38.

56   Hoyte DAN, Enlow DH. Wolff's Law and the problem of muscle attachment on resorptive surfaces of bone. *American Journal of Physical Anthropology*, 1966: **24**: 205–214.

57   Niepel GA, Sit'aj S. Enthesopathy. *Clinics in Rheumatic Diseases* 1979; **5**: 857–872.

58   Resnick D, Niwayama G. Entheses and enthesopathy: anatomical, pathological and radiological correlation. *Radiology* 1983; **146**: 1–9.

59   Kaur H, Jit I. Brief communication: coracoclavicular joint in Northwest Indians. *American Journal of Physical Anthropology* 1991; **85**: 457–460.

60   Cunha E, Umbelino C. What can bones tell about labour and occupation: the analysis of skeletal markers of occupational stress in the Identified Skeletal Collection of the Anthropological Museum of the University of Coimbra (preliminary results). *Anthropologia Portuguesa* 1995; **13**: 49–68.

61   Shaibani A, Workman R, Rothschild BM. The significance of enthesopathy as a skeletal phenomenon. *Clinical and Experimental Rheumatology* 1993; **11**: 399–403.

62   Stirland AJ, Waldron T. Evidence for activity related markers in the vertebrae of the crew of the *Mary Rose*. *Journal of Archaeological Science* 1997; **24**: 329–335.

63   Hawkey DE, Merbs CF. Activity-induced musculoskeletal stress markers (MSM) and subsistence strategy changes among ancient Hudson Bay Eskimos. *International Journal of Osteoarchaeology* 1995; **5**: 324–338.

64   McGhee R. Disease and the development of Inuit culture. *Current Anthropology* 1994; **35**: 565–594.

65   Munson Chapman NE. Evidence for Spanish influence on activity induced musculoskeletal stress markers at Pecos Pueblo. *International Journal of Osteoarchaeology* 1997; **7**: 497–506.

66   Lai P, Lovell N. Skeletal markers of occupational stress in the fur trade: a case study from a Hudson's Bay Company fur trade post. *International Journal of Osteoarchaeology* 1992; **2**: 221–234.

67   Molleson T. The eloquent bones of Abu Hureyra. *Scientific American* 1994; **271**: 70–75.

68   Molleson T. Seed preparation in the Mesolithic: the osteological evidence. *Antiquity* 1989; 63(239): 356–362.

69   Ubelaker DH. Skeletal evidence for kneeling in prehistoric Ecuador. *American Journal of Physical Anthropology* 1979; **51**: 679–686.

70   Trinkaus E. Squatting among the Neanderthals: a problem in the behavioural interpretation of skeletal morphology. *Journal of Archaeological Science* 1975; **2**: 327–351.

71   Samanta A, Chatterjee BB. A physiological study of manual lifting of loads in Indians. *Ergonomics* 1981; **24**: 557–564.

72   Kelley MA. Intervertebral osteochondrosis in ancient and modern populations. *American Journal of Physical Anthropology* 1982; **59**: 271–279.

73   Hoshina H. Spondylolysis in athletes. *The Physician and Sports Medicine* 1980; **8**: 75–79.

74   Waldron T. Variation in the rates of spondylolysis in early populations. *International Journal of Osteoarchaeology* 1991; **1**: 63–65.

75   Jackson DW, Wiltse LL, Circincione RJ. Spondylolysis in the female gymnast. *Clinical Orthopaedics* 1976; **117**: 68–73.

76   Weatherley CR, Mehdian H, Vanden Berghe L. Low back pain with fracture of the pedicle and contralateral spondylolysis: a technique of surgical management. *Journal of Bone and Joint Surgery* 1991; **73B**: 990–993.

77   Hardcastle P, Annear P, Foster DH, Chakera TM, McCormick C, Khangure M, Burnett A. Spinal abnormalities in young fast bowlers. *Journal of Bone and Joint Surgery* 1992; 74B: 421–425.

78   McCarroll JR, Miller JM, Ritter MA. Lumbar spondylolysis and spondylolisthesis in college football players: a prospective study. *American Journal of Sports Medicine* 1986; **14(5)**: 404–405.

79   Merbs CF. *Patterns of Activity-Induced Pathology in a Canadian Inuit Population*. Mercury Series no. 119. Ottawa: National Museums of Canada, 1983.

80   Merbs CF. Spondylolysis and spondylolisthesis: a cost of being an erect biped or a clever adaptation. *Yearbook of Physical Anthropology* 1996; **39**: 201–228.

81   Farfan HF, Osteria V, Lamy C. The mechanical etiology of spondylolysis and spondylolisthesis. *Clinical Orthopaedics and Related Research* 1976; **117**: 40–55.

82   Venable JR, Flake RE, Kilian DJ. Stress fracture of the spinous process. *Journal of the American Medical Association* 1964; **190**: 103–107.

83   Merbs CF. Incomplete spondylolysis and healing: a study of ancient Canadian Eskimo skeletons. *Spine* 1995; **21**: 2328–2334.

84   Steele J. Skeletal indicators of handedness (Chapter 19 – this volume).

85   Peterson J. The Natufian hunting conundrum: spears, atlatls, or bows? *International Journal of Osteoarchaeology* 1998; **8**: 378–389 .

86   Mays S. A biomechanical study of activity patterns in a medieval human skeletal assemblage. *International Journal of Osteoarchaeology* 1999; **9**: 68–73.

87   Mays S, Steele J, Ford M. Directional asymmetry in the human clavicle. *International Journal of Osteoarchaeology* 1999; **9**: 18–28 .

88   Nag PK, Sebastian NC, Mavlankar MG. Occupational workload of Indian agricultural workers. *Ergonomics* 1980; **23**: 91–102.

89   Herrick RT. Clay-shoveler's fracture in power-lifting. *American Journal of Sports Medicine* 1981; **9**: 29–30.

90   Meyer PG, Hartman JT, Leo JS. Sentinel spinous fractures. *Surgical Neurology* 1981; **18**: 174–178.

91   Knüsel CJ, Roberts CA, Boylston A. When Adam delved ...: an activity-related lesion in three human skeletal populations. *American Journal of Physical Anthropology* 1996; **100**: 427–434.

92   Stroud G, Kemp RL. *Cemeteries of St. Andrew, Fishergate*. The Archaeology of York: The Medieval Cemeteries 12/2, York: Council for British Archaeology for York Archaeological Trust, 1993.

93   Freivalds A. The ergonomics of shovelling and shovel design – an experimental study. *Ergonomics* 1986; **29**: 19–30.

94   Herring SW. Epigenetic and functional influences on skull growth. In: Hanken J, Hall BK (eds), *The Skull*, vol. **1**: *Development*. Chicago: University of Chicago Press, 1993: pp. 153–206.

95   Lieberman DE. How and why humans grow thin skulls: experimental evidence for systemic cortical robusticity. *American Journal of Physical Anthropology* 1996; **101**: 217–236.

96   Washburn SL. The relation of the temporal muscle to the form of the skull. *Anatomical Record* 1947; **99**: 239–248.

97   Hohl TH. Masticatory muscle transposition in primates: effects on craniofacial growth. *Journal of Maxillofacial Surgery* 1983; **11**: 149–156.

98   Ingervall B, Bitsanis E. A pilot study of the effect of masticatory muscle training on facial growth in long-face children. *European Journal of Orthodontics* 1987; **9**: 15–23.

99   Kiliaridis S. Masticatory muscle influence on craniofacial growth. *Acta Odontologica Scandinavica* 1995; **53**: 196–202.

100   Carlson DS, van Gerven DP. Masticatory function and post-Pleistocene evolution in Nubia. *American Journal of Physical Anthropology* 1977; **46**: 495–506.

101   Jurmain RD. The pattern of involvement of appendicular degenerative joint disease. *American Journal of Physical Anthropology* 1980; **53**: 143–150.

102   Felson DT. Epidemiology of hip and knee osteoarthritis. *Epidemiologic Reviews* 1988; **10**: 1–28.

103   Panush RS, Inzinna JD. Recreational activities and degenerative joint disease. *Sports Medicine* 1994; **17(1)**: 1–5.

104   Waldron T. Changes in the distribution of osteoarthritis over historical time. *International Journal of Osteoarchaeology* 1995; **5**: 385–389.

105   Lane NE, Bloch DA, Jones HH, Marshall WH, Wood PD, Fries JF. Long-distance running, bone density, and osteoarthritis. *Journal of the American Medical Association* 1986; **255**: 1147–1151.

106   Puranen J, Ala-Ketola L, Peltokallio P, Saarela J. Running and primary osteoarthritis of the hip. *British Medical Journal* 1975; **2**: 424–425.

107   Panush RS, Brown DG. Exercise and arthritis. *Sports Medicine* 1987; **4**: 54–64.

108   Waldron T. Osteoarthritis in a Black Death cemetery in London. *International Journal of Osteoarchaeology* 1992; **2**: 235–240.

109   Bridges PS. Degenerative joint disease in hunter-gatherers and agriculturalists from the southeastern United States. *American Journal of Physical Anthropology* 1991; **85**: 379–392.

110   Knüsel CJ, Bridges PS. Comment and reply to 'On the biomechanical and osteoarthritic differences between hunter-gatherers and agriculturalists'. *American Journal of Physical Anthropology* 1993; **91**: 523–527.

111   Bridges PS. Vertebral arthritis and physical activities in the prehistoric southeastern United States. *American Journal of Physical Anthropology* 1994; **93**: 83–93.

112   Knüsel CJ, Göggel SC, Lucy DJ. Comparative degenerative joint disease of the vertebral column in the medieval monastic cemetery of the Gilbertine Priory of St. Andrew, Fishergate, York, England. *American Journal of Physical Anthropology* 1997; **103**: 481–495.

113   Waldron HA, Cox M. Occupational arthropathy: evidence from the past. *British Journal of Industrial Medicine* 1989; **46**: 420–422.

114   Anderson JAD. Arthrosis and its relation to work. *Scandinavian Journal of Work, Environment and Health* 1984; **10**: 429–433.

115   Sairanen E, Brüshaber L, Kaskinen M. Felling work, low-back pain and osteoarthritis. *Scandinavian Journal of Work, Environment and Health* 1981; **7**: 18–30.

116   Lovell NC. Spinal arthritis and physical stress at Bronze Age Harappa. *American Journal of Physical Anthropology* 1994; **93**: 149–164.

117   Brumfiel EM, Earle TK. Specialization, exchange, and complex societies: an introduction. In: Brumfiel EM, Earle TK (eds), *Specialization, Exchange, and Complex Societies*. Cambridge: Cambridge University Press, 1987: pp. 1–9.

118   Hadler NM. Industrial rheumatology: clinical investigations into the influence of the pattern of usage on the pattern of regional musculoskeletal disease. *Arthritis and Rheumatism* 1977; **20**: 1020–1025.

119   Knüsel CJ, Chundun ZC, Cardwell P. Slipped proximal femoral epiphysis in a priest from the medieval period. *International Journal of Osteoarchaeology* 1992; **2**: 109–119.

24

THE ANALYSIS OF CREMATED BONE

Jacqueline McKinley

INTRODUCTION

Cremated bone represents not only the physical remains of one or more individuals, but also is the product of a series of ritual acts that comprise the disposal of the dead by the mortuary rite of cremation. Consequently, the analysis of cremated bone encompasses a number of aims in addition to the usual osteological research objectives of ascertaining demographic and pathological data, seeking to deduce evidence pertaining to pyre technology and indications of the rites and rituals attendant on funerary practice.

This chapter will outline the process of cremation, comparing modern crematoria with pyre cremation, and review experimental work and analysis of the characteristic form and nature of cremated bone. Methods of analysis for the recovery of demographic, anthropological and pathological data specific to cremated remains will be discussed. The final section will consider how data may be assessed in order to ascertain aspects of the technology, rites and rituals involved in the mortuary rite of cremation.

CREMATION

An understanding of the process of cremation is essential. Observations at modern crematoria provide monitored controls against which to assess archaeological material, and information on efficient and effective cremation technology. Detailed observations of the cremation process, including variables relating to different cadavers and slightly differing working conditions within British crematoria (e.g. different types of cremator) or between different operatives (e.g. the level of vigour in raking-out)[1-4] are augmented by descriptions of specific technical details.[5,6] Observations from other countries further demonstrate variations in the functioning of modern crematoria.[7,8]

Cremation is a process of dehydration and oxidation of the organic components of the body, including the about 30% organic component of the skeleton.[9] Modern British crematoria aim to effect full oxidation of all the organic components by monitored control of the temperature and oxygen input;[3] although this was not necessarily considered a prerequisite of cremation in the past, nor is it in other contemporary cultures. The heat-retentive nature of the Cremator means the external heat source is not always necessary to maintain the working temperature (*about* 700–1000°C). Airflow is used to circulate heat within the chamber but, inevitably, a uniform temperature may not be attained across the whole corpse due to the position of the gas jets[3] and the different density distribution of soft tissues within the body. Cremation generally takes 1–1.5 hr to complete, though there may be rare, inexplicable exceptions taking a much shorter (about 30 min)[10] or longer (> 3 hrs). Soft tissues must be removed (burnt away) from individual bones before they will burn; body tissues are not good heat conductors and without sufficient oxygen supply, oxidation cannot occur. The stage at which individual skeletal elements cremate is, therefore, dependent on their soft tissue coverage, and the temperature within any given part of the Cremator. In about the first 45 minutes of cremation, the heat produced by the burning soft tissues increases the temperature within the Cremator; thereafter, although some soft tissues will continue to burn for some time, there is a dramatic fall-off in temperature.[3]

At the end of cremation there remains a recognizable skeleton, this is also true for neonatal/young infant skeletons.[3,11,12] The latter are obviously fragile and in modern crematoria coffins may be placed on a metal tray and airflow reduced to ensure the remains are not pulverized and lost within the Cremator. The weight of bone recovered from an adult cremation varies between *about* 1000 and 3600 g.[2,5] It has been observed that few articular surfaces and generally less spongy bone survives among the raked-out remains of some elderly individuals (> 80 years), particularly females of obviously gracile build. This is believed to reflect the destruction of osteoporotic bone during cremation.[2] The familiar fine-fraction ashes from modern cremations are the product of deliberate pulverization of cremated bone within a 'cremulator'.[3]

Detailed study of the thermodynamics of modern cremation included calculations of combustion rates, gas volumes, air and fuel requirements, conditions of combustion and the calorific values of various species of wood.[8] It was concluded that the energy used is roughly equal to 146 kg of pinewood for a pyre, but that a considerably greater amount of fuel is often necessary.[8] Open pyres do not, for instance, retain and circulate hot gases as in a modern Cremator. It was also found that the time, temperature and amount of oxygen affect grade of burning.[8] These three factors, and the relationship between them, represent the necessary criteria for cremating a corpse. For example, insufficient oxygen supply may create reducing rather than oxidizing conditions, resulting in the bone being charred rather than burnt (oxidized), and a corpse burning for too short a time, even at the required temperature, will not fully cremate.

FORM AND NATURE OF CREMATED BONE

Cremated bone (from the Latin *cremare*; to burn 'to consume by fire ... to reduce (a corpse) to ashes'[13]) may be described as 'burnt', 'calcined' or 'oxidized'. However, cremated bone is often not fully calcined/oxidized and not all burnt bone has been subject to cremation. The macroscopic and microscopic form and nature of cremated bone has been subject to much investigation and discussion, with several reviews and summaries.[3,7,14]

The macroscopic appearance is altered as dehydration causes shrinkage, fissuring and sometimes twisting of the bone. Fissuring generally follows a distinctive pattern dictated by bone morphology (shape, size, density, etc.), e.g. characteristic 'U-shaped' fissures develop along the anterior femur and humerus shafts, with concentric fissuring in the proximal heads (Figure 1). Small bones, such as carpals and phalanges, often survive whole. Laboratory experiments to identify differences in appearance between bone burnt before or after the loss of water and organic content,[15–19] found that the already dehydrated condition of the latter rendered impossible the development of fissures so characteristic in the former. Cremation of dissection-room cadavers (where much of the soft tissues has already been stripped from the bone) results in the same visual end product as with fleshed cadavers, the only observable difference being the decrease in the time taken for the bone itself to cremate.[3]

Cremated bone may range in colour from brown/black (slightly charred), through hues of blue and grey, to buff/white (oxidized).[20–22] It is not unusual to see a range of colours among the remains from a single cremation (even modern), reflecting that within a limited time span, bone with dense soft tissue cover will not cremate as fully as bone with less cover. Also, some bone has a higher infiltration of organic components than others, e.g. compact as compared with 'spongy' bone, and consequently takes longer to oxidize. Experiments have found a correlation between temperature and bone colour,[20–22] and have shown a relationship between the temperature attained in the bone and the radial distance from the outer cortical bone surface.[21] The maximum temperature indicated by the

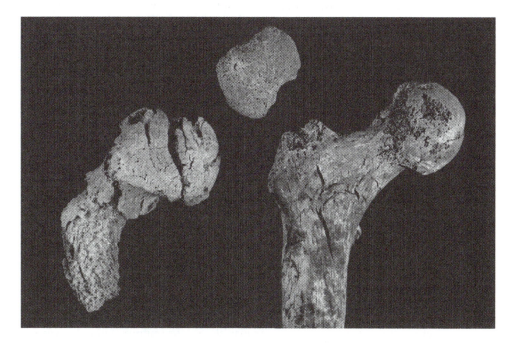

Figure 1 – Fragments of proximal femora showing the rare recovery of the whole femoral head (right), classic concentric fissuring (left) and commonly recovered fragment size (centre).

condition of a single bone fragment does not necessarily reflect the temperature attained across the entire corpse.

Bone shrinkage during cremation has been subject to laboratory investigations using parts of cadavers, with varying results.[8,14,20,23] Proposed shrinkage factors include; an overall factor of 12%,[23] maximum mean percentage shrinkage of about 15%,[20] a cross-sectional shrinkage of 25–30% for femur shafts, 5% longitudinal shrinkage of long bones, and 12% for a femoral head;[14] and variations of between 0 and 25%.[8] Preliminary experiments using dissection-room cadavers indicated 1.9–2.5% cross-sectional shrinkage in the radius shaft and 3.8–5.0% in the head. These figures imply that there is no reliable overall shrinkage factor; they suggest variability not only between individuals, but also between different skeletal elements. Since shrinkage is related to changes in the crystal structure, a factor affected by temperature (see below), it is probable that one will find variability in the degree of shrinkage in cremation as different bones may be subject to different temperatures. It had been noted, for example,[22] that a greater degree of shrinkage occurs at $> 600°C$ than at lower temperatures. Biological age also has an influence, reflecting the cross-linking of collagen with age, which provides resistance to movement.[22] The variability in shrinkage is likely to increase in pyre cremation (see below).

The 70% mineral component of bone comprises hydroxyapatite, a calcium phosphate, $Ca_{10} (PO_4)_6(OH)_2$. Changes in crystal structure have been linked to specific temperatures, although experimental results are not always in full agreement as to the nature of these changes, or when they occurr.[14,20,21] Shipman et al.[20] observed that following a break in the hydroxy bonds during dehydration, the crystals reformed in a larger size, first gradually up to 525°C, with a large increase to 645°C and almost no change beyond (maximum of 940°C). Lange et al.[14] record a reduction in crystal volume as a result of dehydration; slight between 150 and 300°C, followed, at about 800°C, by a 'sintering' process (localized melting) leading to increased reduction due to fusion of the crystal units. Holden et al.[21] observed recrystallization of the mineral commencing at 600°C, with crystal growth between 600 and 1000°C, the sintering process occurring at about 1000°C, and up to 1400°C, leading to fusion of the crystals (this sintering temperature is noted to give a standard minimum form by other workers[24,25]). A range of crystal structures was observed,[21] the changes being linked not just with temperature, but also the duration of heating and the age of the deceased, within three broad bands of young (< 22 years), adult (22–60) or old (> 60). During heating, pyrophosphate is produced at temperatures $> 600°C$, which, during the sintering process, leads to the formation of tricalcium phosphate in a variety of crystal forms.[14,22]

A knowledge of the mechanics of the cremation process, together with the methods which may be employed for ascertaining the 'efficiency' of cremation, provide the osteoarchaeologist with the potential for assessing pyre technology from cremated remains. It should be clear, however, that the relationship between factors affecting cremation is not a simple one, and even in modern crematoria there may be inexplicable variations from the norm. The effect of these factors on the body may also not be uniform, either between cremations or across individual cadavers.

PYRE CREMATION

Textual accounts and pictorial representations of ancient cremations[3,8,26] together with anthropological data[27–31] provide us with some information on the funerary procedure and beliefs.

Basic pyre structure appears to have remained relatively constant. It generally comprises a rectangle, which can vary in size, formed of layers of spaced timbers set at right angles and infilled with brushwood. The pyre performs two basic functions, being a fuel source and a stable support for the corpse and pyre goods (i.e. items placed on the pyre not just in the grave[11]) while allowing circulation of oxygen. Construction may be on a flat surface, such as in the cremation *ghat*s of India, or over a shallow scoop or pit[29] to provide an under-pyre draught.

Observation of experimental pyre cremations has demonstrated the temperatures which may be attained within the pyre (> 1000°C), the time taken to cremate, how the pyre collapses and the efficiency of cremation.[11,32–35] Although the basic process is the same as in modern crematoria, additional factors may affect an open pyre, and thereby, the efficiency of the cremation. For example, heat cannot be retained and circulated as in modern crematoria.[8] The highest temperatures are concentrated in the centre of the pyre[33] and parts of the corpse or pyre goods close to the peripheries will experience much lower temperatures. In addition to its cooling effect, a strong wind may cause the pyre to burn and collapse unevenly, potentially affecting the efficiency of cremation. A heavy downpour may curtail the process completely. The duration, and thereby the potential efficiency of cremation, is affected by the quantity of wood used to build the pyre. That the quantity of wood may vary, often according to the wealth of the deceased, is demonstrated in accounts of ancient cremations, e.g. that of Patroclos[36] or Imperial Romans,[26] and in reports from present day India.[3]

Duration has variously been quoted as 3 hrs (modern India), 7–8 hrs,[32] or 7–10 hrs for the pyre to cool sufficiently to collect the bone;[7] completion of cremation partly depends on how fully cremated the remains are required to be. Pyres that have largely burnt down after about 3 h may still be too hot to allow manual recovery of bone 10 hrs after lighting. Both the bone and, more significantly, the thoracic and abdominal soft tissues will continue to burn slowly on the remnants of the pyre for many hours in favourable weather conditions. This probably explains the common reference to bones being recovered the day after cremation.[7,28,29] The pyre gradually collapses down upon itself during cremation and, provided there was no manipulation during cremation and the body was placed on the top of the pyre, the skeletal remains (which appear just as those in modern crematoria before cremulation) will retain anatomical order and be clearly visible in the final stages.[11,35,37]

Interpretation of ancient pyre technology from cremated remains requires consideration of the additional potential variables of pyre cremation; including body position, location of the body on the pyre and the inhibition of oxygen supply to the corpse due to other inclusions on the pyre.[3,7,8]

AIMS AND METHODS OF ANALYSIS

The quantity and quality of retrievable demographic and pathological information is dependent on two factors: the degree of fragmentation and the level of skeletal recovery.

The size of bone fragments varies considerably, the identification of specific skeletal elements becoming harder with decreasing size, although specific skull elements are easily recognizable even as very small fragments and are useful since they often occur singly or in pairs (Figure 2). The major difficulty however, arises from the characteristic incomplete recovery of skeletal remains from pyres.[11] Frequently, 50% or less of the bone remaining after cremation was included in the burial, and of that only 30–50% may be identifiable to a specific skeletal element. While there is nothing intrinsically more difficult in ageing and sexing cremated human remains than those of unburnt skeletons, and the same criteria[38,39] may potentially be applied, inevitably, at least some of the elements of greatest use for assessment of age and sex will not be available for examination.

Number of individuals

The number of individuals within a deposit is demonstrated either by obvious age-related differences in bone size and development or by the duplication of identifiable bone fragments (Figures 2 and 3). The condition and integrity of the context must always be considered, e.g. a disturbed burial within a cemetery may be contaminated by bone from an adjacent burial.

It has been suggested that weights > 2141–2500 g are indicative of multiple burials.[8,14,23] However, greater weights have been recorded from single modern cremations; weights

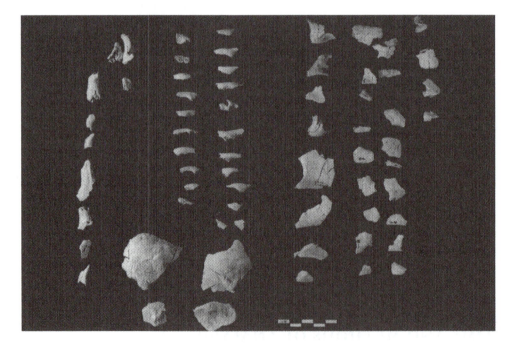

Figure 2 – Frequently recovered skull fragments; right and left malar processes (left), right and left zygomatic arches and tubercles (centre top), external occipital protuberances (centre bottom), left and right supra-orbits (right). Bronze Age cist grave, Trelowthas Barrow, Cornwall.

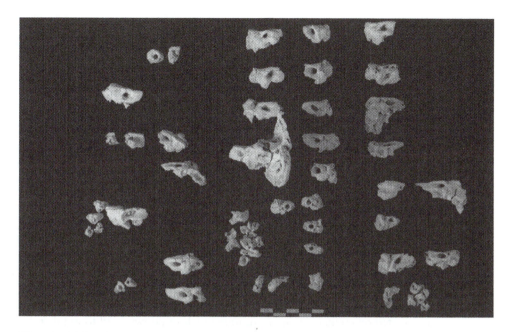

Figure 3 – Adult and immature petrous temporals from the Bronze Age cist grave, Trelowthas Barrow, Cornwall.

ranging from 57 to 3000 g have been recorded from undisturbed, archaeological burials of single adults, and multiple burials of two adults comprising < 2000 g are not infrequent, with far less being recorded from those of an adult and immature individual. A rare occasion where weight was indicative of multiple burials was the 9584.8 g, representing the remains of at least 19 individuals (duplicate petrous temporals) from a cist grave in Cornwall[11] (Figures 2 and 3). The use of different colours (see above[11]) is unreliable unless observed in duplicated bones. Apparent contradictions in sexual dimorphic traits between different skeletal elements are also unreliable, certainly within British populations where there can be great variability between groups and dimorphism of different traits within individual assemblages.[39] The suggested use of histological analysis of diaphyseal bone structures,[40] while having some possible potential, should be viewed with caution given the current levels of reliability of this method with respect to ageing cremated remains[41] (see below).

Age

Unerupted tooth crowns frequently survive cremation intact, protected within the supportive structure of the mandible or maxilla. The development and fusion of growth centres are often visibly detectable. However, since entire long bones are only very rarely recovered, recorded patterns of growth[42] cannot be applied, although diaphyseal diameters are sometimes used.[8,23]

Some methods for ageing adults[38] may only very rarely be applied to cremated remains, including dental attrition, and the morphology of the pubic symphysis, rib end and auricular surface of the ilium. The enamel of erupted teeth shatters during cremation, the only recognizable fragments often being the tooth roots; where enamel is recovered, insufficient generally remains from which to assess occlusal attrition. Pubic symphyses are uncommon (e.g. maximum 4% burials from an about 4000 sample), the sternal ends of ribs never having been noted.[8] Small parts of the auricular surface of the ilium are occasionally noted, but are rarely of sufficient size for assessment.

Cranial suture fusion is often relied on in the absence of any other criteria, skull vault being frequently recovered, usually with at least one fragment having evident sutures.[8,34] Broad age bands are applied (30+ years), but progressive suture fusion with age is only a general trend to which there will always be exceptions, and in the absence of any additional supportive evidence even broad groups are open to question.[38]

Application of histological ageing methods[38,43,44] has the potential to overcome the problems of fragmentation and the frequent lack of visible morphologically diagnostic features. Initial consideration of the specific potential for histological analysis of cremated diaphyseal bone[45,46] concluded that at < 700–800°C shrinkage would be minimal and the internal structures maintained intact. However, methods were developed for specific skeletal elements that may be missing or unidentifiable within cremation burials. Experiments conducted on cremated bone from individuals of known age[41] found that the best results were obtained using the qualitative method (comparison of a cross-section with unburnt reference material of known age) rather than quantitative (number of osteons within a given area). However, both tended to over-age young individuals (by up to 20 years) and underage the older ones (by up to 19 years), particularly at either end of the range; the average difference between chronological age and assessed age was 8.4 ± 6.5 years. It was concluded that the results with cremated bone were not as good as with unburnt material.[41]

The detrimental affect of shrinkage on any form of quantitative analysis is accepted[8,46,48] (see above). Recent experiments[22] concluded that because of shrinkage and fusion at > 600°C, microscopic ageing techniques relying upon measurements of the number of structural subunits within a given area (e.g. the packing density of osteons) were inappropriate. These observations support the consensus that quantitative methods should not be employed with cremated material.

The frequent recovery of tooth roots renders them a useful area of investigation. They are not subject to pathological changes in the same way as bone, and although potentially subject to variable shrinkage[47] the basic structure remains intact after cremation. Early attempts to apply the analysis of incremental lines in the dental cementum[43] to cremated remains failed to produce any useable sections,[8] however, recent analyses claim greater success.[48] The technique is time consuming (200× conventional light microscope, 100 μm thin sections), requiring 20 cross-sections/tooth to cover a representative area and overcome potential problems of insufficient light permeability.[48] Accuracy decreases where the sex is unknown and when it is unclear exactly which tooth is being analysed, both frequent problems with cremated remains (see below).[47] The effect of this is to reduce estimates from a potential ± 3.2 to ± 6.2 years.[48] It was concluded, however, that the method should not be used in isolation,[48] that potential problems include doubling of lines in 10% of cases and that the reliability of the technique decreases with age.[43]

It has been noted[22] that the structural changes occurring during heating are affected by the age of the individual (see above), and that broad age groups of adult (22–60 years) or old (60+) can be obtained by microscopic analysis. The lack of reliable results for older adults using other histological methods[22] illustrates the potential usefulness of this technique.

While offering the potential to provide closer ageing for many adult burials than with macroscopic techniques, the results currently available from histological analysis are of variable reliability. It is still preferable to use broad adult age groups, rather than stating a specific age in years,[38] even if this does lead to a restriction in demographic interpretation, to avoid basing any such analysis on potentially erroneous data.

Sex

Tests in modern crematoria, where the full skeletal remains of individuals of known sex were examined, have shown a high rate of accuracy in sexing using visual methods. In archaeological deposits, pelvic fragments are uncommon and often too small to enable confident sexing (Figure 4). Skull fragments are frequently found, and even small

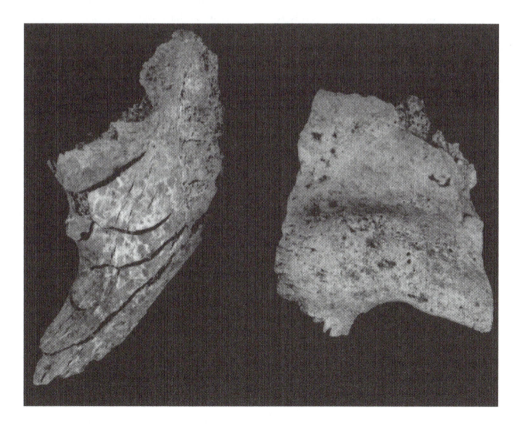

Figure 4 – Sexing; rare recovery of the pubic symphysis (left) and commonly occurring supra-orbital (right), both male.

fragments of, for example, supra-orbit, mastoid process, mandible, etc. (Figures 2–4) may assist in attribution of sex. Metric analysis of the teeth[39] is not possible other than with unerupted crowns in immature individuals. While general observation of size and robusticity might give further indication of the individual's sex, much of the usual metric analysis[39] is not possible with cremated remains due to fragmentation and incomplete skeletal recovery.

Schemes of measurements have been devised specifically for use in sexing cremated remains,[49–52] criteria being developed using cremated remains from modern crematoria (known sex and age). Gejvall's method[49,50] includes up to seven measurements taken from the skull vault, humerus, radius and femur. Using these criteria, Schutkowski and Herrmann[53] assigned a sex to a further 25% of previously unsexed adults in three assemblages of cremation burials. However, it has been suggested that the variability in skull vault and diaphyseal thickness is not sufficiently significant,[8] and the potential problems resulting from age and variable shrinkage have been highlighted. Further potential difficulties lay in correctly identifying the required bone fragments.[54] For example, one measurement, at the external occipital protuberance, is easily distinguished but another encompasses a large area of the vault within which maximum thickness is required. If only a few fragments from this area are recovered one cannot guarantee the thickest part is present, potentially biasing the results. Measurement of the humeral head would not be open to errors of identification, but the whole head is rarely recovered from archaeological cremation burials (about 4%). Similar problems of non-recovery or fragmentation also apply with respect to van Vark's 57 suggested measurements.[51,52]

The petrous temporal bone is frequently recovered, is easily identified even when fragmentary (Figure 3), and maintains its form in cremation. The high potential for application of a sexing technique based on this bone led Wahl to devise a series of five measurable variables.[7] The sample group of 125 comprised a non-homogeneous assemblage (about 1200-year span) of unburnt skeletal remains, the potential problem of shrinkage being countered by adjustments of 1.5–12% for the different variables (see above). The results demonstrated sexual dimorphism in the range of measurements for each variable, with suggested correct classification rates of 91.4% for unburnt bones and 80% for cremated bone, though large areas of overlap are apparent within some variables.[7] Lower correct classification rates of 70.2–76.6% for unburnt bones and 67.0–73.4% for cremated bones were produced on application of the technique to 94 individuals of known sex.[55]

Metric methods require a minimum dataset to be statistically viable. Van Vark[56] advocated a minimum assemblage size of ten for calculation of dimorphism, using more than one (preferably five) comparable measurements per burial.[51,52] Consequently, the practical application of some of these methods is, unfortunately, often limited. The potential problem of variable shrinkage[8] must always be considered. The most secure results are likely to be obtained via a combination of morphometric methods; the use of a single trait of either form being unreliable. All identifications should be accompanied by a confidence rating.

Currently, little has been attempted with respect to the possible application of DNA analysis to cremated remains. The technique requires the retention of sufficient organic components in a suitable condition for analysis,[57,58] and the successful extraction of protein (albumin) from archaeological cremated bone[59] suggests that this may occur in some cases. Complete oxidation of the bone was not always attained in ancient cremations (see above) and certain skeletal elements (those with the greatest soft tissue coverage) may prove suitable for analysis. The occasional survival of charred soft tissue fragments[3,35,60] also offers analytical potential, although the suitability of this material has yet to be investigated.

Skeletal Indices

Most standard skeletal indices cannot be calculated, though there are very exceptional circumstances where calculation of cranial indices has been achieved.[61] Stature estimates using standard regression equations[62] have been made from the estimated lengths of radii, humeri and femora calculated from the diameters of the respective articular heads.[63–66] Databases of variable size were used to calculate correlations between head diameter and long bone length.[63,64] Varying shrinkage factors are advocated (e.g. 12%,[23] 1.4%,[63] or none[64]). Rösing's conversion tables[23] (diameter of heads to estimated stature for both sexes) are derived from combined regression equations,[64,66] noting the 'considerable statistical error' of ± 6.9 to ± 8.6 cm. Müller[63] claims accuracy of ± 7.5 cm for individuals of known sex, increasing to ± 10 cm for those of indeterminate sex.

The potential inaccuracies, chiefly resulting from shrinkage and high statistical error, are discussed by Holck.[8] Failure to take shrinkage into account will inevitably result in the under-estimation of stature.[7] The characteristic problems of incomplete skeletal recovery and fragmentation leads to limited applicability.[3,8] For example, in > 4000 British cremation burials analysed by the writer, the complete femoral head was recovered in < 0.5% (and in some of these the characteristic concentric fissuring of the head rendered measurement impossible; Figure 1), the complete humeral head in < 1%, and the radial head in about 5%.

Pathology

Reliable diagnoses of pathological conditions require full (or close to full) skeletal recovery, consequently the limitations with cremated remains will be self-evident. The same range of pathological lesions can be observed as in unburnt bone[3,7,8,67] but the observance of lesions is as, if not more, dependant on the condition of the bone as it is on the prevalence of diseases. For example, the 6.4% of burials containing bones with lesions from a Norwegian sample of 1082,[8] compared with the 30.6% from an English sample of 2284,[3] is likely to reflect bone preservation rather than genuine frequency of lesions.

Some conditions, for example osteoporosis, predispose bone to disintegrate during cremation.[2] Identifiable dental diseases tend to be limited to those affecting the supportive structure, but carious lesions may be recognized where they have affected the roots.[3] Cuts, to both human and animal bone, have been recognized,[8,68] but the numbers of fractures and other injuries noted are relatively low, probably as a direct consequence of cremation.[8] Some rarer conditions have been noted in cremated remains, e.g. trepanation,[69] weapon injuries,[70] calcified lymph nodes,[3,71] gallstones[3,72] and DISH.[73]

Interpretation of pyre technology and ritual

Not all deposits containing cremated bone represent the remains of a cremation burial. Pyre sites, cleared or uncleared of their debris, are found[74–77] and clearance of pyre sites resulted in redeposition of pyre debris.[11,78,79] Each of these ritual acts bore significance to the mortuary rite, and their physical remains need to be excavated and analysed appropriately if we are to expand our understanding of funerary practices and beliefs.[11,80,81]

All cremation-related deposits should be subject to whole-earth recovery; the level of division of individual deposits into subcontexts during excavation will depend on the type (i.e. pyre site, burial, redeposited pyre debris) and size of the deposit, and the level of disturbance.[80,82] Different types of deposit may comprise similar archaeological components (i.e. cremated bone, fuel ash, pyre goods, etc.), often it is only the physical and stratigraphic relationships between the components that hold the clue to the nature of the deposit and the formation processes. At minimum, contexts should initially be half-sectioned to enable the vertical distribution of archaeological components to be recorded, the relative three-dimensional distribution being noted throughout. Disturbance may affect the original order of deposition of remains, bone fragment size[2] and, in cases of heavy truncation, some loss of bone may occur. Recording the pre-excavation maximum bone fragment size provides a check against which to compare the maximum size noted during osteological analysis. Cremated bone is very brittle and, even where great care is exercised, on lifting it tends to fracture along dehydration fissures formed in cremation;[2] because the broken surfaces are engrained with the burial matrix, the amount of fragmentation occurring post- rather than pre-excavation may be difficult to deduce. Following floatation for the recovery of material such as charred plant remains where appropriate, the whole-earth 'samples' should be *carefully* wet-sieved to 1 mm fraction-size;[81,82] this serves to ensure complete recovery of all the bone and is the easiest way of cleaning bone before analysis. It is essential that the osteologist considers both the context and its integrity during analysis, as both may affect interpretation, e.g. was the burial urned/unurned, soil pH, level of disturbance, etc.[7,80]

The positions in which a corpse may have been placed on the pyre are illustrated from anthropological sources (see above).[7] They may also be inferred from the distribution of cremated remains within *in situ* combined pyre/grave,[33,74] and the adherence of pyre goods to specific skeletal elements.[3] The formation processes attendant on subsequent parts of the mortuary rites may also be illustrated.[11,83]

Efficiency of cremation and potential technical problems may be deduced using knowledge gained from modern crematoria, experimental work, and anthropological sources (see above). Temperatures attained in different areas of the pyre during cremation may be gauged using the visual and microscopic criteria discussed above, as well as the appearance of pyre goods and pyre debris.[3] Geographic and temporal variations in efficiency have also been noted.[8,35]

References to pyres being deliberately extinguished[7] are not entirely corroborated by experimental work[35] and, in the absence of any urgency over access to the pyre site, this would not have been necessary. There are also references to 'quenching' or ritual 'washing'[35] and these practices are likely to have been more common. Experiments have demonstrated the naturally 'clean' appearance of bone at the end of cremation[35,37], indicating that washing the bone[7] was probably for ritual rather than practical purposes.

The weight of bone collected for burial varied both geographically and temporally. Average weights from Norway,[8] for example (269.7 g single burials, 985.2 g dual burials) are relatively low compared with those from British burials (see above), suggesting that in general the entire cremated remains were not collected. The reasons for variations in bone weights are unclear. Evidence to suggest male burials on average incorporated larger quantities of bone than female ones[7] are not necessarily statistically significant, and there are large overlaps in the weight ranges. Suggestions such as only the largest fragments or only about half the cremated remains were collected for burial,[7] are not supported by the skeletal elements recovered or the bone weights recorded from individual burials (see above). Possibly of relevance is the *consistently* high weights of bone recovered from British Bronze Age 'primary' burials (average weight 1525.7 g[11]) the 'status' of the deceased possibly being reflected in the time expended collecting bone for burial.

An apparently random selection of skeletal elements generally appears to be represented in deposits.[7] What may appear to be a predominance of skull fragments is, in most cases, indicative of preferential survival and the ease with which skull fragments may be recognized. Rare cases where skull is absent from an assemblage are likely to represent deliberate exclusion. One observation (a single site[84]) that specific skeletal elements were more common in burials of one or other sex is currently uncorroborated.

The size of bone fragments is affected by several factors.[3,4,7] In Wahl's[7] review, 80% of fragments were between 10 and 50 mm in length and he suggested that bones had been ritually broken to fit the burial container. Other studies indicate an absence of conclusive evidence for deliberate bone breakage and show that much fragmentation occurs after burial along the dehydration fissures formed during cremation.[4] Temporal and geographic variations in practice are possible, with slight differences in modes of tending and collection affecting bone fragment size.

There has been relatively little attention as to how bone was collected from the pyre for burial, the general assumption being that individual fragments were recovered manually once the pyre had cooled.[7] This would have been a relatively simple task, the buff/white cremated bone being easily visible and accessible at the end of cremation (see above), but time consuming (estimated up to 4 hrs person-time for complete recovery[35]). Other possible modes of recovery have been suggested, such as raking-off of bone and winnowing.[3,11] Again, it is likely that practices varied both over time and between different geographical areas. The deposition of pyre debris after collection of the bone for formal burial may take a variety of forms.[11] Analysis of material from these deposits and comparison with that recovered from contemporaneous burials and pyre sites is increasing our understanding of mortuary rites.[11,79,83,85]

Although the ordered deposition of skeletal elements in burials has been observed in rare instances, the overwhelming majority show random deposition.[7] Not only skeletal elements, but also multiples of individuals and animal bones (pyre goods) within a burial have been mixed throughout.[3,35,54]

A distinction needs to be made between multiple cremations (corpses cremated on the same pyre), multiple burials (one vessel/grave used for simultaneous burial of remains from separate cremations) and multiple graves (remains of separate cremations and burials made in one grave). The two former categories may be difficult to distinguish from each other. Several studies have shown similar frequencies of dual cremations/burial, for example 4.4%[8] and 3%[34] from Scandinavian assemblages, the majority being of two adults (usually a female and a male), concluding that burials including immature individuals were under-estimated. About 5% of burials in British assemblages are dual, usually comprising an immature individual with an adult of either sex, but most frequently with a female.[11] Theories regarding dual cremations/burials include possible instances where an urn may have remained unburied until the bones from a second pyre were included,[7] as, for example, in a Bronze Age burial from Hampshire[11,86] where the remains of one of the identified adults were confined to the lower half of the urn and those of the second adult to the upper half. In most cases, however, thorough mixing of the remains suggests dual cremation occurred, rather than just dual burial. Whatever the reasons behind the practice, the physical proximity in death is likely to mirror close relations (friend, relative, etc.) in life,[3] though some theories favour sacrifice for cases of males and females buried/cremated together.[7]

Cremation burials commonly include cremated animal bone, distinguishable from the human bone in terms of size, density and morphology.[3,7,8] However, there are rare occasions, where fragments are very small and/or the visible morphology eroded, where conclusive identification is difficult. In these cases, differences in the microstructure of the bone could be used.[8,40,87] Cremated animal bone may be encountered in burials of all periods, although there is a change in the frequency of occurrence, quantity, number and type of species over time. There is a progressive increase from the Bronze Age (about 16% of British burials, little bone, one to two species) to the Anglo-Saxon period (about 50% of burials, > 100 g of bone, one to five species[3]). The remains generally represent pyre goods, for example food, amuletic, pets or indicators of status,[3,8,34,68,88–92] though some are believed to be remnants of funeral feasts.[7] A variety of contemporaneous accounts gives insights into the role of animals in the rites and rituals of cremation[26,36,93] where they invariably represent offerings to, or companions for the dead.

CONCLUSION

The development of more reliable, applicable and accessible methods of ageing and sexing will have a major impact on cremation cemetery studies, both from the point of new demographic research and to aid the interpretation of status and gender as reflected through pyre goods and grave goods. Advances have undoubtedly being made in metric and microscopic methods, but the latter often follow in the wake of developments aimed at unburnt material. The immense potential of DNA analysis has yet to be realised, almost nothing having yet been done with respect to cremated remains.

It is necessary to focus on devising methods which will be commonly applicable to cremated remains, using fragments which occur frequently and are of distinctive appearance.[7,48] Microscopic methods would benefit from more detailed research concentrating on cremated remains and preferably using reference material of known age and sex, enabling the specific problems of cremated remains to be tackled directly, rather than being tagged on as an after-thought. The formation of more extensive reference collections based on such data, including specimens produced at different temperatures, should help in overcoming potential problems arising from comparing burnt material with unburnt specimens. Laboratory instrumentation techniques also need to be made more accessible in terms of cost, equipment and expertise, certainly in the UK (this type of analysis being already routinely undertaken in some countries); the answer may lie in the development of laboratories that can provide specialist services. Meanwhile we need to be realistic and accept the limitations imposed by the material and the reliability of our means of analysing it. Better this than potentially misleading ourselves and others.

Myriad unanswered questions remain with respect to specific facets of the rites and rituals of cremation. The growing detailed data assemblages being accumulated from different periods over large geographic areas mean that more detailed comparison of specific rituals should now be possible, moving beyond the past focus on the pyre goods with which an individual was cremated or the grave goods with which they were buried (the significance of even this distinction has yet to be fully realised). Pyre technology may be compared, together with individual facets of ritual as reflected in the mode of deposition and condition of the cremated remains. For this, data records need to be of a comparable nature and, equally important, primary data recovery on site needs to ensure full recovery and recording.

ACKNOWLEDGEMENTS

I thank Elaine Wakefield of Wessex Archaeology for producing the Figures, and Jacqueline Nowakowski of the Cornwall Archaeological Unit for permission to reproduce Figures 2 and 3.

REFERENCES

1   McKinley JI. Cremations: expectations, methodologies and realities. In: Roberts CA, Lee F, Bintliff J (eds), *Burial Archaeology; Current Research, Methods and Developments* British Archaeological Reports, British Series 211. Oxford: British Archaeological Reports, 1989: pp. 65–76.

2   McKinley JI. Bone fragment size and weights of bone from modern British cremations and its implications for the interpretation of archaeological cremations. *International Journal of Osteoarchaeology* 1993; **3**: 283–287.

3   McKinley JI. *The Anglo-Saxon Cemetery at Spong Hill, North Elmham Part VIII: The Cremations.* Report No. 69. Dereham: East Anglian Archaeology, 1994.

4   McKinley JI. Bone fragment size in British cremation burials and its implications for pyre technology and ritual. *Journal of Archaeological Science* 1994; **21**: 339–342.

5   Evans WED. *The Chemistry of Death.* Springfield: Charles C Thomas, 1963.

6   Polson CJ, Marshall TK. *The Disposal of the Dead* (3rd edn). London: English Universities Press, 1975.

7   Wahl J. Leichenbranduntersuchungen. Ein überblick über die bearbeitungs- und aussagemöglichkeiten von Brandgräbern *Prähistorische Zeitschrift* 1982; **57**: 1–125.

8   Holck P. *Cremated Bones: A Medical–Anthropological Study of an Archaeological Material on Cremation Burials.* Anthropologiske skrifter Nr.1. Oslo: Anatomisk Institutt, University of Oslo, 1986.

9 Glorieux FH. Mineral. In: Cruess RL. *The Musculoskeletal System* Edinburgh: Churchill Livingstone, 1982: pp. 97–106.

10 Anon., personal communication.

11 McKinley JI. Bronze Age 'barrows' and funerary rites and rituals of cremation. *Proceedings of the Prehistoric Society* 1997; **63**: 129–145.

12 Holck P. Why are small children so seldom found in cremations? In: Smits E, Iregren E, Drusini AG (eds), *Cremation Studies in Archaeology* (Symposium Proceedings) Saonara: Logos, 1997: pp. 33–38.

13 Oxford English Dictionary. Oxford: Clarendon, 1973.

14 Lange M, Schutkowski H, Hummel S, Herrmann B. *A Bibliography on Cremations* (PACT) Rixensart: Hackens, 1987.

15 Krogman WM. *A Guide to the Identification of Human Skeletal Material*. FBI Law Enforcement Bulletin, vol. 8, no. 8. Washington, DC: Federal Bureau of Investigation, 1939.

16 Webb WS, Snow CE. *The Adena People*. Reports in Archaeology and Anthropology 6. Lexington: University of Kentucky, 1945.

17 Baby RS. *Hopewell Cremation Practices*. Papers in Archaeology 1. Columbus: Ohio Historical Society, 1954.

18 Binford LR. An analysis of cremations from three Michigan sites. *Wisconsin Archaeologist* 1963; **44**: 98–110.

19 Thurman MD, Wilmore LJ. A replicative cremation experiment. *North American Archaeologist* 1981; **2**: 275–283.

20 Shipman P, Foster G, Schoeninger M. Burnt bones and teeth, an experimental study of colour, morphology, crystal structure and shrinkage. *Journal of Archaeological Science* 1984; **11**: 307–325.

21 Holden JL, Phakey PP, Clement JG. Scanning electron microscope observations of incinerated human femoral bone: a case study. *Forensic Science International* 1995; **74**: 17–28.

22 Holden JL, Phakey PP, Clement JG. Scanning electron microscope observations of heat-treated human bone. *Forensic Science International* 1995; **74**: 29–45.

23 Rösing FW. Methoden und aussagemöglichkeiten der anthropologischen leichenbrandbearbeitung. *Archäologie und Naturwissenschaeften* 1977; **1**: 53–80.

24 Williams RAD. *Basic and Applied Dental Biochemistry*. Edinburgh: Churchill Livingstone, 1979.

25 Pollard M, personal communication.

26 Toynbee JMC. *Death and Burial in the Roman World*. London: John Hopkins, 1996.

27 Wahl J, Wahl S. Zur Technik de Lichenverbrennung: I. Verbrennungsplätze aus ethnologischen quellen. *Archäologisches Korrespondenzblatt* 1983; **13**: 513–520.

28 Dubois JA, Beauchamp HR. *Hindu Manners, Customs and Ceremonies* Oxford: Clarendon, 1943.

29 Hiatt B. Cremation in aboriginal Australia. *Mankind* 1969; **7**: 104–115.

30 Pautreau JP. Quelques aspects des cremations contemporaries en Asie de Sud-Est. In: Lambot B, Friboulet M, Méniel P. *Le site Protohistorique D'Acy-Romance (Ardennes) – II; Les Necropoles dans ler contexte régional* Reims: Memoire de la Societe Archeologique Champenoise 8, 1994: pp. 306–315.

31 Downes J. Cremation: a spectacle and a journey. In: Downes J, Pollard T (eds), *The Loved Body's Corruption*. Glasgow: Cruithne, 1999: pp. 19–29.

32 Piontek J. The process of cremation and its influence on the morphology of bones in the light of results of experimental research. *Archeologica Polski* 1976; **21**: 247–280.

33 Lambot B, Friboulet M, Méniel P. *Le Site Protohistorique D'Acy-Romance (Ardennes) – II; Les Necropoles dans ler Contexte Régional* Reims: Memoire de la Societe Archeologique Champenoise 8, 1994.

34 Sigvallis B. *Funeral Pyres. Iron Age Cremations in North Spånga*. Theses and papers in Osteology 1. Stockholm: Stockholm University, 1994.

35 McKinley JI. The cremated human bone from burials and cremation-related contexts. In: Fitzpatrick AP. *Westhampnett, West Sussex, vol. 2: The Iron Age, Romano-British and Anglo-Saxon Cemeteries Excavated in 1992*. Report No. 12. Salisbury: Trust for Wessex Archaeology, 1997: pp. 55–72.

36 Homer. *Iliad*, translated by Rieu EV. Harmondsworth: Penguin, 1966.

37   Méniel P. Les restes animaux du bucher. In: Lambot B, Friboulet M, Méniel P. *Le site Protohistorique D'Acy-Romance (Ardennes) – II; Les Necropoles dans ler contexte régional* Reims: Memoire de la Societe Archeologique Champenoise 8, 1994: pp. 283–286.

38   Cox M. Ageing adults from the skeleton (Chapter 5 – this volume).

39   Mays S, Cox M. Sex determination in skeletal remains (Chapter 8 – this volume).

40   Cuijpers SAGFM. Possibilities of histological research on diaphyseal fragments in cremated remains. In: Smits E, Iregren E, Drusini AG (eds), *Cremation Studies in Archaeology* (Symposium Proceedings). Saonara: Logos, 1997: pp. 73–86.

41   Hummel S, Schutkowski H. Approaches to the histological age determination of cremated human remains. In: Grupe G, Garland AN (eds), *Histology of Ancient Human Bone: Methods and Diagnosis.* London: Springer, 1993: pp. 111–123.

42   Bass W. *Human Osteology: A Laboratory and Field Manual* (3rd edn). Special publication 2. Columbia: Missouri Archaeological Society, 1987.

43   Whittaker D. Ageing from the dentition (Chapter 6 – this volume).

44   Bell LS, Piper K. An introduction to palaeohistopathology (Chapter 16 – this volume).

45   Herrmann B. Möglichkeiten histologischer untersuchungen an leichenbränden. *Mitteilungen der Berliner Gesellschaft für Anthropologie, Ethnologie und Urgeschicte* 1973; **2**: 164–167.

46   Herrmann B. On histological investigations of cremated human remains *Journal of Human Evolution* 1977; **6**: 101–103.

47   Chandler NP. Cremated teeth. *Archaeology Today* 1987; August: 41–45.

48   Grosskopf B. Counting incremental lines in teeth – a valid method for age determination in cremations. In: Smits E, Iregren E, Drusini AG (eds), *Cremation Studies in Archaeology* (Symposium Proceedings). Saonara: Logos, 1997: pp. 87–94.

49   Gejvall NG. Cremations. In: Brothwell D, Higgs E (eds), *Science in Archaeology* (2nd edn). London: Thames & Hudson, 1969: pp. 468–479.

50   Gejvall NG. Determination of burned bones from prehistoric graves: Observations on the cremated bones from the graves at Horn. *Ossa, Letters* 1981: 2.

51   Van Vark GN. The investigation of human cremated skeletal material by multivariate statistical methods, I. Methodology. *Ossa* 1974; **1**: 63–95.

52   Van Vark GN. The investigation of human cremated skeletal material by multivariate statistical methods, II. Measures. *Ossa* 1975; **2**: 47–68.

53   Schutkowski H, Herrmann B. Variabilitätsvergleich von wandstärken für die geschlechts-zuweisung an leichenbränden. *Anthropologischer Anzeiger* 1987; **45**: 43–47.

54   McKinley JI. Cremated Bone. In: Timby J, Sancton I. Anglo-Saxon cemetery excavations carried out between 1976 and 1980. *Archaeological Journal* 1993; **150**: 243–365.

55   Schutkowski H, Herrmann B. Zur möglichkeit der metrischen geschlechtsdiagnose an der pars petrosa ossis temporalis. *Zeitschrift für Rechtsmedizin* 1983; **90**: 219–227.

56   Van Vark GN, personal communication.

57   Brown KA. Gender and sex – what can ancient DNA tell us? *Ancient Biomolecules* 1998; **2**: 3–15.

58   Brown KA. Ancient DNA applications in human osteoarchaeology: achievements, problems and potential (Chapter 27 – this volume).

59   Cattaneo C, Gelsthorpe K, Sokol RJ, Phillips P. Immunological detection of albumin in ancient human cremations using ELISA and monoclonal antibodies. *Journal of Archaeological Science* 1994; **21**: 565–571.

60   Buikstra JE, Swegle M. Bone modification due to burning: experimental evidence. In: Bonnichern R, Sorg MH (eds), *Peopling of the Americas.* University of Maine: Centre for the Study of the First Americans, Institute of Quaternary Studies, 1989: pp. 247–258.

61   Wiercinka A. The methods of anthropological investigations of cremated bones in Poland. *Actes di VII Congrès International des Sciences Préhistoriques et Protohistoriques, Prague, 21–22 ao–t 1966.* Academia, Praha: l'Academie Tchécoloslovaque des Sciences, 1970.

62   Olivier G, Tissier H. Détermination de la stature et de la capacité cranienne. *Buletins et Mémoires du Société d'Anthropologie de Paris* 1975; **2**: 297–306.

63   Müller C. Schätzung der köperhöhe bei funden von leichenbränden. *Ausgrabungen und Funde* 1958; **2**: 52–58.

64   Gralla G. Próba Rekonstruckcji Wzrostu ze szczatków ciaopalnych. *Materiaty Prace Antropologiczne* 1964; **70**: 95–98.

65   Strzalko J. O odtwarzaniu dlugosci kosci ramiennej, i udowej na podstawie pomiarów ich głów. *Przeglad Antropologiczny* 1966; **32**: 261–268.

66   Malinowski A. Synthéses des recherches polonaises effectuées jus qud présent sur les os des tombes à incineration *Przeglad Antropologiczny* 1969; **35**: 141.

67   von Grimm H. Palaeopathology in a series of cremated bones. *Humanbiologia Budapestinensis* 1982; **10**: 81–89.

68   Bond J. The cremated animal bone. In: McKinley JI. *The Anglo-Saxon Cemetery at Spong Hill, North Elmham Part VIII: The Cremations*. Report No. 69. Dereham: East Anglian Archaeology, 1994: pp. 121–135.

69   von Grimm H. Anthropologische Ergebnisse der Untersuchung von Leichenbrandresten der Schönfelder, Einzelgrab- und Kugelamphorenkultur. *Jahresschrift für Mitteldeutsche Vorgeschichte* 1974; **58**: 265–274.

70   Musgrave JH. The skull of Philip II of Macedon. In: Lisney SJW, Matthews B (eds), *Current topics in Oral Biology*. Bristol: University of Bristol Press, 1985: pp. 1–16.

71   Garland N. Histological analysis of the calcined masses. In: McKinley JI. *The Anglo-Saxon cemetery at Spong Hill, North Elmham Part VIII: The Cremations*. Report No. 69. Dereham: East Anglian Archaeology, 1994: p. 135.

72   Schutkowski H, Hummel S, Gehner S. Case report 8 (cremated urinary calculi). *Palaeopathology Newsletter* 1986; **55**: 11–12.

73   Smits E, Verhart LMB, Cuijpers SAGFM, Grosskopf B. The chieftain's grave of Oss. In: Smits E, Iregren E, Drusini AG (eds), *Cremation Studies in Archaeology* (Symposium Proceedings). Saonara: Logos, 1997: pp. 95–102.

74   Sjosvard L, Vretemark M, Gustavson H. *Vendal Warrior from Vallentuna*. Stockholm: Vendal Period Studies 2, 1983.

75   Downes J. Linga Fold. *Current Archaeology* 1995; **142**: 396–399.

76   Downes J. *Linga Fold, Sandwick, Orkney; Excavation of a Bronze Age Barrow Cemetery 1994*. GUARD 59.2. Glasgow: Glasgow University Archaeological Research Division, 1995.

77   Fitzpatrick AP. *Westhampnett, West Sussex*, vol. 2: *The Iron Age, Romano-British and Anglo-Saxon Cemeteries Excavated in 1992*. Report No. 12. Salisbury: Trust for Wessex Archaeology, 1997.

78   Wenham LP. *The Romano-British Cemetery at Trentholme Drive, York*. London: HMSO, 1968.

79   Polfer M. La nécrople gallo-romaine de Septfontaines-Deckt (Grand-Duché de Luxembourge) et son *ustrinum* central: analyse comparative de matériel archéologique. In: Fredière A (ed.), *Monde des Mortes, Monde des Vivants en Gaule Rurale*. Tours: Acytes des colloque AGER/ARCHEA 1993: pp. 173–176.

80   McKinley JI. Archaeological manifestations of cremation. *The Archaeologist* 1998; **33**: 18–20.

81   McKinley JI. Putting cremated human remains in context. In: Roskams S (ed.), *Interpreting Stratigraphy*. York (in press).

82   McKinley JI, Roberts C. *Excavation and Post-Excavation Treatments of Cremated and Inhumed Human Remains*. Technical Paper 13. Birmingham: Institute of Field Archaeologists, 1993.

83   Schucany C. *Eine Grabanlage im Römischen Gutshof von Biberist-Spitalhof*. Basel: Archäologie der Schweiz, 1995.

84   Robertson D, personal communication.

85   Cosack E. *Das sachsische Graberfeld bei Liebenau*, vol. 1. Berlin: Mann, 1983.

86   McKinley JI. Human bone and funerary deposits. In: Walker KE, Farwell DE. *Twyford Down, Hampshire. Archaeological Investigations on the M3 Motorway Bar End to Compton 1990–1993*. Monograph 9. Salisbury: Hampshire Field Club, 1999: pp. 85–117 (in press).

87   Harsanyi L. Differential diagnosis of human and animal bone. In: Grupe G, Garland AN (eds), *Histology of Ancient Human Bone: Methods and Diagnosis*. Berlin: Springer 1993: pp. 79–94.

88   Sigvallis B. Animals in Iron Age cremations in Central Sweden. In: Smits E, Iregren E, Drusini AG (eds), *Cremation Studies in Archaeology* (Symposium Proceedings). Saonara: Logos, 1997: pp. 39–49.

89   Bond J. Cremated Animal Bone. In: Timby J, Sancton I. Anglo-Saxon cemetery excavations carried out between 1976 and 1980. *Archaeological Journal* 1993; **150**: 300–308.

90   Lepetz S. Les restes animaux dans les sépultures Gallo-Romaines. In: Ferdière A. *Monde des Morts, Monde des Vivants en Gaule Rural*. Tours: FERACF, 1993.

91   von Sten S, Vretemark M. Osteologische analysen knochenreicher Brandgräber der jüngeren Eisenzeit in Schweden. *Zeitschrift fuer Archaeologie* 1992; **26**; 87–103.

92   Müller HH. Tierreste in brandnestattungen unf ihre bedeutung für die rekonstruktion der bestattungssitten. In: Horst F, Keiling H (eds), *Bestattungswesen und Totenkult*. Berlin: Akademie, 1991: pp. 377–380.

93   Brøndsted J. *The Vikings*. Harmondsworth: Penguin, 1965.

Section VI

Microscopic, biochemical and analytical approaches

This final section comprises a group of contributions examining specific aspects of osteological analysis and research.

Stable isotope analysis of skeletal remains is examined by Simon Mays. He begins by explaining the background science, before moving on to consider the archaeological applications of stable isotope analysis using both bone collagen and apatite. Such analyses can explore ancient dietary practices, and through this, changes in subsistence strategies, weaning practices in earlier populations, and questions of differential access to foodstuffs according to gender or social position. Isotope ratios can also reflect local geology so can be used to investigate mobility of past human groups, and they can also provide insights into past climates.

Christina Nielsen-Marsh and colleagues introduce the reader to aspects of bone diagenesis. While acknowledging the role of autolysis and microorganisms on fleshed cadavers in the early post-mortem period, they focus on the transition of bone from its immediate post-mortem state, with a high lipid content and intact collagen, to that devoid of both. The authors consider some of the key variables determining bone survival including bone porosity and the hydrological regime of the burial environment.

Keri Brown explores the scientific principles, methodological issues and the history of the study of DNA from human skeletal remains. She discusses the application of analysis of human DNA for sex identification and kinship analysis, and the identification of disease by the detection of traces of DNA left in the bones by infecting microorganisms that were present in the body at time of death. Both the potential and the limitations of DNA work are considered.

John Robb examines the analysis of osteological data starting from the all too true premise that, for many osteologists 'hell is statistics'. His lucid exposition clearly demonstrates that without appropriate analytical tools, data collection is a futile exercise. He discusses the nature of osteological data and provides us with a brief guide to selecting the correct techniques for data analysis. He stresses the importance of incorporating the needs of data analysis into research designs.

In the final chapter in this volume Sue Black examines the demanding requirements of forensic osteology. She gives a brief tour of the particular requirements of the judicial process and the pitfalls which may await the unwary. She compares the nascent state of the subject in the UK with its status in the USA, where it makes an important contribution to the legal process. She points out that although forensic osteology is still in its infancy in the UK, it is likely that it will in future assume a greater role in the judicial system.

25

NEW DIRECTIONS IN THE ANALYSIS OF STABLE ISOTOPES IN EXCAVATED BONES AND TEETH

Simon Mays

INTRODUCTION

Isotopes are atoms of an element having different masses. Most elements exist naturally as mixtures of two or more isotopes. Some isotopes, such as carbon–14, are radioactive and hence steadily decay, transmuting into other elements. Others are not radioactive, but are stable. For example, the elements that together make up about two-thirds of bone collagen by weight, carbon and nitrogen, each occur in two stable isotopic forms. Those of carbon have mass 12 and 13 (written as ^{12}C and ^{13}C), those of nitrogen mass 14 and 15 (^{14}N and ^{15}N). Their different masses mean that isotopes fractionate in natural processes, so stable isotope ratios may differ in different parts of the natural environment and in different biological materials. Differences in isotopic ratios are generally quite small, so stable isotope ratios are not normally written simply as a ratio of one isotope to another, but are measured in δ units and expressed as parts per thousand (‰). Delta units measure the deviation in the isotope ratio from that in an accepted standard material. Most biological materials contain less ^{13}C than the mineral used as the standard; hence $\delta^{13}C$ is generally negative. The majority of biological tissues contains more ^{15}N than the standard (air), so $\delta^{15}N$ is usually greater than zero.

In the cases of carbon and nitrogen, different classes of food differ in their stable isotope ratios. For carbon isotope values there are two groups of plants: those which use the C3 photosynthetic pathway (most temperate zone vegetation) are more depleted in ^{13}C (i.e. have more negative δ) than do those using the C4 pathway (some tropical and subtropical vegetation, including important cultigens such as maize). Marine organisms differ from terrestrial ones; their $\delta^{13}C$ is intermediate between those of C3 and C4 terrestrial foods. Marine and terrestrial foods also differ in $\delta^{15}N$, the former being enriched with ^{15}N compared with the latter. Carbon and nitrogen stable isotope values for different foods are shown in Figure 1.

Stable carbon and nitrogen isotope ratios of animal tissues show a firm relationship with those in foods eaten: the $\delta^{13}C$ of human bone collagen is about 5‰ less negative than diet;

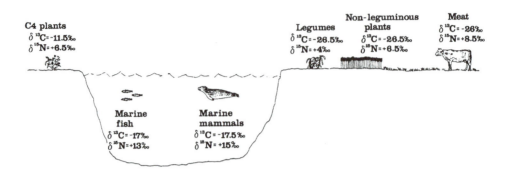

C3 environment

Figure 1 – Approximate mean carbon and nitrogen stable isotope values for some major food classes. Values are estimates of those obtaining in antiquity, i.e. they are adjusted to take into account the effects of fossil fuel burning and chemical fertilizers on modern values. Reproduced from Mays.[1]

the $\delta^{15}N$ of collagen is 2–3‰ greater than diet.[2,3] Hence, bone stable isotope ratios can be used to study ancient diets. Most of the carbon stable isotope work using human remains has focused on investigation of marine or C4 contributions to early diets. Nitrogen isotope values may be utilized to investigate the importance of marine foods, or can be used in conjunction with carbon values to elucidate diets which potentially have both C4 and marine components (Figure 2).

Bone collagen is slowly turned over throughout life. Turnover rates are poorly documented, but complete replacement may take 10–30 years in the adult.[2] For an adult skeleton, collagen stable isotope determinations therefore give a long-term indication of diet. Carbon in collagen comes mainly from protein but there may be some contributions from other foods, particularly when diets are low in protein. Collagen $\delta^{13}C$ therefore largely reflects dietary protein.[4,5] Virtually all nitrogen in diet comes from protein, so nitrogen stable isotope values tell us about dietary protein.

Intact collagen preserves *in vivo* isotope ratios (which is why it has always been the bone component of choice for radiocarbon determinations). It has been shown[6] that during diagenesis a collagen-like amino acid profile (implying the presence of intact collagen) persists until about 5% of the original protein content remains. Workers using collagen therefore generally either restrict dietary analyses to bone retaining at least 5% of its original protein, or else verify the presence of intact collagen using amino acid analysis.[7]

ARCHAEOLOGICAL APPLICATIONS OF STABLE ISOTOPE WORK

Studies using bone collagen

A major application of the carbon isotope work has been the study of the rise of maize agriculture in North America.[8] For example, in eastern North America maize cobs start

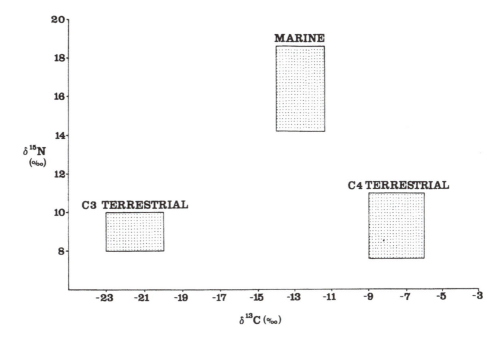

Figure 2 – Approximate human bone collagen carbon and nitrogen stable isotope ratios expected for archaeological populations consuming pure C3, C4 and marine diets. Reproduced from Mays.[1]

appearing on settlement sites from about 200 AD. However, stable isotope work has revealed that maize did not in general begin to make a significant contribution to human diets until about 800 years after this.[7] In most of Europe there is no natural C4 vegetation, so before significant importation of C4 foods, such as sugar cane, began during post-medieval times, diets lacked a terrestrial C4 component. Most carbon stable isotope work on European archaeological remains has focused on the relative contribution of marine resources to ancient diets. As in North America, much carbon and nitrogen stable isotope work in Europe has centred on the introduction of agriculture and its effects on human diet. A pioneer in this respect in Europe was Henrik Tauber.[9,10] He showed that Mesolithic man in Denmark was heavily reliant on marine foods, but with the introduction of agriculture at the transition to the Neolithic an abrupt change occurred, so that even coastal Neolithic people ate little or no seafood. In southern Sweden, coastal Neolithic people continued to show a marine component in their diets, albeit to a lesser extent than did their Mesolithic predecessors.[11] Looking at sites in Portugal, Lubell *et al.*[12] concluded that Mesolithic diets consisted of a balance of marine and terrestrial resources, whereas Neolithic people consumed a terrestrial diet. In Britain, the paucity of Mesolithic human remains limits the potential of stable isotope analysis for the study of the effect on human diets of the advent of agriculture here. However, recent work by Richards and Mellars, who had access to small amounts of Mesolithic and Neolithic material from coastal sites, generally indicates a size-able seafood component in Mesolithic diets, but an abrupt change to a terrestrial diet at the transition to the Neolithic.[13,14]

Although to date, most carbon and nitrogen stable isotope work has concentrated on the effects of subsistence change on human diet, other archaeological questions are now also being tackled. An important area of study is the investigation of variations in diet between the sexes and between status and other social subgroups. Some workers examining Mesoamerican material have reported status differences in diets. In Belize, at the Mayan site at Pacbitun, high-status individuals (identified by grave goods and interment type) showed less negative $\delta^{13}C$ than other burials,[15] suggesting higher maize consumption among the elite. Ubelaker *et al.*[16] also found elevated (i.e. less negative) carbon isotope ratios in high-status individuals from a prehistoric site in the Ecuadorean Highlands. They suggest that this may have been due to the greater consumption of maize beer by the elite (although, given the propensity of collagen stable isotope ratios to reflect dietary protein, elite beer consumption would have had to have been prodigious to make much impact on isotopic values!).

Some work on dietary differences between different social groups has been carried out on British material. At Poundbury Camp Roman cemetery, Dorset, England, Richards *et al.*[17] found that those individuals interred in mausolea (inferred high-status) showed greater consumption of marine foods than did those in simple earth-cut graves. Turning to the medieval period, isotopic work has revealed dietary differences between layfolk and monastic brethren. At a site in York, individuals from a monastic community showed greater consumption of marine resources than did layfolk.[18] Dietary rules of many medieval religious houses proscribed the consumption of meat, but fish could be substituted. It would seem that brethren in this monastic community were consuming a distinctive diet, in accordance with religious edicts of the time.

Occasionally, stable isotope work reveals dietary differences by sex. For example, in the Pacbitun study referred to above, White *et al.*[15] found that males had less negative $\delta^{13}C$ than females, indicating greater maize consumption by men. Given the evidence that maize was a high-status food at Pacbitun, this was possibly indicative of generally elevated socio-economic status for males and preferential access to valued food resources.

Recent work has enabled the analysis of collagen carbon and nitrogen stable isotopes to be extended beyond questions of C3/C4 or terrestrial/marine contributions to diets. Some of this work has involved the closer investigation of sources of dietary protein, particularly the use of freshwater fish. Freshwater resources generally show similar $\delta^{13}C$ to terrestrial foods,[19–21] although those from carbonate-rich waters may give a marine-like signal,[22] as may those of anadromous fish (those which migrate from marine to freshwater environments to breed). Nitrogen stable isotope ratios in freshwater systems are highly variable.[20,21,23] In some instances, stable isotopes may be used to investigate the importance of riverine resources in ancient diets, although interpretation of results is aided if faunal remains too are analysed and if both carbon and nitrogen determinations are used.

Bonsall *et al.*[24] studied material of Mesolithic and Neolithic date from Lepinski Vir and other sites in the Iron Gates region of the Danube in Serbia. Food remains from these sites revealed no evidence for consumption of seafood, although river fish were caught. Isotopic analysis of faunal remains showed that local aquatic resources had higher $\delta^{15}N$, and to a lesser extent less negative $\delta^{13}C$, than terrestrial animals. Mesolithic human remains showed elevated $\delta^{15}N$, and to some extent $\delta^{13}C$, indicating that riverine resources made a major contribution to dietary protein. By contrast, skeletons from Neolithic contexts indicated a marked increase in terrestrial foods.

Pate[21] studied material from Roonka Flat, South Australia, an inland site that lies on the lower Murray River where it transects a semi-arid plain. He found elevated $\delta^{15}N$ in the human remains from the site, despite the fact that the $\delta^{13}C$ confirmed the absence of a major dietary seafood component. Analysis of faunal remains indicated that both terrestrial animals and freshwater fish were enriched in ^{15}N (it seems generally true that animals from arid regions tend to show higher ^{15}N levels[25]). Pate interpreted his results as indicating that animals hunted from the local area and fish caught nearby provided substantial contributions to the protein parts of Roonka diet.

Flesh has a $\delta^{15}N$ some 2–3‰ higher than diet.[3] This means that there is an increase in $\delta^{15}N$ as one ascends a food chain. Some have suggested that because of this, nitrogen stable isotope values might be of use in investigating meat:vegetable ratios in ancient diets.[26] However, the trophic level effect is fairly modest, and a variety of other factors affect precise $\delta^{15}N$ even if seafood consumption can be excluded; these include consumption of leguminous plants, the application of natural fertilizers such as guano, and local environmental factors such as temperature, altitude, rainfall and soil salinity.[25] This makes study of dietary meat: vegetable ratios using nitrogen values rather difficult. However, the trophic level effect has enabled the use of nitrogen isotope values to investigate weaning practices in earlier populations. A newborn infant has a $\delta^{15}N$ similar to that of its mother. Breast-fed infants are in effect consuming their mother's tissues and so are at a higher trophic level. During breast-feeding their $\delta^{15}N$ rises, as the $\delta^{15}N$ signal from the milk is incorporated into their bone collagen. During the weaning process, as mother's milk is gradually replaced by other foods, $\delta^{15}N$ normally declines.[27] Katzenberg and Pfeiffer[28] studied nitrogen isotopes in infants from the colonial cemetery at Newmarket, Ontario. They observed a decline in the $\delta^{15}N$ of bone collagen after about 12 months of age, suggesting that weaning occurred a few months before the end of the first year. At another Ontario colonial site, Belleville, Herring *et al.*[29] likewise found a decline in $\delta^{15}N$ in collagen from about 1 year of age. Schurr[30] found that breast-milk provided most dietary nitrogen up to about 2 years of age in Native American material from the Angel site, Indiana. At another Native American site, MacPherson in Ontario, $\delta^{15}N$ started to decline from an age of about 9 months,[31] indicating much earlier weaning than at Angel. In addition to allowing investigation of age at weaning, isotope studies may also provide insights into the duration of the weaning process, as the rapidity with which other foods replace breast-milk influences the rate of decline in $\delta^{15}N$ during weaning. The colonial material from Newmarket showed a rapid decline in $\delta^{15}N$, indicating abrupt weaning; the Belleville and the two Native American groups showed more gradual declines, indicating that in these populations weaning was a more protracted process.[29,31]

Diet during childhood can also be investigated by analysing dental hard tissues. These are not turned over as is bone, and so even in adult individuals their isotopic signature enables the investigation of diet during that part of the individual's childhood when the tooth was growing. Enamel contains little organic material, so collagen work perforce uses dentine. Analysis of bone and dental tissues in the same individual may potentially indicate instances where individuals have migrated between environmental zones during their life-times. For example, Sealey et al.[32] found a trend towards less negative $\delta^{13}C$ and more posi-tive $\delta^{15}N$ in a series through first incisor dentine, third molar dentine, cortical bone and cancellous bone in a skeleton of a European buried at a Dutch East India Company outpost on the South African coast. This was consistent with a change from a terrestrial diet in childhood in a C3 environment, presumably Europe, to a much more marine diet during adolescence and adulthood.

As well as investigating new archaeological questions, bone collagen stable isotope work has also seen some recent methodological developments. Some workers have begun to take apart the collagen molecule to look at the intra-molecular distribution of $\delta^{13}C$ and $\delta^{15}N$. Hare et al.[33] showed that the constituent amino acids of collagen differ in their carbon and nitrogen isotope values, and that this may perhaps, in future, be a source of additional dietary information. In addition, they pointed out that in instances where intact collagen is not preserved, individual amino acids may yet be present so that isotopic determinations can be carried out. Potentially this may allow dietary inferences to be made when intact collagen does not survive. However, perhaps due to the time and expense involved in isolating individual amino acids from skeletal remains, little further archaeological work appears to have been carried out in this direction.

Keeling et al.[34] took a slightly different approach to intra-molecular analysis of collagen stable isotopes. They studied $\delta^{13}C$ at a specific location, the carboxyl carbon, in the amino acids that make up collagen. The carboxyl carbons were generally isotopically heavier than the total carbon in collagen. There also appeared to be a trophic level effect: the difference between carboxyl and total collagen $\delta^{13}C$ was less for organisms at higher trophic levels. This suggested that analysis of carboxyl carbon $\delta^{13}C$ could potentially provide additional information on protein sources in ancient diets. However, as Keeling et al. point out, a great deal of further work is needed firmly to establish the origin of differences in carboxyl carbon and total collagen $\delta^{13}C$.

Alternatives to collagen for stable isotope work

The mineral component of skeletal hard tissues

Recent work has centred on the potential of stable isotope analyses of the mineral parts of bones and teeth. Carbon stable isotope ratios in the carbonate component have been studied, as have oxygen isotopes in phosphate and to a lesser extent, carbonate. Isotope ratios of trace elements such as strontium and lead have also been investigated.

The hydroxyapatite of mineralized tissues contains about 2–4% carbonate (CO_3^{2-}).[35] Animal feeding experiments[4,5] have shown that $\delta^{13}C$ in carbonate varies with that in diet, the offset between diet and carbonate values being about 9–10‰.[5] For an adult skeleton, the rate of turnover of bone mineral varies between different skeletal elements or parts thereof, but on average a complete replacement cycle takes about 7–10 years.[36] Bone carbonate therefore gives a long-term indication of adult diet, albeit averaged over a somewhat shorter period than appears to be the case for collagen. Analysis of dental enamel (or dentine) carbonate gives an indication of diet in childhood, when the tooth was forming.

A potential problem in using carbonate analyses to investigate past diets is that the mineral part of bone may be vulnerable to post-depositional changes in its chemical composition. So, for example, neither ^{14}C dating based on the carbonate fraction of bone mineral, nor much of the bone mineral trace element work done for dietary reconstruction, are generally accepted as reliable.[37,38] Some factors contribute to the propensity of bone mineral (and dentine) for diagenetic change. Bone and dentine have a very small crystal size, and so present a high surface area for chemical exchange. They are also highly porous (this is particularly so for bone), facilitating post-depositional penetration by soil water. Their high levels of organic material make them targets for attack by soil-dwelling microorganisms. However, some diagenetic material, including contaminative carbonates, can be removed from archaeological bone by washing with dilute acetic acid,[39] and this pre-treatment has become routine in isotopic analyses of the carbonate component of skeletal material.[40]

Dental enamel has larger crystals than bone mineral and they have fewer defects.[41,42] In addition, it contains little organic material, and so does not appear to be decomposed by soil-dwelling microorganisms, unlike bone.[43] One might therefore expect that enamel may be less subject to diagenetic change than bone mineral or dentine, and there is ample empirical evidence to support this. For example, Koch et al.[41] studied various Pleistocene and Holocene specimens and found that the carbonate isotope ratios of bone and dentine were unreliable for palaeodietary reconstruction, despite acetic acid pre-treatment. By contrast, enamel and bone collagen gave consistently reliable results. In a natural experiment, Kruger[44] analysed mastodon teeth dredged from the seabed of the continental shelf of the eastern USA. These represented the remains of land-dwelling creatures submerged for 11 000 years when the continental shelf was inundated at the end of the Pleistocene. Dental enamel carbonate δ^{13}C determinations gave values typical of terrestrial animals, with no indication of contamination of biological apatite with marine carbonate. Hedges et al.[37] studied tooth enamel specimens dating from 11 000 to 200 000 BP. Although they found that radiocarbon dates on the apatite were all too young, indicating post-depositional exchange with carbonate in the burial environment, the degree of contamination was too slight to affect significantly δ^{13}C. It would seem that reliable δ^{13}C signals can be obtained from enamel carbonate; however, more caution is required in the case of bone and dentine.

The dietary information from δ^{13}C in carbonate differs somewhat from that obtained from collagen, and for this reason allows other aspects of early diets to be elucidated. The animal feeding experiments referred to above indicate that in contrast to bone collagen, carbonate δ^{13}C reflects the carbon stable isotope values in whole diet not just protein. Carbonate δ^{13}C enables the study of ancient diets to be extended to investigating whole diet. So, for example, there is important potential here for shedding additional light on the introduction of maize cultivation into North America. Maize is low in protein, and therefore consumption of it has to be considerable before it will be evident in the collagen δ^{13}C signal. However, as apatite δ^{13}C reflects whole diet it will be a more sensitive indicator of maize consumption. In the 800 years between the first findings of maize cobs on settlement sites in eastern North America and the evidence of the adoption of maize as a dietary staple, it has been suggested[45] that it may have been used as a ceremonial food. Carbon isotope determinations on apatite may help to clarify whether it was indeed eaten in small quantities during this period, and if so by whom.

Apatite is more persistent in the archaeological record than collagen, so that carbonate $\delta^{13}C$ determinations, particularly from dental enamel, also provide a means by which dietary analyses using carbon stable isotope values can be extended back into the more remote past. For example, Lee-Thorpe et al.[46] investigated the diet of australopithecines using apatite carbon stable isotope analysis. They found that these creatures ate both C3 and C4 foods. Given that studies using dental wear and comparative tooth morphology indicate that direct consumption of grasses is unlikely, the investigators argue that Australopithecus was omnivorous, the C4 component in diet coming from consumption of herbivores grazing on C4 grasses.

As was discussed above, carbon stable isotope analysis of bones and teeth from the same individual can potentially be used to detect instances where a person has migrated between different environmental zones (areas with or without C4 foods or marine versus inland areas). However, even when migrations do not involve movement between different ecological zones, movement of peoples can potentially be detected using other stable isotopes, such as $^{87/86}Sr$. Strontium stable isotopes do not fractionate in food webs, but rather reflect local geology. Strontium in diet is incorporated into apatite in trace amounts, so the strontium stable isotope ratio in skeletal material can be used as an indicator of place of residence. Diagenetic problems with bone strontium are well known,[38] and the acetic acid pretreatment method is routinely used for preparation of excavated skeletal material for strontium isotope analysis.

Grupe and co-workers.[47,48] compared strontium isotope ratios in bone and tooth enamel from Bell-Beaker burials in Bavaria. This produced evidence for considerable mobility in this group, with about one-fifth to one-quarter of individuals being migrants from regions of different geology. The general direction of migration in the study area appeared to be from north-east to south-west and involved distances of up to about 220 km.

Patterns of migrations in the vicinity of Grasshopper Pueblo, Arizona, have been investigated by Price and co-workers[49,50] with strontium stable isotopes, using a slightly different strategy. They used modern rodent remains to give an indication of isotope ratios expected in the Grasshopper Pueblo locale and further afield. Interpreted against this background, analysis of dental enamel from human remains from the Pueblo site indicated that between about one-third and one-half of individuals analysed were non-locals, having migrated to the site since childhood from areas with different geology. Immigrants appeared to originate from two geological areas, those underlain by Precambrian rocks to the south and west and those underlain by Phanerozoic strata to the north and east. In addition, locals and non-locals were interred in different areas of the site at Grasshopper.

Analysis of the isotopic composition of skeletal lead can also be used to investigate movements of people in ancient times. Naturally occurring lead is a mixture of four stable isotopes, of mass 204, 206, 207 and 208, and different geological deposits may differ in their isotopic composition. Lead isotopes were used to identify a possible migrant at Poundbury Roman cemetery.[51] Four individuals were analysed, and determinations from three of them matched those expected if the sources of their skeletal lead burden were purely local. The isotopic values for the fourth individual, a child, lay outside this range, and a match was found with an ore source in Greece. That the skeletal value matched the Greek ore so well, and showed no drift towards local values, suggested that the child might have died soon after its arrival in England.

Cultural differences may be revealed by lead isotope work. Carlson,[52] looking at skeletal material from western Canada, found that European fur-traders and Native Americans differed in their lead isotope values. The values from the remains of the fur traders resembled those from contemporary lead artefacts, suggesting that contamination of food and drink was the principal source of lead ingestion in these individuals. The isotope values of the Indians grouped with those from contemporary animal bones, indicating that their lead intake derived from the natural environment rather than anthropogenic food contamination.

Analyses of stable isotopes in biological materials, including human remains, have been used to investigate ancient climate. In biological materials both carbon[53] and nitrogen[25] stable isotope ratios vary with climatic conditions; however, these variations are rather small relative to those caused by dietary and other factors and this limits their use for reconstructing climates and climate change in Holocene times. Oxygen isotope ratios ($\delta^{18}O$), however, are valuable for this purpose. It has been known for some time that $\delta^{18}O$ in meteoric water varies with climate,[54] and in most regions a firm relationship exists between $\delta^{18}O$ and temperature, lower temperatures meaning a lower δ. Oxygen isotope values in body water are, for most larger mammals, directly related to their drinking water.[55] In the mineral fraction of bones and teeth, oxygen is present in both carbonate and phosphate. It has been confirmed that both phosphate[56] and carbonate[57] $\delta^{18}O$ reflect ingested values. Phosphate is less vulnerable to diagenetic exchange than carbonate[40] and has attracted more attention for oxygen isotope work on biological apatites. As with other apatite work, dental enamel is the sample material of preference, due to its delimited formation time and lesser vulnerability to diagenesis. Fricke et al.[56] indicate that it should, in principle, be possible to resolve temperature changes of $< 1°C$ using $\delta^{18}O$ analysis of dental enamel phosphate. Studies using dental enamel, both from modern animals and from ancient faunal remains, have shown that by careful sampling along the length of a single tooth, it is even possible to detect seasonal climatic variations.[58–60]

Although most palaeoclimatic $\delta^{18}O$ work on excavated biological remains has been done on faunal material[61] some has been conducted on human remains. Fricke et al.[56] analysed human tooth enamel from skeletons excavated in Denmark and Greenland and found a good relationship between phosphate $\delta^{18}O$ and the latitude of the site. They also examined change in oxygen isotope ratios over time. In material from the Julianehaab Bay area of Greenland they observed a fall in $\delta^{18}O$ in the early post-medieval period, corresponding to the climatic deterioration known as the Little Ice Age. In a comment on Fricke et al.'s paper, Bryant and Froelich[62] raised some points that are relevant not just to Fricke et al.'s work, but which also have a bearing on the general potential of oxygen isotope work using human skeletal remains for the investigation of past climates. Breast-feeding and its duration are likely to have an important effect on $\delta^{18}O$ in tooth enamel. Breast milk is rich in ^{18}O relative to the water imbibed by the mother, and in the suckling child this will be incorporated into dental enamel forming during this time. Thus, enamel $\delta^{18}O$ will tend to be increased to a degree dependent upon the extent to which crown formation time overlaps with breast-feeding (indeed, looking at enamel $\delta^{18}O$ has been suggested as another way of investigating weaning in earlier human populations[63]). Bryant and Froelich also point out that marine foods are richer in ^{18}O than terrestrial ones, and boiling water for beverages tends to enrich it with ^{18}O by preferential evaporation of ^{16}O. An additional factor that should be considered is the source of water for human consumption. Water from perennial springs, groundwater or large lakes will reflect local precipitation averaged over decades,[64] but water collected for human consumption from rain or snow fall, or from small bodies of water such as pools or ponds, will reflect climate variations over shorter periods.

Another archaeological example which illustrates that the interpretation of $\delta^{18}O$ signals from human remains is not straightforward, is that of Stuart-Williams *et al.*[65] They looked at phosphate $\delta^{18}O$ from skeletal material from the Mexican sites at Monte Alban in the Oaxaca Valley and Teotihuacan. Material from the latter was richer in ^{18}O. Teotihuacan lies at a greater elevation and so has a cooler climate than Monte Alban, so the $\delta^{18}O$ results were the opposite of those which might have been anticipated. The writers point out that because of the direction of the prevailing winds during the season of high rainfall, Monte Alban is in the rainshadow of the mountains, so that it receives precipitation which is already depleted in ^{18}O.

Because $\delta^{18}O$ may vary between geographical regions, oxygen isotope analysis is potentially another means of shedding light on ancient migrations. For example, the Mexican material studied by Stuart-Williams *et al.* included skeletons from Tlailotlacan, an enclave of Oaxacan culture in Teotihuacan. They found that the $\delta^{18}O$ of this group clustered with other Teotihuacan material rather than with that from the Oaxacan site at Monte Alban.[66] Although precise interpretation was difficult, the results were thought to support the idea that there was little or no further inflow from the Oaxaca region into Tlailotlacan subsequent to the founding of the community.

Lipids

It has recently been shown[67] that lipids, particularly cholesterol, survive regularly in ancient bones. Feeding experiments using pigs[68] indicate that $\delta^{13}C$ of lipids reflects that of diet. Cholesterol, for example, shows a regular depletion of about 3‰ compared with diet,[68] giving about –28‰ for an animal on a pure C3 diet. Cholesterol $\delta^{13}C$ appears to reflect the isotopic content of bulk diet rather better than does collagen $\delta^{13}C$.[68,69] In addition, lipids cycle over a much shorter period than does collagen or bone apatite,[70,71] so lipid carbon stable isotope values represent diet over the last few weeks of an individual's life rather than a long-term average. When lipids are extracted from ancient remains, the structure of the molecule can be confirmed unambiguously in the laboratory, so one can be sure that there has been no diagenetic alteration to its isotopic chemistry. Little archaeological work has yet been done on bone lipid stable isotopes; however, Stott and Evershed[69] report a pilot study in which $\delta^{13}C$ determinations were carried out on some medieval skeletons from

Barton-on-Humber, North Lincolnshire, England. The site lies on the Humber estuary, giving ready access to coastal waters. The $\delta^{13}C$ from cholesterol from the burials confirmed the presence of a sizeable seafood component in local diets.

SUMMARY

Since the first palaeodietary stable isotope studies were performed more than 20 years ago, isotopic analyses of carbon and nitrogen from bone collagen have made a major contribution to our understanding of ancient diets, in particular the importance or otherwise of sea-food or C4 terrestrial components. Classically, the archaeological focus of this work has been on subsistence change, particularly the adoption of agriculture and its effects on human diets. However, in recent years, researchers have applied collagen isotopic analyses to a wider range of questions, including the study of differential access to foodstuffs according to gender or social position, and the study of weaning practices in ancient times. As well as addressing new questions, researchers have started to analyse different skeletal components. Carbon stable isotope analysis of the mineral component of skeletal remains has allowed investigations to be expanded to looking at whole diets rather than just the protein part. Work has particularly concentrated on dental enamel, as this is less susceptible to diagenesis than bone mineral. Skeletal mineral is much more persistent in the archaeological record than is collagen, so it offers the opportunity to extend the isotope work back into the very remote past. Furthermore, expansion of isotopic work to the mineral component permits the analysis of isotopic ratios of other elements, be they bulk elements such as oxygen, or trace elements such as strontium or lead. These investigations are providing fascinating new information on aspects as diverse as ancient climates, population movements and cultural affiliation. Both bone collagen and apatite give summaries of diets averaged over many years; however, the isotope work on bone lipids, although still in its infancy, may offer a means of gaining insights into short-term rather than long-term dietary habits.

REFERENCES

1   Mays S. *The Archaeology of Human Bones*. London: Routledge/English Heritage, 1998.

2   Ambrose SH. Isotopic Analysis of palaeodiets: methodological and interpretative considerations. In: Sandford MK (ed.), *Investigations of Ancient Human Tissue*. Reading: Gordon & Breach, 1993; pp. 59–130.

3   DeNiro MJ, Epstein S. Influence of diet on the distribution of nitrogen isotopes in animals. *Geochimica et Cosmochimica Acta* 1981; **45**: 341–351.

4   Ambrose SH, Norr L. Experimental evidence for the relationship of the carbon isotope ratios of whole diet and dietary protein to those of bone collagen and carbonate. In: Lambert JB, Grupe G (eds), *Prehistoric Human Bone – Archaeology at the Molecular Level*. Berlin: Springer, 1993; pp. 1–37.

5   Tieszen LL, Fagre T. Effect of diet quality and composition on the isotopic composition of respiratory CO_2, bone collagen, bioapatite and soft tissues. In: Lambert JB, Grupe G (eds), *Prehistoric Human Bone – Archaeology at the Molecular Level*. Berlin: Springer, 1993; pp. 121–155.

6   Stafford TW, Hare PE, Currie L, Jull AJT, Donahue DJ. Accelerator radiocarbon dating at the molecular level. *Journal of Archaeological Science* 1991; **18**: 35–72.

7   Schwarcz HP, Schoeninger MJ. Stable isotope analysis in human nutritional ecology. *Yearbook of Physical Anthropology* 1991; **34**: 283–321.

8   Schoeninger MJ, Moore K. Bone Stable isotope studies in archaeology. *Journal of World Prehistory* 1992; **6**: 247–296.

9   Tauber H. ¹³C Evidence for dietary habits of prehistoric man in Denmark. *Nature* 1981; **292**: 332–333.

10   Tauber H. Analysis of stable isotopes in prehistoric populations. In: Herrmann B (ed.), *Innovative Trends in Prehistoric Anthropology*. Berlin: Mitteilungen der Berliner Gesellschaft für Anthropologie, Ethnologie und Urgeschichte, Band 7, 1986; pp. 31–38.

11   Lidén K. Megaliths, agriculture, and social complexity: a diet study of two Swedish Megalithic populations. *Journal of Anthropological Archaeology* 1995; **14**: 404–417.

12   Lubell D, Jackes M, Schwarcz H, Knyf M, Meiklejohn C. The Mesolithic–Neolithic transition in Portugal: isotopic and dental evidence of diet. *Journal of Archaeological Science* 1994; **21**: 201–216.

13   Richards MP. *Palaeodietary Studies of European Human Populations Using Bone Stable Isotopes*. PhD thesis, University of Oxford, 1998.

14   Richards MP, Mellars PA. Stable isotopes and the seasonality of the Oronsay middens. *Antiquity* 1998; **72**: 178–184.

15   White CD, Healy PF, Schwarcz HP. Intensive agriculture, social status, and Maya diet at Pacbitun, Belize. *Journal of Anthropological Research* 1993; **49**: 347–375.

16   Ubelaker DH, Katzenberg MA, Doyon LG. Status and diet in precontact highland Ecuador. *American Journal of Physical Anthropology* 1995; **97**: 403–411.

17   Richards MP, Hedges REM, Molleson TI, Vogel JC. Stable isotope analysis reveals variations in human diet at the Poundbury Camp cemetery Site. *Journal of Archaeological Science* 1998; **25**: 1247–1252.

18   Mays SA. Carbon stable isotope ratios in medieval and later human skeletons from northern England. *Journal of Archaeological Science* 1997; **24**: 561–567.

19   Schwarcz HP. Some theoretical aspects of isotope palaeodiet studies. *Journal of Archaeological Science* 1991; **18**: 261–275.

20   van der Merwe NJ, Lee-Thorpe JA, Raymond JS. Light stable isotopes and the subsistence base of formative cultures at Valdivia, Ecuador. In: Lambert JB, Grupe G (eds), *Prehistoric Human Bone – Archaeology at the Molecular Level*. Berlin: Springer, 1993; pp. 63–97.

21   Pate FD. Bone chemistry and palaeodiet: reconstructing prehistoric subsistence–settlement systems in Australia. *Journal of Anthropological Archaeology* 1997; **16**: 103–120.

22   Day SP. Dogs, deer and diet at Starr Carr: a reconsideration of C-isotope evidence from early Mesolithic dog remains from the Vale of Pickering, Yorkshire, England. *Journal of Archaeological Science* 1996; **23**: 783–787.

23   Katzenberg, MA. Stable isotope analysis of archaeological faunal remains from southern Ontario. *Journal of Archaeological Science* 1989; **16**: 319–329.

24   Bonsall C, Lennon R, McSweeney K, Stewart C, Harkness D, Boroneant V. Mesolithic and early Neolithic in the Iron Gates: a palaeodietary perspective. *Journal of European Archaeology* 1995; **5**: 50–92.

25   Ambrose SH. Effects of diet, climate and physiology on nitrogen isotope abundancies in terrestrial food webs. *Journal of Archaeological Science* 1991; **18**: 293–317.

26   Schoeninger MJ. Trophic level effects on $^{15}N/^{14}N$ and $^{13}C/^{12}C$ ratios in bone collagen and strontium levels in bone mineral. *Journal of Human Evolution* 1985; **14**: 515–525.

27   Katzenberg MA, Herring DA, Saunders SR. Weaning and infant mortality: evaluating the skeletal evidence. *Yearbook of Physical Anthropology* 1996; **39**: 177–199.

28   Katzenberg MA, Pfeiffer S. Nitrogen isotope evidence for weaning age in a nineteenth century skeletal sample. In: Grauer AL (ed.), *Bodies of Evidence*. New York: Wiley, 1995; pp. 221–235.

29   Herring DA, Saunders SR, Katzenberg MA. Investigating the weaning process in past populations. *American Journal of Physical Anthropology* 1998; **105**: 425–439.

30   Schurr MR. Stable nitrogen isotopes as evidence for the age of weaning at the Angel site: a comparison of isotopic and demographic measures of weaning age. *Journal of Archaeological Science* 1997; **24**: 919–927.

31   Schurr MR. Using stable nitrogen isotopes to study weaning behavior in past populations. *World Archaeology* 1998; **30**: 327–342.

32   Sealey J, Armstrong R, Schrire C. Beyond lifetime averages: tracing life histories through isotopic analysis of different calcified tissues from archaeological human skeletons. *Antiquity* 1995; **69**: 290–300.

33   Hare PE, Fogel ML, Stafford TW, Mitchell AD, Hoering TC. The isotopic composition of carbon and nitrogen in individual amino acids isolated from modern and fossil proteins. *Journal of Archaeological Science* 1991; **18**: 277–292.

34   Keeling CI, Nelson DE, Slessor KN. Stable carbon isotope measurements of the carboxyl carbons in bone collagen. *Archaeometry* 1999; **41**: 151–164.

35   Hillson S. *Dental Anthropology*. Cambridge: Cambridge University Press, 1996; Table 10.1.

36   Lowenstam and Weiner, cited in Price *et al.*[49]

37   Hedges REM, Lee-Thorpe JA, Tuross NC. Is tooth enamel carbonate a suitable material for radiocarbon dating? *Radiocarbon* 1995; **37**: 285–290.

38   Radosevich SC. The six deadly sins of trace element analysis: a case of wishful thinking in science. In: Sandford MK (ed.), *Investigations of Ancient Human Tissue*. Reading: Gordon and Breach, 1993; pp. 269–332.

39   Sillen A. Biogenic and diagenetic Sr/Ca in Plio-Pleistocene fossils of the Omo Shungura Formation. *Palaeobiology* 1986; **12**: 311–323.

40   Wright LE, Schwarcz HP. Infrared and isotopic evidence for diagenesis of bone apatite at Dos Pilas, Guatemala: palaeodietary implications. *Journal of Archaeological Science* 1996; **23**: 933–944.

41   Koch PL, Tuross N, Fogel ML. The effects of sample treatment and diagenesis on the isotopic integrity of carbonate in biogenic hydroxylapatite. *Journal of Archaeological Science* 1997; **24**: 417–429.

42   Ayliffe LK, Chivas AR, Leakey MG. The retention of primary oxygen isotope compositions of fossil elephant skeletal phosphate. *Geochimica et Cosmochimica Acta* 1994; **58**: 5291–5298.

43   Hackett CJ. Microscopic focal destruction (tunnels) in exhumed bone. *Medicine, Science and the Law* 1981; **21**: 243–265.

44   Kruger HW. Exchange of carbon with biological apatite. *Journal of Archaeological Science* 1991; **18**: 355–361.

45   Smith BD. Origins of agriculture in eastern North America. *Science* 1989; **246**: 1566–1571.

46   Lee-Thorpe JA, van der Merwe NJ, Brain CK. Diet of *Australopithecus robustus* at Swartkrans from stable carbon isotopic analysis. *Journal of Human Evolution* 1994; **27**: 361–372.

47   Grupe G. Reconstructing migration in the Bell Beaker period by $^{87}Sr/^{86}Sr$ isotope ratios in teeth and bones. In: Radlandski RJ, Renz H (eds), *Proceedings of the Tenth International Symposium on Dental Morphology*. Berlin: Brunne, 1996; pp. 339–342.

48   Price TD, Grupe G, Schröter P. Migration in the Bell Beaker period of central Europe. *Antiquity* 1998; **72**: 405–411.

49   Price TD, Johnson CM, Ezzo JA, Ericson JA, Burton JH. residential mobility in the prehistoric southwest United States: a preliminary study using strontium isotope analysis. *Journal of Archaeological Science* 1994; **21**: 315–330.

50   Ezzo JA, Johnson CM, Price TD. Analytical perspectives on prehistoric migration: a case study from east-central Arizona. *Journal of Archaeological Science* 1997; **24**: 447–466.

51   Molleson TI, Eldridge D, Gale N. Identification of lead sources by stable isotope ratios in bones and lead from Poundbury Camp, Dorset. *Oxford Journal of Archaeology* 1986; **5**: 249–253.

52   Carlson AK. Lead isotope analysis of human bone for addressing cultural affinity: a case study from Rocky Mountain House, Alberta. *Journal of Archaeological Science* 1996; **23**: 557–567.

53   Richards MP, van Klinken GJ. A survey of European human bone stable carbon and nitrogen isotope values. In: Sinclair A, Slater E, Gowlett J (eds), *Archaeological Science 1995*. Oxford: Oxbow, 1997; pp. 363–368.

54   Dansgaard W. Stable isotopes in precipitation. *Tellus* 1964; **16**: 436–468.

55   Bryant JD, Froelich PN. A model of oxygen isotope fractionation in body water of large mammals. *Geochimica et Cosmochimica Acta* 1995; **59**: 4523–4537.

56   Fricke HC, O'Neill JR, Lynnerup N. Oxygen isotope composition of human tooth enamel from medieval Greenland: linking climate and society. *Geology* 1995; **23**: 869–872.

57   Bryant JD, Koch PL, Froelich PN, Showers WJ Genna BJ. Oxygen isotope partitioning between phosphate and carbonate in mammalian apatite. *Geochimica et Cosmochimica Acta* 1996; **60**: 5145–5148.

58   Koch PL, Fisher DC, Dettman D. Oxygen isotope variation in the tusks of extinct proboscideans: a measure of season of death and seasonality. *Geology* 1989; **17**: 515–519.

59   Stuart-Williams HLeQ, Schwarcz HP. Oxygen isotope determination of climatic variation using phosphate from beaver bone, tooth enamel and dentine. *Geochimica et Cosmochimica Acta* 1997; **61**: 2539–2550.

60   Sharp ZD, Cerling TE. Fossil isotope records of seasonal climate and ecology: straight from the horse's mouth. *Geology* 1998; **26**: 319–322.

61   Koch PL. Isotopic reconstruction of past continental environments. *Annual Review of Earth and Planetary Sciences* 1998; **26**: 573–613.

62   Bryant JD, Froelich PN. Oxygen isotope composition of human tooth enamel from medieval Greenland: linking climate and society: comment and reply. *Geology* 1996; **24**: 477–479.

63   Wright LE, Schwarcz HP. Stable carbon and oxygen isotopes in human tooth enamel: identifying breast-feeding in prehistory. *American Journal of Physical Anthropology* 1998; **106**: 1–18.

64   Reinhard E, de Torres T, O'Neil J. $^{18}O/^{16}O$ ratios of Cave Bear tooth enamel: a record of climate variability during the pleistocene. *Palaeogeography, Palaeoclimatology, Palaeoecology* 1996; **126**: 45–59.

65   Stuart-Williams HLeQ, Schwarcz HP, White CD, Spence MW. The isotopic composition and diagenesis of human bone from Teotihuacan and Oaxaca, Mexico. *Palaeoclimatology, Palaeobiology, Palaeoecology* 1996; **126**: 1–14.

66   White CD, Spence MW, Stuart-Williams HLeQ, Schwarcz HP. Oxygen isotopes and the identification of geographical origins: the Valley of Oaxaca versus the Valley of Mexico. *Journal of Archaeological Science* 1998; **25**: 643–655.

67   Evershed RP, Turner-Walker G, Hedges REM, Tuross N, Leyden A. Preliminary results for the analysis of lipids in ancient bone. *Journal of Archaeological Science* 1995; **22**: 277–290.

68   Stott AW, Davies E, Evershed RP. Monitoring the routing of dietary and biosynthesised lipids through compound-specific stable isotope (δ13C) measurements at natural abundance. *Naturwissenschaften* 1997; **84**: 82–86.

69   Stott AW, Evershed RP. δ13C Analysis of cholesterol preserved in archaeological bones and teeth. *Analytical Chemistry* 1996; **68**: 4402–4408.

70   Sabine, JR. *Cholesterol*. New York: Dekker, 1977.

71   Guo ZK, Luke AH, Lee WP, Schoeller D. Compound-specific carbon isotope ratio determination of enriched cholesterol. *Analytical Chemistry* 1993; **65**: 1954–1959.

26

THE CHEMICAL DEGRADATION OF BONE

Christina Nielsen-Marsh, Angela Gernaey, Gordon Turner-Walker,
Robert Hedges, Alistair Pike and Matthew Collins

INTRODUCTION

The general view of bone diagenesis is that biologically controlled degradation is the key factor governing the survival of archaeological bone in the burial environment. Many publications emphasize the importance of the role of water on the attack of the bone by microorganisms.[1-4] It is unquestionable that in the early stages of taphonomic change, while the body is still fleshed, microorganisms will play an important role in the cadaver's decomposition.[5] *Skeletal* remains, however, require a different approach if we are to unravel the processes which determine their survival in the archaeological record.

Bone can survive differentially, even across one archaeological site, and a bewildering array of different factors have been suggested to be involved in this apparently random survival.[6-9] Osteologists and archaeologists are both aware of the *physical changes* arising from bone diagenesis, and that the transition from so called 'green' to 'dry' bone has important taphonomic implications. These terms are not properly defined, but reflect a transition from bones with high residual lipid contents (waxy to the touch) and intact collagen (residual flexibility) to bones which have lost lipid and collagen and gained an increase in porosity (see below) and are therefore much more brittle.[10]

This transition is fundamental to bone survival, and highlights the importance of defining the process that initiates such alteration. Originally, it was assumed that bone degradation was primarily related to destruction of the mineral phase,[11] but later studies[12] have focused mainly on the loss of the organic phase. Essential to unravelling this dichotomy is an understanding of the relationship between the mineral and the protein, which gives modern bone the tensile strength and elasticity usually lacking in archaeological specimens.[10]

Organization of bone

Living bone is made up of water, mineral and organics and its density varies according to the relative proportions of these three components.[13,14] The proportions of water, mineral and organics are governed by species and age and are different for compact and cancellous bone; the principle component of the organic phase is collagen.

Bone collagen

In bone, about 90% of the organic matrix is composed of long fibrils of Type I collagen.[14] Type I collagen molecules have a high degree of organization, comprising three stretched helical amino acid chains twisted into a triple helix. These triple-helices are grouped into bundles (fibrils) and the bundles grouped into fibres. Under physiological conditions, Type I collagen is insoluble, because of:

- The highly ordered three-dimensional arrangement of fibres.
- The ionic and hydrophobic interactions with adjacent chains.
- The extent of cross-linking.

If the helix is denatured, either by heating or chain scission, the stretched amino acid chains relax, causing the fibrils to shrink lengthways but expand in diameter. This leads to an unravelling of the helix and the production of soluble gelatine. The temperature at which collagen 'shrinks' or melts (the melt temperature, T_m), is an important property of the material and can be increased by stabilizing the helix, for example, by tanning.[15]

Both bone and skin comprise predominantly Type I collagen, however, in bone the collagen has enzymatically mediated covalent cross-links (lysyl or hydroxylysyl) between adjacent amino acid chains. These cross-links do not increase the T_m significantly, but the presence of bone apatite physically restricts the ability of the helix to expand. This means that the T_m in bone is much higher (> 150°C) than in unmineralized collagen (about 68°C).[16]

Following death, non-enzymatic cross-linking can be expected to occur. Collagen will form cross-links with sugars,[17] and these reactions have been assumed to be important in the formation of 'humics',[18] which have been reported in bone.[19] Accelerated damage and concomitant shrinking of collagen (e.g. by ultraviolet irradiation) may disrupt the mineral packing and be responsible for the cracking and spalling of the mineral observed in weathered bones.

Bone mineral

The building blocks of bone mineral are extremely small, plate-shaped crystals of a carbonated form of non-stoichiometric hydroxyapatite, $Ca_5(PO_4)_3OH$.[20,21] A more suitable term would be bone apatite, which is more ambiguous, but reflects the uncertainty that surrounds the structure of bone mineral and its intimate association with collagen. Although the nature of this collagen-mineral association has yet to be satisfactorily explained, studies investigating bone mineral organization have shown that the crystals are embedded within the collagen fibres with their c-axes aligned parallel to the long axis of the fibre. These fibres are, in turn, arranged in parallel to form successive lamellae, in which the fibre orientation forms a 'twisted or rotated plywood structure'.[22,23] The strength of a calcified tissue is dependent, in part, on the molecular structure and organization of its constituent mineral crystals in the organic matrix.[23–26] The exceptionally small size of the crystals (typical values for human bone are $2–3 \times 5 \times 35$ nm) gives bone mineral a very high surface area (between 85 and 170 m^2g^{-1}).[21] Maturity and species determine the size and shape of bioapatitic crystals *in vivo.* In all species the average crystal size increases with age, often in correlation with fluoride content, until maturity is reached, at which point the bone, and therefore the crystals, continue to be remodelled, although the average crystal size remains constant.[27] The crystals of bone apatite have highly reactive surfaces, where either Ca^{2+} or $PO_4{}^{3-}$ ions are exposed.[28] After death, the biologically formed mineral becomes unstable, and because it is still highly reactive, this makes it very susceptible to alteration by the burial environment.[29]

Hydroxyapatite is isomorphous with a range of other apatites, therefore it can undergo complete replacement of some of its ions without changing its structure, for example, replacement of OH^- with F^- leads to the formation of fluorapatite. It is also possible to replace Ca^{2+} with Sr^{2+}, Ba^{2+}, Pb^{2+}, Cd^{2+} or Sn^{2+} and partial substitution of Ca^{2+} occurs with Zn^{2+}, Cu^{2+}, Co^{2+}, Ni^{2+} and Mn^{2+}, and many other ions including lanthanides and actinides can also substitute into the lattice.[30]

Biological degradation of the protein fraction

The main arguments in this chapter concern the *chemical* degradation of mineral and protein. Currently, these can only be modelled in isolation from the microbial influences, since all the variables for this latter diagenetic pathway are unknown. Here we present, for completeness, an overview of microbial degradation; the emphasis lies not on the mechanisms of degradation, which are already reviewed elsewhere,[1,31,32] but on the mechanisms of suppression of microbial activity, allowing study of the chemical factors alone.

During early diagenesis of a corpse, the role of microorganisms must be the key driving force, and microbial transformations following death have been discussed.[1] The loss of soft tissue is predominantly microbially mediated, with some autolytic component, but the presence of the mineral phase in bone means that other processes must be involved – because fully mineralized collagen is resistant to microbial attack. This resistance is due to the absence of pores with diameters of > 8 nm. Collagenases are large, between 60 and 130 kDa,[33] so that their access will be physically restricted by the micro-pores present in bone. These micro-pores have diameters <8 nm[8] so that not only will collagenase access be inhibited, but also that of other bacterial and fungal exo-enzymes.[34] Enzymes of this size would require that the bone mineral is first removed, and enzyme studies support this hypothesis.[35]

Diagenetic alterations that remove the mineral will permit access of collagenases, as well as disrupt the integrity of the collagen. Chemical processes (see below) will also change the collagen, rendering it more amenable to proteolysis by non-specific enzymes. Only a small proportion of extracted archaeological 'collagen' is enzymatically sensitive,[19] therefore chemical diagenetic effects will eventually limit microbial activity; supression of enzyme action is usually ascribed to interference by 'humic substances'.

The following sections focus upon the continuous chemical diagenetic processes, namely non-enzymatic hydrolysis of bone collagen and bone demineralization which, we believe, are fundamental to an understanding of the survival of archaeological bone.

CHEMICAL DIAGENESIS OF THE PROTEIN FRACTION – NON-ENZYMATIC HYDROLYSIS

There is a lack of detailed understanding of the long-term diagenesis of proteins in the archaeological record, however, in environments protected from enzymatic degradation, the most significant process is hydrolysis of the peptide bond.[36] Unlike enzymatic hydrolysis, the intimate association of mineral and collagen cannot prevent chemical hydrolysis, since there will always be available water.[37]

Degradation of bone collagen lowers the T_m and leads to the production of soluble peptide fragments that can then be lost from the bone. Some of the authors (MJC, AMG, GTW) have earlier proposed a model of collagen degradation based upon random chain scission leading to destabilization of the helix and an increase in soluble components.[38] Although the model predicts the observed weight loss at extremes of pH, recent results in our laboratory suggests that it does not adequately describe bone collagen decomposition. Investigations by others,[39,40] and unpublished results by ourselves have revealed the relationship between temperature and collagen degradation. The results from these studies display similar temperature dependence, but estimates for the survival of collagen vary. The results from our study suggest that in the absence of mineral dissolution (and resulting microbial decomposition) there should be no significant loss of collagen over archaeological time in temperate environments. Nitrogen yields measured in bones from Gough's Cave, Somerset (12 kyr) were close to modern values. This suggests that the estimates by Ortner et al.[39] for the rates of collagen loss are probably too rapid, but whether our estimates are too low is as yet unclear (Table 1). In warmer climates, however, both studies agree that the loss of collagen will be significant. Ambrose[41] comments that in open sites in Africa, collagen is lost in < 3000 years, while in rockshelters, which are typically cooler, collagen survives until about 7000 years.

CHEMICAL DIAGENESIS OF THE MINERAL FRACTION

In general, most studies measuring structural and chemical alterations in archaeological bone mineral, do so only as verification that data derived from surviving collagen are reliable as a scientific resource,[9,42] but the factors that govern mineral degradation may turn out to be crucial to bone survival. Understanding which factors are key to sustaining mineral in the burial environment will help to establish how and why certain environments produce better bone preservation than others, and may lead to a more comprehensive theory of bone survival.

Dissolution of bone apatite – effects on mineral structure

In the simplest terms, mineral alterations are determined by the extent of dissolution of bone apatite. In the burial environment, it is the action of groundwater on the bone that

Table 1 – Predicted survival of collagen at 10 and 20°C.

Author	Method	Estimated $t_{1/2}$ of collagen (years)	
		at 10°C	at 20°C
Ortner et al.[39]	release of soluble nitrogen (140–100°C)	7000	1000
Collins et al. (unpublished data)	survival of insoluble protein (95–55°C)	110 000	20 000

dissolves and then leaches the mineral component. The alterations caused by groundwater can be measured, and diagenetic indices have been defined which indicate the preservation state of archaeological bones. Most of these indices have now become recognized parameters of diagenesis; Table 2 briefly outlines the analytical techniques available for assessing both mineral and protein preservation.

There are three important alterations to bone apatite that can be used as indicators of diagenetic change: porosity increase, crystallinity increase and inclusion of exogenous ions. Although the chemical mechanisms that control these alterations are, as yet largely unknown, unlike the biodegradation of bone, these chemical processes can be modelled. Mineral diagenesis, therefore, has the potential to allow predictions to be made for bone survival under particular burial conditions.[8,43]

Porosity

The most common change resulting from mineral dissolution is the increase in the porosity of archaeological bones, in comparison to modern bone. Modern bone is a very porous material, about 12% of fresh cortical bone is occupied by pore spaces. Hedges and Millard[44] have outlined the main reasons for investigating porosity in archaeological bone. The pore structure (i.e. the distribution of porosity for a given pore radius) of bone influences the extent of diagenetic alteration which can occur, and an increase in this porosity will, subsequently, increase the rate of mineral dissolution processes, which will, in turn, lead to greater porosity, etc.

Although investigations into porosity changes are still relatively new, the studies carried out so far suggest that porosity has the potential to be one of the most useful indicators of diagenetic change.[7,8,43,45,46] The novel use of mercury intrusion porosimetry,[46] as a technique for analysing porosity changes in archaeological bones, has greatly enhanced the ability to record these alterations, especially with respect to creating realistic dissolution models. Early results using this technique have shown that pore ranges affected by biological degradation processes can be determined.[8,46] Figure 1 illustrates the obvious differences in porosity between modern bone and a poorly preserved archaeological bone using mercury intrusion porosimetry.

Crystallinity

One of the most consistent, but ambiguous, changes recorded in archaeological bone is the increase in the 'crystallinity' relative to fresh bone.[29,47] Although the exact processes behind this phenomenon are still unknown, it is recognized as an important alteration, and understanding its occurrence could be useful for interpretation of other diagenetic processes. Two mechanisms are often proposed to explain the increases measured in the crystallinity of archaeological bone:

- Dissolution of the smallest crystallites.
- Dissolution and subsequent recrystallization to larger, more thermodynamically stable crystals of bone apatite.

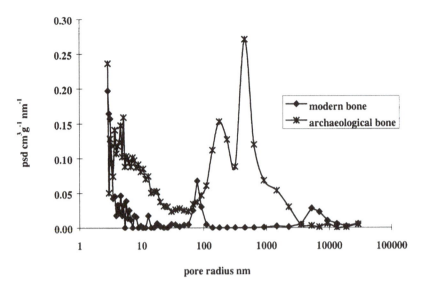

Figure 1 – Mercury intrusion porosimetry traces for modern and diagenetically altered archaeological bone. psd = pore size distribution

The second of these mechanisms will lead to incorporation of *diagenetic ions* (see below), which will affect the mineral structure and the size of bone apatite crystals. During diagenesis, exogenous ions such as Sr^{2+} and CO_3^{2-} can adsorb to the surface of bone apatite, or exchange with its ions.[29,48] If recrystallization takes place, these ions may be incorporated deeper into the mineral structure. If, on the other hand, the change in crystallinity is due to the differential dissolution of the crystallite population (with preferential loss of the less stable, less crystalline material),[49] exogenous ions associated with dissolving bone apatite may simply be re-adsorbed.[50]

While different processes can contribute to crystallinity increases during diagenesis, it may be possible to distinguish between those that act by dissolution (preferentially removing the less stable components) and those that act by recrystallization (forming a population of more stable crystallites). As discussed above, these two mechanisms have different implications for diagenetic change, and for methods that aim to remove diagenetic alteration.[50,51] Crystallinity changes are an important process in diagenetic alteration of archaeological bone, not least because they are relevant to understanding bone dissolution processes and accompanying porosity changes.

Incorporation of exogenous ions

The reactivity of the ions in bone apatite and the ready accommodation of its structure makes bone apatite a good absorbent for many ionic species.[28] Elements present in the surrounding soil or groundwater can be taken up by buried bones, as observed increases in fluorine, carbonate and uranium content of archaeological bones, relative to modern bones show.[52–54] The exchange of PO_4^{3-} and CO_3^{2-} ions between bone and the environment can also lead to altered $\delta^{13}C$ and $\delta^{18}O$ in the bone mineral (see Mays, chapter 25, in this volume).[51,52,55]

Table 2 – Analytical methods available for assessment of mineral and proteinaceous preservation in archaeological bones.

Method	Measured parameter	Advantages/disadvantages	Amount of sample required	References
Mercury intrusion porosimetry	Mesoporosity, pores of 2.8-36 444 nm radii	Destructive and relatively expensive technique. However, the information obtained is of great value in the assessment of overall bone preservation.	Between 500 and 700 mg fragment	8, 78
Water sorption★	Macroporosity, pores of > 4 nm radii. Microporosity, pores of < 4 nm radii. Total porosity, pores including (0–∞)	Less informative than mercury intrusion porosimetry; however, the technique is not destructive and the necessary equipment can be easily set-up and used in any location at no great cost. Large margin for error above certain pore sizes. However, reproducible values for total porosity and the distribution of macro– and microporosity within both archaeological and modern bones are obtained.	Between 300 and 500 mg fragment	8
Fourier transform infrared spectroscopy (FTIR)★	Increases in crystallinity (IRSF), diagenetic carbonate content (C/P) and presence of diagenetic minerals, e.g. calcite, fluorapatite, etc.	Quick and efficient, though costly, method that can provide semiquantitative measures for several important mineral alterations. Results also provide a qualitative indication of surviving collagen	1 mg powdered bone	6, 42
Optical microscopy★	Assessment of transverse section using the Oxford histological scale	Time-consuming preparative method, but analyses are quick and easy. Samples are destroyed	Between 200 and 500 mg fragment	7, 8
Differential scanning calorimetry (DSC)	Melt temperature for transition from helical collagen to randomly coiled gelatine (T_m)	Expensive technique that has yet to be satisfactorily proven as an indicator of collagen preservation. Preparation of samples is very time-consuming	Between 300 and 600 mg fragment	16
Mass spectrometry★	Protein content (%N). Carbon to nitrogen ratio (C/N). Stable isotopic data ($\delta^{13}C$, $\delta^{15}N$)	Costly and destructive analysis. Badly preserved material will result in less accurate data	10 mg bone powder for %N; 10 mg collagen for C/N, $\delta^{13}C$, $\delta^{15}N$	7, 41
Acid dissolution	% insoluble fraction (collagen)	Cheap, destructive analysis – moderately time-consuming. Can be compared with model that predicts survival[72]	100 mg fragment	38, 75
Immunology	Small regions of protein (collagen)	Specific to targeted protein. Costly and prone to ambiguous results	10 mg powder	76, 77

★Used for determining the preservation of archaeological bones featured in Figure 2.

Exogenous carbonate is a particularly important contaminant of bone apatite and there is an appreciable amount of controversy concerning the validity of using carbonate in bone apatite as an alternative to collagen for stable isotopic analyses.[56] In bone apatite there is a natural level of biogenic carbonate (between 2 and 5%), of which a large proportion is assumed to be adsorbed onto the surface of the mineral.[57] During burial, this carbonate is either decreased via dissolution processes, or increased via different mechanisms that introduce exogenous CO_3^{2-} ions (usually from the surrounding groundwater) into the mineral lattice.

Uptake of diagenetic CO_3^{2-} may occur via the following processes:

1. Addition via absorption/exchange with the mineral surface.[58]
2. Addition via substitution into the mineral lattice, usually for PO_4^{3-} groups.[51]
3. Exchange with the original CO_3^{2-} via either points 1 or 2 – overall CO_3^{2-} content may not be increased.
4. Recrystallization of the bone apatite matrix; possibly reducing the contribution of CO_3^{2-} from surface adsorption or exchange due to loss of mineral surface area.
5. Crystallization of calcite into the pore spaces.

In the burial environment, incorporation of exogenous carbonate into buried bone may occur simultaneously, via these various mechanisms. This variability makes it hard to distinguish and remove diagenetic carbonate from the original, biogenic carbonate, if this still remains, thereby decreasing the chances of obtaining reliable biogenic CO_3^{2-} from archaeological bone.[51,56] In experiments on archaeological human remains, Wright and Schwarcz[54] removed carbonate substitution from apatite where carbonate had been adsorbed onto the surface (case 1), but found it harder to remove carbonate which had been substituted into the lattice (case 2).

Key environmental parameters controlling bone apatite dissolution

The rates of dissolution of bone mineral once in the burial environment, will, we argue, depend on three key environmental parameters:

- pH.
- How saturated the water is with respect to Ca^{2+} and PO_4^{3-} ions.
- The rate of groundwater movement.

Effects of pH

In the majority of soils, bone mineral is only one of a number of calcium-phosphate species which can exist (e.g. brushite, $CaHPO_4.2H_2O$; fluorapatite, $Ca_5(PO_4)_3F$), depending upon environmental conditions, such as the chemical composition of the surrounding soil and groundwater, and the pH.[29,59,60] In general, all of the calcium phosphates become more soluble with reduction in pH. The following equation shows the role of the hydrogen ion on the solubility of hydroxyapatite:

$$Ca_5(PO_4)_3OH + 7H^+ \rightleftharpoons 5Ca^{2+} + 3H_2PO_4^- + H_2O.$$

An increase in the hydrogen ion concentration forces the reaction to the right and hydroxyapatite dissolves. In more alkaline conditions therefore, hydroxyapatite is increasingly stable, but, in the presence of CO_2, calcium will precipitate out of solution as bicarbonate. In such an environment, the solubility of hydroxyapatite can increase under alkaline conditions, but this will be limited by the concentration of CO_2. When hydroxyapatite dissolves, it consumes H^+ ions and pushes the reaction to the left, reducing the acidity. Using this equation and known chemical constants, the solubility of hydroxyapatite, and therefore bone apatite, at different pH can be calculated.[8,43]

Except for its fluoridated form, bone apatite is one of the most stable calcium phosphate phases, at pH levels that characterize most groundwater.[59] Hydroxyapatite is most stable about pH 7.8 and has low solubility in alkaline aqueous systems (pH > 7.5), while in an acidic environment (pH ≤ 6.0), its solubility is relatively high.[59,60] Bone tends, therefore, to survive better in alkaline environments, as the bone apatite is less likely to dissolve; however, soils low in phosphate will also promote demineralization.[61]

The pH of the surrounding groundwater also determines the nature of the ions present for ionic exchange reactions. This has important consequences for attempts to reconstruct palaeodiet from trace elements in the inorganic component of archaeological bone.[62] Groundwater can lie within a pH range of 2.8–10; wet soils ranging from 3.7 to 8.5; and waterlogged soils from 5.0 to 8.0: the acid limits of each type corresponding to component mineral differences.[63] Gordon and Buikstra[64] carried out a survey that investigated how the soil pH at mortuary sites in west central Illinois, USA, influenced bone preservation. They found a very high correlation between soil pH and bone preservation ($r = -0.92$) in both mature and immature skeletal remains.

Importance of Ca^{2+} and PO_4^{3-} in bone apatite dissolution

The simple dissolution model for bone apatite, envisaged by Hedges and Millard,[44] assumes that mineral loss occurs via *diffusion*, where the movement of Ca^{2+} and PO_4^{3-} ions away from the surface of the bone apatite is believed to be the rate-limiting step. Before their work, Whitmer *et al.*[65] had already discussed the value of diffusion models in providing plausible accounts of bone diagenesis, in spite of the potentially complex chemical processes that characterize most burial environments. Review of subsequent literature provides evidence to suggest that diffusion of some sort is responsible for the transport of matter away from enamel and hydroxyapatite surfaces under controlled laboratory conditions.[66–70] Groundwater movement, or hydrology, therefore becomes a determining factor in mineral dissolution, as it controls the extent to which the immediate groundwater surrounding the bone is saturated with respect to Ca^{2+} and PO_4^{3-} ions. Saturated solutions will retard, and may even halt the process of dissolution. The introduction of 'fresh, unsaturated groundwater', will in contrast, increase the rate of dissolution. Dissolution of Ca^{2+} and PO_4^{3-} ions into the surrounding groundwater solution, however, will be extremely limited in environments where bone apatite solubility is low.

Importance of groundwater activity (hydrology)

The importance of groundwater activity, or hydrology, on bone diagenesis has been discussed in various studies.[44,52,53,55,71] In particular, Hedges and Millard[44] defined three specific hydrological environments (or regimes): recharge, diffusion and hydraulic flow. Using both the principles of water movement and the factors that govern bone apatite solubility, subsequent studies have extended their ideas and led to the development of quantitative models of bone dissolution.[8,43] The following sections outline the important elements of these regimes and how they are expected to affect bone apatite dissolution.

Diffusive regime

In the simplest form, a bone is buried in an environment where water movement is limited or negligible. In this case there is no net flow of water into or out of the bone, therefore the hydraulic potential (the free energy required to move water from its state in the soil to a standard state[72]) is constant in both time and space. Solutes can still move under the influence of diffusion gradients, but dissolution will become increasingly limited as the groundwater surrounding the bone becomes saturated with respect to bone apatite (Ca^{2+} and PO_4^{3-} ions). Diffusive environments may be represented by waterlogged conditions; however, diffusion may also apply in soils that are not permanently saturated (e.g. clay).

Recharge regime

Once a bone establishes equilibrium with its surroundings, a *fluctuating* hydraulic potential, such as that generated by a wetting-drying cycle, will drive water into and out of the bone. The effect of this water cycling will create a situation where dissolution effects become much more extreme, leading to significant increases in the bone porosity and the formation of very large pores, which in turn will increase the effects caused by water cycling. A recharge environment can be represented by bones buried close to the surface, in soil which possesses high hydraulic conductivity (the ease with which water can flow through a porous medium), such as gravel-based soils. Bones buried in such an environment are expected to undergo relatively extreme alterations, such alterations were measured in Anglo-Saxon bones from the site of Yarnton, Oxfordshire, buried on a gravel terrace above a floodplain.[8]

Flow regime

Under a hydraulic gradient there will be a flow of water through the soil and also through the bone. This will occur, for example, following infiltration after rainfall in unsaturated soils. The magnitude of the flow through a bone buried in such an environment, will depend upon the hydraulic conductivities of both the soil and the bone, and the total volume of water available to flow (mainly due to rainfall), which in reality will be seasonal and sporadic. As for the recharge regime, water fluctuation, i.e. a constant supply of ground water, unsaturated with respect to bone apatite, will lead to a faster rate of dissolution than experienced in a diffusion environment; again, formation of large pores will result in poorly preserved bones.[8,43]

BONE SURVIVAL; THE INFLUENCE OF THE BURIAL ENVIRONMENT

Using the above observations, we believe that groundwater is likely to be the most influential agent of bone diagenesis. It is the medium in which nearly all other diagenetic processes we have discussed occur. Dissolution and recrystallization, hydrolysis, microbiological attack and ion exchange all require water in some form to be present. Based on the arguments above, a simple diagenetic model can be built up for bone survival in different burial environments.

Bone buried in a soil where water movement is limited and Ca^{2+} or PO_4^{3-} concentrations are relatively high can, in principle, survive for an indefinite period, since the mineral structure is likely to remain unaltered by dissolution. If the mineral is dissolved to any significant extent, however, then the accompanying porosity increase will augment the rate of dissolution, concomitantly making the organic component of bone available for microbial assimilation. A drop in the Ca^{2+} (and/or PO_4^{3-}) content of soil water, accompanied by a greater movement of soil water, will lead to an increase in the rate of mineral dissolution, and the survival potential for the bone, in contact with such fluid conditions, will decrease dramatically. Thus, it can be foreseen that a combination of all three (increase in porosity, a low Ca^{2+} or PO_4^{3-} soil concentration and a fluctuating water content) will produce conditions where bone will dissolve very rapidly, even at alkaline pH levels. Bone porosity is, therefore, one of the major determining factors in bone dissolution; any changes which lead to its increase will greatly decrease the prospect of bone survival in the burial environment.

Three different hydrological mechanisms (diffusion, recharge and flow) have been described, but principle components analysis performed on diagenetic measurements from archaeological bones buried in different environments (Table 2),[8] suggest that bone preservation can be more simply classified by two basic hydrological conditions (Figure 2):

- Saturated or dry conditions, which experience very little, or no oscillation in ground water content (diffusion).
- Fluctuating conditions, where there is substantial oscillation in groundwater content around buried bones (recharge and flow).

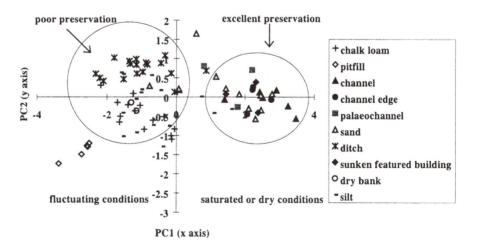

Figure 2 – Influence of hydrological environment over bone preservation (data from [8]).

The expected effects of these two environments have been discussed above. However, it becomes obvious after analysis of the results in Figure 2, that the hydrological environment has an important role in bone preservation patterns.

The points discussed above show that, both in theory and in the archaeological record, clear distinctions can be made between saturated and unsaturated environments. In most archaeological samples, however, the structural and chemical alterations are far too extreme to make any conclusions about whether protein or mineral loss is the *initiating* process. Recent analyses of bones buried for 32 years in the experimental earthworks project set up at Overton Down and Morden Bog, England,[73] have gone some way to answering this question. The results show that, in almost every case, the mineral had undergone a degree of alteration normally measured in much older samples,[8] but the proteinaceous component, with the exception of one sample that had been cooked before burial, was generally unaltered. The results from these bones illustrate that in the early stages of diagenesis, in these samples, dissolution of the mineral had occurred *before* any significant protein loss.

In a temperate climate, bones may lie within a burial environment for a very long period of time, with little change to either their mineral or proteinaceous components. This statement is supported by the excellent preservational standard of Bronze Age material from the site of Yarnton, Oxfordshire, and Neolithic remains from Bercy, Paris.[8,9] As the bones from the Overton Down site have shown, however, certain burial environments encourage mineral dissolution, greatly reducing the likelihood of bones buried in these conditions to survive into the archaeological record.

CONCLUSIONS

Removing the ambiguity surrounding archaeological bone survival will be enormously beneficial in this complex field, where the variability of bone preservation has, in the past, impeded any significant steps forward. Previously, most research has focused on the biological degradation of the proteinaceous component in archaeological bone. Increasingly, however, more studies are focusing on bone apatite alteration. The question of which component is most influential in determining bone survival is becoming more compelling. It is the intimate association between collagen and mineral in bone that underpins all bone preservation mechanisms. If the mineral remains intact then, arguably, microbial attack is prevented; we believe that the initial step in degradation is partial dissolution of the mineral phase exposing collagen to microbial attack.

The use of mercury intrusion porosimetry to examine porosity increase in archaeological bone, coupled with the concept of hydrologically influenced dissolution processes, will lead to the development of predictive models to identify sites prone to bone dissolution and subsequent biodeterioration. Site hydrology will play a leading role in these models. A unified theory of bone degradation will enable those researchers working in this field to recognize why and where the best surviving bones can be found. This knowledge can be used to identify bones from which reliable scientific data may be gained. Recognition of environments in which bones are at risk is equally important, in order that such bones can be made a priority for excavation and conservation.

ACKNOWLEDGEMENTS

This work was supported financially by the European Union, Directorate General No. XII, project number ENV4-CT98–0712 and the NERC grants GST/02/824 and GT4/94/11/B.

REFERENCES

1   Child AM. Microbial taphonomy of archaeological bone. *Studies in Conservation* 1995; **40**: 19–30.

2   Hanson DB, Buikstra JE. Histomorphological alteration in buried human bone from the lower Illinois valley: implications for palaeodietary research. *Journal of Archaeological Science* 1987; **14**: 549–563.

3   Nicholson RA. Bone degradation in a compost heap. *Journal of Archaeological Science* 1998; **25**: 393–403.

4   Mays S. *The Archaeology of Human Bones*. London: Routledge/English Heritage 1998.

5   Henderson J. Factors determining the state of preservation of human remains. In: Boddington A, Garland AN, Janaway RC (ed.), *Death, Decay and Reconstruction: Approaches to Archaeology and Forensic Science*. Manchester: Manchester University Press, 1987: pp. 127–148.

6   Weiner S, Bar-Yosef O. States of preservation of bones from the prehistoric sites in the Near East: A survey. *Journal of Archaeological Science* 1990; **17**: 187–196.

7   Hedges REM, Millard AR, Pike AWG. Measurements and relationships of diagenetic alteration of bone from three archaeological sites. *Journal of Archaeological Science* 1995; **22**: 201–211.

8   Nielsen-Marsh CM. Studies in archaeological bone diagenesis. Unpublished doctoral dissertation, University of Oxford, 1997.

9   Bocherens H, Tresset A, Wiedemann F, Giligny F, Lafage F, Lanchon Y, Mariotti, A. Diagenetic evolution of mammal bones in two French Neolithic sites. *Bulletin de la Société Géologique de France* 1997; **168**: 555–564.

10 Turner-Walker G, Parry TV. The tensile strength of archaeological bone. *Journal of Archaeological Science* 1995; **22**: 185–192.

11 Chaplin E. *The Study of Animal Bones from Archaeological Sites*. London: Seminar, 1971: pp. 13–19.

12 Beeley JG, Lunt DA. The nature of the biochemical changes in softened dentine from archaeological sites. *Journal of Archaeological Science* 1980; **7**: 371–377.

13 Eastoe JE, Eastoe B. The organic constituents of mammalian compact bone. *Biochemical Journal* 1954; **57**: 453–459.

14 Triffitt JT. The organic matrix of bone. In: Urist MR (ed.), *Fundamental and Clinical Bone Physiology*. Philadelphia: Lippencott, 1980: pp. 45–82.

15 Covington AD. Chromium in the leather industry. *Chromium Review* 1985; **5**: 2–9.

16 Kronick PL, Cooke P. Thermal stabilisation of collagen fibres by calcification. *Connective Tissue Research* 1996; **33**: 275–282.

17 Kent MJC, Light ND, Bailey AJ. Evidence for glucose-mediated covalent cross-linking of collagen after glycolysation *in vitro*. *Biochemical Journal* 1985; **72(6)**: 1189–1194.

18 Collins MJ, Westbroek P, Muyzer G, de Leeuw JW. Experimental evidence for condensation reactions between sugars and proteins in carbonate skeletons. *Geochimica et Cosmochimica Acta* 1992; **56**: 1539–1544.

19 Van Klinken GJ, Hedges REM. Experiments on collagen–humic interactions: speed of humic acid uptake, and effects of diverse chemical treatments. *Journal of Archaeological Science* 1995; **22**: 263–270.

20 LeGeros RZ. Apatites in biological systems. *Progress in Crystal Growth and Characterization of Materials* 1981; **4**: 1–45.

21 Lowenstam HA, Weiner S. *On Biomineralization*. Oxford: Oxford University Press, 1989.

22 Giraud-Guille, MM. Twisted plywood architecture of collagen fibrils in human compact bone osteons. *Calcified Tissue International* 1988; **42**: 167–180.

23 Weiner S, Traub W. Bone structure: from angstroms to microns. *Federation of American Societies for Experimental Biology (FASEB) Journal* 1992; **6**: 879–885.

24   Weiner S, Traub W. Organisation of hydroxyapatite crystals within collagen fibrils. *Federation of European Biochemical Societies (FEBS) Letters* 1986; **206**: 262–266.

25   Landis WJ, Hodgens KJ, Song MJ, Arena J, Kiyonaga S, Marko M, Owen C, McEwen BF. Mineralization of collagen may occur on fibril surfaces: evidence from conventional and high-voltage electron microscopy and three-dimensional imaging. *Journal of Structural Biology* 1996; **117**: 24–35.

26   Ziv V, Sabanay I, Arad T, Traub W, Weiner S. Transitional structures in lamellar bone. *Microscopy Research and Technique* 1996; **33**: 203–213.

27   Vaughan J. *The Physiology of Bone* (3rd edn). Oxford: Clarendon, 1981.

28   Kibby, Hall. Surface properties of calcium phosphates. In: Hair ML (ed.), *The Chemistry of Biosurfaces*, vol. 2. New York: Dekker, 1972: pp. 686–727.

29   Piepenbrink H. Examples of chemical change during fossilisation. *Applied Geochemistry* 1989; **4**: 277–280.

30   Valsami-Jones E, Ragnarsdottir KV, Putnis A, Bosbach D, Kemp AJ. The dissolution of apatite in the presence of aqueous metal cations at pH 2–7. *Chemical Geology* 1998; **151**: 215–233.

31   Child AM, Gillard RD, Pollard AM. Microbially induced promotion of amino acid racemization in bone: isolation of the micro-organisms and detection of their enzymes. *Journal of Archaeological Science* 1993; **20**: 159–168.

32   Child AM. Towards an understanding of the decomposition of bone in the archaeological environment. *Journal of Archaeological Science* 1995; **21**: 165–174.

33   Bond MD, Van Wart HE. Characterisation of the individual collagenases from *Clostridium histolyticum*. *Biochemistry* 1984; **23**: 3085–3091.

34   Mayer LM. Surface area control of organic carbon accumulation in continental drift shelf sediments. *Geochimica et Cosmochimica Acta* 1994; **58**: 1271–1284.

35   Krane S. Degradation of collagen in connective tissue diseases. Rheumatoid arthritis. In: Burleigh, PMC, Poole AR (eds), *Dynamics of Connective Tissue Macromolecules*. Amsterdam: North Holland, 1970: pp. 309–326.

36   Hare PE, Hoering TC. The organic constituents of fossil mollusc shells. *Carnegie Institute of Washington Year Book* 1977; **76**: 625–631.

37   Pineri MH, Escombes M, Roche G. Water–collagen interactions: calorimetric and mechanical experiments. *Biopolymers* 1978; **17**: 2799–2815.

38   Collins MJ, Riley M, Child AM, Turner-Walker G. A basic mathematical simulation of the chemical degradation of ancient collagen. *Journal of Archaeological Science* 1995; **22**: 175–183.

39   Ortner DJ, von Endt DW, Robinson MS. The effect of temperature on protein decay in bone: its significance in nitrogen dating of archaeological specimens. *American Antiquity* 1972; **37(4)**: 514–520.

40   von Endt DW and Ortner DJ. Experimental effects of bone size and temperature on bone diagenesis. *Journal of Archaeological Science* 1984; **11**: 247–253.

41   Ambrose SH. Preparation and characterisation of bone and tooth collagen for isotopic analysis. *Journal of Archaeological Science* 1990; **17**: 431–451.

42   Sillen A, Parkington J. Diagenesis of bones from Eland's Bay cave. *Journal of Archaeological Science* 1996; **23**: 353–542.

43   Pike AWG, Nielsen-Marsh CM. Modelling bone dissolution and hydrology. In: Millard AR (ed.), *Proceedings of Archaeological Sciences '97*. British Archaeological Reports. Oxford: Archaeopress (in press).

44   Hedges REM, Millard AR. Bones and groundwater: towards the modelling of diagenetic processes. *Journal of Archaeological Science* 1995; **22**: 155–165.

45   Pike AWG. Bone porosity, water and diagenesis: towards a grand unifying theory of bone diagenesis. Part 2. Unpublished undergraduate dissertation, University of Bradford, 1993.

46   Nielsen-Marsh CM, Hedges REM. Bone porosity and the use of mercury intrusion porosimetry in bone diagenesis studies. *Archaeometry* 1999; **41(1)**: 165–174.

47   Pate FD, Hutton JT, Norrish K. Ionic exchange between soil solution and bone: toward a predictive model. *Applied Geochemistry* 1989; **4**: 303–316.

48   Pate D, Brown KA. The stability of bone strontium in the geochemical environment. *Journal of Human Evolution* 1985; **14**: 483–491.

49   Weiner S, Price PA. Disaggregation of bone into crystals. *Calcified Tissue International* 1986; **39**: 365–375.

50   Sillen A, Sealy JC. Diagenesis of strontium in fossil bone: a reconsideration of Nelson *et al*. *Journal of Archaeological Science* 1995; **22**: 313–320.

51   Koch PL, Tuross N, Fogel ML. The effects of sample treatment and diagenesis on the isotopic integrity of carbonate in biogenic hydroxylapatite. *Journal of Archaeological Science* 1997; **24**: 417–429.

52   Millard AR. Diagenesis of archaeological bone: the case of uranium uptake. Unpublished DPhil thesis, University of Oxford, 1993.

53   Millard AR, Hedges REM. The role of the environment in uranium uptake by buried bone. *Journal of Archaeological Science* 1995; **22**: 239–250.

54   Wright LE, Schwarcz HP. Infrared and isotopic evidence for diagenesis of bone apatite at Dos Pilas, Guatemala: palaeodietary implications. *Journal of Archaeological Science* 1996; **23**: 933–944.

55   Wang Y, Cerling T.E. A model of fossil tooth and bone diagenesis: implications for palaeodiet reconstruction from stable isotopes. *Palaeogeography, Palaeoclimatology, Palaeoecology* 1994; **107**: 281–289.

56   Lee-Thorp JA, van der Merwe NJ. Aspects of the chemistry of modern and fossil biological apatites. *Journal of Archaeological Science* 1991; **18**: 343–354.

57   Eanes ED. A note on the crystal growth of hydroxyapatite precipitated from aqueous solutions. *Materials Research Bulletin* 1970; **5**: 377–384.

58   Krueger HW. Exchange of carbon with biological apatite. *Journal of Archaeological Science* 1991; **18**: 355–361.

59   Lindsay WL. *Chemical Equilibria in Soils*. New York: Wiley, 1979.

60   White EM, Hannus LA. Chemical weathering of bone in archaeological soils. *American Antiquity* 1983; **48**: 316–322.

61   Rottlander RCA. Variation in the chemical composition of bone as an indicator of diagenetic change. *Journal of Archaeological Science* 1976; **3**: 83–88.

62   Sillen A, LeGeros RZ. Solubility profiles of synthetic apatites and of modern and fossil bones. *Journal of Archaeological Science* 1991; **18**: 385–397.

63   Baas Becking LGM, Kaplan IR, Moore D. Limits of the natural environment in terms of pH and oxidation–reduction potentials. *Journal of Geology* 1960; **68**: 243–284.

64   Gordon CC, Buikstra JE. Soil pH, bone preservation and sampling bias at mortuary sites. *American Antiquity*, 1981; **46**: 566–571.

65   Whitmer AM, Ramenofsky AF, Thomas J, Thibodeaux LJ, Field SD, Miller BJ (eds), *Stability or Instability: The Role of Diffusion in Trace Element Studies*. Tuscon: University of Arizona Press, 1989.

66   Christoffersen J, Christoffersen MR, Kjaergaard N. The kinetics of dissolution of calcium hydroxyapatite in water at constant pH. *Journal of Crystal Growth* 1978; **43**: 501–511.

67   Gramain PH, Voegal JC, Gumpper M, Thomann JM. Surface properties and equilibrium kinetics of hydroxyapatite powder near the solubility equilibrium. *Journal of Colloid and Interface Science* 1987; **118**: 148–157.

68   Thomann JM, Voegal JC, Gramain P. Kinetics of dissolution of calcium hydroxyapatite powder: III: pH and sample conditioning effects. *Calcified Tissue International* 1990; **46**: 21–129.

69   Gray JA. Kinetics of the dissolution of human dental enamel in acid. *Journal of Dental Research* 1962; **41**: 353–359.

70   Gramain PH, Voegal JC, Gumpper M, Thomann JM. Dissolution kinetics of human enamel powder: 1. Stirring effects and surface calcium accumulation. *Journal of Colloid and Interface Science* 1989; **128**: 370–381.

71   Millard AR. The survival and alteration of bones: a hydrogeochemical approach. *Universities of Newcastle-upon-Tyne and Durham Archaeological Reports* 1996; **19**: 78–82.

72   Ward RC and Robinson M. *Principles of Hydrology* (3rd edn). London: McGraw-Hill, 1990.

73   Bell M, Fowler PJ, Hillson SW (eds), *The Experimental Earthwork Project 1960–1992*. Research Report 100. York: Council for British Archaeology, 1996.

74   Miles CA, Durjanadze TV, Bailey AJ. The kinetics of the thermal-denaturation of collagen in unrestrained rat tail tendon determined by differential scanning calorimetry. *Journal of Molecular Biology* 1995; **245**: 437–446.

75   Collins MJ, Galley P. Towards and optimal method of archaeological collagen extraction; the influence of pH and grinding. *Ancient Biomolecules* 1999: **2**; 209–222.

76   Collins MJ, Child AM, Van Duin ACT, Vermeer C. Is osteocalcin stabilised in ancient bones by adsorption to bioapatite? *Ancient Biomolecules* 1999: **2**; 223–238.

77   Hodgins GWL, Hedges REM. On the immunological characterisation of ancient collagen. In: Millard AR (ed.), *Proceedings of Archaeological Sciences 1997*. British Archaeological Reports. Oxford: Archaeopress (in press).

78   Portsmouth RL and Gladden LF. Mercury porosimetry as a probe of pore connectivity. *Chemical Engineering Research and Design* 1992; **70**: 63–70.

27

ANCIENT DNA APPLICATIONS IN HUMAN OSTEOARCHAEOLOGY: ACHIEVEMENTS, PROBLEMS AND POTENTIAL

Keri Brown

INTRODUCTION

The discovery of the structure of DNA in 1953 heralded a new era in biological sciences and has had profound implications for many other disciplines. The double helix structure explained how gene replication occurs, while the order of the nucleotides in DNA showed how biological information could be encoded. This discovery revolutionized genetics, led to the development of molecular biology (the study of biological processes at the molecular level) and provided a mechanism for Darwin's theory of evolution (Neo-Darwinism, the study of evolution at the level of the gene). Other disciplines owing their origins to DNA include population genetics, molecular ecology and biotechnology. Diseases can be studied and conquered by analysing the DNA of bacteria, viruses and faulty genes. DNA is used by forensic scientists to identify criminals and corpses; there need never again be an 'Unknown Warrior' in future conflicts. Now DNA has been found to be relevant in archaeology, in areas such as human evolution, population movements, palaeodisease and the domestication of plants and animals. Ancient DNA extracted from human skeletal remains can be analysed to uncover aspects of past social organization which were previously unknowable or difficult to ascertain using conventional archaeological techniques.

This chapter reviews the achievements of ancient DNA that are applicable to human osteoarchaeology. It does not intend to raise unreasonable expectations in the archaeological community. There are many problems to be overcome before ancient DNA analysis becomes routine with human remains. These problems, and the prospects of future improvements in methodology and sampling procedures, will be discussed.

WHAT IS DNA?

DNA stands for deoxyribonucleic acid. It is a polymer made up of repeated units called nucleotides. Each nucleotide consists of a ring structure (the 'base') attached to the sugar

2′-deoxyribose and a phosphate group. The sugar and phosphate groups are linked together to form the 'backbone' of the polynucleotide chain which forms one-half of the double helix (Figure 1). There are four bases present in DNA, called adenine, thymine, guanine and cytosine, but always referred to as A, T, G and C, and these can be linked together in any order. It is this nucleotide sequence that defines the property of each gene (Figure 2). Chemical links between the bases facing each other on the opposing chains of the double helix hold the halves of the molecule together. This base pairing follows strict rules, A always pairing with T, G always pairing with C. Because of these rules, the two chains in a double helix have 'complementary' sequences, the sequence of one dictated by the sequence of the other. The length of a DNA molecule is described in terms of the number of the base pairs (bp) it contains.

Every one of the 10^{13} cells in the adult human body (with a few exceptions such as red blood cells) has a nucleus that contains a set of chromosomes. Inside each chromosome there is a single DNA molecule between 55 and 250 million bp in length. The normal number of chromosomes in human each cell is 46; 22 pairs of autosomal chromosomes, and one pair of sex chromosomes, the latter being XX or XY. Twenty-two chromosomes and one sex chromosome are inherited from each parent. There are about 200 000 genes in human nuclear DNA, each present as two copies, one on each of a pair of chromosomes. Another type of DNA is present outside the nucleus in small structures (organelles) called

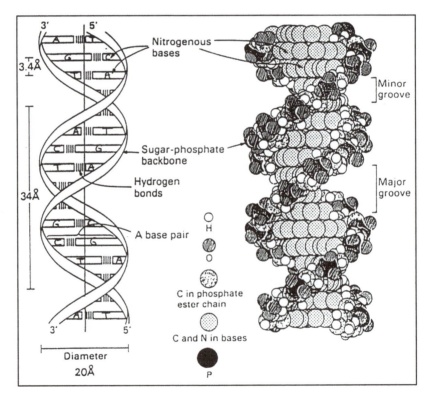

Figure 1 – Structure of DNA.

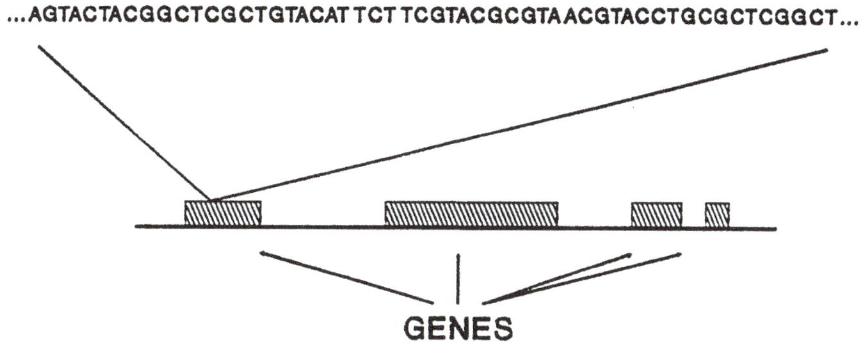

...AGTACTACGGCTCGCTGTACAT TCT TCGTACGCGTAACGTACCTGCGCTCGGCT...

GENES

Figure 2 – A DNA sequence is formed by the order of the bases.

mitochondria. Mitochondrial DNA is relatively short, only 16 569 bp long, and codes for just 37 genes. It has been completely sequenced (the order of the bases has been worked out) and is very well studied and understood by molecular biologists. There are about 800 mitochondria present in each cell, and each mitochondrion contains about ten DNA molecules, so mitochondrial genes have a high copy number. Mitochondrial DNA is inherited from the mother only.

So far about 5000 of the 200 000 human genes have been sequenced. Only 30% of the human genome (all the DNA in a cell) consists of genes and other regions of DNA needed to make the genes work. The rest is made up of non-coding DNA ('intergenic regions') that does not seem to code for biological information. In the past, molecular biologists called these sequences 'junk DNA'. We now know that these sequences change relatively quickly because they accumulate mutations (single nucleotide changes in the DNA sequence) and rearrangements (deletions, insertions and duplications of part of a DNA sequence). This fact makes non-coding DNA very useful for studying populations and even identifying individuals, more of which is discussed below.

A single gene can exist as two or more versions, each with a slightly different nucleotide sequence, but with the same function. These variations on a gene are called alleles. The study of allele frequencies can be used to help define a population, and to identify kinship between individuals.

STUDYING ANCIENT DNA

'Ancient DNA' is the term used to describe the DNA fragments that are found in some types of preserved biological material. The very nature of ancient DNA dictates which methods can be used to study it; modern DNA molecules, which are long intact chains with no chemical damage to the bases, can be studied in many different ways. Ancient DNA, however, is fragmented into short pieces, a few hundred bp at most, possibly much shorter.[1] Some of the bases may have undergone chemical changes, and the amounts of DNA that survive are extremely small, perhaps less than ten molecules per g bone.[2] These factors (fragment length, damage and limited quantity) dictate that just two methods from the total repertoire can be used with ancient DNA.

Hybridization analysis

Hybridization analysis is a long established method in molecular biology.[3] A short piece of artificial DNA is synthesized, usually about 20 bp long, the sequence of bases in this 'probe' being complementary to a 'target' sequence that is being sought, a male-specific sequence for example. DNA extracted from the material under investigation is bound to a piece of filter paper and washed with a solution containing the probe DNA. If the complementary sequence is present in the DNA extract, the probe binds to it; if absent, the probe does not bind and can be washed off the filter. The probe DNA can be labelled with a radiochemical or fluorescent tag so that positive results, the binding of probe to target, are indicated by a signal of some sort (Figure 3).

Hybridization analysis is used in diagnostic medical testing and can discriminate just 1 bp difference between probe and target. It is therefore highly specific and can be used to test for the presence or absence of a particular DNA sequence in a DNA extract. It is not affected by impurities in the extract or the length of ancient DNA molecules, and perhaps could be used more widely than at present in ancient DNA analysis.

Polymerase chain reaction (PCR)

The reason that hybridization analysis is not widely used is because it does not have the sensitivity needed to detect the small numbers of DNA molecules present in many ancient extracts. The more sensitive technique used for most ancient DNA work is PCR. This is an enzymatic reaction that copies a defined sequence of DNA (the 'template') many times.[4] PCR works with very small amounts of template DNA, just a single molecule under ideal conditions. The technique was invented in the late 1980s and has had a huge impact on molecular biology, and its inventors were awarded the Nobel Prize in 1993 (surprisingly, this was for Chemistry, not Physiology and Medicine).

Two short pieces of DNA, called primers, are used to define the limits of the DNA sequence to be copied (Figure 4). It follows from this that PCR can only be used when the sequence of the DNA to be studied is known in advance. It cannot be used with genes that have not previously been studied in some other way, but this is not a problem in archaeology as plenty of interesting and informative genes are known.

PCR results in an exponential copying of the template referred to as 'amplification', the resulting molecules being called the PCR product. The product is usually examined by gel electrophoresis. A sample is placed in a well in an agarose gel and a current passed through. The DNA molecules, which have negative charges, move through the gel towards the positive electrode. How fast they move depends on their lengths, shorter DNA molecules moving faster through the gel than longer ones. This means that PCR products of different lengths separate into bands, and appear like the rungs of a ladder when the gel is stained and

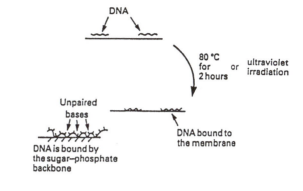

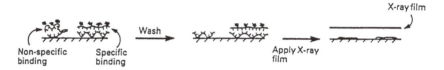

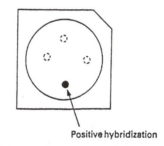

Figure 3 – How hybridization analysis works.

examined under ultraviolet irradiation (Figure 5). Often the lengths of the PCR products, as indicated by the band positions, are informative; alternatively the molecules can be sequenced.

ANCIENT DNA – IN THE BEGINNING

Ancient DNA research began before PCR was invented, in 1984 when mitochondrial DNA from a 140-year-old skin of a quagga, an extinct member of the horse family, was sequenced by the slower and less sensitive cloning method. The results showed that quaggas were related to the zebra.[5] The following year, Svante Pääbo cloned and sequenced the first ancient human DNA, from a 2400-year-old Egyptian mummy.[6] At this time ancient DNA

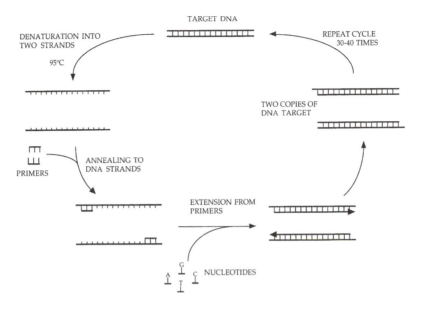

TARGET DNA

DENATURATION INTO
TWO STRANDS

95°C

REPEAT CYCLE
30-40 TIMES

TWO COPIES OF
DNA TARGET

PRIMERS

ANNEALING TO
DNA STRANDS

EXTENSION FROM
PRIMERS

NUCLEOTIDES

Figure 4 – Polymerase chain reaction. The target DNA molecule is denatured by heating to 95°C – this separates the two strands of the double helix so that the primers can anneal to each strand as shown. The primers define the stretch of DNA that is to be copied, and the DNA sequence is formed from the four nucleotides present in the reaction mixture (extension). This results in two copies of the target DNA sequence. The cycle is repeated 30–40 times, with double the number of DNA sequences being copied each time (1, 2, 4, 8, 16, 32, 64, 128, etc.) until eventually there are millions of copies of the original DNA molecule.

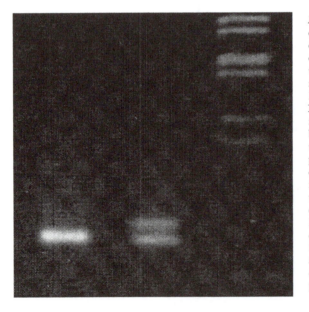

Figure 5 – Products of a PCR experiment can be visualized on an electrophoresis gel. DNA is stained with ethidium bromide that fluoresces under ultraviolet irradiation. This gel shows the results from an experiment to amplify DNA from the amelogenin genes on the X and Y chromosomes. Looking from right to left: the first lane shows multiple bands, these represent the DNA marker used to check the sizes of the PCR products. The middle lane shows two clear bands, these are the PCR products from a human male DNA sample. The upper band comes from the Y chromosome and is 112 bp long, the lower band comes from the X chromosome and is 106 bp long. The last lane shows just one clear band from a female DNA sample, where the two X chromosomes give rise to one PCR product of 106 bp.

seemed to be a scientific curiosity, with no real applications. This was mainly because it was thought that DNA would only survive in exceptionally preserved remains which had a high degree of biological and structural integrity, such as mummies, bog bodies, museum skins, frozen mammoths, etc. The invention of PCR overturned this assumption. In 1989 Erika Hagelberg, with Brian Sykes and Robert Hedges, used PCR to amplify DNA from human bones ranging in date from Neolithic to medieval, demonstrating that ancient DNA could be obtained from the sort of material found on typical archaeological sites.[7]

A wide range of materials have yielded ancient DNA (Table 1), including not just animal and human remains but also plant material and preserved microbes. Little is known about the optimum preservation conditions; but temperature, pH and moisture levels are probably the most important factors, as well as the degree of protection from the external environment. Low pH (acidic conditions) is not conducive to ancient DNA survival (no ancient human DNA has been detected in Lindow Man), though high pH (alkaline) may not be so detrimental as DNA has been reported from bones recovered from quicklime.[8] Burial in wet soil may be unsuitable for DNA survival, leading to extreme fragmentation of the DNA, and microbial activity and microenvironmental variation around the bones must also play important roles. Part of the reason for the lack of information on preservation conditions is that there is no method in place for the rapid screening of bones for indications of

Table 1 – Material from which ancient DNA has been obtained.

Human material	Oldest so far (years)
Bones and teeth	about 60 000
Mummies	5000
Bog bodies	7500
Hair	2
Fingernails	fresh
Embedded tissue specimens	80
Animal material	
Bones	25 000
Frozen mammoths	40 000
Naturally preserved skins	13 000
Museum skins	140
Feathers	130
Hair	2
Faeces/coprolites	20 000
Amber specimens★	135 million
Dinosaur bones★	80 million
Plant material	
Herbaria specimens	118
Charred seeds and cobs	3000
Desiccated seeds	1800
Mummified seeds and embryos	44 600
Fossil leaves★	16 million

★Results are unrepeatable and should be treated with caution.

DNA survival. There is no direct correlation between DNA content and the age of a bone, though Colson *et al*. suggest that there might be a correlation with the quality of the bone microstructure.[9,10]

ANCIENT DNA APPLICATIONS IN HUMAN OSTEOARCHAEOLOGY

Ancient DNA is just another tool, a new form of evidence that has great potential to give archaeologists information about past societies, but it also has limitations. DNA cannot, as yet, tell us about attributes such as hair and eye colour, intelligence and personality. DNA from bones will not tell us anything about identity or ethnicity as defined by theoretical archaeologists. We can only look for DNA sequences that are already known from modern research. Most of this research has been concerned with identifying genes involved in genetic diseases or biochemical pathways. Some of the research has thrown up unexpected sidelines that have been explored by biomolecular archaeologists, as for example with the work on the amelogenin gene (see below). Major research efforts at the moment in molecular biology include the various genome-sequencing projects, whereby the total DNA of an organism is sequenced. The organisms where this has been completed include *Mycobacterium tuberculosis*, and ongoing projects include *Plasmodium falciparum* (the causative agent of malaria) and *Homo sapiens*. The results of these projects will increase the utility of ancient DNA to biomolecular archaeologists in the years ahead.

At the moment, the major applications of ancient DNA analysis in human osteoarchaeology lie in three main areas: the sex identification of human remains, kinship analysis, and the study of palaeodisease via the DNA of the causative agent. Other areas of research such as population affinities and human evolution will undoubtedly come to use ancient DNA from human remains to add time depth to these studies. It must be remembered, however, that up to now that the vast majority of the DNA data used to study populations and their movements around the globe are derived from present day populations and their gene distributions. In fact, nearly all of the genetic data relevant to the debate on the origins of anatomically modern humans has been obtained from existing populations of humans (with the sole exception of the Neanderthal DNA sequence). It is probable that in the future ancient DNA will be used to test hypotheses derived from studies of modern DNA, and indeed several scientists have advocated this use of ancient DNA.

DNA-based sex identification of human remains

This subject has recently been reviewed in detail and is only briefly discussed here.[11] In strongly sexually dimorphic samples, observation of secondary sex characteristics can usually be used to provide a reliable assessment of sex in adult material (see Mays and Cox, chapter 8, in this volume). This reliability is directly proportionate to the survival of both skull and pelvis and assumes no pathology affecting the morphology of either. But in an archaeological scenario, the skeletal remains are often neither complete nor unambiguous. In addition, morphological and morphometric standards used to identify the sex of skeletal remains are derived from reference collections from modern populations. The application of such standards to earlier samples has to be undertaken with some caution as we cannot predict which intrinsic and extrinsic variables affect levels of dimorphism in both modern and ancient assemblages. Determination of sex in juveniles and infants[12] is a notoriously contentious subject (see Mays and Cox, chapter 8, in this volume) and it is generally presently considered that neither may be sexed with any degree of confidence. Cremations have their own difficulties, which include the cracking, shrinking and distortion of diagnostic bones; it has also been shown that Bronze Age cremation burials contain only a proportion of the total cremated bone originally present.[13,14] Thus, a cremation may lack the diagnostic bones necessary for sex identification. Osteoarchaeologists themselves recognize the need for an independent, accurate and reliable method of identifying the sex of human remains. Several PCR-based methods have been developed and applied with varying success to DNA extracted from human bones.

In humans, maleness is conferred by the presence of the Y chromosome; males have one X and one Y chromosome, while females have two X chromosomes (the exceptions to this rule are the very rare sex-reversed individuals who are XX males and XY females). Even in cases of sex chromosome aneuploidy (abnormal numbers of sex chromosomes) the presence of the Y chromosome indicates a male phenotype. PCR has been used to amplify a repetitive DNA sequence from the Y chromosome, but in this experimental system a negative result is interpreted as indicating a female.[15] This is unsatisfactory as negative PCRs can be due to many different factors, not just absence of template DNA. A better system is one where DNA sequences are amplified from both X and Y chromosomes. The amelogenin gene, which is present on the X and Y chromosomes, is useful for this purpose because the X and Y versions are non-identical, which means that a PCR system can be designed to utilize the differences, with the resulting PCR products showing sex-specific size differences. After gel electrophoresis, two bands of different lengths indicate a male, while only one band indicates a female (Figure 5) Three different PCR systems based on the amelogenin gene have been used with ancient human DNA samples (Figure 6). The first system uses three primers in a single reaction.[16] Primers 1 and 2 anneal to the X chromosome, while primers 1 and 3 anneal to the Y chromosome, which has a 64 bp deletion. Therefore, the PCR product from the X chromosome is larger (195 bp) than that from the Y chromosome (132 bp), these sizes being routinely amplifiable from modern DNA samples, though with ancient DNA there may be partial amplification failure, only one band being seen with male samples. A similar PCR system was used by Faerman et al. to investigate the infant remains recovered from a 4th century AD bathhouse in Roman Ashkelon.[17] The hypothesis was that the infant remains were victims of infanticide, which was widely practised in the past, and usually involved the disposal of unwanted female offspring. The sex of the infants could only be identified by molecular methods. Of the 43 individuals tested, only 19 yielded PCR products. Fourteen were males and only five were females, according to the PCR results. These results are significant at the 5% level of confidence; one more male result would have given 1% confidence. It was therefore concluded that male infanticide was practised at this site, in contrast to the expected female infanticide. Even though PCR was unsuccessful with many of the infant remains, enough results were obtained to gain important insights into the practice of infanticide. Whether males or females were disposed of depended on particular cultural and economic contexts.

Method 1 (Gotherstrom *et al.* 1997)[16]

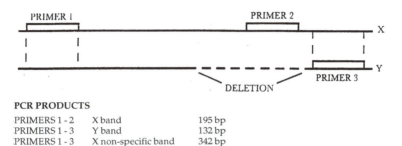

PCR PRODUCTS

PRIMERS 1 - 2	X band	195 bp
PRIMERS 1 - 3	Y band	132 bp
PRIMERS 1 - 3	X non-specific band	342 bp

Method 2 (Sullivan *et al.* 1993)

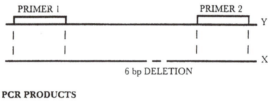

PCR PRODUCTS

X band	106 bp
Y band	112 bp

Method 3 (Stone *et al.* 1996)

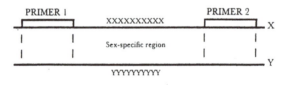

PCR PRODUCTS

X and Y bands are both 112 bp. Males and females are distinguished by hybridisation analysis with probes specific for the sex-specific regions:

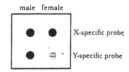

Figure 6 – PCR-based methods of sex identification using the amelogenin gene on the X and Y chromosomes.

The second PCR system is more widely used by forensic scientists and biomolecular archaeologists. The size difference between the PCR products is due to a 6 bp deletion in the X chromosome and, in the standard test, results in a 112 bp Y product and 106 bp X product.[18] This system is also subject to partial amplification failure of either the X or the Y template DNA.

The third PCR system does not make use of a size difference. Instead, a 112 bp portion of the amelogenin gene which has sequence differences on the X and Y chromosomes is amplified. The products are analysed by hybridization with probes specific for the X or Y sequences. This method was used by Stone et al.,[19] firstly on 20 DNA samples of known sex from a modern population, then on 20 burials that had been sexed morphologically from a 700-year-old Native American site in Illinois. This method showed impressive accuracy with both the modern and ancient samples, but more recent results have apparently encountered the same problems with partial amplification failures experienced by other researchers.[20]

It is clear from this brief outline that amelogenin PCRs have the potential to remove the uncertainties of sex identification of human remains, but that the methods currently used have their own uncertainties, and the test has not been completely successful with archaeological samples. In a survey of four recent papers, it was found that less than two-thirds of all samples tested gave PCR results that enabled the sex of the sample to be identified (Table 2). These four papers suggest that DNA-based sex identification is applicable to less than two-thirds of human burials and has a confidence limit of 85%, no better than the traditional methodology based on bone morphology. It may be necessary to move away from PCR-based methods to explore new techniques, such as those based on hybridization probing.

Kinship analysis

There is no indisputable method in human osteoarchaeology for determining kinship within a group of burials. Although the genetic basis for the expression of non-metric skeletal traits in the phenotype is not known (indeed one might question the assumption that all non-metric skeletal traits have a hereditary basis), molecular biology has in the last decade uncovered the existence of DNA sequences that have proved to be of great value in kinship studies. These genetic fingerprinting techniques have been employed in the identification of criminals, murder victims, paternity disputes, etc. In short, it can be employed in any question involving doubts over the identity or relationship between individuals.

Table 2 – Success rates for amelogenin-based sex identification of human remains.

Reference	No. of specimens	Sex identification possible	Sex identification not possible	Success rate %
Lassen et al.[39]	34	29	5	85
Faerman et al.[17]	43	19	24	44
Evison[40]	27	13	14	48
Vernesi et al.[41]	45	30	15	66
Total	149	91	58	61

The DNA sequences used in these applications are called short tandem repeats (STR) or microsatellites. They are found in the intergenic regions (the stretches of DNA between the genes) and their function is unknown. A typical STR consists of a 2, 3, 4 or 5 bp sequence repeated five to 30 times: CACACACACACACA is an example of dinucleotide repeat. There are > 10 000 STRs in the entire human genome. Several versions of each STR exist in the human population, each of these alleles having a different number of repeats and so its own diagnostic length. For example the STR called HUMTHO1 is the tetranucleotide TCAT repeated five to 11 times, each number of repeats representing one allele. PCR primers can be designed for each STR, yielding PCR products of 100–300 bp, ideal for ancient DNA analysis. No two humans alive today have exactly the same combination of STR alleles (except for monozygotic twins), so if enough STRs are examined then a unique genetic fingerprint can be established for every person. In a court of law, in order to identify an individual beyond doubt, the Forensic Science Service uses a total of 12 STRs. With this number, there is only one in a 10^{15} chance that two individuals will have the same combination of alleles. It is important to have detailed knowledge of the frequency of STR alleles in various populations in order to calculate the statistical likelihood of the chances of these 12 combined alleles occurring more than once. This may be a problem when using STRs for individual identification in an archaeological setting because the present-day frequencies may not be the same as those from so many years ago.

Recently the remains of the Romanovs were given a state funeral in Russia. These remains were identified via DNA extracted from the bones.[21] The circumstance of the recovery of the remains and their identification resembles an archaeological scenario, and thus can serve as an example of the elucidation of kinship within a burial group. In this case STRs were used to test the hypothesis that of the nine skeletons recovered from a shallow grave in Ekaterinburg, the three children in the burial group were the offspring of two of the six adults, this group being the Tsar, the Tsarina and three of their daughters. Five tetranucleotide STRs were amplified from DNA extracted from the bones. Table 3 shows that two of the adults could indeed be the parents of the three children. At the STR called HUMVWA/31, all three children have the same alleles, 15 and 16. The adults are more varied, but the ones with 14,20 and 17,17 cannot be the parents because these alleles do not

Table 3 – STR results from the Romanov remains.[21]

Skeleton	HUMVWA/31	HUMTHO1	STR locus HUMF13A1	HUMFES/FPS	HUMACTBP2
1. Male adult	14,20	9,10	6,16	10,11	nd
2. Male adult	17,17	6,10	5,7	10,11	11,30
3. Child	15,16	8,10	5,7	12,13	11,32
4. Male adult	15,16	7,10	7,7	12,12	11,32
5. Child	15,16	7,8	5,7	12,13	11,36
6. Child	15,16	8,10	3,7	12,13	32,36
7. Female adult	15,16	8,8	3,5	12,13	32,36
8. Male adult	15,17	6,9	5,7	8,10	nd
9. Female adult	15,17	6,6	6,7	11,12	nd

nd, No data.

appear in the children. However, there are four adults who could have contributed their alleles to the children; one adult has 16,17, one has 15,17 and two have 15,16. By looking at the other results, we see at HUMFES/FPS the children are all 12,13, while three adults are 10,11 and 8,10, so they cannot be parents. One adult has 12,13, one has 12,12 and one has 11,12. The one with 11,12 cannot be a parent because at HUMTHO1 this person has 6,6. The other two individuals have 8,8 and 7,10 while the children all have combinations of 7,8 and 10. The parents are therefore skeletons number 4 (the Tsar) and number 7 (the Tsarina).

STRs are a powerful tool for kinship analysis but so far applications with archaeological material are limited. They have been used in Japan to investigate the possibility of kinship among human remains from the 5th century AD (Kofun era) and the 1st century BC–1st century AD (Yayoi era).[22] Archaeologists have suggested that close relatives were buried together in tombs at the Kofun site of Hirohata. The DNAs of two individuals from the same tomb were tested, one juvenile and one mature male. Nine STRs were used, seven of which were dinucleotide repeats, one a trinucleotide and one a pentanucleotide. The results did not disprove the kinship hypothesis (Table 4). With the second site, Hanaura, another two individuals were tested with the same STRs. These were two females, one mature, the other juvenile, buried in jar-coffins halfway up a hill, which contained 27 other burials. These two female burials alone had about 20 cone-shell bracelets on their arms. The archaeologists suggested that these two were members of the same family, probably mother and daughter, who had ruled the area as shaman or leader. Unfortunately the STR data did not support this hypothesis, but nevertheless a more distant kinship, that of grandmother and granddaughter, could not be ruled out. Mitochondrial DNA from the two females was therefore tested, but again showed no support for kinship through maternal descent.

There are many archaeological scenarios where investigators would like to know whether groups of burials represent related individuals. Identifying kinship in past societies is

Table 4 – STR results from Kurosaki *et al.*[22]

Repeat unit and locus	Hirohata		Hanaura	
	ST16–1	ST16–2	SJ4	SJ5
Dinucleotide				
APOA2	133,131	133,131	133,131	133,131
GSN	127,127	127,111	127,127	131,131
CYP2D	nt	nt	110,104	108,98
HMG14	193,189	189,189	189,189	193,189
D6S105	134,128	128,128	122,122	128,128
D15S87	176,174	176,170	nt	nt
D16S266	168,166	168,168	nt	nt
D18S34	130,130	132,130	nt	nt
Trinucleotide				
PLA2	131,122	131,122	137,134	137,134
Pentanucleotide				
CD4	108,108	108,108	108,108	108,108

nt, Not tested.

fundamental for understanding many aspects of social organization. As social anthropologists have demonstrated, a person's status may depend on their position in a complex network of lineage and kin obligation. Up to now, this dimension of prehistoric society could only be based on speculation. In later societies, status becomes institutionalized and hierarchical, wealth and power are inherited, ruling elites becoming dynasties. The use of ancient DNA to uncover the existence of kinship could add greatly to our understanding of the past.

Palaeodisease

This is a research area with huge potential for interdisciplinary cooperation. Molecular evolutionists are interested in such questions as the origins, spread and development of disease organisms, and how they have changed at the molecular level, for instance, whether virulence has been acquired or lost over time. The prevalence of disease in past populations, and how and when defence mechanisms at the genetic level arose, are questions that are not just academic, but have real relevance in today's world. The input from archaeology into the study of palaeodisease is vital; osteoarchaeologists have the material remains that can add a new temporal dimension to these research questions.

There are, very broadly, two types of disease that can be studied via ancient DNA:

- *Infectious diseases, caused by bacteria or parasites, which leave a DNA signature in the bones or bloodstream.* Examples include tuberculosis, syphilis, leprosy and malaria. In these examples the DNA of the causative organism is targeted by PCR. Even remains that are show no bony signs of disease may contain the causative agent's DNA. A truer picture of disease prevalence in past populations may therefore be obtained.

- *Inherited or genetic illnesses caused by a faulty gene,* such as cystic fibrosis, thalassaemia, Marfan's syndrome and colour blindness. Of interest to those studying the evolution of disease is whether some of these mutations occurred as a response to the incidence of parasitic-borne disease. For example, it has been suggested that the thalassaemias and sickle-cell anaemia may have conferred some protective advantage against malaria. Ancient DNA analysis could help to pinpoint where and when a mutation in a DNA sequence leading to a faulty protein resulting in a genetic disease occurred. Some populations contain higher frequencies of particular genetic diseases than others. Past populations of the same geographical region can be tested through time, and the frequency of a particular mutation compared with its present day population frequency.

The following sections expand on some examples of the applications of ancient DNA analysis in palaeodisease.

Ancient tuberculosis

Recently there has been a spate of publications on ancient tuberculosis DNA from archaeological human remains.[23–28] Only a minority of present-day tuberculosis victims (5–7%) develop visible lesions on their bones. Was this also the case in medieval times? Or was the tuberculosis bacterium more virulent then? Did tuberculosis confer some protection against the closely related *Mycobacterium leprae*, the microorganism responsible for leprosy?

These are questions that a research programme incorporating ancient DNA extracted from tubercular and non-tubercular skeletons could attempt to answer. A PCR-based system for identifying the microbial agent, *Mycobacterium tuberculosis*, has now been developed which does not amplify DNA from related soil bacteria. However, it also amplifies *Mycobacterium bovis* DNA, which is why many papers on this topic refer to *Mycobacterium tuberculosis* complex DNA, as the disease in humans may be the result of infection by either organism. It has been suggested that human tuberculosis may have originated from bovine tuberculosis in prehistoric times, with the advent of farming and close proximity to cattle in the Neolithic.[29] However, Salo[24] and Braun *et al.*[28] have shown the presence of *Mycobacterium tuberculosis* DNA in pre-Columbian human remains from both South and North America respectively. This would suggest that the origins of New World tuberculosis might be even more ancient, if one assumes it was originally carried over the Bering land bridge by the first colonizers. Alternatively, pre-Columbian Europeans, such as the Vikings, may have introduced tuberculosis. DNA sequence analysis of the Old and New World strains of the microorganism might reveal significant differences between the two.[28]

The PCR-based system used to detect ancient tuberculosis complex DNA amplifies sequences from a repetitive insertion called IS6110. This sequence occurs 0–20 times per bacterium (depending on type of bacterial strain), and the target within this is 123 bp long. Many workers use two rounds of PCR, re-amplifying the 123 bp product with primers designed for a 92 bp portion. It is important that soil samples from around the burials are also tested by PCR to eliminate the possibility that there is cross-contamination from other remains or soil bacteria; otherwise there may be an element of doubt over positive results from remains showing no bony signs of disease.[27,28] The detection of ancient tuberculosis DNA in remains which otherwise show no gross signs of disease means that the true prevalence of this disease in past societies, and hence its impact on local economies, settlements and demography can be assessed in conjunction with other forms of archaeological evidence.[†]

Ancient malaria

Like tuberculosis, malaria is a disease of huge importance in global human health today. Until fairly recently it was widespread in the Mediterranean region and was also present in more northerly countries, such as England and Sweden, albeit in a milder form. Whether malaria leaves its mark on bone tissue is debatable. Porotic hyperostosis and/or cribra orbitalia have sometimes been interpreted as resulting from the chronic anaemia associated with malarial infection.[30] More recent interpretations have suggested that the chronic anaemia resulted from iron-deficient diets, as might have been experienced in early farming societies. Other causes of anaemia could also include the genetic diseases of thalassaemia and sickle-cell anaemia, which occur in Mediterranean and African populations respectively. Research has shown that the anaemia question is complex, as lower levels of iron in the body may actually function as a defence mechanism against pathogenic invasion.[31] It has been hypothesized that thalassaemia and sickle-cell anaemia are evolved

---

[†] Note added in proof: Since this was written it has become apparent that it is possible to distinguish M. bovis from M. tuberculosis, and to investigate the evolution of tuberculosis at the genetic level, using ancient DNA (Taylor et al. Microbiology 1999; 145: 899–904).

responses to malarial parasites. These genetic mutations are advantageous when heterozygous, but deleterious when homozygous. Therefore, there are three possible causes of porotic hyperostosis (dietary, disease or genetic) and two of out of these three can be detected by ancient DNA.

It is now possible to use ancient DNA extracted from bones to detect the presence of the four *Plasmodium* species that can cause malaria. The four species are *P. falciparum*, *P. vivax*, *P. ovale* and *P. malariae*. A PCR system has been designed based on the 18S ribosomal DNA sequence, which is present in the Plasmodium genome in high numbers.[32] The PCR target is 147 bp long, with a second PCR carried out with the initial PCR product to give a 138–135 bp product to confirm the authenticity of the ancient malarial DNA. This second round PCR product is sequenced to identify the particular species of *Plasmodium* responsible for the infection. The samples used by Taylor *et al.*[32] included a 60-year-old rib bone of an individual known to have had malaria-induced anaemia. This gave PCR products of the expected size, but another specimen known to have had malaria failed to produce positive results. Actual amounts of bone used in this study were limited, and it may be that there simply was no parasite DNA in the latter. It is important in ancient DNA investigations that several bone samples from different parts of the skeleton are available for repeat extractions and amplifications.

Thalassaemia

Research on the incidence of malaria in the Mediterranean region is relevant to the evolution and frequency of thalassaemias in prehistoric and later populations. Thalassaemia (from *thalasso* – of the sea) or *anaemia mediterranea* is the result of a faulty protein involved in the formation of haemoglobin, the oxygen carrying component of red blood cells. Haemoglobin consists of an iron-containing haem group and two α-globin protein subunits and two β-globin subunits. Each type of globin subunit is coded by its own gene, mutations in which affect or prevent the formation and function of the relevant globin, and hence impair the oxygen-carrying capacity of the red blood cells. Thalassaemias result from mutations, or more commonly deletions, in either the α-or β-globin gene.

Porotic hyperostosis, indicative of severe anaemia, may in some cases be the result of thalassaemia. Ancient DNA has recently been used to identify this genetic disease.[33] The skull of a child from an Ottoman grave (16th–19th centuries AD) in Israel had porotic hyperostosis, including cribra orbitalia and thickening of the diploe. The dental evidence suggested an age of 7–8 years at death, which is highly unusual in cases of thalassaemia major in children. Filon *et al.*[33] therefore extracted ancient DNA from the skull and carried out PCRs aimed at a 232 bp portion of the β-globin gene. Sequence analysis of the PCR products revealed a rare single base change, which is present in 13% of Mediterranean β-thalassaemias. This change does not affect the globin protein, but a second mutation was also found, this one being a deletion of two bases (the FS8 mutation); PCR products obtained from the ancient DNA were tested for these mutations by hybridization analysis. The FS8 mutation is found at a frequency of 2–10% of all thalassaemia genes in the Mediterranean region, but in modern Israel today is present almost exclusively in Arabs (frequency of 2.3%). The FS8 mutation results in no β-globin production. The foetus and infant survives because of the production of foetal haemoglobin, but the child is dependent on blood transfusions from an early age. Transfusions were not an option for the Ottoman child, but he or she still survived until 8 years of age. How was this possible? The answer is that the single nucleotide change noted in the PCR sequence is associated with persistence of foetal globin production into childhood. It was the continued presence of foetal haemoglobin that enabled the Ottoman child to live longer than is usual in such cases.

β-Thalassaemia mutations persist in present-day populations around the Mediterranean, the highest frequency for one particular mutation being in Sardinia (95.7%). In a heterozygous form, it confers some protection against malaria. Unfortunately for the biomolecular archaeologist, β-thalassaemia major can be caused by any of 200 mutations in the β-globin gene. Obviously the target for PCR needs to be narrowed down. Filon *et al.*[33] were successful because they knew the frequency of β-globin mutations in the present-day Arab population in Israel, and the child whose DNA was being analysed was buried in Moslem fashion, and thus could be cautiously assigned to the same population. Although theoretical archaeologists may decry their naivety, in assuming that a child of the 16th–19th centuries AD belonged to the same population as present-day Arabs, nevertheless some assumptions have to be made and tested if progress in the study of genetic palaeodisease is to be made. In investigating thalassaemias and other genetic diseases, the frequency of gene mutations in present-day populations can give valuable clues as to which DNA sequences to target in ancient DNA from past populations.

ANCIENT DNA – PROBLEMS AND POTENTIAL

The full potential of ancient DNA as a new tool in archaeology will only be realised once some basic problems have been overcome. Biomolecular archaeology is perhaps the only area of research where the publication of negative results is seen as an important means of assessing the reliability and validity of a project. This reflects the difficulty of working with ancient DNA. There is still much basic research that needs to be carried out to understand the survival of ancient DNA and the reasons for amplification failures. Because ancient human DNA is the same as modern human DNA, contamination of bones by handling during or after excavation is a serious concern; recommendations have been given in other publications[34,35] for avoiding contamination of newly excavated material.

Fully realising the potential of ancient DNA depends on four factors:

- *The improvement of current techniques and the development of new ones.* Areas where improvements may be expected include DNA extraction, with perhaps the use of monoclonal antibodies specific for ancient human DNA; greater use of hybridization analysis, including the development of DNA chip technology for forensic and ancient DNA analysis; methods to 'repair' ancient DNA and thus provide longer sequences for analysis (as proposed in reconstructive PCR, for example); and a wider choice of PCR targets with the completion of the Human Genome Project.[36,37]
- *Improved sampling strategies for ancient DNA must be incorporated into excavations to minimize contamination.* The use of sterile gloves should be routine on all excavations. Other biomolecules, such as lipids absorbed into ceramics, are also prone to problems with contamination from handling.[38]

- *The widespread application of ancient DNA analysis to human bone samples over wide geographical and temporal scales, as well as single site analysis.* In the future it may be possible that ancient DNA analysis will be offered as a service to archaeologists, like radiocarbon dating. Sex identification of human remains seems to be a prime candidate, although kinship analysis is another area of potential.[39–41]

- *Close collaborations between archaeologists and molecular biologists so that interpretations of ancient DNA results are fully integrated with archaeological evidence and theory.* It must be remembered that ancient DNA analysis is another tool for understanding the past. Its potential can best be realised by using it to test hypotheses formulated from archaeological evidence, where those hypotheses are resolvable via ancient DNA. New interdisciplinary bonds need to be forged. For example, ancient DNA could make a valuable contribution to the study of disease and its evolution at the molecular level, but only if archaeologists talk to genetic epidemiologists and molecular evolutionists.

ACKNOWLEDGEMENTS

Many thanks to Dr Terry Brown for reading and commenting on this chapter.

REFERENCES

1   Allaby RG, O'Donoghue K, Sallares R, Jones MK, Brown TA. Evidence for the survival of ancient DNA in charred wheat seeds from European archaeological sites. *Ancient Biomolecules* 1997; **1**: 119–129.

2   Krings M, Stone A, Schmitz RW, Krainitzki H, Stoneking M, Pääbo S. Neanderthal DNA sequences and the origin of modern humans. *Cell* 1997; **90**: 19–30.

3   Brown TA. *Gene Cloning: An Introduction* (3rd edn). London: Chapman & Hall, 1995.

4   Saiki RK, Gelfland DH, Stoffel S, Scharf SJ, Higuchi R, Horn GT, Mullis KB, Erlich HA. Primer-directed enzymatic amplification of DNA with a thermostable DNA polymerase. *Science* 1988; **239**: 487–491.

5   Higuchi R, Bowman B, Freiberger M, Ryder OA, Wilson AC. DNA sequences from the quagga, an extinct member of the horse family. *Nature* 1984; **312**: 282–284.

6   Pääbo S. Molecular cloning of ancient Egyptian mummy DNA. *Nature* 1985; **314**: 644–645.

7   Hagelberg E, Sykes B, Hedges R. Ancient bone DNA amplified. *Nature* 1989; **342**: 485.

8   Evison MP, Smillie DM, Chamberlain AT. Extraction of single-copy nuclear DNA from forensic specimens with a variety of postmortem histories. *Journal of Forensic Sciences* 1997; **42(6)**: 1032–1038.

9   Brown KA, Brown T. Amount of human DNA in old bones. *Ancient DNA Newsletter* 1992; **1(1)**: 18–19.

10   Colson I, Bailey JF, Vercauteren M, Sykes B, Hedges REM. The preservation of ancient DNA and bone diagenesis. *Ancient Biomolecules* 1997; **1**: 109–118.

11   Brown KA. Gender and sex – what can ancient DNA tell us? *Ancient Biomolecules* 1998; **2**: 3–15.

12   Schutkowski H. Sex determination of infant and juvenile skeletons. I. Morphognostic features. *American Journal of Physical Anthropology* 1993; **90**: 199–205.

13   McKinley JI. Bone fragment size in British cremation burials and its implications for pyre technology and ritual. *Journal of Archaeological Science* 1994; **21**: 339–342.

14   McKinley JI. Bronze Age 'barrows' and funerary rites and rituals of cremation. *Proceedings of the Prehistoric Society* 1997; **63**: 129–145.

15   Hummel S, Herrmann B. Y-chromosome-specific DNA amplified in human bone. *Naturwissenschaften* 1991; **78**: 266–267.

16   Gotherstrom A, Liden K, Ahlstrom T, Kallersjo M, Brown TA. Osteology, DNA and sex identification: morphological and molecular sex identifications of five Neolithic individuals from Ajvide, Gotland. *International Journal of Osteoarchaeology* 1997; **7**: 71–81.

17   Faerman M, Kahila G, Smith P, Greenblatt CL, Stager L, Filon D, Oppenheim A. DNA analysis reveals the sex of infanticide victims. *Nature* 1997; **385**: 212–213.

18   Sullivan KM, Manucci A, Kimpton CP, Gill P. A rapid and quantitative DNA sex test: fluorescence-based PCR analysis of X–Y homologous gene amelogenin. *Biotechniques* 1993; **15**: 636–641.

19   Stone AC, Milner GR, Pääbo S, Stoneking M. Sex determination of ancient human skeletons using DNA. *American Journal of Physical Anthropology* 1996; **99**: 231–238.

20   Stone AC, Stoneking M. Analysis of ancient DNA from a prehistoric Amerindian cemetery. *Philosophical Transactions of the Royal Society of London, Series B* 1999; **354**: 153–159.

21   Gill P, Ivanov PL, Kimpton C, Piercy R, Benson N, Tully G, Evett I, Hagelberg E, Sullivan K. Identification of the remains of the Romanov family by DNA analysis. *Nature Genetics* 1994; **6**: 130–135.

22   Kurosaki K, Matsushita T, Ueda S. Individual DNA identification from ancient human remains. *American Journal of Human Genetics* 1993; **53**: 638–643.

23   Spigelman M, Lemma E. The use of the polymerase chain reaction (PCR) to detect *Mycobacterium tuberculosis* in ancient skeletons. *International Journal of Osteoarchaeology* 1993; **3**: 137–143.

24   Salo WL, Aufderheide AC, Buikstra J, Holcomb TA. Identification of *Mycobacterium tuberculosis* DNA in a pre-Columbian Peruvian mummy. *Proceedings of the National Academy of Sciences, USA* 1994; **91**: 2091–2094.

25   Baron H, Hummel S, Herrmann B. *Mycobacterium tuberculosis* complex DNA in ancient human bones. *Journal of Archaeological Science* 1996; **23**: 667–671.

26   Taylor GM, Crossey M, Saldanha J, Waldron T. DNA from *Mycobacterium tuberculosis* identified in mediaeval human skeletal remains using polymerase chain reaction. *Journal of Archaeological Science* 1996; **23**: 789–798.

27   Faerman M, Jankauskas R, Gorski A, Bercovier H, Greenblatt CL. Prevalence of human tuberculosis in a medieval population of Lithuania studied by ancient DNA analysis. *Ancient Biomolecules* 1997; **1**: 205–214.

28   Braun M, Cook DC, Pfeiffer S. DNA from *Mycobacterium tuberculosis* complex identified in North American, pre-Columbian human skeletal remains. *Journal of Archaeological Science* 1999; **25**: 271–277.

29   Manchester K. Tuberculosis and leprosy in antiquity: an interpretation. *Medical History* 1984; **28**: 162–173.

30   Angel JL. Porotic hyperostosis, anemias, malarias, and marshes in the prehistoric Eastern Mediterranean. *Science* 1966; **153**: 760–763.

31   Stuart-Macadam P. Anemia in past human populations. In: Stuart-Macadam P, Kent S (eds), *Diet, Demography and Disease: Changing Perspectives on Anemia*. New York: Aldine de Gruyter, 1992: pp. 151–170.

32   Taylor GM, Rutland P, Molleson T. A sensitive polymerase chain reaction method for the detection of *Plasmodium* species DNA in ancient human remains. *Ancient Biomolecules* 1997; **1**: 193–203.

33   Filon D, Faerman M, Smith P, Oppenheim A. Sequence analysis reveals a β-thalassaemia mutation in the DNA of skeletal remains from the archaeological site of Akhziv, Israel. *Nature Genetics* 1995; **9**: 365–368.

34   Brown TA, Brown KA. Ancient DNA and the archaeologist. *Antiquity* 1992; **66**: 10–23.

35   Brown KA. Keeping it clean: the collection and storage of ancient DNA samples from the field. *The Archaeologist* 1998; **33**: 16–17.

36   Ramsay G. DNA chips: state of the art. *Nature Biotechnology* 1998; **16**: 40–44.

37   Deakin WJ, Rowley-Conwy P, Shaw CH. The sorghum of Qasr Ibrim: reconstructing DNA templates from ancient seeds. *Ancient Biomolecules* 1998; **2**: 117–124.

38   Evershed RP. Biomolecular archaeology and lipids. *World Archaeology* 1993; **25(1)**: 74–93.

39   Lassen C, Hummel S, Herrmann B. PCR based sex identification of ancient human bones by amplification of X- and Y-chromosomal sequences: a comparison. *Ancient Biomolecules* 1996; **1(1)**: 25–34.

40   Evison MP. Ancient HLA: a preliminary survey. *Ancient Biomolecules* 1999; **3(1)**: 1–28.

41   Vernesi C, Caramelli D, Carbonelli S, Ubaldi M, Rollo F, Chiarelli B. Application of DNA sex tests to bone specimens from two Etruscan (VII–III century BC) archaeological sites. *Ancient Biomolecules* 1999; **2(4)**: 295–305.

28

ANALYSING HUMAN SKELETAL DATA

John Robb

INTRODUCTION

To existentialist philosophers, hell is other people. To most of us, however, hell is statistics. Aside from a handful of wizard-like experts, archaeologists seem to deal with statistics by taking a course somewhere during the educational process, forgetting it all, and then relearning the specific bits required by one's dissertation advisor, journal reviewers or, rarely, data. This is, of course, a caricature that does little justice to the many statistics-friendly archaeologists on both sides of the Atlantic, but it contains a grain of truth. For many, data analysis is equated with a body of specific, standard and often unpleasant statistical techniques borrowed wholesale from other fields.

The result is that data analysis is something of a black hole in the osteoarchaeological literature. Nobody really talks about *how* we go about interpreting bones, whether we do it through a paragraph of text or a fiendishly complex multivariate analysis. In major introductions to human osteology,[1-7] only Ubelaker and especially Mays get beyond data collection to discuss what can be done with osteological data. This lack of explicit discussion also characterizes much, but not all, advanced literature.[8-12] There have been few reviews of statistical methodology in human osteology beyond Waldron's elegant *Counting the Dead*.[13] The exceptions are palaeodemography,[14,15] biodistance studies,[16] and quantitative morphometrics.[17-19] However, the highly technical methods involved in these fields have had little influence in general osteoarchaeology, since statistical methods do not always fit bioarchaeological problems, bioarchaeologists often lack mathematical training, time or resources, and 'the complexity of mathematical multivariate methodology tends to generate a certain fear among anthropologists' (p. 254).[19]

Our silence on data analysis does not mean that it is not important. Quite the contrary: data analysis is really the central linkage between the bones in the laboratory and whatever we think we can learn from them. What determines which observations we collect, how we produce graphs, tables and summaries from them, and how we pursue patterns within the data? This disciplinary lore is rarely written about; instead, it is taught practically by example, by apprenticeship, and by institutional rites such as refereeing of journal articles. There are three reasons for a review of data analysis in human osteology. The first is to understand human osteology as a theoretical endeavour with specific research traditions. The second is to review standard practices of data analysis in human osteology. The third is to foresee creative developments emerging in archaeological studies of human skeletons.

The goal of this paper is to discuss the *process* of data analysis. It would be superfluous to write for experienced data analysts[20] or to review standard statistical methods, since textbook presentations of them for archaeologists are readily available.[21–23]. Rather, my goal is to show when, how and why we use such methods, for those taking their first plunge into data analysis. How do we select appropriate analytical tools, use them to cope with the specific nature of human skeletal data, and build a research strategy around the requirements of data analysis? By taking a straightforward approach to such questions, I hope to show that the water is not so deep and cold as many fear.

STANDARD PRACTICE: THE INFLUENCE OF DISCIPLINARY TRADITIONS

As post-processual archaeologists have pointed out,[24] there are no neutral methods: *how* one carries out an archaeological study is intimately related to *why* one does so, both theoretically and institutionally. Post-processual critique has had little impact in human osteology, but as the history of physical anthropology on matters such as racial classification shows,[25] disciplinary traditions can be deeply influenced by structural, institutional and cultural practices and at the same time be executed within the methodology of "objective" science. It is worth considering disciplinary traditions briefly here since data analysis is a key locus where research traditions are created, deployed and reproduced through the questions researchers consider worth asking, the answers they look for, and the methods they use.

Perhaps the clearest portrait of disciplinary traditions is anecdotal. In 1990 I was preparing a description of Neolithic skeletons for an Italian journal, focusing upon their pathologies and archaeological context.[26] Italian anthropologists who read my first draft advised me that many older colleagues would regard the publication of a skeleton as incomplete without an extensive list of often esoteric metrics and classifications such as 'platycephalic' and 'cryptozygoid' drawn from Martin and Saller,[27] even though such data were rarely actually used for any interpretative purpose.[28] The data were duly included. This situation reflects the social and historical aspects of Italian osteology: its origin in the natural sciences, its legitimization of status via the amassing and control of data, the importance placed upon expert classification, and the particular Italian archaeological concept of 'palaeoethnology' (*paletnologia*).[29] These features coalesced into a paradigm of racial craniology, and with the postwar decline of 'race' as a master concept for understanding human variation, one result was the habitual collection of traditional data in an interpretative void. This, of course, reflects a particular historical moment; in the last two decades this framework has been rapidly expanded by new and creative research directions.[30]

American bioarchaeology from the 1980s provides another case of a tradition with specific historical and theoretical groundings. Stereotypically, the American bioarchaeologist would go forth to demonstrate a New Archaeology-inspired 'Big Social Problem'; after all, what *I* was doing in Italy in 1990 was trying to explain the 'evolution of social inequality' through the study of several hundred miscellaneous, often highly fragmented skeletons! This tradition, too, has its preferred methods (the cross-cultural comparative study using biosocial 'indicators') and its preferred data analysis techniques, such as formal hypothesis testing. American bioarchaeology has often been ambitious and creative, especially in recognizing and investigating skeletal phenomena such as enamel hypoplasia and creating methodologies for comparative analyses. But the American approach, as critics of New Archaeology in general have pointed out,[31] has often relied upon quite blunt-edged rather than nuanced research questions, for instance, in the case of studies comparing 'agriculturalists' and 'hunter-gatherers,' or 'egalitarian' and 'stratified' societies as homogeneous categories with straightforward skeletal signatures.[32] In the rush to do social science, biological features were sometimes shoehorned into interpretative roles. 'Generalized stress,' for example, was sometimes employed as a concept for coping with the indeterminacy of many palaeopathologies, but sometimes regarded as a social phenomenon in its own right. Several other 'social indicators' (e.g. Harris lines and trace element profiles) have since been largely deconstructed for comparative purposes. As Larsen[11] notes, American bioarchaeology has matured greatly in the last several decades.

British osteoarchaeology has a quite different tradition. In America, where archaeology has evolved in a colonial situation, the research agenda has been set by anthropological questions. In Britain, historical ones have set it. American researchers have looked to the social sciences for methods, whereas in the UK, the main inspiration has traditionally been clinical. This is hardly surprising since most British osteoarchaeologists have begun their careers with medical or anatomical training. As Mays' recent bibliographic review[33] shows, the result is that British researchers focus heavily on palaeopathology, and a far greater proportion of their output consists of 'case studies'. Data analyses correspondingly downplay statistics and multivariate analysis, and focus instead upon detailed documentation; congruence with historical and clinical sources, rather than statistical significance, is the gold standard for establishing truth. Furthermore, while American palaeopathology often aims to outline the distribution of pathologies within populations, in British work reaching a differential diagnosis is often the primary end in itself. Like the American tradition, the British tradition has its pros and cons, though (as this volume itself demonstrates) we must recognize a rapidly developing field. Palaeopathological diagnosis reaches a very high standard, methodology is strong, and historical studies attain impressive levels of detail. However, there is little spur to interpretative creativity, and often, active resistance to it. Most work focuses upon periods with historical information and large numbers of complete skeletons, with surprisingly few bioarchaeological studies of prehistoric material. Finally, there is a tendency to give up on problems that do not yield a clear diagnosis rather than to work out creative strategies to make the best of bad data.

As these three traditions show, there is an intimate link between how we collect and analyse skeletal data, the research tradition we work in and the historical moment we are working at. We thus have a situation common in the sciences, with internationally standardized techniques for observation and measurement deployed in very different ways within distinct traditions of inquiry. Indeed, one goal of drawing the linkage between research contexts and methods explicitly is to make us realise that alternative methods and questions are possible.

THE NATURE OF OSTEOLOGICAL DATA

A second major influence on osteological data analysis is the nature of skeletal data, which shapes our strategies for answering research questions. It is worth reviewing briefly some aspects that we must take into consideration.

Human skeletal data come from dead people. Thus, the palaeopathological record, derived from a death sample, cannot be read as a straightforward record of health in a living population.[13,34-36] As a result of this, healthier populations may appear in worse health skeletally because they survive longer to suffer mild, chronic skeletal pathologies. Also, samples of any particular age group, such as children, consist of people who died at that age rather than a representative cross-section of a living population.

Human skeletal data come from a social context formed by meanings and social relations as well as biological and taphonomic forces. Thus, regardless of our osteological expertise, biosocial analyses can only be as reliable as our theoretical understanding of society, and social theory as well as biological studies can prove a source of exciting research questions.

Skeletal data are organized at several levels. We can analyse the prevalence of pathology in a subregion of a bone (e.g. the distal femur shaft), in a bone (e.g. the femur) or in a multi-element area (e.g. the knee joint). We can also analyse prevalences in a skeleton, in a subgroup of the skeletal sample, in an entire sample or in several pooled samples. Particular collections may allow analysis at only some levels. In collective burials or disarticulated bones, for example, analysis may have to be conducted at the region-by-region or bone-by-bone level. One technical implication of multi-level data is that the units we analyse are often *not* the biologically operative units. For example, in studying caries in two dentitions, the sample size may be 64 total teeth, but in reality only two independent data points are effectively represented, since dental health in one tooth from a dentition is likely to be partially correlated with dental health in the other teeth. This can pose problems in using methods that require independent observations, such as most significance tests. A second implication is that we have to collect and report data so as to allow interconvertability between levels. To go from the individual skeleton to the population level, for example, we need to have consistently collected data on the absence of pathologies as well as their presence.

Most skeletal phenomena involve many factors. Hence, bivariate methods (relating x to y) really work only in tightly controlled situations, as there are always variables z, a, b and c lurking in the background. A common (and commonly disregarded) example is age-related phenomena. Since dental caries increases with age, one cannot realistically compare dental caries rates among different samples without first considering whether they have similar age structures. In practical terms, we usually have two strategies for dealing with multivariate situations: to build complex, multivariate models, or to use simple benchmarks and demonstrate that other factors are equal or control for their differences.

Virtually all relationships in skeletal data are non-linear. For example, stature reconstructions using linear regressions usually work well for most individuals but distort estimates for very small and very large people.[37] The progression of dental wear with age provides another common example of non-linearity. Thus, we should use methods such as linear regression cautiously, since they will always be valid for only part of the range of variability; alternatively, non-linear methods can be tried.

The structure of biological variation itself can vary from population to population. One common example is sexual dimorphism: the criteria that best distinguish European males and females may not be identical to those which distinguish the sexes in non-Europeans. Stature regression models, which are based on a specific reference group's body proportions, are another example. Hence, our models may have to be group-specific as well as multivariate.

On the practical level, much of our data is fragmentary and/or commingled; it is rare to study a skeleton with no missing data at all. Missing data frequently forces us to find alternative analyses or strategies, since many multivariate analyses (especially cluster analysis and factor analysis) require complete data matrices. More generally, we have to collect and present our data so as to allow comparison between dissecting-room quality specimens and shoebox samples by anyone ultimately using the data. This is usually done by rigorously collecting data at a finer level than the entire skeleton or whole bone, such as regions of bones.[12]

These characteristics of human skeletal data affect two key aspects of data analysis: how we incorporate data analysis into an overall research design, and which analytical tools we use.

BUILDING DATA ANALYSIS INTO THE RESEARCH PROCESS

Because of the nature of archaeological skeletal data, palaeopathology is not simply pathology applied to dead people. Much of the practice of palaeopathology is structured by the needs of the data analysis at the end of the process. Once we have a research question and possible samples, the next step is planning the research.

In designing a skeletal research project, to avoid finishing empty handed or having to repeat data collection, data analysis must be built into research designs from the start. This is all the more so since skeletal research almost always requires striking a practical balance between the number of specimens studied, the amount of detail recorded, and research time and money. Some basic questions to consider include:

- What kinds of data are needed to answer the research questions? What statistical techniques will be used to analyse them?
- What collateral data are necessary to allow other analyses, for complete documentation, or to control for possible intervening factors such age, sex or social group?
- Does answering the research question require either complete or articulated skeletons (e.g. to control for age and sex)?
- Is the necessary information about archaeological context available (a problem with many older museum collections)?
- What social and taphonomic biases affect the sample? How can they be minimized, taken into account, or studied as interesting phenomena in their own right?

- How many specimens are needed to answer the research questions using the appropriate statistical techniques? Too few will yield inconclusive results, but too many will be costly with little additional information gained. Shennan,[22] Thomas[23] and other texts give methods for estimating adequate sample sizes.
- How many observations per specimen are necessary? Too few may leave important questions unanswered; too many may cost research time with little additional information gained.
- Since measurements are typically more time-consuming to collect than categorical observations, what level of measurement does the analysis require?
- How will the data be computerized? How can data collection be set up to make data entry and analysis convenient and error-free?
- Can the analysis be done with standard methods or will it require novel methods? Is a pilot study of methods needed to establish their reliability, practicality or speed? Are controls for intra- and inter-observer error needed?
- What level of detail will the research be published at? Broad basic documentation of a collection? Specialized restudy of a narrow topic? What other documentation (such as maps and photos) is necessary?

Once we have actually collected our data, the analysis itself is typically a lengthy, recursive process (Figure 1). The first results to emerge rarely present a clear picture, but they frequently suggest questions for further analysis, alternative ways to group and analyse the data, and so on. Figure 2 presents a simple example. All of these histograms represent the same dataset: which one portrays its variation best? Coming to understand one's data requires re-interpreting them, often many times, cycling between statistical analysis and our knowledge of the sample, the methods, the biological phenomenon and the archaeological

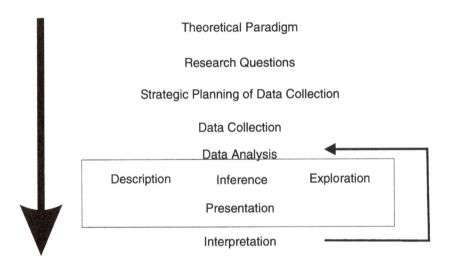

Figure 1 – Data analysis in the research process.

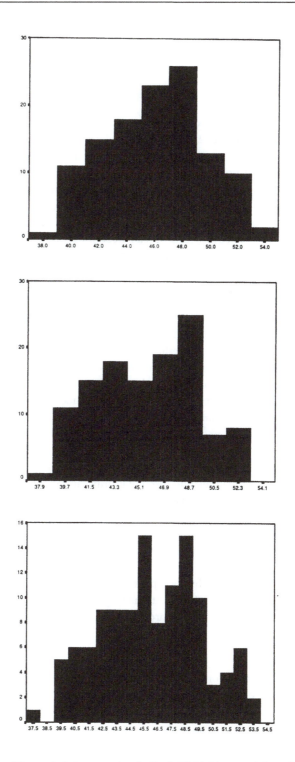

Figure 2 – Example of data analysis-interpretation feedback. Which histogram is better?

context. (In this case, the data are femur head diameters, and a bimodal histogram with bars > 1 mm wide is probably most useful).

CHOOSING TOOLS OF DATA ANALYSIS

Once data has been collected, it is typically entered first into a database or spreadsheet program. In dealing with multi-level skeletal data, the most important recent technical advance has been the spread of relational database programs such as Paradox and Access, which allow automatic error checking, economical data entry and flexible reporting of results. A relational standard osteological database designed to accommodate data collected according to Buikstra and Ubelaker[12] is available from the Center for Advanced Spatial Technologies at the University of Arkansas. Subsequent tabulations and analyses can often be carried out within spreadsheet or database programs, though many statistical tests and manipulations are much easier to perform by exporting the data into a dedicated statistics package.

Data analysis techniques *per se* fall into three categories: descriptive, exploratory and inferential. *Descriptive* methods begin with creating and presenting data, based upon visual filtering of information ('seeing') by the analyst, trained observation and verbal descriptions ('noting') and formalized methods of data collection (such as measuring, drawing and photographing). Descriptive methods also include summarizing data visually through graphs and charts, and numerically through basic summaries such as percentages, the mean, median and standard deviation. *Exploratory* methods aim at revealing patterns in the data. Simple exploratory methods, such as cross-tabulations of data, are an extension of data description. More complicated exploratory methods[38,39] include regression, or fitting linear and non-linear mathematical models to data; log-linear modelling of multivariate categorical data; cluster analysis to produce tree diagram classifications; discriminant functions for classifying items into discrete groups; and various forms of factor analysis, which reduces many covarying variables such as skull measurements into a few axes representing shared dimensions of size and shape. Some recent statistics packages include semi-automated data exploration techniques under rubrics such as 'data mining'. *Inferential* methods (or 'hypothesis testing') include tests used to verify the reality of possible patterns in the data by deciding whether a given proposition is 'statistically significant'. 'Significance' here technically means that the observed pattern is improbable enough that it is unlikely to have arisen purely by chance. Conventionally, patterns with < 1:20 chance of arising through random fluctuations ($p < 0.05$) are regarded as representing a genuine finding.

The standard toolbox

Inferential statistics form the substance of most statistics courses and texts, and a well-developed suite of methods exists. Table 1 presents an overview of the standard toolbox of inferential methods. In choosing a method, the most basic consideration is what kind of data are to be analysed. Many skeletal data are numerical, such as measurements. But many consist of non-numerical categories, either dichotomous (such as sex or presence-absence data) or with several variants (as when we compare three archaeological sites). An intermediate kind of data is ordinal, or ranked categories which are graded but which do not necessarily represent uniformly spaced intervals (as when osteoarthritis or muscle markings are scored as 'mild' 'moderate' or 'severe'). Methods have been developed specifically for analysing ordinal data, as it usually makes little sense to calculate 'average' muscle marking or osteoarthritis grades.[40] A second consideration in choosing a method is that most have inherent conditions which must be met to give meaningful results. For instance, the popular chi-square analysis of categorical data requires a minimal sample size and distribution, and the Student's t-test usually requires that the data approximate to a normal distribution. Before using a method, one should check that the data meet such conditions.[22,23]

To test or not to test? inferential versus exploratory methods

Perhaps no aspect of statistical practice shows more variation than significance testing. American osteoarchaeologists routinely carry out such tests, while they are far less frequent in European work. It is worth considering the logic and justification for significance testing.[20,41] Inferential statistics carry the cachet of 'hard science' and are the most readily available 'off the shelf' methods, but they are crude instruments for exploring complex situations. In many analyses, the result from a significance test depends largely upon the data exploration and preparation taking place before the test is carried out. Significance tests are designed to reject most novel ideas conservatively, and they often require unrealistic assumptions about the data. Important patterns may be missed if one simply reads the output from the first round of tests, declares anything with $p < 0.05$ to be a new fact, and discards the rest. Hypothesis testing is especially inappropriate as a tool for screening large numbers of variables, as is sometimes done, since by definition five of every 100 tests will yield 'significant' results even with purely random data. Moreover, the results of a hypothesis test need to be interpreted carefully. In particular, p provides a poor measure of how strong a relationship or difference is, as it is strongly dependent upon sample sizes. Rather, additional measures of the strength of relationship are needed.[22] For similar reasons, when a test fails to demonstrate a significant relationship or result, this does *not* mean that the groups compared are homogeneous or the variables are independent (an interpretation often encountered in osteoarchaeological reports).

Inferential statistics really belong to a second round of data analysis; they are useful primarily for *verifying* specific patterns, usually in simplified and groomed datasets, rather than for *discovering* patterns in the early stage of analysis, which is often better accomplished through exploratory methods. However, for this specific purpose, they are invaluable and should rarely be omitted.

What can be done with human skeletal data?

The research questions central to osteoarchaeological traditions, the available statistical methods, and the nature of human skeletal data have combined to create measures and procedures commonly used for analysing specific skeletal data (Table 2). (An in-depth review of skeletal data analyses is impossible here, but refer to other chapters in this volume and to Larsen[11] and Mays[4].) Most involve standard methods; a few involve tools adapted for particular problems such as the 'minimum number of individuals' (MNI), the 'decayed-

Table 1: **a)** One- and **b)** Two variable methods for data description and inference (after Blalock[58], with modifications)

a) One-Variable Procedures

Nature of Variable			
2 categories (e.g. male/female)	>2 Categories (e.g. comparing three sites)	Ranked Categories (e.g. mild, moderate, severe)	Numerical (e.g. measurements)
Proportions, percentages, ratios; χ^2 Goodness of Fit	Proportions, percentages, ratios; χ^2 Goodness of Fit	Medians, percentiles; Kolmogorov-Smirnov Goodness of Fit	Means, medians, standard deviations

b) Two-Variable Procedures

Nature of Second or Dependent Variable	Nature of First or Independent Variable			
	2 categories (e.g. male/female)	>2 Categories (e.g. comparing three sites)	Ranked Categories (e.g. mild, moderate, severe)	Numerical (e.g. measurements)
2 categories (e.g. male/female)	χ^2 Test of Independence; measures of association (ϕ, V, etc); difference of proportions; Fisher's Exact Test	χ^2 Test of Independence; measures of association (ϕ, V, etc.)		
>2 Categories (e.g. comparing three sites)	χ^2 Test of Independence; measures of association (ϕ, V, etc.)	χ^2 Test of Independence; measures of association (ϕ, V, etc.)		
Ranked Categories (e.g. mild, moderate, severe)	Mann-Whitney, runs test, Kolmogorov-Smirnov, signed-ranks, Wald-Wolfowitz	Rank-order ANOVA (Kruskal-Wallis H)	Rank-order correlation (Spearman's r), Kendall's tau, gamma, etc	
Numerical (e.g. measurements)	Difference of means (Student's-test)	ANOVA		Correlation and regression

missing ratio' and other parameters for estimating dental disease,[42,43] demographic analysis,[44] parameters for functional analysis of long bone architecture,[45] various multivariate analyses for biodistance,[16,18] and the 'mean measure of divergence' for analysis of non-metric traits.[46] Many other creative analyses have been carried out without becoming part of a routinely used corpus of methods.

Much more work remains to be done in developing methods for coping with archaeological skeletal data in all their imperfect and peculiar glory. One major problem in osteological analysis is avoiding preservation bias: how to compare pathology rates in a well-preserved cemetery and a poorly preserved commingled ossuary. Standard practice[12,47] involves comparison at the level of the small regions of bones. A complementary approach would be to develop standard benchmark figures such as the estimated prevalence in complete skeletons, which can be derived using simple probability calculations[48] and which may be more intuitively and socially interpretable. Estimation of dental pathology rates in incomplete dentitions may be amenable to similar solutions. A third approach for use with age-related pathologies is to convert their observed prevalences into estimates of individuals affected in each age category, and by extension to estimate how these pathologies accumulated in the skeleton throughout the life span. Though it requires sizeable well-aged samples, this allows comparison of samples with different age structures as well as an understanding of the risks people ran at each stage of their lives.

To understand complex biosocial situations, multivariate methods provide an under-used, open field of research. Muscle markings, non-metric traits and osteoarthritis data are all potentially amenable to methods such as factor analysis and correspondence analysis, since each skeleton provides us with many observations which presumably share underlying axes of variability. Methodologically, the major barrier to work around is missing data, since most methods require complete data for each specimen. Another useful pattern recognition tool is cluster analysis,[49] which can be used on almost any kind of data to shed light upon groupings within it.[40] New possibilities in multivariate pattern recognition may arise with the development of user-friendly artificial intelligence programs. Neural network programs, for instance, deal with classification problems of the kind we routinely face in sexing skeletons; they can also be used to analyse visual as well as numerical data (such as scanned images). Other artificial intelligence methods include classification tree routines for classifying items according to multiple, shifting criteria, which may be applicable in problems such as palaeopathological diagnosis.

One of the most useful ways to understand complex situations is by building models of them. Regression analysis allows us to use both linear and non-linear models. An alternative tack is to use simulations, which can be extremely simple. Simulations may be especially useful for working back from the skeletal record to a reconstructed biological or social world, taking into account the sensitivity of skeletal indicators to develop boundary conditions for specific problems. For instance, what conditions would have to hold in order for us actually to detect genetically a major migration? Can we reconstruct the distribution of diseases such as tuberculosis in ancient populations, given the prevalence of skeletal lesions and estimates of the proportion of exposed people actually developing the disease and the proportion of those developing skeletal lesions?

Spatial analysis has rarely been applied in osteoarchaeology, but GIS techniques could potentially be applicable to study pathologies, metric and non-metric variation, and taphonomy both at the regional level and within individual cemeteries. This would be an efficient way to relate biological variation to distance and to integrate archaeological, osteological and environmental data, for instance, in understanding the social and biological structure of large cemeteries or in relating geographical factors to disease patterns.

CONCLUSIONS

Human skeletal data analysis has many strengths, including a robust set of internationally accepted methods and standards for data collection,[12] and a critical mass of sophisticated analyses of many important topics.[11] Evaluation of the field must be somewhere between

Table 2 – Data analysis in human skeletal studies: some commonly used techniques and estimates.

Problem	Result
Demography	Age estimates and sex estimates for individuals Discriminant functions for metric sex estimation Age profile and sex ratio Life tables and associated indicators (average age at death, life expectancies, etc.) Minimum number of individuals (MNI)
Growth	Stature estimates via linear regression Average statures and associated variation Growth curves in juveniles
Dental disease	Prevalence of caries, ante-mortem loss and other pathologies by tooth (e.g. % of teeth affected) Decayed-missing ratio (% affected by caries plus % lost ante-mortem) Number of lesions per dentition Distribution patterns within subgroups Significance testing using numerical methods (for percentages) and categorical methods (for presence/absence)
Pathology and trauma	Presence/absence in an individual skeleton Percentage of individuals affected Prevalence by bone or region Distribution patterns within subgroups Significance testing using numerical methods (for percentages) and categorical methods (for presence/absence)
Osteoarthritis and muscle markings	Presence and severity at specific locations Percentage of joint surfaces affected in an individual or sample Percentages of individuals affected Distribution within skeletons and samples Significance testing using ordinal statistics
Metrics	Tabulation Averages, standard deviations and other summary statistics Discriminant function for assignment to biological groups Significance testing using numerical statistics Multivariate analyses of function Multivariate analyses of biodistance
Non-metrics	Presence/absence/tabulation of individuals by category Percentages for each category for samples Significance testing using categorical statistics Multivariate biodistance models (e.g. mean measure of divergence)
General	Photos, charts and written descriptions Summary statistics (mean, median, SD, etc.) Significance testing of summary statistics

'dire' and 'glowing'. Many osteoarchaeologists use statistics capably and comfortably. However, even work published in major journals shows distinct areas for improvement. Many analyses rely heavily upon a narrow subset of statistical tools, rather than using the full range available. For example, we often summarize data through the mean rather than considering sometimes more appropriate measures such as the median. It is common to publish summarized data only as averages, without measures of variability that allow the reader to evaluate them. In bivariate and multivariate situations, we should perhaps rethink the balance between data exploration and inference. Especially with the development of new modelling tools, there is little reason to rely heavily upon hypothesis testing as the single most important statistical manoeuvre. Rather it should be used tactically to answer specific questions within the context of an overall analysis. We need to branch out from relying upon simple description and inference to data exploration and model building, especially when developing techniques and strategies for dealing with the specific characteristics of human skeletal data.

One challenge remains largely unanswered. Both American and British researchers have tended to use skeletal analysis to deal with a relatively narrow range of questions set by specific, sometimes unimaginative theoretical traditions. In order that we do not study skeletons and palaeopathologies purely for their own sake, we must draw inspiration from theoretical views of society. Conversely, we have much to contribute to interpretations of ancient societies; some of the most exciting developments in human skeletal analysis require ideas more than computers. Some avenues of thought are well explored, although far from exhausted. Studies of trauma, for instance, provide a starting point for understanding violence, which is an important symbolization of social relations.[50] Many pathologies have a class, occupational or economic dimension in both historical and prehistoric societies.[51] Particularly in economic studies, it has rarely been appreciated that skeletal studies are almost unique in their ability to provide information on actual patterns of behaviour and consumption and their effects upon specific individuals of known age and sex. For instance, few other branches of archaeology are as well placed to address the question of the 'Secondary Products Revolution'.[52]

In addition, we also have points of contact with 'post-processual' and other archaeologies. Osteoarchaeology is essential for accurately studying burial taphonomy and ritual, an important theme in much recent Neolithic and Bronze Age archaeology.[53] Much recent theorization has dealt with the human body as a social operator, as a gendered phenomenon, and as the locus of human experience and hence of social reality.[54] Here the effect of disciplinary boundaries is clear, for instance, in the fact that palaeopathologists have rarely discussed the experience and social understanding of illness, of disability or of healing, even when studying maladies with well-defined aetiologies. Skeletal studies provide an essential dimension to gender archaeology, as they provide one of the few fixed reference points associating particular symbols, lifestyles, and activities with sexed individuals. They may also supply direct evidence upon gender relations.[55-57] Instances of intentional bodily modification are far from rare, nor is skeletal evidence for experienced processes such as growth and ageing. How we make use of the wealth of possibilities for theoretical interpretation is limited only by our imagination.

ACKNOWLEDGMENTS

I am grateful to Mary Lucas Powell, Giorgio Manzi and two anonymous reviewers for helpful comments. Any viewpoints, errors, and omissions remain my own work.

REFERENCES

1   Bass W. *Human Osteology* (3rd edn). Columbia: Missouri Archaeological Society, 1987.

2   Steele D, Bramblett C. *The Anatomy and Biology of the Human Skeleton*. College Station: Texas A & M University Press, 1988.

3   Brothwell DR. *Digging Up Bones: The Excavation, Treatment and Study of Human Skeletal Remains* (3rd edn). Ithaca: Cornell University Press, 1981.

4   Mays S. *The Archaeology of Human Bones*. London: Routledge, 1998.

5   Schwartz JH. *Skeleton Keys: An Introduction to Human Skeletal Morphology, Development, and Analysis*. New York: Oxford University Press, 1995.

6   Ubelaker D. *Human Skeletal Remains: Excavation, Analysis, Interpretation* (2nd edn). Washington, DC: Taraxacum, 1989.

7   White TD. *Human Osteology*. San Diego: Academic Press, 1991.

8   Kennedy K, Isçan M. *Reconstruction of Life from the Skeleton*. New York: Alan R Liss, 1989.

9   Krogman W, Isçan M. *The Human Skeleton in Forensic Medicine* (2nd edn). Springfield: Charles C Thomas, 1986.

10 Ortner D, Putschar W. *Identification of Pathological Conditions in Human Skeletal Remains*. Washington, DC: Smithsonian Institution Press, 1981.

11 Larsen CS. *Bioarchaeology: Interpreting Behavior from the Human Skeleton*. New York: Cambridge University Press, 1997.

12 Buikstra J, Ubelaker D. *Standards for Data Collection from Human Skeletal Remains*. Research Series, 44. Fayetteville: Arkansas Archaeological Survey, 1994.

13 Waldron T. *Counting the Dead: the Epidemiology of Skeletal Populations*. New York: Wiley, 1994.

14 Buikstra J, Konigsberg L. Paleodemography: critiques and controversies. *American Anthropology* 1985; **87**: 316–333.

15 Meindl RS, Russell KF. Recent advances in method and theory in paleodemography. *Annual Review of Anthropology* 1998; **27**: 375–399.

16 Buikstra J, Frankenberg S, Konigsberg L. Skeletal biological distance studies in American physical anthropology: recent trends. *American Journal of Physical Anthropology* 1990; **82**: 1–7.

17 Richtsmeier JT, Cheverud JM, Lele S. Advances in anthropological morphometrics. *Annual Review of Anthropology* 1992; **21**: 283–305.

18 Van Vark GN, Howells WW (eds), *Multivariate Statistical Methods in Physical Anthropology: a Review of Recent Advances and Current Developments*. Dordrecht: Reidel, 1984.

19 Van Vark GN, Schaafsma W. Advances in the quantitative analysis of skeletal morphology. In: Saunders S, Katzenberg MA (eds), *Skeletal Biology of Past Peoples: Research Methods*. New York: Wiley-Liss, 1992: pp. 225–258.

20 Thomas DH. The awful truth about statistics in archaeology. *American Antiquity* 1978; **43**: 231–244.

21 Drennan R. *Statistics for Archaeologists*. New York: Plenum, 1996.

22 Shennan SJ. *Quantifying Archaeology* (2nd edn). Edinburgh: Edinburgh University Press, 1997.

23 Thomas DH. *Refiguring Anthropology* (2nd edn). Prospect Heights: Waveland, 1986.

24 Shanks M, Tilley C. *Re-Constructing Archaeology: Theory and Practice* (2nd edn). London: Routledge, 1992.

25 Gould SJ. *The Mismeasure of Man* (2nd edn). New York: WW Norton, 1996.

26   Robb J, Mallegni F, Ronco D. New human remains from the Southern Italian Neolithic: Ripa Tetta and Latronico. *Rivista di Antropologia* 1991; **69**: 125–144.

27   Martin R, Saller K. *Lehrbuch der Anthropologie in systematischer Darstellung*. Stuttgart: Fischer, 1956.

28   Borgognini Tarli S, Masali M. Osteometria e morfoscopia dello scheletro. In: Borgognini Tarli S, Pacciani E (eds), *I Resti Umani nello Scavo Archeologico*. Rome: Bulzoni, 1993: pp. 107–169.

29   Guidi A. *Storia della Paletnologia*. Bari: Laterza, 1988.

30   Borgognini Tarli S, Pacciani E (eds), *I Resti Umani nello Scavo Archeologico: Metodiche di Recupero e Studio*. Rome: Bulzoni, 1993.

31   Trigger BG. *A History of Archaeological Thought*. Cambridge: Cambridge University Press, 1989.

32   Powell M. *Status and Health in Prehistory: A Case Study of the Moundville Chiefdom*. Washington, DC: Smithsonian Institution Press, 1988.

33   Mays SA. A perspective on human osteoarchaeology in Britain. *International Journal of Osteoarchaeology* 1997; **7**: 600–604.

34   Wood JW, Milner GR, Harpending H, Weiss K. The osteological paradox: problems in inferring prehistoric health from skeletal samples. *Current Anthropology* 1992; **33**: 343–370.

35   Cohen MN. The osteological paradox reconsidered. *Current Anthropology* 1995; **35**: 629–637.

36   Cohen MN. Does paleopathology measure community health? a rebuttal of the 'osteological paradox' and its implication for world history. In: Paine RR (ed.), *Integrating Archaeological Demography: Multidisciplinary Approaches to Prehistoric Populations*. Carbondale: Southern Illinois University, 1997: pp. 242–260.

37   Formicola V. La ricostruzione della statura dalle ossa degli arti. Valutazioni sull'attendibilità dei risultati in campioni neolitici. *Rivista di Antropologia* 1989; **67**: 307–318.

38   Baxter MJ. *Exploratory Multivariate Analysis in Archaeology*. Edinburgh: Edinburgh University Press, 1994.

39   Hartwig F, Dearing BE. *Exploratory Data Analysis*. Beverly Hills: Sage, 1979.

40   Robb JE. The interpretation of skeletal muscle sites: a statistical approach. *International Journal of Osteoarchaeology* 1998; **8**: 363–377

41   Cowgill GL. The trouble with significance tests and what we can do about it. *American Antiquity* 1977; **42**: 350–368.

42   Lukacs J. Dental paleopathology. In: Kennedy K, Isçan M (eds), *Reconstruction of Life from the Skeleton*. New York: Alan R Liss, 1989: pp. 261–286.

43   Powell M. The analysis of dental wear and caries for dietary reconstruction. In: Gilbert R, Mielke J (eds), *The Analysis of Prehistoric Diets*. New York: Academic Press, 1985: pp. 307–338.

44   Chamberlain A. Problems and prospects in palaeodemography (Chapter 7 – this volume).

45   Ruff C. Biomechanical analyses of archaeological human skeletal samples. In: Saunders S, Katzenberg MA (eds), *Skeletal Biology of Past Peoples: Research Methods*. New York: Wiley-Liss, 1992: pp. 37–58.

46   Ossenberg N. Within and between race distances in population studies based on discrete traits of the human skull. *American Journal of Physical Anthropology* 1976; **45**: 701–716.

47   Paleopathology Association. *Skeletal Database Committee Recommendations*. Detroit: Paleopathology Association, 1991.

48   Robb J. Violence and gender in early Italy. In: Frayer D, Martin D (eds), *Troubled Times: Osteological and Archaeological Evidence of Violence and Warfare*. New York: Gordon & Breach, 1997: pp. 108–141.

49   Aldenderfer MS, Blashfield RK. *Cluster Analysis*. Beverly Hills: Sage, 1984.

50   Frayer DW, Martin D (eds), *Troubled Times: Archaeological and Osteological Evidence of Violence and Warfare*. New York: Gordon & Breach, 1997.

51   Cohen MN. *Health and the Rise of Civilization*. New Haven: Yale University Press, 1989.

52   Sherratt A. Plough and pastoralism: aspects of the secondary products revolution. In: Hodder I, Isaac G, Hammond N (eds), *Pattern of the Past: Studies in Honour of David Clarke*. Cambridge: Cambridge University Press, 1981: pp. 261–305.

53   Tilley C (ed.), *Interpretative Archaeology*. Oxford: Berg, 1993.

54   Shilling C. *The Body and Social Theory*. London: Sage, 1993.

55   Cohen M, Bennett S. Skeletal evidence for sex roles and gender hierarchies in prehistory. In: Miller B (ed.), *Sex and Gender Hierarchies*. Cambridge: Cambridge University Press, 1993: pp. 273–294.

56   Holliman S. Health consequences of the sexual division of labor among prehistoric Native Americans: the Chumash of California and the Arikira of the North Plains. In: Claassen C (ed.), *Exploring Gender through Archaeology: Selected Papers from the 1991 Boone Conference*. Madison: Prehistory Press, 1992: pp. 81–89.

57   Shermis S. Domestic violence in two skeletal populations. *Ossa* 1984; **11**: 143–152.

58   Blalock HM. *Social Statistics* (2nd edn). New York: McGraw-Hill, 1979.

29

FORENSIC OSTEOLOGY IN THE UNITED KINGDOM

Sue Black

Within the past 5 years, the word 'forensic' seems to have been catapulted into media appro-bation, and sneaking in under the hem of its surgical greens lurks the supporting role of the 'bone expert'. Consider the impact of popular television programmes such as *Silent Witness* and *McCallum*, or the role of the scientific experts in fictional series such as *Taggart* and *Morse*. Or indeed examine their involvement in factual programmes such as *Meet the Ancestors*, *Time Team* and *The Coroner* let alone the coverage given in popular novels by authors such as Patricia Cornwell, Kathy Reichs and Val McDermid – and suddenly we are trendy and have come of age. It has been a long road and a huge fashion revolution since the ground breaking days of *Quincy*.

Or maybe not! In a recent questionnaire to every police force in the UK (55 in all, 75% of which have so far responded), > 98% of respondents said that they had never required the services of a forensic osteologist (FO) or bone expert. This came as a bit of a blow to some-body who has spent the past 13 years in that field and worked extensively for many forces up and down the length of the country. How then can this be explained? One needs firstly to examine the means whereby an expert is initially brought into an investigation. In most instances the role of identifying a suitable specialist often lies with the forensic pathologist, procurator fiscal or coroner, and so police officers may not have any direct line of contact with the bone expert. It must be said that in addition to this, much of the routine osteolog-ical work is in fact carried out by the forensic pathologist. However, many do appreciate that this is a specialized field of expertise and do tend to have a favoured contact, who may work in a local museum, anthropology, archaeology or anatomy department and a few even employ a part time in-house forensic osteologist.

However, it is also true to say that many police officers are unaware of the services that a FO can provide and even if they did know, often they are unsure of where to actually find one. Of course this is grossly unfair to the many forward thinking police forces who do regularly consult osteologists, odontologists, archaeologists, facial reconstruction experts and profes-sionals in many other areas of anthropological expertise. Should the need arise, a police officer can of course contact the National Crime Faculty (NCF) at Bramshill but unfortu-nately they have very few experts listed in the field of forensic osteology. However, they can be assured that if the individual is indeed listed with the NCF then they have been closely monitored and deemed to be of a high professional standard in all aspects of the occupation.

Who then, is to blame for the seemingly sporadic co-operative investigations between the FO and the judicial system? Unfortunately we can probably only blame ourselves. In our own defence though, we have always suffered from a paucity of formal training, lacked any regulation regarding competence, been devoid of an organizational body and so have generally appeared as a fragmented body of uncertified, self-appointed experts. This is terribly unjust, however, as there are many well qualified UK scientists working in this field who are engaged in ground-breaking research and whose services are requested all over the world. So therefore our science, as it stands today in the UK, can best be described as in a state of discordant flux. On the one hand it lacks the respect and power of a professional cohesive organization but on the other it is composed of some eminent and extremely capable scientists.

In the USA and also in many European countries, forensic anthropology is a well-recognized field of investigative expertise.[1] The American Academy of Forensic Sciences was established in 1949, with a separate physical anthropology section being recognized in 1972. By 1977 the American Board of Forensic Anthropologists[2] was established which now boasts over 40 members at Diplomate status. Why then is there such an apparent chasm between the level of professional organization in this subject in the USA and the seemingly amateurish approach often found in the UK? The answer, with a somewhat optimistic note, is probably historical. The relatively lower level of crime in the UK in conjunction with the smaller geographical area and population size has meant that we have never had the workload to sustain full-time specialists in this area. Even those who work regularly for police forces in the UK will tell you that the caseload is best described as 'feast or famine'. It is not a predictable occupation in terms of time management and as a result the experts must have alternative means of sustaining income. Many find their way to this subject through medicine or preclinical training, anatomy, anthropology, archaeology and many other surprisingly tortuous routes.

Until very recently there has been no formal training in forensic anthropology in this country, although most students would probably agree that it is a fascinating subject that they would enjoy studying. However, in realistic and practical terms we have an obligation to ensure that they are fully aware that we may be preparing them for a job which they may never be required to perform. The reality is that full-time employment as a FO in the UK is at present untenable. Therefore, forensic skills often have to be viewed as an alternative string to one's bow.

I am aware of only three educational institutions in the UK that offer training courses in forensic anthropology. Bournemouth University runs an MSc course in forensic archaeology of which 25% is given over to the teaching of anthropological skills. University College London offers a MSc course in forensic archaeological science, which has a large, although optional, anthropological component. The Universities of Bournemouth and Bradford seem to be the only academic institutions in the UK to run a postgraduate qualification that is exclusively dedicated to forensic anthropology; they offer a one-year MSc/Postgraduate diploma. While these courses do laudably attempt to bridge the chasm in our meagre teaching curriculum, many former students have been quick to state that they have subsequently found themselves to be woefully unprepared for the rigours of the real world of forensics.

Forensic osteology is a small branch of the much larger discipline of forensic anthropology, although the two terms are sometimes used interchangeably and often incorrectly. The FO tends to be concerned with the initial investigative procedures of the corpse/skeletal remains before a wider range of more advanced technical assistance is explored and requested within the field of forensic anthropology. The principal aim of the FO is to attempt to provide hitherto unknown information that may be of value in attempting to ascertain the identity of the deceased. Occasionally, information may also be deduced with regards to the circumstances surrounding the death or indeed to the actual cause of death. This work may involve homicides, suicides, mass disasters, war graves, unexplained deaths and of course natural deaths, as not all forensic work has a criminal element. Regardless of the nature of the material, the legal requirements of our judicial system state that every reasonable attempt must be made to identify the remains of the deceased, regardless of the possibility of criminal involvement.

The skills of the FO are normally only sought when the police have no further lines of inquiry to follow and have exhausted all other avenues of investigation. Therefore, we begin our work at a disadvantage. In moments of despair, I often feel that we are sometimes considered to be the last vestige of hope, almost the proverbial scraping at the bottom of the barrel. This invariably means that the FO rarely attends the crime scene and although the remains will probably find their way to the bone laboratory, it is likely to be quite some considerable time after their initial discovery. For example, in a recent case I did not become involved until more than 2 years after the discovery of the remains and then only by accident as I had been to primary school with the investigative officer and found myself in conversation with his mother. It seems in many cases to be merely fortuitous if the correct specialist is found for a specific job. We have a responsibility to both the public and the legal profession to attempt to provide a national professional network of competent experienced practitioners. Such a national register of experts in forensic anthropology is long overdue and, thankfully, is now underway with the guidance of the Council for the Registration of Forensic Practitioners. If the services of forensic osteology are to be taken seriously and utilized to their full potential in the UK, then we have some very major amendments to make at the grass roots level concerning how human remains should be excavated and processed before presentation to the appropriate judicial authorities.

What then is the difference between a FO and any other scientist who works on human bone? Do they have any extra exceptional skills that set them apart? Of course not, but it has to be said that there are probably one or two character traits that most adequately describe the FO. First, they tend to have a highly suspicious temperament that rarely accepts the obvious. A decomposed body found wearing a pair of panties and a matching lace bra will not always be indicative of the biological sex of the deceased. There is a quote by Giovanni Morgagni (1682–1771) that captures this sentiment beautifully: 'Those who have dissected or inspected many bodies have at least learned to doubt, while those who are ignorant of anatomy and do not take the trouble to attend to it, are in no doubt at all'. Anybody who works in forensic sciences will agree that fact is often much stranger than fiction and it is only after exposure to several absurd cases that one really begins to develop a honed sense of scepticism. There is no doubt that if we were to write a novel based on the details of some forensic cases we have been involved in, any publishing house would probably deem many of them to be too outrageous and far-fetched.

Second, a strong stomach is an absolute necessity. There are many osteologists who prefer not to work on forensic material unless they can be assured that the remains are entirely dry and odourless. Although some forensic work may indeed involve dry skeletal remains, much is often less pleasant to handle. The FO rarely has to work with fresh remains, as the identity of the deceased is seldom in question in such circumstances. More commonly the material may necessitate dissection of decomposing (often maggot ridden) remains and so the ability to dissect is an extremely valuable asset. In all honesty, anosmia would probably be the ideal clinical condition to suffer from in this job.

Third, the FO must be willing to attend scenes of crime wherever and whenever they should arise. Three years ago I was requested to attend a crime scene in Kent where small parts of a murdered victim were thought to have been flushed into the sewerage system. The senior police officer failed to inform us that there was indeed no formal sewerage system in that area and it would necessitate the excavation of a cesspit. I suppose one should be grateful that it occurred in mid-December and not mid-July, when the contents might have been less amenable to a shovel and a slurry pump might have been more desirous.

The final character trait that is essential, is an almost obsessive fixation with detailed administrative organization. This is absolutely necessary to ensure the smooth progression of a case through the processes of continuity of evidence, confidentiality, case reporting and the *terminus ante quem* – evidence in court. There is no place in current day forensic science for the somewhat eccentric, absent minded, disorganized, bumbling academic.

The first task for the FO is usually to ensure that the remains that are presented are indeed human. A murder investigation based on the remains of a Saturday night carry out are unlikely to lead to a conviction for murder! While this sounds obvious, it is not always easy to establish. Given a set of rib fragments recovered from a refuse tip many experienced workers would be reluctant to say with any conviction whether they are human or porcine at a first glance. It is worthwhile remembering in such circumstances that the sense of smell can be a wonderfully simplistic scientific tool. Domestic refuse tends to contain a high proportion of cooked animal bones and so the remains placed in a sealed plastic bag on a radiator for a few minutes may smell like the cooked foodstuff. Sheep bones will smell like lamb, pig bones will smell like pork and while perhaps not terribly scientific (or indeed always appropriate or possible), it is worth remembering.

Indeed not all bones are in fact 'bone'. I have been presented with a scapula from a student's anatomical teaching skeleton that was polymer resin based, and while the morphology was indeed human, the subject had assuredly never drawn a single breath. Once the remains have been established as human then the next question that is always asked is 'How long has the individual been deceased?' Unfortunately, this is probably the most difficult question to answer and the one that can prove to be the most pivotal to the future success of the investigation. In legal terms the temporal cut off point between forensic and archaeological provenance is arbitrarily set at between 70 and 75 years before the present. This allows for the passage of the purported three score years and ten of mortal existence and almost certainly ensures that the perpetrator of the crime is unlikely to be brought to justice. Also, it is unlikely that any living relatives could be found who could identify either the remains or any associated artefacts. In reality, however, the distinction is rarely so clear cut. For example, the passage of time will be almost irrelevant if juvenile remains are ever found on Saddleworth Moor, Yorkshire, as such matters will always fall into forensic territory, albeit eventually historical. It is of course in situations like this that the field of forensic archaeology would come to the fore.

Assigning a precise post-mortem interval is extremely difficult and can rarely be done on site without the presence of circumstantial evidence. In the laboratory it tends to require precise analytical procedures (see below) which are rarely accurate, tend to take some time to complete and can be costly. However, the investigating officer usually wants the answer as soon as possible so that the case can be processed in an appropriate manner. Unquestionably, being present at the scene of retrieval (not necessarily synonymous with the scene of crime) is likely to reveal the first clues regarding the period of interment. Surface concealments tend not to be archaeological just as deep graves tend not to be forensic in nature. The presence of a burial receptacle can be useful; a coffin is unlikely to be forensic (unless the perpetrator was an undertaker), while a carpet or plastic sheeting will not be archaeological. The presence of a Bronze Age pot will be as clearly indicative of a time period as will the retrieval of a coin of the realm. It is the absence of circumstantial evidence that is most detrimental to the accurate determination of the time since death. For example, last year a local council employee discovered some human bones about 100 m from the site of an ancient churchyard near Crawfordjohn, Strathclyde. It was known that workers repairing the road in the 1950s had found human bones and had reburied them on the other side of a low wall next to a stream. There was no supporting evidence regarding the date of interment and on first inspection the assemblage seemed archaeological but when one of the femora was sectioned, adipocere was found filling the medullary cavity. Although adipocere has been found in archaeological material it is frequently associated with more recent death. In the absence of that adipocere, there would have been little uncertainty in assigning the remains to an archaeological provenance, but its presence raised a doubt, albeit fleeting.

In some circumstances the assignment of a time since death is almost irrelevant. For example, a skull with hook and rivet attachments for the skull cap or holes in a parallel line down the anterior ends of consecutive ribs, caused by articulation wires, will all strongly indicate the previous teaching nature of the material, the provenance of which was probably not even known at the date of purchase. Yet it is amazing just how many medical specimens do turn up buried in gardens, usually because the family of the deceased academic had not known what else to do with them.

Although archaeological bone experts have a veritable battery of techniques available for estimating time since death, the forensic scientist has few that are of any truly noteworthy reliability that operate within their narrow temporal framework. Obviously the presence of soft tissue is generally an indication of relatively recent death but the variability in tissue preservation is notoriously unreliable. It is not the first time that a body has been exhumed from boggy areas even with eyes intact only to eventually discover that they may even predate the current millennium. In an effort to establish the interval since time of death, forensic scientists have examined many potential indicators including the equilibrium between ^{210}Po and ^{210}Pb levels, ^{90}Sr levels, ^{14}C levels, ultraviolet fluorescence, nitrogen content, benzidine reaction, immuno-electrophoresis, paper chromatography and many others.[3–10] Knight and Lauder did caution that 'Frequently the pronouncement of the age (time since death) is made with a confidence inversely proportional to the experience of the examiner' (p. 338).[9] Time since death is probably the most difficult decision that the FO has to make when the remains are reduced to dry bone and not associated with circumstantial evidence. For these very reasons, remains that are washed up on the shoreline, caught in fishing nets or found floating in the harbour are notoriously difficult to assign. Ultimately, if the remains are considered to be outside the temporal realms of the forensic examiner then they are usually passed on to the appropriate county archaeologist or a university department of archaeology. Even so, it is prudent for the FO to write a full report on the specimen to complete the police file on the investigation.

If, however, the remains are deemed to be of forensic concern then a chain of judicial events is set in motion. At the back of one's mind must always be the little nagging voice of doubt that warns of caution and double checking at all successive stages. A tragic scenario could ensue if the case came to court and was subsequently dismissed on the grounds of lack of continuity of evidence or some other avoidable technicality. Being assigned to a forensic case carries an inordinate burden of moral responsibility and the FO must at all times maintain an unbiased stance. While the easiest way to achieve this would be to remain entirely detached and not become involved with the case, in practise this is often an impossible role to play. The handling of a person's mortal remains seems to insidiously percolate an element of unshakeable personal contact and respect that can intensify into an almost unconscious necessity to achieve closure and even justice on their behalf. That is not to say that the FO will go out and stalk the perpetrator, as is often seen on television programmes, but there is an urgency to perform to the best of one's abilities and not to fail. There is a true sense of guilt and failure if, after every possible effort has been made, the deceased remains unidentified. The responsibility that one feels resides at many levels. Initially it is usually to the deceased who deserves a name and an appropriate and fitting burial and of course to his or her relatives. But there is also a sense of responsibility to the police as their investigation and perhaps the eventual apprehension of a suspect will rely heavily on assigning a name to the deceased. Without a positive identification of the deceased, police investigations usually cannot be taken to a successful conclusion.

When the remains are skeletonized, the FO will sign for them and they will duly pass into his or her custody where their security must be ensured at all times. When passed on to other experts for their opinion, the remains are still technically under the guardianship of the original signatory on the evidentiary inventory. Therefore, the paranoia that can surround the location of forensic specimens is understandable. Recently I received a frantic phone call from Italy to ask if I still had a particular skull from a recent multiple murder case in my possession, as it could not be found. It was eventually located in a box on a shelf in the laboratory proving that it is equally important to obtain a signature on returning evidence as it is upon receiving it.

While a case is in process, any information pertaining to it must be considered to be confidential as it is sub judice. If one should be unlucky enough to become involved in an investigation that attracts intense media attention then extreme care must be exercised not only with regards to the passing on of verbal information, but also to any written material that may be placed in the refuse for disposal. It should also be borne in mind that following the Criminal Proceedings and Investigations Act (1996) every piece of evidence (even notes on scraps of paper) may be required to be disclosed and ultimately subjected to the critical examination of the defence experts. It is not surprising, therefore, that many experts are extremely cautious in revealing any information on a current case, given the detailed level of scrutiny that they may face. Even if a case does not come to court at the present time, it should be borne in mind that it may yet appear at a later date. Inappropriate dissemination of information pertaining to that case could seriously jeopardise its future judiciary outcome.

Unquestionably the biggest impact on forensic skeletal analysis and incontrovertible identification of the deceased has come with the ability to extract DNA from bone. It is important to bear this in mind at the outset of an investigation, as it may be the final means whereby an individual can be positively identified especially if samples can be obtained from living relatives. For this very fact, all due care and attention must be paid towards the prevention of contamination of the sample at the retrieval scene. If soft tissue is present then it is a relatively simple procedure to remove a sample and store it in isolated conditions should matching be considered appropriate at a later date. When only skeletal remains are presented then it is advisable that a relatively small sample of bone (metacarpals or metatarsals are ideal) should be isolated as soon as possible for future genetic matching. It is worth bearing in mind that the selection of the actual bone specimen is important. There is some evidence to suggest that DNA may have a greater chance of survival in protected areas such as the root canals of teeth, but of course areas of the skeleton that will prove important in the initial identification stages of the investigation should not be selected. It would not be wise to choose the pubic bone for example. Although a major breakthrough in scientific procedures, DNA analysis only has some bearing on confirming the identity of the deceased when a possible suspect is isolated. I remember being asked by a coroner at a press conference whether we believed that DNA would sound the death knell for the forensic anthropologist. DNA is not the panacea to solve all criminal investigations and I believe that many non-scientific personnel are unaware of this. In a recent case in the Scottish Highlands, the investigating officer asked me whether DNA would allow us to identify the deceased. If we could only find a genetic sequence for name, address and date of birth perhaps it would indeed be so. Until such times DNA analysis must remain as a tool to aid in the confirmation of identity only once a victim has already been tentatively identified.

From this stage onwards the procedures and techniques adopted are very similar to those followed in any archaeological skeletal investigation. The initial process will be dependent upon the number of bodies that are interred. In multiple burial situations, the first step in the analysis is to assign, where possible, the appropriate skeletal elements or body parts to specific individuals. A mixture of adult and juvenile remains is readily separated on the basis of size and degree of skeletal development. The separation of commingled juvenile remains relies heavily on a sound appreciation of complex juvenile osteology.[11] For example, the presence of three distinct components to a thoracic vertebra in conjunction with a distal radial epiphysis will automatically alert the expert to the presence of two juvenile individuals. The separation of commingled adult remains is dependent on many factors including size, robusticity, consistency of pathological conditions and the identification of the four basic parameters of biological identity: race, sex, age at death and height.

The evaluation of race or ethnic origin is among the most contentious issues in forensic osteology. The almost arbitrary separation of human races into Caucasoid, Negroid and Mongoloid is terribly outdated. The term Caucasoid originated from individuals who lived in the region of the Caucasus Mountains in Eastern Europe! It is generally taken to mean 'white' but it must by definition include such disparate racial groups as those found in the Asian subcontinent and therefore such terminology is clearly nonsensical. Given the degree of racial admixture in our cosmopolitan world it is also clear that there is little so called 'purity of race' and so in many ways this has to be the most difficult trait to establish. Often the geographical location of the specimen is used as a possible indicator of race but this is a very dangerous precedent. A FO working in the British Midlands may be more alert to the potential of Asian material but then so must the investigator in the Outer Hebrides where there is a large Asian population particularly around the town of Stornaway. We are guilty of being more wary of racial assignation in large cities but we must be equally alert in any part of the country, however much it may feel like a sleepy backwater. It is, however, true to say that most osteologists in the UK rarely encounter skeletal remains that are not north-west European in origin and as a result are often inexperience in racial assignation from other parts of the world. Several years ago I was asked to look at a skeleton that had been sent to a London department of forensic medicine for facial reconstruction. The osteologist who had originally examined the remains reported that they were from a white female of between 20 and 25 years of age. Accordingly, the police had sent photographs of missing persons who conformed to this description in the hope that a positive identification would ensue. On examining the remains, it was clear that they were neither 'white' nor indeed female but in fact male and Asian in ethnic origin. Subsequently the individual was identified as the victim of a caste murder who had paid inappropriate attentions to a specific young lady. Understandably the gracile nature of the bones had led the original osteologist to assume they were female, but the best training that an FO can give himself or herself, is to spend time examining as many varied documented specimens as possible.

If soft tissue is present the task of assigning race can be easier given the degree of skin pigmentation and hair type and colour. However, it is not the first body that has been dredged from the sea and been pronounced 'black' due to the skin colour only to be told that this is a normal stage of 'white' body putrefaction.

It has never ceased to amaze me when I have heard experienced bone specialists claim that the identification of sex is easy and relatively straightforward to establish. Anybody who has worked on skeletal collections of documented sex will agree that this is an absurd statement.

It is true to say that in the majority of the population, sex is a discrete dichotomous variable. However, there are genetic conditions, surgical interventions and hormonal influences (sometimes artificial) to be considered which can technically result in an individual being precisely neither one sex nor the other. Such a gender crisis has been brought to light in the recent case of a transsexual convicted for a crime and sentenced to incarceration. Genetically he is male but externally in terms of appearance and secondary sexual characteristics she is female. The social quandary is, can a man be placed in a woman's prison and for her own safety and therefore on humanitarian grounds, could she justifiably be condemned to a man's prison? It is important to bear in mind the fact that even at the most basic level of cellular organization, sex can be unclear.

Population specific levels of sexual dimorphism show considerable degrees of variation and as the genetic origin of the individual is rarely known in forensic investigations one cannot assume that the textbook stereotype form will apply. It is also important to remember that most of the techniques that we use to establish the identity of the deceased were originally derived on relatively large sample sizes where an accuracy of 85% was considered eminently acceptable. However, in a forensic situation, this amounts to almost one in every seven individuals being incorrectly assigned and this is certainly a level of inaccuracy that will be utilized to great effect by the defence experts. Therefore, acceptable levels of accuracy in other osteological fields may not be tolerated in forensic work.

There is a vast array of techniques available for the identification of sex (see Mays and Cox, chapter 8, in this volume) but it is probably one of the most difficult biological factors to ascribe to juvenile remains. While there are some techniques that purport to identify sex differences, the degree of accuracy falls far short of the more stringent forensic requirements. It is likely that only genetic identification of the sex chromosomes will permit the unequivocal identification of sex for the juvenile skeleton.

The identification of age at death is relatively reliable when considering juvenile remains but becomes less dependable with more advanced years (see Scheuer and Black, chapter 2, and Cox, chapter 5, in this volume). Bearing in mind that the average life span is about 70–75 years and most of our techniques lose their accuracy before 40 years of age, there is close to half the human life span during which individuals cannot be aged with any degree of confidence. This is not a reassuring fact to pass on to the police officer in charge of the investigation who perceives there to be a significant discrepancy between saying that the deceased was 50 or 65. Unfortunately this is one of the drawbacks of adult human ageing, that it does not occur at either a regular or a predictable rate.

Although the identification of stature has its own problems, it still remains one of the most relatively straightforward parameters that can be established. Of course this is only true if the ethnic origin of the individual, and their sex, is known and if the long bones are both present and relatively intact. As I have found to my cost, the estimation of stature from a decapitated, dismembered, decomposed torso is not particularly accurate but perhaps this best illustrates the dogged determination of forensic scientists. They are painfully aware that they have no control over which elements of the corpse will be presented for analysis and so have endeavoured to establish the viability of almost every skeletal element for the purposes of identification of biological identity. One might ask why you would want to calculate stature from a metacarpal, but if that is all that is present then the best must be made out of that situation.

Despite all these pitfalls, most individuals can be assigned to a biological profile (e.g. male, between 20 and 25 years, white and between 173 cm (5 foot 8 inches) and 178 cm (5 foot 10 inches) in height). The establishment of 'biological identity' allows the police to narrow the potential number of individuals from a missing persons list, and so forms a sort of starting platform from which the process of identification can truly begin. From here the next step is to attempt to establish personal identity and hopefully assign a name to the deceased. This has to be the ultimate rationale of our profession. In the vast majority of cases it is not identifying the murder weapon or establishing a cause of death that is at issue, it is being able to provide incontrovertible evidence that the remains are that of somebody's next of kin. It is often only then, when the deceased has been positively identified, that the family can accept the bereavement, pay their respects and begin closure to allow them to continue with their own lives. For many, the acceptance of death can only begin when its rituals have been attended to. Having spoken to some of the widows of the Piper Alpha oil platform disaster, it is clear that while the majority have fully accepted the loss of their partner, a few still cling to the hope that maybe they are still alive somewhere but perhaps suffering from amnesia, and that one day they will come home. In these circumstances we have to ask whether the fictitious world of television, film and trashy novels really prepares us for the reality of our world. Without a body to place in the ground and allow the grieving process to begin, they cannot truly be in control of the rest of their lives. However, it is vital that the FO is not pressurized into making a false identification but must be 100% certain before agreeing to the identification. Positive identification should never be made if there is even the slightest doubt as it is always possible that the named deceased may still be alive. Therefore, the FO carries a heavy social burden, as the future path of an entire family can be dependent upon the positive identification of the deceased.[12]

Personal identity often relies on the presence of idiosyncratic features that separate one person from another even if they share the same biological profile. It may be a particular form of dental work, a previous fracture, a developmental anomaly, evidence of surgical intervention or perhaps a pathological condition. To establish a positive identity requires that the evidence obtained from the remains must, within reason, match secure information known about the deceased from pre-mortem sources. This information may come from relatives, friends, general practitioners, dentists, previous X-rays, military records, school records, etc. It might be of little value to note in isolation that the skeletal remains showed bony resorption of the metatarsals but it becomes highly informative if one of the potential matches was a long-term diabetic. Often, however, even this information is not without its problems. In one case we were asked to confirm identity from the decapitated remains of a microlight pilot who had ditched his aircraft in the sea off the coast of Inverbervie, Aberdeenshire. His girlfriend stated that he had a very prominent mole below his left nipple while his mother who stated that she should know best because she had seen him naked from the day he was born, assured us he had never had any kind of skin blemish. To make things even more complicated in this case, the pilot was known to have been in hospital 2 years previously suffering from injuries that included multiple broken ribs. The hospital records revealed that he had fractured ribs five to eight on the left side while we found evidence of healed fractures in ribs six to eight on the right side. This serves as a warning that even if medical or dental records are available they can only ever be as accurate as the individual who initially recorded the information.

One of the most useful tools for either discarding or including individuals as possible matches is facial superimposition.[13] Given a photograph of the missing person (preferably smiling with the teeth exposed) an image of the skull can be superimposed and a match either confirmed or rejected in most instances. If at the end of this process the deceased still remains unidentified then a facial reconstruction may be commissioned. This is generally approached by one of two methods: anatomical modelling using clay or computer generated best-fit images (see Neave, chapter 20, in this volume). While facial reconstruction does not purport to present a true image of the deceased, it does seek to nudge the memory of the public into admission of absence.

The FO will ultimately submit his or her final report to the body that commissioned the work and this may be the forensic pathologist, procurator fiscal (in Scotland), coroner (in England and Wales) or police force. In the majority of cases, the FO is not required to attend an inquest or trial, as by that stage in the proceedings the identity of the deceased is rarely in question. However, it does happen and this is when the earlier meticulous attention to detail is so important. It should be borne in mind that the court appearance may not arise until quite some considerable time after the report was written, sometimes several years, so painstaking attention to recording detail is essential so that it can be readily recalled while in court. In a criminal court, the FO usually appears for the Crown (prosecutor), although there is an increasing proportion of experts who are called upon to appear for the defence. I have always maintained that exposure to the courtroom circus often leaves the FO with little more than a personality complex. On one hand the prosecution will call you a foremost expert in your chosen field while the defence will do their utmost to prove you an incompetent amateur. Surviving the rigours of the courtroom is something for which most scientists are woefully unprepared. With time, perseverance, practise and the donning of a thick skin, one can come to accept it but rarely to enjoy or feel comfortable in such surroundings. There are some simple rules that can be employed to minimize the horrors of the event. Ensure that the final report is clear, as free from jargon as possible and that the conclusions can be fully supported by the evidence. Only answer the question that is asked and do not try to be clever. It is always safest to say 'I don't know' than look incompetent. Never offer an opinion on something that is outside your own area of expertise and do not allow yourself to be drawn on such matters. Having given evidence in a foreign court, there is little that can prepare you for the additional problem of loss of meaning in translation and so clear and bold answers are essential. Should an expert be called to give testimony there are two appropriate texts that, although they are American and therefore not directly applicable to the UK courts, do give valuable information in terms of psychological preparation.[14,15]

Forensic osteology is clearly still in its infancy in the UK and I suspect that the next 10 years will see it approach maturity. It is vital therefore that the solid foundations that we put in place today serve us in good stead for the future. There are several valuable texts in this field that can be consulted both for informative[16–19] and entertainment[20,21] purposes. Many police officers, coroners, procurator fiscals and even forensic pathologists have commented on how amazed they are at the amount of information an osteologist can extract from the skeleton. It is vital, therefore, that we constantly strive to improve our professional reputation and skills by increasing the awareness of the services that can be provided. It is critical that we continue to improve the reliability of our existing techniques of identification through constant re-evaluation and testing. It is of course equally important that we continue to develop new methods and ensure their validity and reliability through close working relationships with all fields of osteological research.

ACKNOWLEDGEMENTS

Thanks to Margaret Cox, Simon Hillson and Charlotte Roberts for information on the various courses available in forensic anthropology.

REFERENCES

1   Işcan MY. Progress in forensic anthropology: the 20th Century. *Forensic Science International* 1998; **98**: 1–8.

2   American Board of Forensic Anthropologists. http://www.csuchico.edu/anth/ABFA/

3   Swift B. Dating human skeletal remains: investigating the viability of measuring the equilibrium between 210Po and 210Pb as a measure of estimating the post-mortem interval. *Forensic Science International* 1998; **98**: 119–126.

4   MacLaughlin-Black SM, Herd RJM, Willson K, Myers M, West IE. Strontium–90 as an indicator of time since death: a pilot investigation. *Forensic Science International* 1992; **57**: 51–56.

5   Neis P, Hille R, Paschke M, Pilwat G, Schnabel A, Niess C, Bratzke H. Strontium 90 for determination of time since death. *Forensic Science International* 1999; **99**: 47–51.

6   Taylor RE, Suchery JM, Payen LA, Slota PJ. The use of radiocarbon (C–14) to identify skeletal materials of forensic science interest. *Journal of Forensic Sciences* 1989; **34**: 1196–1205.

7   Zimmerman MR, Angel JL. *Dating and Age Determination of Biological Materials*. London: Croom Helm, 1986.

8   Knight B, Lauder I. Practical methods of dating skeletal remains: a preliminary study. *Medicine, Science and the Law* 1967; **7**: 205–209.

9   Knight B, Lauder I. Methods of dating skeletal remains. *Human Biology* 1969; **41**: 322–341.

10 Bell LS, Skinner MF, Jones SJ. The speed of post mortem change to the human skeleton and its taphonomic significance. *Forensic Science International* 1996; **82**: 129–140.

11 Scheuer L, Black S. *Developmental Juvenile Osteology*. London: Academic Press (in press).

12 Cox M. Forensic archaeology in the UK: Questions of socio-intellectual context and socio-political responsibility. In: Lucas G, Bucchli V (eds), *The Archaeology of the Contemporary Past*. London: Routledge, 1999.

13 Clement JG, Ranson DL. *Craniofacial Identification in Forensic Medicine*. London: Arnold, 1998.

14 Froede RC. *The Scientific Expert in Court: Principles and Guidelines*. Washington, DC: American Association for Clinical Chemistry, 1997.

15 Becker RF. *Scientific Evidence and Expert Testimony Handbook: A Guide for Lawyers, Criminal Investigators and Forensic Specialists*. Springfield: Charles C Thomas, 1997.

16 Fazekas IG, Kósa F. *Forensic Fetal Osteology*. Budapest: Akadémiai Kiadó, 1978.

17 Krogman WM, Işcan MY. *The Human Skeleton in Forensic Medicine* (2nd edn). Springfield: Charles C Thomas, 1986.

18   Hunter J, Roberts C, Martin A. *Studies in Crime: An Introduction to Forensic Archaeology.* London: Batsford, 1996.

19   Reichs KJ. *Forensic Osteology: Advances in the Identification of Human Remains* (2nd edn). Springfield: Charles C Thomas, 1998.

20   Ubelaker D, Scammel H. *Bones: A Forensic Detective's Casebook.* New York: HarperCollins, 1992.

21   Stern C. *Dr Iain West's Casebook.* London: Warner, 1996.

INDEX

A

abdomen, weapon-related trauma, 365
abdominis rectus muscle, 135–137
Abingdon, Oxon., multiple myeloma, 205
abortion, spontaneous, 45
abrasion, teeth, 232
abscesses, periapical, 87, 231
Abu Hureyra, Syria, activity-related changes, 389–390
acetabulum/pubis index, 119
acetic acid washing, for isotope studies, 431, 432
acid dissolution (technique), diagenesis assessment,
        (Table) 445
actinomycetes, 245
activity, bone adaptation, 381–401
adamantinoma, (Table) 212
adaptation, response to activity, 382–385
Addingham, W. Yorks., weapon-related trauma, (Table) 370
adenoma, (Table) 203
adipocere, 495
adolescence, 9, 10
    growth spurt, 29
adult size attained
    Denver and London Crypt samples, 33–35
    percentage, 29
Africa, collagen loss, 442
African-American slaves, dental enamel hypoplasia, 47
age
    cultural significance, 61–64
    at death
        bone dimensions, 385
        cremated bone, 406, 409–411
        data analysis, 478
    determination
        forensic science, 499
        see also dental age determination; skeletal age determin-
            ation
        fractures, 345
        non-metric traits, bias, 299
age structure, populations, 102–103
ageing, bone, 64
agriculture
    caries, 230, 233

Europe, 280
    long bone size changes, 386
    maize, isotope studies, 426–427, 428, 431–432
    non-specific infection, 147
    osteoarthritis, 394
    skull shapes, 393
Ailcey Hill, Ripon, weapon-related trauma, (Table) 370
alanine, dental age determination, 95
Alaska, Aleuts, Western Eskimos, skeletal growth studies,
        (Table) 25
alginate moulds, 330–331
Altenerding, skeletal growth studies, (Table) 25
aluminium foil, archaeological skull moulding, 330
amelogenin gene, PCR sexing, 463–465
America
    maize agriculture, isotope studies, 426–427, 428,
        431–432
    skeletal asymmetry, 317
    syphilis, 153
    tuberculosis DNA, 469
    see also United States
American football, spine, 391
amino acids
    isotope distribution, 430
    protein survival and, 241
    racemization, dental age determination, 94
amplification, polymerase chain reaction, 458–459
amputations, 344
    Marion 'Peg Leg' Brown, 386–387
anadromous fish, isotope ratios, 428
anaemias, 469–470
    see also iron deficiency anaemia
anatomical approach, facial reconstruction, 327, 332
anatomy, knowledge requirement, 139–140
Ancaster, Lincs., weapon-related trauma, (Table) 368
ancient DNA, 455–473
    cremated remains, 412–413
    sexing, 126
anencephaly, 217–218
aneurysmal bone cysts, 266
Anglo-Saxon period
    frequency of congenital and neoplastic diseases, 217

weapon-related trauma, 369–371
weapons, 358, 366
angular transformation, mean measure of divergence, 302
animals
  cemental annulations *vs* age, 92–93
  cremation, 416
  forensic anthropology, remains pitfall, 494
  isotope ratios, 425–426
    climate, 433
    marine (Fig.), 426
  trait inheritance, 297
anisotropism, bone, 383
ankylosing spondylitis, 175–176
ankylosis, (Fig.) 164
Annett, M., on handedness, 307–308
annulations, cemental, dental age determination, 92–94
Anscombe transformation, mean measure of divergence,
  301–302
antibodies, stains, 257
apatite *see* calcium hydroxyapatite
apical translucency, dental age determination, 89–91
Apple Down, Chichester, congenital anomalies, 204
arachnoid granulation, age determination, 74
archers, *Mary Rose*, 385
Arikara, skeletal growth studies, (Table) 25
armature, skull as, 325–326, 328
Arras culture, Yorkshire, 283–284
arthritis *see* joints
arthritis mutilans, 177
arthrogryposis multiplex congenita, (Table) 201, (Table) 216
artificial bones, 494–495
artificial intelligence, 485
Ashkelon (Roman), PCR sexing studies, 463–465
aspartic acid, dental age determination, 94, 95
asymmetry, 314–316
  archers, 385
  compensatory, 386–387
  non-metric traits, 299–300
  population prevalences, 316–317
  see also handedness
asymptotes, and polynomial equations, 32
athletes
  arm asymmetry, 311
  osteoarthritis, 393–394
  spondylolysis, 391
Atlas of occupational markers on human remains (Capasso *et al*),
  382
atrophic arthritides, 163
attrition, teeth, 87–89, 232
auricular surface of ilium
  age determination, 70–71, 74
  sexing of immature skeleton, 122–123
australopithecines, isotope diet studies, 432
autopsies (forensic), 108–109
averages, 487
avulsion fractures, 339

B
Bach, J.S., facial reconstruction, 326

backscattered electron mode SEM, 257
bacterial diseases, 245–249
Baldock, Herts.
  decapitation, 368
  weapon-related trauma, (Table) 368
bamboo spine, 176
Barlow's disease, 51
Barma Grande 2 remains, Liguria, skeletal asymmetry, 387
Barrington, Cambs., weapon-related trauma, (Table) 370
basal cell naevus syndrome, 265
bases, DNA, 456
Bateman, T., early skeletal collection, 2
battered baby syndrome (child abuse), 48, 51 (Fig.), 342
battles
  sharp force injury, 361, 374–375
  of Towton, 374–375
  of Wisby, 366
Bayesian estimation, age structure elimination, 107–112
Beaker people, 281–283
  Bell-Beaker burials, Bavaria, strontium isotope studies,
    432
  influx, 3
  Stonehenge, weapon-related trauma, 366
beer, maize, 428
bejel, 153
Belkin *et al*, environment on age signs, 75
Bell-Beaker burials, Bavaria, strontium isotope studies, 432
benign tumours, *vs* malignant tumours, 214
Bergfelder, T., Hermann, B., pubic tubercle extension, 138
Berry, A.C., Berry, R.J., epigenetic variants, 291–292
Berwick St John, Wilts., weapon-related trauma, (Table) 367
bevelling, cranial injuries, 367, 373
bias
  age determination, 63
  demography, 104–105
  non-metric trait studies, 298–300
biceps brachii muscle, handedness, 311
biocultural matrices, 258
biocultural population approach
  infections, 147
  trauma, 337–356
biodistance
  craniometry, 277–288
  non-metric traits, 301–302
biological identity, forensic science, 500
biomarkers, 239–249
Biometrika (Pearson), 2–3
biometry, occupational adaptations, 282–283
birth rates, 102
bivariate methods, limitations, 478
Blackfriars cemetery, Ipswich, weapon-related trauma,
  371
blood groups, cancers, 209
blunderbuss wound, 365
blunt trauma
  battle of Towton, 374
  long bones, 365
  Ofnet, Bavaria, 366
  skull, 361–364

Bocquet-Appel, J.P, Masset, C., age determination, 63

bodkin arrow wound, 373

body mass, 396

bog bodies
ancient DNA destruction, 461
forensic science and, 496
Lindow II body, Schmorl's nodes, 4
Lindow Man, ancient DNA destruction, 461

boiled water (drinking), isotope studies, 434

bone, 439–441
cremated, 404–407
density, 192
development, 13–16
diagenesis, 439–452
dynamics, 64, 183–184
pregnancy and lactation, 137–138
turnover rates, 184
histomorphometry, 72–73
infection, juvenile, 42
mineral distribution, handedness, 309–314
see also collagens

'boneformers', 171

Boxgrove, palaeolithic finds, 2

brain
asymmetry, 316
lateralization, 307
trauma, 364

Bramshill, National Crime Faculty, 491–492

breast carcinoma, 209
metastasis frequency, 217

breast-feeding, stable isotopes, 429, 433–434

Brick Earth, Halling skeleton, 2

Britain
diets, isotope studies, 427
non-adult pathology, 47–48
non-metric traits, 292–293
osteoarchaeology, 477
osteoarthritis, 167 (Table)
population history, craniometry, 280–285
weapon-related trauma, 357–380

Britons, Pleistocene, 1–2

Bronze Age
dual burial, 416
skulls, 281–283
weapon-related trauma, 366
weight of bone from burials, 415

Brooks, S., Suchey, J.M., age determination, Bayesian analysis, 108–109

Brothwell, D.R.
dental age determination, 87, 88–89
recording dental disease, 234
weapon trauma classification, 359

Brown, Marion 'Peg Leg', 386–387

brown tumours, 266

brushite, 446

bruxism, 232

bubonic plague, 246

buccolabial erosion, 232

Buckland, Kent, weapon-related trauma, (Table) 370

Buikstra, J.E., Ubelaker, D.H., recording dental disease, 234

Burgh Castle, Norfolk, weapon-related trauma, (Table) 370

burial customs
Arras culture, 283
Bronze Age, 366
children, 10–11, 40–42, 104–105
congenital deformities, 218–219
decapitation, 367–368
Neolithic–Bronze Age transition, 280–281

burial environment, 448–450
on biomarkers, 239–240
experimental, 450
forensic vs archaeological remains, 495
skull, 359–360

Burton Fleming, E. Yorks., weapon-related trauma, (Table) 367

Butler's Field, Lechlade, weapon-related trauma, (Table) 370

C

C4 plants, 425, 426

caf1, Yersinia pestis V antigen, 246

Caffey's disease, 51
rediagnosed as child abuse, 48

Caister-on-Sea, Norfolk, weapon-related trauma, (Table) 370

calcium
dental age determination, 94
soil, bone mineral dissolution, 447, 449

calcium hydroxyapatite, 240, 440–441
chemical diagenesis, 442–448
cremated bone, 406
isotope studies, 430–434

calculi, renal, hyperparathyroidism, 266

calculus, dental, 227–228

California, skeletal growth studies, (Table) 26

canalized structures, epigenetic development, 294

cancer see neoplastic disease

cancer (Old English), 219

Candida albicans, 244

cane sugar, caries, 230

canine teeth, sexing, 124

Capasso, L. et al, Atlas of occupational markers on human remains, 382

carbohydrates, as biomarkers, 242

carbon, stable isotopes, 425–426

carbonate
exogenous, 446
isotope studies, 430–432
oxygen, 433

carboxyl carbon, stable isotopes, 430

caribou hunting, entheseal changes, 389

caries, 229–230, 233
cremation, 413
data analysis, 478

Carston Annis Bt-5, Kentucky, skeletal growth studies, (Table) 25

cart burials, Arras culture, 283, (Fig.) 284

cartilage
  ossification, age determination, 71–72
  osteoarthritis, 166
Castillon sword, 374
Castledyke, N. Lincs., osteoarthritis, 167 (Table), 169
casts
  facial reconstruction, 329–331
  non-metric trait recording, 300
catch-up growth, 44
Caucasoid skeletons, medial clavicular epiphyseal fusion, 66
cemental annulations, dental age determination, 92–94
cementoblastoma, 267–268
cemento-enamel junction, caries, 230
cemento-ossifying fibroma, 268, (Fig.) 269
cemeteries
  for children, 41–42
  skeletal asymmetry studies, 318
central chondrosarcoma, 205
central giant cell granuloma, 266, (Fig.) 267
Chelmsford, Essex, weapon-related trauma, (Table) 372
chemical palaeopathology, 239–253
chemotaxonomy, 245
Chester, weapon-related trauma, (Table) 372
Chichester, Sussex
  congenital anomalies, 204
  skeletal growth studies, (Table) 26
child abuse, 48, 51 (Fig.), 342
child labour, 62
child worth, Crawford on, 48
childbirth see parturition
children
  burial customs, 10–11, 40–42, 104–105
  diastasis, skull trauma, 363
  fractures, 345–346
  isotope studies, 429–430
  see also juvenile skeletons
chimeric sequences, 241
chimney sweeps, scrotal carcinoma, 209
China, dental age determination, 88–89
chlamydia, 244
cholesterol, isotope studies, 434–435
chondroblastoma, (Table) 211
chondromyxoid fibroma, (Table) 211
chondrosarcoma, (Table) 212
  central, 205
chordoma, (Table) 212
Christ Church, Spitalfields, 12
  age determination
    cranial suture closure, 68
    rib ends, 70
  infections, 148
  obstetric histories, 135, 138
  osteoarthritis, 394–395
  sexing from skulls, 123
  suicide case, 365
  super-eruption of teeth, 229
  tuberculosis, 50
  see also London crypt sample

chromosomes, 456
  see also X chromosome; Y chromosome
cicatrization, 364
Cirencester
  gout, 173
  weapon-related trauma, 366–367, (Table) 368
cist graves, Trelowthas Barrow, 408 (Fig.) 409
classification tree routines, 485
classifications
  disease, 256
  weapon trauma, 359
    blunt trauma, 363–364
clavicle
  age determination, 66, 72
  handedness, 310
clay modelling, facial reconstruction, 326, 332
clay shoveller's fracture, 342, 391, 392
cleft palate/lip, 204 (Fig.)
  cases, (Table) 201, (Table) 208
  factors affecting, (Table) 213
  frequency, (Table) 216
  treatment, 202
  vitamin A deficiency, 208
cleidocranial dysplasia, (Table) 213
climate
  hand bone age, 75
  isotope studies, 433, 434
  skulls, 282–283
clinical literature
  congenital and neoplastic diseases, 210
  dental disease, 234–235
close range photogrammetry, 193
closed populations, 102
club foot, (Table) 201, (Table) 213, (Table) 216
cluster analysis, data analysis, 485
clusters, endocranial vascular variation, 215
coefficient of racial likeness (Pearson), 3
collagenases, microbial, 441
collagens, 440
  isotope studies, 426–430
  post-mortem loss, 359–360
Colles' fracture, prevalence, 346
colonial sites, Ontario, weaning practices, 429
colour
  cremated bone, 405
  multiple burials, 409
comminuted fractures, 339
Complex Method, age determination, 73
  cranial suture closure, 68
compound fractures, 339
compression fractures, vertebrae, 339, 340
computed tomography
  facial reconstruction, 328
  fractures, 350
computers
  artificial intelligence, 485
  digital facial reconstruction, 327–328
confidentiality, forensic science, 497
confocal reflecting scanning laser light microscope, 257

congenital conditions, 199–204, (Table) 213–214
  archaeological *vs* present-day frequency, 215–217
  publication, 207, 208–210
  see also genetic diseases
congenital dislocation of hip, 200, (Table) 201, (Table) 213
  frequency, (Table) 216
congenital syphilis, 153, (Table) 214
conjoined twins, (Table) 208
connective tissue diseases
  genetic matrix disorders, 243
  see also rheumatoid arthritis
continuing eruption, 228–229
contractures, 350
contrecoup fractures, 361, (Fig.) 362
coroners
  material, pubic pitting, 135
  see also medical examiners
cortical bone, 184
  pregnancy and lactation, 137–138
Corynebacterium diphtheriae, 247–248
costoclavicular ligaments, handedness, 310
court appearances, 501
Cox Lane, Ipswich, weapon-related trauma, 370–371
Crania Britannica (Davis and Thurnam), 2
cranial suture closure, age determination, 66–68, 410
craniodiaphyseal dysplasia, (Table) 214
craniofacial robusticity, 125–126
craniometry, biodistance, 277–288
Crawford, S., on child worth, 48
Crawfordjohn, Strathclyde, forensic remains, 495
cremation, 403–421
  sexing of skeletons, 411–413, 463
cribra
  pregnancy and lactation, 137–138
  see also orbits, cribra
cricket, spine, 391
cross-linkages, collagen, 440
cross-sectional areas, long bones
  activity on, 384, 386
  age at death, 385
crystallinity, bone change, 443–444
crystals, bone mineral, 440–441
  cremated bone, 406
cultures
  and age, 61–64
  congenital diseases, 217–219
  handedness, 307–308
  infectious diseases, 145–162
  lead isotope studies, 433
  see also biocultural population approach
Cunha, E., Umbelino, C., on manual labour, 396
custody, forensic specimens, 496–497
cuts (sharp force injury), 361, 369

D
Danebury
  cranial injuries, 366
  weapon-related trauma, (Table) 367
Danes' Graves, Driffield

Arras burial, 284
  weapon-related trauma, (Table) 367
data analysis, 475–490
databases
  computer programs, 482
  congenital and neoplastic diseases, 209–210
date of death, forensic anthropology, 494–496
Davis, B., Thurnam, J., *Crania Britannica*, 2
decapitation, 367–368
deciduous teeth
  age determination, 84–87
  sexing, 123–124
degeneration, bone, 64
dehydration, cremated bone, 405, 406
delta units, isotope ratios, 425
demography, 101–115
  data analysis methods, (Table) 486
Denmark
  dental age determination, medieval skulls, 88
  diets, isotope studies, 427
dental age determination, 12–13
  adults, 87–95
  children, 83–87
  vs maturation delay, 29–30
  population studies, 27
  vs size, developmental stress, 28
dental disease, 227–237
  nutritional stress, 48
  see also caries
dental enamel *see* enamel
dentinal tubules, age determination, 91–92
dentine
  root translucency, 90–91
  secondary deposition, 89–90
dentistry, 229
Denver, bone growth study, 30
  vs London Crypt sample, 31–35
depressed fractures, 363–364
descriptive methods, data analysis, 482
desmoplastic fibroma, (Table) 211
development
  embryonic, factors affecting, 293–296
  juvenile skeletons, 9–21, 64
  see also maturation, delay
developmental instability, fluctuating asymmetry, 314
developmental stress indicators, 28–30
developmental thresholds, 290
DEXA *see* dual energy X-ray absorptiometry
diagenesis
  ancient DNA, 461–462
  biomarkers, 243
  bone, 439–452
  carbonate, isotopes, 431
  collagen, 426
  exogenous ions, 444–446
  histology, 260
    Paget's disease, 261–263, (Fig) 264
diagnosis, osteoarthritis, 168

diaphyseal aclasia, (Table) 201, 202
diaphyseal dysplasia, (Table) 214
diaphyseal measurements, activity on diameters, 384
diastasis, skull trauma, 363
diet
    caries, 229–230
    isotope studies, 425–432, 434–435
    neoplasms, 209
    prostatic carcinoma, 209
    on skull, 125
    tooth erosion, 232
differential scanning calorimetry, (Table) 445
diffuse idiopathic skeletal hyperostosis, 170
    vs ankylosing spondylitis, 176
diffusion, bone mineral dissolution, 447
diffusive regime, hydrology, 448, 449–450
digital facial reconstruction, 327–328
diphtheria, 247–248
directional asymmetry, 315
disease
    ancient DNA, 468–471
    British populations, 3–5
    classification, 256
    on post-mortem change, 240
    see also pathology
DISH see diffuse idiopathic skeletal hyperostosis
dislocations, 342
    see also congenital dislocation of hip
distance matrix concordance, 296–297
disuse atrophy, 316
DNA, 112–113, 240–241, 455–457
    genetic fingerprinting, 465–467, 497
    see also ancient DNA
documentation see recording
Dordrecht, Holland, osteoarthritis, (Table) 167
Down's syndrome, (Table) 201, (Table) 213, (Table), 216
dual cremation/burials, 416
dual energy X-ray absorptiometry, 192
    standards development, 194
Dunstable, Beds.
    mutilation, 368
    weapon-related trauma, (Table) 368
Dutour, O., on study of occupational changes, 382
dyschondrosteosis, (Table) 213
dysplasias, 268–269

E
early childhood, definition, (Table) 10
ears
    facial reconstruction, 332
    infections, 149
eburnation, 166
    congenital dislocation of hip, (Fig.) 200
Eccles, Kent, weapon-related trauma, 369, (Table) 370
Ecuador, status and diet, 428
edged weapons, sharp force injury, 361, 369
EDLAXS (energy dispersive low angle X-ray scattering), 192
Eggelling, von, facial reconstruction experiment, 326
Eggington, Beds., weapon-related trauma, (Table) 367

Ekaterinburg, Romanov family, 466–467
elasticity, bone, 383
elderly people, under-representation, 62–63, 105
electron microscopy, 256–257
elephant man (J. Merrick), 218
embryology, 293–296
embryos, (Table) 10
enamel (dental)
    environmental stress, 27–28
        hypoplasias, 46–47
    isotope studies, 431, 433–434
enchondroma, (Table) 202, (Table) 211
endochondral bone formation, 13, 183
endocranial lesions, new bone formation, 43, 48–49, (Fig.) 155
endocranial suture closure, 67
endocranial vascular variation, 214–215
endosteal hyperostosis, (Table) 214
energy dispersive low angle X-ray scattering, 192
England, osteoarthritis, (Table) 167
entheses
    activity-related change, 387–388, 389
    data analysis methods, (Table) 486
enthesophytes, 387–388
envelopes, viruses, 244–245
environmental stress factors, on growth, 23–24, 39
enzymes, microbial, 441
epigenetic factors, non-metric traits, 3, 292, 293
epiphyses, 13–14
    clavicle, age determination, 66
epitopes, 241
erosion of teeth, 232
erosive arthropathies, 171–174
erosive osteoarthritis, 172
Eskimo, Western, skeletal growth studies, (Table) 25
Eskimo-Inuits, skeletal asymmetry, 317
ethics, non-metric trait studies, 303
ethnicity
    arachnoid granulation, age determination, 74
    coefficient of racial likeness, 3
    forensic science, 498
Europe
    agriculture, 280
    C4 food imports, 427
    mitochondrial DNA, 280
    syphilis, 52
evidence (forensic), disclosure, 497
Ewing's sarcoma, (Table) 212
exogenous ions, diagenesis, 444–446
exotoxin A, Streptococcus pyogenes, 247
experimental burial environments, 450
exploratory methods, data analysis, 482, 483
expressed fractures, 363
extracellular matrix, genetic matrix disorders, 243
eyeballs, facial reconstruction, 331

F
face
    activity-related bone remodelling, 392–393

leprosy, (Fig.) 157
  reconstruction, 325–333, 501
  sex differences, 119, 123
  superimposition identification method, 501
  trauma, 365–366
  treponemal infection, (Fig.) 156
Falconer, D.S., developmental thresholds, 290
Fazekas, I.Gy., Kósa, F., foetuses, age development, 13
fecundity, 131
Feik, S.A. *et al*, bone cross-sections, age determination, 72
femora
  cremated remains, 413
  cross-sections, image analysis, 72
  dimensions, 386
    Denver study and London Crypt sample, 31–35
  fractures, (Fig.) 351
    osteoporosis, 191–192
  King site, Georgia, 385
  pregnancy and lactation, 137
  sexing, 120–121
fertility, 131
  age-specific rates, 102
fibrosarcoma, (Table) 212
fingerprinting, genetic, 465–467, 497
Finglesham, Kent, weapon-related trauma, 370 (Table)
firearms, 359
  gunshot wounds, 364, 365
fish, isotope ratios, (Fig.) 426, 428
Fishergate, St Andrew, weapon-related trauma, 371
Fishergate, York, osteoarthritis, (Table) 167
fissuring, cremated bone, 405
Five Knolls barrows, 3
flexion contracture, 350
florid cemento-osseous dysplasia, 269, (Fig.) 270
flour, caries, 230
flow regime, hydrology, 448, 449–450
fluctuating asymmetry, 314
fluorapatite, 441, 446
foetal alcohol syndrome, (Table) 213
foetal haemoglobin, thalassaemia case, 470–471
foetuses
  definition, (Table) 10
  dental age determination, 84–85
  development *vs* age, 13–14
  directional asymmetry, 315
  pathology and, 44–45
  testosterone, 121
Folly Lane, St Albans, ritual cranial trauma, 368
Fong's syndrome (osteo-onychodysplasia), 201, 202, Table 213, (Table) 216
Food Vessel people *see* Beaker people
foramen of Hüschke, sex differences, 298
foramina, moulds from skull, 330
force
  on bone, 383–384
  fractures, 360
forensic science, 491–503
  dental age determination, 83–84
  DNA fingerprinting, 466

facial reconstruction, 329
  handedness, 317–318
Forestier's disease *see* diffuse idiopathic skeletal hyperostosis
Fourier transform infrared spectroscopy, (Table) 445
fourth rib
  finding, 69–70
  sexing, 120
Foxhall, Red Crag sands, 1
Fraction 1 protein, *Yersinia pestis*, 246
fractures, 339–341
  age at death, 345
  children, 345–346
  Colles', prevalence, 346
  computed tomography, 350
  contrecoup, 361, (Fig.) 362
  force required, 360
  green-stick, 44
  humerus, 350
  metal-dippers, 392
  non-union, (Fig.) 348, (Fig.) 349
  osteoporosis, 191–192, 350
  post-mortem, 346, 359, 376
  prevalence rates, 346, 350
  radiology, 349
  radius, (Fig.) 347, (Fig.) 348
  recording, 346–350
  ribs, (Fig.) 349
  shoveller's, 342, 391, 392
  skull, 363–364
  stress fractures, 346
  treatment, 343
  ulna, (Fig.) 347, (Fig.) 348
  upper limb, lateralization, 312
  see also femora, fractures; Looser's zones
fragments
  long bones, growth studies, 11
  size, cremation burials, 415
freshwater fish, isotope ratios, 428
Fricke, H.C. *et al*, isotope studies on enamel, 433
Frisian Islands, *vs* Netherlands, mitochondrial DNA, 113
FS8 mutation, thalassaemia, 470
F_{ST}(genetic diversity), 112
fungal diseases, 244
fur traders
  entheseal changes, 389
  lead isotope studies, 433

G
Galen (b. A.D. 129), on bones, 325
Galley Hill, Thames terrace, 1–2
Garton Slack, E. Yorks., weapon-related trauma, (Table) 367
Gejvall, N.G., sexing cremated skeletons, 412
gender, *vs* sex, 117
genes, 457
genetic diseases
  ancient DNA, 468
  see also congenital conditions
genetic fingerprinting, 465–467, 497
genetic matrix disorders, 243

genetics
craniometry, 278–279
demography, 112–113
non-metric traits, 290–291, 296–298
genomes, 457
sequencing projects, 462
genotypic variance, *vs* phenotypic variance, 296
geology, strontium migration studies, 432
Gerasimov, M.M., facial reconstruction, 327
Germany, 5th century migration from, 285
giant cell granuloma, central, 266, (Fig.) 267
giant cell tumour, (Table) 202, (Table) 212
gigantiform cementoma, 269, (Fig.) 270
GIS techniques, data analysis, 485
Glasgow Cathedral cemetery, suicide case, 365
glenoid fossa, extensor facet, 309
glutamic acid, dental age determination, 95
Goat's Hole, Paviland, 1
God, wrath of, 218
Gorlin–Goltz syndrome, 265
Gough's Cave, Somerset, collagen loss, 442
gout, (Fig.) 164, 172–173
vs hallux valgus, 174
Gram-negative bacteria, 246–247
Gram-positive bacteria, 247–249
Grant collection, skeletal age determination, 74
granulomas
bacterial diseases, 245
periapical, 231, 265
Grasshopper Pueblo, Arizona, strontium isotope studies, 432
Grattan, J., osteometry, 2
gravidity, 131
Great Chesterford, Essex, weapon-related trauma, (Table) 370
greater sciatic notch, sexing, 118, 119
juvenile, 121–122, 126
greenstick fractures, 44, 339
grip strength, handedness, 309
groundwater, on bone mineral, 442–443, 447–448
growth
cessation *see* maturation, delay
data analysis methods, (Table) 486
disorders, and skeletal sexing, 125
long bone measurement, 13
rates, and bone tumours, 209
studies, populations, 23–38
variation, 11–12
growth curves, 45
growth plates, 13
Grüneberg, H., non-metric traits, 290
Guale (people), scurvy, 186
gunshot wounds, 364, 365
Gussage All Saints, Dorset, weapon-related trauma, (Table) 367
Gustafson, G., dental age determination, 89
gutter fractures, 363

H
haemangioma, (Table) 203, (Table) 211

haemoglobin, 470
hallux valgus, 174
Hamann–Todd collection
age determination, 63, 66, 67
pubic pitting, 134
hamulus, hypoplasia, 204
Hanaura, Japan, DNA kinship analysis, 467
handball players, 309–310
handedness, 307–323
population prevalences, 316–317
hands
asymmetry, 313–314
bone age, environmental factors, 75
injuries and handedness, 314
Harris lines
British populations, 4
environmental stress, 27, 39, 47
'Harrying of the North' (William I), 371
Haversian systems, 184
heads, weight-bearing, osteoarthritis, 395
healing, fractures, 340, 374–375
cranial, 364–365
height *see* stature
hemihypertrophy, 315–316
hemivertebrae, (Table) 201
heritability, non-metric traits, 296–298
hibernation, cemental annulations *vs* age, 93
Hillson, S., Bond, S., tooth enamel, environmental stress, 27–28
Hirohata, Japan, DNA kinship analysis, 467
His, W., facial reconstruction of J.S. Bach, 326
histograms, compared, 480–482
histology
cremated bone, 416–417
age, 410–411
vs histopathology, 258–260
histomorphometry of bone, 72–73
histopathology, 255–274
osteomalacia, 190
Holocene populations, 2–3
homicide *see* forensic science; infanticide
Homo erectus, 2
Homo ergaster (Nariokotome boy), asymmetry, 316
hormones, sex differences from, 117
horsemen, weapons, 357–358
Hulton Abbey, Staffs., weapon-related trauma, (Table) 372
humerus
cremated remains, 413
sexing, 412
foetal asymmetry, 315
fractures, 350
handedness, 309–310, 310–311
humidity, hand bone age, 75
hunchback deformity, 152
hunter-gatherers
humeral asymmetry, 312
osteoarthritis, 394
Hutton, C., evolution of joints, 166
Huxley, T.H., 2

hyaline cartilage, ossification, age determination, 71–72
hybridization analysis, ancient DNA, 458, (Fig.) 459
hydrocephaly, 200, (Table) 201
    frequency, (Table) 216
hydrology, 447–449
hydrolysis, non-enzymatic, bone protein, 441–442
hydrophobicity, biomarkers, 242
hydroxyapatite *see* calcium hydroxyapatite
hyoid bones, recovery, 16
hypercementosis, 228
hyperostotic traits, age variation, data bias, 299
hyperparathyroidism, 266
hypersphere, trait frequencies, 302
hypertrophic arthritides, 163, 165–171
hypertrophy, from exercise, 385
hypostotic traits, age variation, data bias, 299
hypothesis testing, 482–483
hypothyroidism, Britain, 4

I
Iberia, Mesolithic–Neolithic cranial change, 280
identification (forensic), 500–501
iliac crest, age determination, 65
ilium *see* auricular surface of ilium
illegitimacy, 41–42
Illinois Valley, skeletal growth studies, (Table) 25
image analysis
    bone cross-sections, age determination, 72
    sexing, 126–127
imaging, medical, 257
immature skeletons *see* juvenile skeletons
immunology, diagenesis assessment, (Table) 445
impacted fractures, 339
Indian Knoll, skeletal growth studies, (Table) 25
industrialization, juvenile skeletons, 49–50
infanticide, 45
    PCR sexing studies, 463–465
infantile cortical hyperostosis *see* Caffey's disease
infants
    decapitation, 368
    definition, (Table) 10
    dental age determination, 85–87
    isotope studies, 429
    wet-nursing, 42
infectious diseases
    biomarkers, 243–249
    cultural aspects, 145–162
    DNA from organisms, 468
inferential methods, data analysis, 482–483
Infirmary site *see* Newcastle, England
influenza, 244, 245
inguinal ligament, 136
intergenic sequences, 457
intersex, 125
intertubercular sulcus, humerus, handedness, 311
intervertebral osteochondrosis, 169, 390–391
intra-cranial haemorrhage, 43
intramembranous bone formation, 13, 183–184
intra-molecular distribution, isotopes in collagen, 430

Inuits
    skeletal asymmetry, 317
    spondylolysis, 391
involution, skeletal age determination, 72–73
ions, exogenous, diagenesis, 444–446
Ipswich, weapon-related trauma, (Table) 372
Iraq, upper limb asymmetry, 312
Iron Age
    Arras culture, Yorkshire, 283–284
    weapon-related trauma, 366
iron deficiency anaemia, 45, 469
    pregnancy and lactation, 138
IS6110 (tuberculosis complex DNA), PCR, 469
isotopes, stable, 425–438
Italy, anthropology, 476

J
Japan
    DNA kinship analysis, 467
    skeletal asymmetry, 317
        upper limbs (modern), 312
jaws, scurvy, 187
Jewbury, York, weapon-related trauma, 371, (Table) 372
joints
    age determination, 66–71
    disabilities on, 384–385
    pathology, 163–182
        handedness, 313–314
jugular growth plate, age determination, 65–66
Julianehaab Bay, Greenland, isotope climate studies, 433
junk DNA (intergenic sequences), 457
juvenile skeletons
    activity on, 384
    development, 9–21, 64
    forensic science, 498
        sexing, 499
    growth, 23–38
    pathology, 39–58

K
kayaking, spondylolysis, 391
Kennedy, K.A.R., publications on occupational stress, 381
Kennewick man, 302
Kent's Cavern, Torquay, 1
keratocysts, odontogenic, 265
Key, C.A. *et al*, cranial suture closure, age determination, 68
kidney stones, hyperparathyroidism, 266
King site, Georgia, pelvic hypertrophy, 385
kinship analysis, ancient DNA, 465–468
Kleinburg, Ohio, arms and handedness, 311
Klippel–Feil syndrome, 210
kneeling, changes from, 390
Kofun era, Japan, DNA kinship analysis, 467
Kollman, J., Buchley, W., neolithic facial reconstruction, 326
Konigsberg, L.W., Frankenberg, S.R., age statistics, 108
Korean War, age determination from soldiers, 69
Krogman, W.M., facial reconstruction, 327
Kulubnarti, Upper Nubia, skeletal growth studies,
    (Table) 25

L

lactation, bone, 137
Larsen syndrome, (Table) 214
laryngeal cartilages
    age determination, 71–72
    retrieval, 16
laser scanning, computer-generated facial reconstruction, 327–328
late childhood, definition, (Table) 10
lateralization, brain, 307
lcrV, *Yersinia pestis* V antigen, 246
lead, isotope studies, 432–433
left-handers, 318
legumes, isotope ratios, (Fig.) 426
leprosy, 4, 149, 150–151, 152, 248
    maxilla, (Fig.) 157
levels, multi-level data, 478
liability, population thresholds and (Falconer), 290
Libben, Ohio
    pregnancy and lactation, 137
    skeletal growth studies, (Table) 25
ligaments, parturition, 132
Liguria, Italy
    Barma Grande 2 remains, skeletal asymmetry, 387
    disuse atrophy, 316
limb reduction deficits, 316
limb shortening, 45, (Fig.) 351
Lincoln Castle, weapon-related trauma, 373
Lindow II bog body, Schmorl's nodes, 4
Lindow Man, ancient DNA destruction, 461
linear measurement, craniometry, 279
linear regressions, limitations, 478–479
lipids
    as biomarkers, 242
    isotope studies, 434–435
load *see* force
London crypt sample, skeletal growth studies, (Table) 26, 31–35
long bones
    activity on, 386–387
    bowing, 210, (Table) 213, 345–346
    foetal asymmetry, 315
    fragments, growth studies, 11
    growth measurements, 13, 30–31
    handedness, upper limb, 310–313
    indices, cremated remains, 413
    new bone formation, (Fig.) 155, (Fig.) 156
    vitamin D deficiency, 189
    weapon-related trauma, 365
longevity, misconceptions, 62–63
Looser's zones, 190
Loth, S.R., age determination from rib ends, 70
Lovejoy, C.O., age determination
    auricular surface of ilium, 70
    multifactorial, 73, 74
LSAMAT (tooth erosion), 232
Lukacs, J., caries correction factor, 230
Lund, Sweden
    gout, 173
    osteoarthritis, (Table) 169

M

M proteins, *Streptococcus pyogenes*, 247
macaques
    pelves and parturition, 135
    trait inheritance, 297
Maiden Castle murder, 371
Maillard reaction products, 242
maize, agriculture, isotope studies, 426–427, 428, 431–432
malaria, 244, 469–470
malignant tumours, *vs* benign tumours, 214
mandible
    facial reconstruction, 331
    scurvy, 187
    sexing, 120
manioc, 232
Maoris, Polynesia, arm asymmetry, 312
Maples, W.R., on age determination, 64
Maresh, M.M., Denver bone growth study, 30
marine organisms, 425, 427
markers (biomarkers), 239–249
Mary Rose (Henry VIII's flagship)
    archers, 385
    arm asymmetry, 312
    vertebrae, osteophytes, 387–388
    weapon-related trauma, 374
mass spectrometry, (Table) 445
Masset, C., cranial suture closure, age determination, 67
masticatory stress, 392–393
mastodon teeth, isotope studies, 431
maternal impressions, congenital deformities, 218
matrix disorders, genetic, 243
maturation
    age determination methods, 65–66
    delay, 28–30
maxilla
    leprosy, (Fig.) 157
    scurvy, 187
maxillary sinuses, infection, 149
maxillary sutures, age determination, 67
maxillo-facial region, histopathology, 263–271
Mayans, status and diet, 428
Mays, S.A., radiogrammetry, 73
McCormick, W.F., Stewart, J.H., age determination from plastron, 71
mean measure of divergence, 301–302
meat:vegetable ratios, isotope diet studies, 429
mechanical stress
    on bone, 383
    fractures, 360
medical examiners, autopsies, 108–109
medical specimens, buried, 495
medicinal plants, cancer, 219
medieval period
    frequency of congenital and neoplastic diseases, 217
    weapons, 358
        trauma, 371–375
Meindl, R.S., Lovejoy, C.O., cranial suture closure, age determination, 67, 68
melt temperature, collagen, 440, 442
meningioma, (Table) 203, (Fig.) 205, 206, (Fig.) 207

diagnosis, 214–215
meningitis, 149
 tuberculosis, 43, 149
mercury intrusion porosimetry, 443, (Table) 445
Merrick, J. (elephant man), 218
mesial drift, 87, (Fig.) 88
Mesolithic groups
 diet, isotope studies, 427, 429
 skeletal asymmetry, 316
 skulls, vs Neolithic, 280
mesomelic dwarfisms, (Table) 213
metabolic bone disease, 183–198
 biomarkers, 243
metacarpals, handedness, 313
metachondromatosis, (Table) 213
metal-dippers, spinal fracture, 392
metals, substitution in bone mineral, 441
metaphyseal dysplasia, 214 (Table)
metastases (secondary tumours), (Table) 203, 204–205, (Fig.)
 206, 217
mice
 non-metric traits, 290
 trait inheritance, 297
microbial degradation, 441
microbial DNA, 241
microcephaly, (Table) 201, (Table) 213, (Table) 216
microfractures, 350
microlight pilot case, identification, 500–501
micro-pores, bone, 441
microscopy, 256–257
 diagenesis, (Table) 445
 see also scanning electron microscopy
microstructure of bone
 histomorphometry, 72–73
 pregnancy and lactation, 137–138
migrations, 277–278, 280–285
 genetics, 112–113
 isotope diet studies, 430, 432, 434
Miles, A.E.W., dental age determination, 87, 88–89
milling, skull copying, 328
mineral distribution, bone, handedness, 309–314
miscarriage, 45
Mississippians, asymmetry, 385
mitochondrial DNA, 112, 113, 457
 inconsistency with European migrations, 280
model life tables, 102–104
model priors, Bayesian estimation method, 109
modelling
 bone, 383
 facial reconstruction, 326
models (data analysis), 485
molecular markers see DNA
Möller–Barlow's disease, 185
monkeys, cemental annulations vs age, 92–93
monks, diet, 428
monoclonal antibodies, stains, 257
Monte Alban, Oaxaca Valley, oxygen isotope studies, 434
Moore, W., Corbett, E., caries, 230
Morden Bog, experimental burial, 450

Morgagni, G., quoted, 493
morphing, computer-generated facial
 reconstruction, 327–328
morphometrics, distance matrices, 297
mortality
 age-specific, 102, (Fig.) 106
 bias in dental sexing, 124–125
 vs burial rates, 40–41
 catastrophic, age distribution, 111–112
moulding, facial reconstruction, 329–330
MTB complex, 248–249
multifactorial age determination, 63, 73–74
multi-level data, 478
multiple burials, 408–409, 416
 forensic science, 497–498
multiple cremations, 416
multiple graves, 416
multiple myeloma, (Table) 212, 267
 Abingdon, Oxon., 205
 cases, (Table) 202
multiple state trait expressions, 300
multivariate methods, data analysis, 485
Murphy, T., recording dental disease, 234
mutations, population growth, 112
mycobacteria, persistence, 245
Mycobacterium bovis, 248–249
 DNA, 469
Mycobacterium leprae, 248
Mycobacterium tuberculosis, 248–249
 DNA, 469
mycolata, 245
mycolic acids
 M. leprae, 248
 M. tuberculosis, 249
myeloma see multiple myeloma
myotonic dystrophy, face, 392, (Fig.) 394

N
nail–patella syndrome (osteo-onychodysplasia), 201, 202,
 (Table) 213, (Table) 216
Nariokotome boy, asymmetry, 316
nasopharyngeal tumours, (Table) 203
National Crime Faculty, Bramshill, 491–492
Native Americans
 lead isotope studies, 433
 PCR sexing studies, 465
 skeletal growth studies, (Table) 25
 weaning practices, 429
Neanderthals
 asymmetry, 316
 upper limb, 386
 replacement by population growth, 101
Negroid skeletons, medial clavicular epiphyseal fusion, 66
Nemeskéri, J. et al, cranial suture closure, age
 determination, 67
neo-Darwinism, 455
Neolithic groups
 Britain, 280
 diet, isotope studies, 427, 429

skeletal asymmetry, 316
weapons, 358
Neolithic–Bronze Age transition, Britain, 280–283
neonatal line, 85, (Fig.) 86
neonates, (Table) 10
asymmetry of long bones, 315
sexual dimorphism, 121
neoplastic disease, 199–200, 204–207, (Table) 211–212,
214–215
archaeological *vs* present-day frequency, 215–217
cases, (Table) 202
factors, 209
histopathology, 266–271
population variation, 208–210
Netherlands, *vs* Frisian Islands, mitochondrial DNA, 113
neural network programs, 485
neurofibroma, (Table) 203
New Archaeology, 476–477
Newcastle, England, Infirmary site
age determination, 111
tuberculosis, 249
nineteenth century, British excavations, 2
nitrogen, stable isotopes, 425–426
non-adult skeletons *see* juvenile skeletons
non-enzymatic hydrolysis, bone protein, 441–442
non-metric traits, 3, 289–306
non-specific infection, 147–149
non-union, fractures, (Fig.) 348, (Fig.) 349
North Elmham Park, Norfolk, weapon-related trauma,
(Table) 370
Nubia, Sudan
sexing from auricular surface of ilium, 123
skull shape and chewing, 392–393
nutrient foramina, humeri, handedness, 311
nutritional stress
dental disease, 48
dental sexing, 124–125

O
Oaxaca Valley, Monte Alban, oxygen isotope studies, 434
obstetric casualties, 44–45
obstetric histories, pelvis studies, 134–135
occipital bone
age determination, 15
new bone formation, (Fig.) 155
occupation
bone adaptation, 381–401
neoplasms, 209
osteoarthritis, 169
shoulder joint, degenerative diseases, 310
social factors, 395–396
tooth wear, 232
odontogenic cysts, 265
odontomes, 208
odontometry, sexing juveniles, 124, 126
Ofnet, Bavaria, blunt trauma, 366
old age, under-representation, 62–63, 105
Ollier's disease, (Table) 214
OM proteins, *Treponema pallidum*, 247

Ontario, colonial sites, weaning practices, 429
optical densitometry, 192
standards development, 194
oral tori, 3
orbits
cribra, 39, 45–46
British populations, 4
scurvy, 186
skull moulding, 330
ordinal categories, 483
os tibiale, 204
Oslo, Dental Faculty, pulp size *vs* age, 92
ossification, hyaline cartilage, age determination, 71–72
ossification centres, 14–16
fusion, 16
osteoarthritis, (Fig.) 164, 165–169
activity on, 393–395
data analysis methods, (Table) 486
erosive, 172
handedness, 313–314
osteoblastoma, (Table) 211
osteoblasts, 184
osteocalcin, 241
osteochondritis dissecans, 179
osteochondroma, (Table) 211
osteochondromatosis, (Table) 201, 202
frequency, (Table) 216
osteoclasts, 184
osteogenesis imperfecta, 201, (Table) 213, (Table) 216
osteoid osteoma, (Table) 202, (Table) 211
osteoma, (Table) 202, 205
osteomalacia, 44, 189–191
osteometry, 2–3
osteomyelitis, 42–43
osteons, bone age determination, 410
osteo-onychodysplasia, 201, 202, (Table) 213, (Table) 216
osteopathia striata with cranial stenosis, (Table) 214
osteopenia
scurvy, 187
WHO definition, 192
osteophytes, 166, (Fig.) 167
vertebrae, *Mary Rose*, 387–388
osteoporosis, 72–73, 191–195
British populations, 4
cremation, 413
fractures, 191–192, 350
parity, 137, 138
scurvy, 187
osteosarcoma, (Table) 202, (Table) 212
maxillo-facial region, 269, (Fig.) 271
Ottoman grave, porotic hyperostosis, 470–471
overprinting, biomarkers, 240
Overton Down, experimental burial, 450
oxygen, isotope studies, 433–434

P
Pacbitun, Belize, gender, status and diet, 428
pachydermia, (Table) 208
Paget's disease of bone, 146

case studies, 260–263
palaeodemography *see* demography
palaeoethnology, 476
Palaeolithic fossils (Pleistocene Britons), 1–2
palaeopathology *see* pathology
pannus, 174
parasites, 244
parathyroid disease, and skeletal sexing, 125
Paré, A., on congenital deformities, 217–218
Parisi, tribes, 283
parity assessment, 132–138
    pubic tubercle, 137
parry fractures, 312
partial aplasias, (Table) 201
parturition, 131–142
    pelvic obstruction, 44–45
patellofemoral joint, osteoarthritis and
        evolution, 166
pathology
    cremated bones, 413
    data analysis methods, (Table) 486
    juvenile skeletons, 39–58
    see also disease
patrilocality, 113
pattern matching, bias detection, 104
Paviland, Goat's Hole, 1
Pearson, K., *Biometrika*, 2–3
pelvis
    exercise hypertrophy, 385
    obstruction at childbirth, 44–45
    sexing, 118–119
        juvenile, 121–122
penetrating injuries, 374
    gunshot wounds, 364, 365
    sharp force injury, 361, 369
People's Republic of China, dental age determination, 88–89
peptides, 241
peptidoglycan, bacteria, 245
periapical lesions, 231, 263–265
    abscesses, 87, 231
    cemental (fibrous) dysplasia, 268–269, (Fig.) 270
    granulomas, 231, 265
peri-mortem trauma, 357
    fractures, 346, 359–360, 376
perinates, (Table) 10
periodontal disease, 228
    apical cysts, 231
periodontal ligament recession, 89
periosteum, juvenile, 42
periostitis, 147, 148
    juvenile, 42–43
    ribs, tuberculosis, 151, 152, 154
petroexoccipital articulation, age determination, 65–66
petrous temporal bones, sexing cremated skeletons, 412
pH
    ancient DNA preservation, 461
    apatite dissolution, 446–447
Phenice, T.W., sexing criteria, 118, 119
phenotypic variance, vs genotypic variance, 296

Phi coefficient, non-metric trait recording, 300
phosphate
    bone mineral dissolution
        groundwater, 447
        soil, 449
    oxygen isotope studies, 433
phosphorus, dental age determination, 94
photogrammetry, close range, 193
photography, recording trauma, 350
Piltdown forgery, 2
pinch strength, handedness, 309
pink teeth, 95
pinta, 153
Piper Alpha disaster, 500
pituitary dwarfism, 149
plague, 145, 246
    leprosy and, 152
plant sterols, 243
plants, isotope ratios, 425
plaque, dental, 227
Plasmodium spp., DNA, 470
plaster of Paris, facial reconstruction, 331
plasticine/plasterline, facial reconstruction, 327
plasticity, bone, 383
plastron, age determination, 71
Pleistocene Britons, 1–2
pneumonic plague, 246
Poland's syndrome, 316
police forces, forensic osteology, 491–492
poliomyelitis, 146
polyclonal antibodies, stains, 257
polyester waste, archaeological skull moulding, 330
polymerase chain reaction, 458–459, (Fig.) 460
    sexing, 463–465
Polynesia, Maoris, arm asymmetry, 312
polynomial equations, population bone growth studies, 32
Pontefract Castle, healed cranial fracture, 364–365
Pontnewydd cave, 1
population thresholds (Falconer), 290
populations
    Britain, craniometry, 280–285
    growth of, genetic signature, 112
    growth studies, 23–38
    see also demography
porosity, bone changes, 443, 449
porotic hyperostosis, 45–46, 470
Portugal, diets, isotope studies, 427
postcranial injuries, 365
posterior probabilities, Bayesian estimation
        methods, 109–110
post-menopausal females, sexing errors, 125–126
post-mortem fractures, 346, 359, 376
post-mortem intervals, 494–496
post-processual archaeology, 278, 476
pottery, Neolithic–Bronze Age transition, 280–281
Pott's disease, spine, (Fig.) 50
Poundbury, Dorset
    juvenile pathology, 47
    migrant, lead isotope study, 433

psoriatic arthropathy, 177
sexing from canines, 124
skeletal asymmetry, 316
skeletal growth studies, (Table) 25
status and diet, 428
super-eruption of teeth, 228–229
weapon-related trauma, (Table) 368
poxviruses, 244, 245
pre-auricular sulci, pelvis, 118
parturition, 132–134, 135, 138
preferences, handedness, 307–308
preservation
juvenile skeletons, 40–42
see also diagenesis
prevalence rates
fractures, 346, 350
handedness, asymmetry, 316–317
non-specific infection, 148
primary centres, bone formation, 13
primates
cemental annulations vs age, 92–93
osteoarthritis and, 166
Princeton University, model life tables, 102–104
prior probabilities, Bayesian estimation
methods, 107–108, 109
probe DNA, 458
projectile trauma, 364
prone burial, 367–368
prostatic carcinoma, 205, (Fig.) 206
metastases frequency, 217
predisposing factors, 209
proteins
abnormal synthesis, 243
as biomarkers, 241–242
see also collagens
Psalm 90, on longevity, 62
pseudopathology, weapon-related trauma, 359–361
pseudo-sinuses, periapical, 231
psoriatic arthropathy, (Fig.) 164, (Fig.) 165, 177–178
puberty, 9, 10
cultural aspects, 62
sex difference, 119
pubic pitting, 118, 132–135, 138
pubic symphysis, age determination, 68–69, 74
Bayesian analysis, 108–109
pubic tubercle, extension, 135–136, 138, 139–140
publication
congenital and neoplastic conditions, 207,
208–210
histology, 260
traditions, 476
trauma, 338–339, 341–342
Pueblo sites
Grasshopper Pueblo, Arizona, strontium isotope
studies, 432
Pecos Pueblo, New Mexico, entheseal changes, 389
pulp chamber, dental age determination, 92
pumice-bone, 185
pycnodysostosis, (Table) 214

Pyle's disease, (Table) 214
pyre cremation, 407, 414–416
pyrophosphate, cremated bone, 406

Q
quaggas, ancient DNA, 459
quarrying, Boxgrove, 2
quasi-continuous development, 290
quenching, after pyre cremation, 414–415

R
race see coefficient of racial likeness; ethnicity
racemization, amino acids, dental age determination, 94
racket sports, arm asymmetry, 311
radicular cysts, 265
radiogrammetry, 73
radiology
bone growth studies, 30
fractures, 349
fusion of epiphyses, 16
osteomalacia, 190
radiolucencies, maxillo-facial region, 265–267
radiopacities, maxillo-facial region, 267–271
radius
cremated remains, 413
foetal asymmetry, 315
fracture, (Fig.) 347, (Fig.) 348
handedness, 310–311
ramus flexure, sexing, 120
randomisation, unilateral trait expression, 300
ranked categories, 483
Raunds, Northants., skeletal growth studies, (Table) 26
reactive arthritis see Reiter's disease
reburial movement, 5, 139, 293
recharge regime, hydrology, 448, 449–450
recording
dental disease, systems, 234
fractures, 346–350
non-metric traits, 292–293, 300
skeletal ages, 17
weapon-related trauma, 375–376
recovery
cremated bone, 407–408
for DNA analysis, 471
hyoid bones, 16
juvenile skeletons, 40–42, 105
from pyres
by archaeologists, 414
by mourners, 415
rectus abdominis muscle, 135–137
Red Crag sands, Foxhall, 1
reference priors, Bayesian estimation method, 109
regression diagrams, foetal age, 13
Reiter's disease, 176–177
vs psoriatic arthropathy, 177–178
relaxin, 132
remodelling, 64, 72, 383–384, 385
craniofacial, activity-related, 392–393
fractures, 340

renal calculi, hyperparathyroidism, 266
research design, data analysis, 479–482
reticulosarcoma, (Table) 212
retrieval *see* recovery
rheumatoid arthritis, 4, (Fig.) 164, (Fig.) 165, 174–175
    handedness, 313
rhomboid fossa, handedness, 310
ribs
    age determination, 72
        ends, 69–70
    fracture, (Fig.) 349
    periostitis, tuberculosis, 151, 152, 154
    rickets, (Fig.) 189
    see also fourth rib
rickets, 43–44, (Fig.) 49, 187–189
    industrial period, 50
    lesion distribution, (Fig.) 51
    skull lesions, 46
rickettsia, 244
Risser's system, iliac crest age determination, 65
rituals
    pyre cremation, 414–416
    see also burial customs
Roberts' syndrome, (Table) 213
Robinow's mesomelic dwarfism, (Table) 213
robusticity, osteoarthritis and, 394
rodents, strontium isotope studies, 432
Rogers, J., Waldron, T., Venn diagrams, diagnosis, 258,
    (Fig.) 259
Roman period, infanticide, 45
Romano-British period, weapon-related trauma, 366–368
Romanov family, 466–467
Roonka Flat, Australia, diets, 429
roots
    dental
        disease, 231
        exposure, 228
    dentine translucency, 90–91
Rösing's conversion tables, cremated
        remains, 413
rRNA genes, 241
rural infections, *vs* urban infections, 147
Russian method, facial reconstruction, 327

S
sabre shin, 210
saccharides, 242
sacrum, osteomalacia, 189
saddle querns, 390
sampling *see* recovery
sands, Pleistocene, 1–2
Sandwell Priory, Paget's disease case, 261, (Fig.) 262, 263,
    (Fig.) 264
Sardinia, thalassaemia, 470–471
Saxons, migrations to Britain, 285
Scandinavia, 5th century migration from, 285
scanning electron microscopy, 256–257
    microfractures, 350
    osteomalacia, 190

scapula, handedness, 309–310
scarlet fever toxin, 247
scars of parturition, 132–135
scenes of crime, 494
Scheuermann's disease, 390
Schmorl's nodes, 4, 169–170, 390
Schwartz-Lélek syndrome, (Table) 213
sciatic notch *see* greater sciatic notch
Scott, E.C., recording dental disease, 234
scrotal carcinoma, 209
scurvy, 46, 51, 184–187
seasonal climate variations, isotope studies on enamel, 433
secondary centres, bone formation, 13
secondary dentine deposition, 89–90
secondary tumours, (Table) 203, 204–205, (Fig.) 206, 217
sections, histopathology, 258
secular trends, handedness, 308
security, forensic specimens, 496–497
senile ankylosing hyperostosis *see* diffuse idiopathic skeletal
    hyperostosis
septic arthritis, 179
Serbia, Iron Gates Region
    diets, 428–429
    Mesolithic–Neolithic cranial change, 280
seronegative spondyloarthropathies, 175–178
sex, *vs* gender, 117
sex differences
    caries, 233
    data analysis, 479
    diet, 428
    handedness, 308
    humeral asymmetry, 312
    juveniles, 40
        dental *vs* skeletal age, 30
        Denver and London Crypt samples, 32–33
    migration rates, 113
    non-metric traits, data bias, 298–299
    osteoarthritis, 394
    see also intersex
sexing of skeletons, 117–130
    cremated, 411–413, 463
    DNA, 462–465
    forensic science, 498–499
    juvenile, 12, 16–17, 121–125, 126
sexual intercourse, prostatic carcinoma, 209
sharp force injury, 361, 369
Sharpey's fibres, juvenile, 42
short tandem repeats, 466
shoulder joint
    bones round, handedness, 309, 313
    definitions, 168
    degenerative diseases, asymmetry, 310
shoveller's fracture, 342, 391, 392
shrinkage, cremated bone, 406
sickle cell anaemia, 469–470
significance, statistical, 482, 483
simulations, data analysis, 485
Singh Index, 193
sintering, cremated bone mineral, 406

sinuses, periapical, 231
sitosterolaemia, 243
size, *vs* dental age determination, developmental stress, 28
skeletal age determination, 12, 13–16
    adults, 61–81
    juveniles, 9–21
        profiles, 45
    statistics, 105–112
skeletal data, nature of, 478–479
skull(s)
    activity-related remodelling, 392–393
    as armature, 325–326, 328
    blunt trauma, 361–364
    burial environment, 359–360
    copying, 328–329
    cranial suture closure, age determination, 66–68, 410
    craniometry, biodistance, 277–288
    holes, 344–345, 361
    Homo erectus, 2
    new bone formation, 43, 48–49, (Fig.) 155
    non-metric traits, 294–295
    rickets, 188
    sexing, 119–120, 125
        cremated skeletons, 412
    treponemal infection, (Fig.) 156
slaves, African-Americans, dental enamel hypoplasia, 47
Slavic remains, skeletal growth studies, (Table) 25
smallpox, 146
smells, forensic anthropology, 494
Smith, B.H., recording dental disease, 234
Snell's Corner, Horndean, weapon-related trauma, (Table) 368
social science, American archaeology, 477
socio-economic class
    cancer types, 209
    see also status
soft tissues
    facial reconstruction
        replication, 331–333
        thickness markers, 327
    neoplasia, 203, (Table) 205
    trauma, 364
soils
    molecules on bone, 240
    pH, 447
Solheim, T., dental age determination, 90
South Africa, immigrant burial, isotope diet studies, 430
South Eastern USA, osteoarthritis, sample, (Table) 167
spatial analysis, data analysis, 485
sphenoid bone, scurvy, 186
spheno-occipital synchondrosis, age at closure, 10, 66
spina bifida cystica, (Table) 208
spine
    activity-related pathology, 390–392
    hunchbacks, 152
    osteomalacia, 190
    Pott's disease, (Fig.) 50
Spitalfields *see* Christ Church, Spitalfields
split moulds, 330

spondylo-epiphyseal dysplasia, (Table) 201, (Table) 213
    frequency, (Table) 216
spondylolysis, 342, 391
spondylosis, 169
squatting, skeletal changes from, 390
squirting cucumber, 219
St Andrew, Fishergate, weapon-related trauma, 371
St Barnabas *see* London crypt sample
St Bride's Church, Fleet Street, 12
    crypt *vs* cemetery, adults *vs* children, 11
    suicide case, 365
    see also London crypt sample
St Helen-on-the-Walls, York
    burial site, 41
    weapon-related trauma, 372
St Margaret *in combusto*, Norwich
    arm asymmetry, 312
    healed cranial fracture, 364
    Paget's disease case, 261–263, (Fig.) 264
    Schmorl's nodes, 390
    weapon-related trauma, (Table) 372, 374
St Merryn, Cornwall, weapon-related trauma, (Table) 367
St Nicholas Shambles, London, weapon-related trauma, 372
St Oswald's Priory, Gloucs., osteoarthritis, (Table)167, (Table) 169
St Peter's, Barton-on-Humber, (Table) 169
    gout, 173
    rheumatoid arthritis, 174
    seronegative arthropathy, 178
stain technology, microscopy, 257
Standlake, Oxon., malignant tumour, 205
statistics, 475–490
stature
    cremated remains, 413
    forensic science, 499–500
    vs long bone length, 31
status
    diet, isotope studies, 428
    DISH, 171
    see also socio-economic class
Staunch Meadow, Brandon, weapon-related trauma, (Table) 370
stereo-lithography, skull copying, 328–329
Stonar, Kent, weapon-related trauma, (Table) 372
Stonehenge, Beaker people, weapon-related trauma, 366
Stratford Langthorne Abbey, London, weapon-related trauma, 371–372
Streptococcus pyogenes, 247
stress, on growth, 23–24, 39
stress fractures, 346
strontium, isotope studies, 432
subgingival calculus, 227–228
subperiosteal haematomas, scurvy, 185, 186
Suchey, J.M., Brooks, S., age determination, Bayesian analysis, 108–109
sugar, caries, 230
suicide cases, gunshot wounds, 365
Sundick, R.I., low retrieval rates for children, 11
sunlight, vitamin D, 187–188, 190

super-eruption of teeth, 228–229
supragingival calculus, 227–228
supra-orbital foramen, age, 299
surface osteophytes, 166
surgical sieve, 256
   radiolucencies, 266
survivorship curves, 103–104
Swanscombe, skull, 2
symmetry, non-metric traits, 299–300
symphalangism, 202
syndromes, 210
synovial joints, 163
syphilis, 153–154
   Britain, 5
   chemistry, 246–247
   congenital, 153, (Table) 214
   Europe, 52
   juvenile skeletons, (Fig.) 51

T

Talbot family, symphalangism, 202
Tauber, H., isotope studies, 427
teeth
   attrition, 87–89, 232
   cremation, 409, 410, 413
   data analysis methods, (Table) 486
   disease, 48, 227–237
   isotope studies, 429–430, 431
   loss, 231, 233–234
   Neanderthals, 386
   non-metric traits, 294–296
   scurvy, 187
   sexing, 123–125, 126
   twin studies, 298
   wear, 232
   see also caries; dental age determination; enamel; maxillo-
      facial region
temperature
   collagen melting, 440, 442
   hand bone age, 75
   vs shrinkage, cremated bone, 406
temporal bones
   ear infection, 149
   sexing cremated skeletons, 412
temporomandibular joint, facial
     reconstruction, 331
tennis players, arm asymmetry, 311
Teotihuacan, oxygen isotope studies, 434
testosterone
   pre-adult levels, 121
   prostatic carcinoma, 209
tetradysmelia, (Table) 208
Thailand, arm asymmetry, 312
thalassaemia, 469–471
Thames terraces, Galley Hill, 1–2
third molars, mice, non-metric traits, 290
three-dimensional coordinate data, craniometry,
   279–280
throwing activities, spine, 391

Thule (Hudson Bay), entheseal changes, 389
thumb
   handedness, 313
   osteoarthritis and evolution, 166
Tilley, C., archaeology as commodification, 61
time of death, forensic anthropology, 494–496
Tlailotlacan, oxygen isotope studies, 434
Todd collection, enthesophytes, 387–388
Todd, T.W., age determination
   cranial suture closure, 68
   pubic symphysis, 68–69
Todd, T.W., Lyon, D.W. Jr., cranial suture closure, age deter-
     mination, 67
toes, hyperdorsiflexion, 389 , 390
torture, 342
Towton, battle of, 374–375
toxic-shock syndrome, 247
trabecular bone, 184
   osteoporosis, 192–195
traction fractures, 339
traditions of archaeology, 476–477
training, forensic anthropology, 492–493
transsexualism, 499
trapezoid ligament, handedness, 310
trauma, 337–356
   data analysis methods, (Table) 486
   skeletal asymmetry after, 386–387
treatment
   cleft palate/lip, 202
   trauma, 342–348
Trelowthas Barrow cist grave, 408, (Fig.) 409
trends, secular, handedness, 308
Trentholme Drive, York, cranial injury, 367
trepanations, 344–345, 367
trephinations, 344–345
Treponema pallidum, 246–247
treponemal diseases, 149, 153–154
   Britain, 4–5
   face, (Fig.) 156
   see also syphilis
Trevor, J., osteometry, 3
trials (court appearances), 501
triangular inequality, mean measures of divergence, 302
tricalcium phosphate, cremated bone, 406
trophic level effects
   carboxyl carbon, 430
   isotope diet studies, 429
Trowbridge, Wilts., osteoarthritis, (Table) 167
Tsar of Russia *see* Romanov family
tuberculosis, 145, 149, 151–152
   ancient DNA, 468–469
   biomarkers, 248–249
   juvenile skeletons, 49–50, (Fig.) 51
   meningitis, 43, 149
tumours *see* neoplastic disease
twins
   conjoined, (Table) 208
   trait inheritance studies, 297–298
two-dimensional facial reconstructions, 327

U

ulcus cancri, 219

ulna
foetal asymmetry, 315
fracture, (Fig.) 347, (Fig.) 348
handedness, 311–312
umiaks (circular rowing boats), entheseal changes
from use, 389
under-ageing, 62–63, 105
uniform priors, Bayesian estimation method, 109
uninformative priors, 108
United States (America)
bioarchaeology, 476–477
forensic science, 492
Upington bone disease, (Table) 213
urban infections, *vs* rural infections, 147
urethritis, arthritis with, 176–177

V

V antigens, *Yersinia* spp., 246
V538 antibody, multiple myeloma, 267
Venn diagrams (Rogers and Waldron), diagnosis, 258,
(Fig.) 259
vertebrae
compression fractures, 339, 340
osteophytes, *Mary Rose*, 387–388
osteoporosis, 192–193, (Fig.) 339
Schmorl's nodes, 4, 169–170, 390
ventral rings, age determination, 65
see also Schmorl's nodes
Victorian period
British excavations, 2
frequency of congenital and neoplastic diseases, 217
violence, 487
viral infections, 146, 244–245
Paget's disease of bone, 261
vitality of teeth, root dentine translucency, 91
vitamin A deficiency, 208
neoplasms, 209
vitamin C, 184–185
see also scurvy
vitamin D deficiency
osteomalacia, 44, 189–191
see also rickets
Volkmann's ischaemic contracture, 350

W

Wadi Halfa, skeletal growth studies, (Table) 25
Waldron, T., on study of occupational changes, 382
Wallin, J.A. *et al*, bone cross-sections, age determination, 72
washing, after pyre cremation, 414–415
water, on DNA, 241
water (drinking), isotope studies, 434

water (groundwater), on bone mineral, 442–443, 447–448
water sorption (technique), (Table) 445
wax, facial reconstruction, 329
weaning practices, isotope diet studies, 429
weapon-related trauma, Britain, 357–380
Weaver, D.S., sexing from auricular surface
of ilium, 122–123
weight of bone
from burials, 408–409
from pyres, 415
Weismann–Netter–Stuhl syndrome, 210, (Table) 213
Wells Cathedral, high-status burials, DISH, 171
Werner's mesomelic dwarfism, (Table) 213
'West' model life curves, 103
wet-nurses, 42
Wetwang Slack, E. Yorks.
Arras burial, 284
weapon-related trauma, (Table) 367
Wharram Percy, N. Yorks.
clavicles, handedness, 310
neonates, asymmetry of long bones, 315
rickets, 188
sexing from face, 123
skeletal asymmetry, 316–317
skeletal growth studies, (Table) 26
Whithorn Church, weapon-related trauma, 372
whole-earth recovery, pyres, 414
William the Conqueror, 'Harrying of the North', 371
Wisby, battle of, 366
World Health Organisation, bone density, 192
'Wound Man', (Fig.) 358
woven bone, skull, 43
wrath of God, 218
wrist extension strength, handedness, 309
WT–15000 (Nariokotome boy), asymmetry, 316

X

X chromosome, 463
tooth growth, 123

Y

Y chromosome, 112, 463
tooth growth, 123
yaws, 153
Yersinia pestis, 246
Yokem Mound, Illinois, skeletal growth studies, (Table) 25
York, weapon-related trauma, 371
York Minster, healed cranial fracture, 364
Yorkshire, Arras culture, 283–284
young adult, definition, 10

Z

zygomatic arches, moulds from skull, 330